GET CONNECTED

To Content Updates, Study Tools, and More!

Meet SIMON 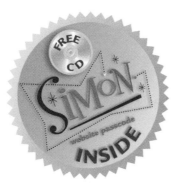 Your free online website companion

sign on at:

http://www.wbsaunders.com/SIMON/Chabner/

what you'll receive:

Whether you're a student or an instructor, you'll find information just for you. Things like:
- Content Updates
- Links to Related Publications
- Author Information . . . and more

plus:

WebLinks

Hundreds of active websites keyed specifically to the contents of this book. The WebLinks are continually updated, with new ones added as they develop.

W.B. Saunders Company

THE
LANGUAGE
OF
MEDICINE

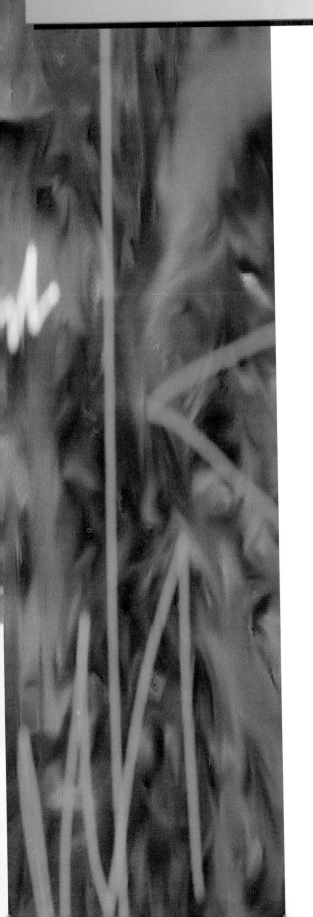

Davi-Ellen Chabner, B.A., M.A.T.

THE
LANGUAGE
OF
MEDICINE

A Write-In Text
Explaining Medical Terms

W.B. Saunders Company
An Imprint of Elsevier Science
Philadelphia   London   New York   St. Louis   Sydney   Toronto

6TH EDITION

W.B. SAUNDERS COMPANY
An Imprint of Elsevier Science

The Curtis Center
Independence Square West
Philadelphia, Pennsylvania 19106

Library of Congress Cataloging-in-Publication Data

Chabner, Davi-Ellen.
The language of medicine: a write-in text explaining medical terms / Davi-Ellen
Chabner.—6th ed.

p. ; cm.

Includes bibliographical references and index.

ISBN 0-7216-8569-2

Medicine—Terminology.   I. Title.   [DNLM: 1. Terminology—Examination
Questions. W 15 C427L 2001]

R123 .C43 2001   610'.1'4—dc2   99-089410

Acquisitions Editor: Maureen Pfeifer
Developmental Editor: Scott W. Weaver
Project Manager: Agnes Hunt Byrne
Production Manager: Frank Polizzano
Illustration Specialist: Lisa Lambert
Book Designer: Ellen Zanolle

THE LANGUAGE OF MEDICINE   ISBN 0-7216-8569-2

Printed in the United States of America

Last digit is the print number: 9   8   7   6   5   4   3

For Bebe (Beatrix Bess) and Solly (Solomon Joseph)
Bringing new life and utmost joy to me
and
For Bruce
Again and always

PREFACE

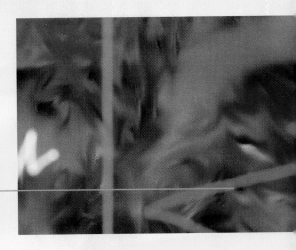

Welcome to the millennium edition of *The Language of Medicine!* I have a special sense of gratitude and pride in its production. First and foremost, I am grateful for the privilege of continuing to teach and write about this fascinating subject into the next century. I also have deep appreciation for the many students and teachers who took the time to write to me with comments and suggestions for this new edition. This is *your* book! I couldn't have done it without you!

The new and dazzling appearance of the sixth edition is its outstanding feature. Starting with the cover and continuing throughout, brilliant color is the keynote of this edition. Every figure in the text was reviewed carefully and redrawn as a full color image. New illustrations were added to enhance your ability to see medical terms in action. This is a reflection of my steadfast philosophy that the best way to study medical terms is to understand them in their proper context . . . the anatomy, physiology, and pathology of the human body.

Not only the images, but also the text itself was reviewed for this new century edition. Medical experts gave valuable suggestions related to updating terminology, in particular for surgical procedures, abbreviations, and drug therapies. In each of the first four chapters, additional Practical Applications sections take the student a step further in understanding terminology. New exercises, testing knowledge of abbreviations and their meanings, have been added to each of the body systems chapters. Since *The Language of Medicine* emphasizes explanation of terminology rather than rote memorization of terms, every chapter was carefully analyzed to meet the criteria of simplicity, practicality, and clarity.*

A new century brings new technology, and this edition now includes a CD-ROM with additional material to test and broaden your knowledge of the medical language.

---

*New to this edition is the omission of the possessive form of all eponyms (e.g., Down syndrome, Tourette syndrome, Alzheimer disease). While the possessive form remains acceptable, I am responding to a growing trend in promoting consistency and clarity. This decision is supported by The American Association for Medical Transcription in their Manual of Style (1995) and the American Medical Association in their Manual of Style, 9th ed. (Williams & Wilkins, 1998), as well as by major medical dictionaries.

The CD-ROM (with images and video clips) contains a wide variety of stimulating questions and answers, examples of medical reports and records using specific terminology learned in each chapter, pronunciation of terms, and analysis of word parts.

In addition, *The Language of Medicine Instant Translator* is now available. It is a pocket-sized medical terminology study reference that contains practical, useful information while providing a quick and valuable resource for the professional. Its contents include a word parts glossary; medical abbreviations, symbols, acronyms and professional designations; definitions of commonly used diagnostic tests and procedures; top 100 medical diagnoses and associated procedures; top 100 prescription drugs and their uses; and full color illustrations of body systems.

For teachers of medical terminology, I have updated *The Language of Medicine Instructor's Manual*. It contains a wealth of information that includes new quizzes, teaching suggestions from other instructors, crossword puzzles, medical reports, and reference materials. An instructor's "ExaMaster" or test bank also is available to complement this sixth edition. It is a CD-ROM program with questions to use in creating examinations for students. The CD-ROM test bank contains a Power Point image collection of 150 figures from *The Language of Medicine*. Instructors may use these figures in quizzes or for classroom teaching.

In this edition, the intrinsic, fundamental features that you depend on in *The Language of Medicine* remain the same. These are:

- Simple, nontechnical explanations of medical terms.
- Workbook format with ample spaces to write answers.
- Organization by body system with additional chapters on specialty medical areas.
- Explanations of clinical procedures, laboratory tests, and abbreviations related to each body system.
- Pronunciation of terms lists with phonetic spellings and spaces to write meanings of terms.
- Practical Applications sections with case reports, operative and diagnostic tests, and laboratory and x-ray reports.
- Comprehensive glossaries and appendices for reference in class and on the job.

Undeniably, the study of medical language requires commitment and hard work, but the benefits are great. You are learning a language that will enable you to interact more effectively in the newly computerized medical workplace and clinically as a health care professional. This book aims at bringing the language alive by making the study logical, interesting, and easy to follow.

Thank you for choosing *The Language of Medicine* and traveling with it into the new century. Please continue to communicate your comments and suggestions so that future editions and students will benefit. You can contact me through my web site (www.Chabner.com) or directly via my e-mail address (MedDavi@aol.com). I am always available for questions and happy to hear from you.

After 28 years of teaching medical terminology, I still feel a thrill and excitement as I begin a new class. I hope my continuing enthusiasm and passion for the medical language is transmitted to you through these pages. Work hard but have fun with *The Language of Medicine!*

Davi-Ellen Chabner

ACKNOWLEDGMENTS

Words are totally inadequate in describing my debt of gratitude to Maureen Pfeifer, Acquisitions Editor at Harcourt Health Sciences. She, most of all, was the driving force behind this new edition and its many ancillary products. A brilliant, dynamic, talented, energetic, and effective leader, Maureen shepherded the edition from its inception to completion. She brainstormed for solutions to any and all problems, nursed me through my computer-ignorant woes, and spent countless hours driving to Boston to work on the CD-ROM and other facets of the edition. Best of all, she is a treasured friend. Thank you, Maureen for your dedication to *The Language of Medicine* and confidence in my work.

The extraordinary talents of Scott W. Weaver, my Senior Developmental Editor, also were invaluable to this new edition. As always, Scott's intelligence, meticulous attention to detail, uncanny good sense, and responsiveness to coping with every aspect of the edition were crucial. I particularly appreciated his excellent organization of *The Language of Medicine Instant Translator*. Thank you, Scott!

I am grateful to the many physicians who read chapters and gave useful suggestions leading to practical and accurate changes in the text. First and foremost, my daughter, Dr. Elizabeth Chabner Thompson, did it all AND at the same time (within 15 months) presented me with two precious grandchildren. Special thanks as well to Dr. Bruce Chabner, Dr. Peter Banks, Dr. Michael J. Curtin, Dr. A.K. Goodman, Dr. Jeremy Coplan, Dr. Jennifer Lawrence, Dr. James Rosenzweig, Dr. Henry Schneiwind, Dr. Daniel Simon, and Dr. Norman Simon.

Many experienced and dedicated medical terminology instructors took the time and effort to communicate with me about classroom experiences and other aspects of *The Language of Medicine*. I appreciated their honesty and astute comments, many of which are reflected in this edition. Thanks to Laura Clark, Judy Aronow, Annalee Collins, Donna Gernert, Leslie Jebson, Kris Lewter, Debra Sweetser, Lisa Stimatz, Lynn White, and Susan Webb.

My family and friends, near and far, have unflaggingly nurtured me and my spirit throughout the years. I will always be grateful to them. Even before beginning the first edition of *The Language of Medicine*, my mother, Estelle Rosenzweig, enthusiastically advocated the project. My long-time friend, Brenda Melson, was particularly encouraging and supportive during the writing of the fifth and sixth editions.

Finally, but certainly not least, an army of loyal and hard-working people at Harcourt Health Sciences tirelessly devoted countless hours to this new edition. Thank you to Andrew Allen, Editor-in-Chief, Health-Related Professions; Agnes Hunt Byrne, Project Manager; Kimberly Coleman, Editorial Assistant; Linn Jeffries, Copy Editor; Lisa Lambert, Illustration Coordinator; Patti Maddaloni, Page Layout; Pat Morrison, Art and Design Director; David Murphy, Production Manager/Electronic Products; Colleen Murray-Lasko, Marketing Manager; Carolyn Naylor, Assistant Director, Book Production; Jim Perkins, Illustrator; Frank Polizzano, Production Manager; Sharon Salomon, Creative Director, Advertising; David Saracco, Manager Electronic Production; and Ellen Zanolle, Designer. Betty Taylor, Director of Production, Editing, and Dictionaries, was my initial editor at W.B. Saunders, and I am forever grateful for her mentorship and loyalty to *The Language of Medicine*.

CONTENTS

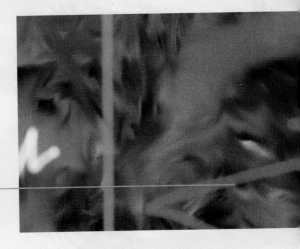

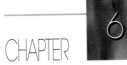

CHAPTER

Additional Suffixes and Digestive System Terminology   179

CHAPTER

Urinary System   203

CHAPTER

Female Reproductive System   241

CHAPTER

Male Reproductive System   293

CHAPTER

Nervous System   319

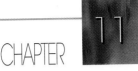

CHAPTER 11

Cardiovascular System   369

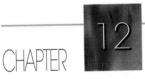

CHAPTER 12

Respiratory System   425

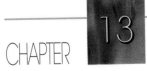

CHAPTER 13

Blood System   465

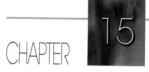

CHAPTER 14

Lymphatic and Immune Systems   505

CHAPTER 15

Musculoskeletal System   533

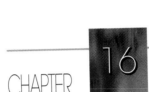

CHAPTER 16

Skin   601

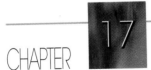

CHAPTER 17

Sense Organs: The Eye and the Ear   637

CHAPTER

Endocrine System

685

CHAPTER

Cancer Medicine (Oncology)

733

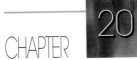

CHAPTER

Radiology, Nuclear Medicine, and Radiation Therapy   775

CHAPTER

Pharmacology   809

CHAPTER 22

Psychiatry   843

Glossary   879

Appendix I   903

Appendix II   905

Appendix III   913

Index   917

CHAPTER

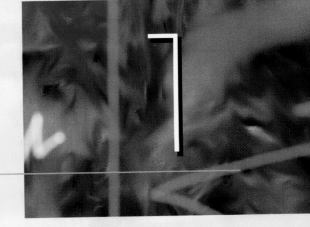

Basic Word Structure

This chapter is divided into the following sections

In this chapter you will

- Become familiar with basic objectives to keep in mind as you study the medical language;
- Divide medical words into their component parts;
- Find the meaning of basic combining forms, prefixes, and suffixes of the medical language; and
- Use these combining forms, prefixes, and suffixes to build medical words.

I. Objectives in Studying the Medical Language

There are three objectives to keep in mind as you study medical terminology.

1. **Analyze words by dividing them into component parts.** Your goal is to learn the *tools* of word analysis that will make the understanding of complex terminology easier. Do not simply memorize terms; think about dividing terms into component parts. This text will show you how to separate both complicated and simple terms into understandable word elements. Medical terms are very much like individual

1

jigsaw puzzles. They are constructed of small pieces that make each word unique, but the pieces can be used in different combinations in other words as well. As you become familiar with word parts and learn what each means, you will be able to recognize those word parts in totally new combinations in other terms.

2. **Relate the medical terms to the structure and function of the human body.** Memorization of terms, although essential to retention of the language, should not become the primary objective of your study. A major focus of this text is to *explain* terms in the context of how the body works in health and disease. Medical terms explained in their proper context will also be easier to remember. Thus, the term **hepatitis,** meaning inflammation **(-itis)** of the liver **(hepat),** is better understood when you know where the liver is and how it functions. No previous knowledge of biology, anatomy, or physiology is needed for this study. Explanations in the text are straightforward and basic.

3. **Be aware of spelling and pronunciation problems.** Some medical terms are pronounced alike but are spelled differently, which accounts for their different meanings. For example, **ilium** and **ileum** have identical pronunciations, but the first term, **ilium,** means a part of the pelvis (hip bone), whereas the second term, **ileum,** means a part of the small intestine. Even when terms are spelled correctly, terms can be misunderstood because of incorrect pronunciation. For example, the **urethra** (ū-RĒ-thrăh) is the tube leading from the urinary bladder to the outside of the body, whereas a **ureter** (ŪR-ĕ-tĕr) is one of two tubes each leading from a single kidney and inserting into the urinary bladder. Figure 1–1 illustrates the difference between the urethra and the ureters.

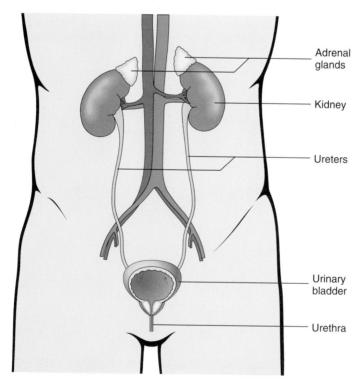

- Adrenal glands
- Kidney
- Ureters
- Urinary bladder
- Urethra

Figure 1–1

Urinary system.

II. Word Analysis

Studying medical terminology is very similar to learning a new language. The words at first sound strange and complicated, although they may stand for commonly known English terms. The terms **otalgia,** meaning ear ache, and **ophthalmologist,** meaning eye doctor, are examples.

Your first job in learning the language is to understand how to divide words into their component parts. The medical language is logical in that most terms, whether complex or simple, can be broken down into basic parts and then understood. For example, consider the following term:

HEMATOLOGY

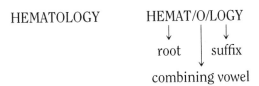

The **root** is the *foundation of the word.* All medical terms have one or more roots. The root **hemat** means **blood.**

The **suffix** is the *word ending.* All medical terms have a suffix. The suffix **-logy** means **study of.**

The **combining vowel** (usually o) *links the root to the suffix or the root to another root.* A combining vowel has no meaning of its own; it only joins one word part to another.

It is useful to read the meaning of medical terms *starting from the suffix and moving back to the beginning of the term.* Thus, the term **hematology** means **study of blood.**

Here is another familiar medical term:

ELECTROCARDIOGRAM

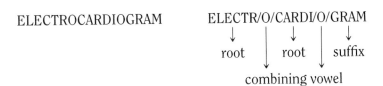

The root **electr** means **electricity.**
The root **cardi** means **heart.**
The suffix **-gram** means **record.**
The entire word means **record of the electricity in the heart.**

Notice that there are two combining vowels in this term. They link the two roots (**electr** and **cardi**) as well as the root (**cardi**) and suffix (**-gram**).

Try another term:

GASTRITIS   GASTR/ITIS
↓   ↓
root suffix

The root **gastr** means **stomach.**
The suffix **-itis** means **inflammation.**
The entire word, reading from the end of the term (suffix) to the beginning, means **inflammation of the stomach.**
Note that the combining vowel, o, is missing in this term. This is because the suffix, **-itis,** begins with a vowel. The combining vowel is dropped before a suffix that begins with a vowel. It is retained, however, between two roots, even if the second root begins with a vowel. Consider the following term:

GASTROENTEROLOGY   GASTR/O/ENTER/O/LOGY
↓ | ↓ | ↓
root | root | suffix
↓   ↓
combining vowel

The root **gastr** means **stomach.**
The root **enter** means **intestines.**
The suffix **-logy** means **study of.**
The entire term means **study of the stomach and intestines.**
Notice that the combining vowel is used between **gastr** and **enter,** even though the second root, **enter,** begins with a vowel. When a term contains two or more roots related to parts of the body, often anatomical position determines which root goes before the other. For example, the stomach receives food first, before the small intestine, thus, **gastroenteritis,** not enterogastritis.

In summary, remember three general rules:
1. Read the meaning of medical terms from the suffix back to the beginning of the term and across.
2. Drop the combining vowel (usually o) before a suffix beginning with a vowel: **gastritis** *not* **gastroitis.**
3. Keep the combining vowel between two roots: **gastroenterology** *not* **gastrenterology.**

In addition to the root, suffix, and combining vowel, there are two other word parts commonly found in medical terms. These are the **combining form** and **prefix.** The combining form is simply the root plus the combining vowel. For example, you are already familiar with the following combining forms and their meanings:

HEMAT/O   means   **blood**
↗   ↗
root + combining vowel = COMBINING FORM

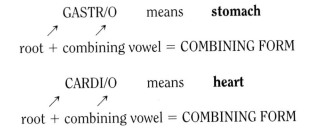

Combining forms can be used with many different suffixes, so it is useful to know the meaning of a combining form to decipher the meaning of a term.

The **prefix** is a small part that is attached to the *beginning of a term*. Not all medical terms contain prefixes, but the prefix can have an important influence on meaning. Consider the following examples:

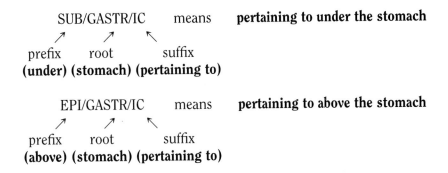

In summary, the important elements of medical terms are:
1. **Root:** foundation of the term
2. **Suffix:** word ending
3. **Prefix:** word beginning
4. **Combining vowel:** vowel (usually o) that links the root to the suffix or the root to another root
5. **Combining form:** combination of the root and the combining vowel

III. Combining Forms, Suffixes, and Prefixes

In previous examples you have been introduced to the combining forms **gastr/o** (stomach), **hemat/o** (blood), and **cardi/o** (heart). The following list contains new combining forms, suffixes, and prefixes with examples of medical words using those word parts. Your job is to write the *meaning* of the medical term in the space provided. As you do this, you may wish to divide the term into its component parts by using slashes (for example: **aden/oma**).

If you have a question about the correct pronunciation of a term, consult the Pronunciation of Terms section at the end of each chapter. In addition, the CD-ROM that accompanies this text contains the pronunciations of all terms on the Pronunciation of Terms lists. Although most medical terms can be divided into component parts and understood, others defy simple explanation. Additional information is provided in the text when those terms are introduced, and you may wish to consult a medical dictionary as well.

To test your understanding of word parts and terminology in this chapter, complete the exercises on pages 14 to 22 and check your answers on pages 22 to 24. Then, as a final review, give the meanings for the combining forms, suffixes, and prefixes on the Review Sheet, pages 29 and 30.

Write the meanings of the medical terms that follow in the spaces provided. The notes in italics below the terms will help you define them. Simple definitions are best. The first one has been filled in as an example.

Combining Forms

Combining Form	Meaning	Terminology	Meaning
aden/o	gland	adenoma _tumor of a gland_	
		The suffix -oma means tumor or mass.	
		adenitis _____	
		The suffix -itis means inflammation.	
arthr/o	joint	arthritis _____	
bi/o	life	biology _____	
		biopsy _____	
		The suffix -opsy means process of viewing. Living tissue is removed from the body and viewed under a microscope.	
carcin/o	cancerous, cancer	carcinoma _____	
		A carcinoma is a cancerous tumor. Carcinomas grow from epithelial (surface or skin) cells that cover the outside of the body and line organs, cavities, and tubes within the body.	
cardi/o	heart	cardiology _____	
cephal/o	head	cephalic _____	
		(sĕ-FAL-ĭk) The suffix -ic means pertaining to.	
cerebr/o	cerebrum (largest part of the brain)	cerebral _____	
		The suffix -al means pertaining to. A cerebrovascular accident (CVA) occurs when damage to blood vessels (vascul/o means blood vessels) in the cerebrum causes injury to nerve cells of the brain. This condition is also called a stroke.	
cis/o	to cut	incision _____	
		The prefix in- means into and the suffix -ion means process.	

excision _____

The prefix ex- means out.

crin/o	secrete (to form and give off)	endocrine glands _____
		The prefix endo- means within; endocrine glands (for example: thyroid, pituitary, and adrenal glands) secrete hormones directly within (into) the bloodstream. Other glands, called exocrine glands, secrete chemicals (saliva, sweat, tears) through tubes (ducts) to the outside of the body.
cyst/o	urinary bladder; a sac or a cyst (sac containing fluid)	cystoscopy _____
		(sĭs-TŎS-kō-pē) The suffix -scopy means process of visual examination.
cyt/o	cell	cytology _____
derm/o **dermat/o**	skin	dermatitis _____
		hypodermic _____
		The prefix hypo- means under, below.
electr/o	electricity	electrocardiogram _____
		The suffix -gram means record. Also called an ECG or EKG.
encephal/o	brain	electroencephalogram _____
		Also called an EEG.
enter/o	intestines (usually the small intestine)	enteritis _____
		The small intestine is narrower but much longer than the large intestine (colon).
erythr/o	red	erythrocyte _____
		The suffix -cyte means cell. Erythrocytes carry oxygen in the blood.
gastr/o	stomach	gastrectomy _____
		The suffix -ectomy means excision or removal.
		gastrotomy _____
		The suffix -tomy means incision or cutting into.
gnos/o	knowledge	diagnosis _____
		The prefix dia- means complete. The suffix -sis means state of. A diagnosis is made after sufficient information has been obtained about the patient's condition. Literally, it is a "state of complete knowledge."

prognosis _____

The prefix pro- means before. Literally, "knowledge before," a prognosis is a prediction about the outcome of an illness, but it is always given after the diagnosis has been determined.

gynec/o   woman, female   gynecology _____

hemat/o   blood   hematology _____
hem/o

hematoma _____

In this term, -oma means a mass or collection of blood, rather than a growth of cells (tumor). A hematoma occurs when blood is lost from blood vessels and collects as clotted blood in a cavity or organ or under the skin.

hepat/o   liver   hepatitis _____

iatr/o   treatment   iatrogenic _____

The suffix -genic means pertaining to producing, produced by, or produced in. Iatrogenic conditions are unexpected side effects that result from treatment by a physician.

leuk/o   white   leukocyte _____

This blood cell helps the body fight disease.

nephr/o   kidney   nephritis _____

nephrology _____

neur/o   nerve   neurology _____

onc/o   tumor   oncology _____

oncologist _____

The suffix -ist means one who specializes in a field of medicine.

ophthalm/o   eye   ophthalmoscope _____

(ŏf-THĂL-mō-skōp) The suffix -scope means an instrument for visual examination.

oste/o   bone   osteitis _____

osteoarthritis _____

This condition is actually a degeneration of bones and joints that occurs as the body ages. It is often accompanied by inflammation.

path/o   disease   pathology _____

pathologist _____

A pathologist examines biopsy samples microscopically and examines a dead body to determine the cause of death.

ped/o   child   pediatric _____

An orthopedist (orth/o means straight) was originally a doctor who straightened children's bones and corrected deformities. Nowadays, an orthopedist specializes in disorders of bones and muscles of people of all ages.

psych/o   mind   psychology _____

psychiatrist _____

radi/o   x-rays   radiology _____

ren/o   kidney   renal _____

Ren/o (Latin) and nephr/o (Greek) both mean kidney. Ren/o is used with -al (Latin) to describe the kidney, whereas nephr/o is used with other suffixes such as -osis, -itis, -ectomy (Greek) to describe abnormal conditions and operative procedures.

rhin/o   nose   rhinitis _____

sarc/o   flesh   sarcoma _____

This is a cancerous (malignant) tumor. A sarcoma grows from cells of "fleshy" connective tissue such as muscle, bone, and fat, whereas a carcinoma (another type of cancerous tumor) grows from epithelial cells that line the outside of the body or the inside of organs in the body.

sect/o   to cut   resection _____

The prefix re- means back. A resection is a cutting back in the sense of cutting out or removal (excision). A gastric resection is a gastrectomy, or excision of the stomach.

thromb/o   clot, clotting   thrombocyte _____

These cells help clot blood and are also known as platelets. A thrombus is the actual clot that forms, and thrombosis (-osis means condition) is the condition of clot formation.

ur/o   urinary tract, urine   urology _____

A urologist is a surgeon who operates on the organs of the urinary tract and the organs of the male reproductive system.

Suffixes

Suffix	Meaning	Terminology	Meaning
-ac	pertaining to	cardiac _____	
-al	pertaining to	neural _____	
-algia	pain	arthralgia _____	
		neuralgia _____	
-cyte	cell	erythrocyte _____	
-ectomy	excision, removal	nephrectomy _____	
-emia	blood condition	leukemia _____	

Literally, this term means a blood condition of white (blood cells). Actually, it is a large increase in the number of cancerous, abnormal white blood cells.

Suffix	Meaning	Terminology	Meaning
-genic	pertaining to producing, produced by, or produced in	carcinogenic _____	

Cigarette smoke is carcinogenic.

pathogenic _____

A virus or a bacterium is a pathogenic organism.

iatrogenic _____

In this term, -genic means produced by.

Suffix	Meaning	Terminology	Meaning
-gram	record	electroencephalogram _____	
-ic, -ical	pertaining to	gastric _____	
		neurological _____	
-ion	process	excision _____	
-ist	specialist	gynecologist _____	
-itis	inflammation	cystitis _____	
-logy	study of	endocrinology _____	
-oma	tumor, mass, swelling	hepatoma _____	

A hepatoma (hepatocellular carcinoma) is a malignant tumor of the liver.

-opsy	process of viewing	biopsy _____
-osis	condition, usually abnormal (slight increase in numbers when used with blood cells)	nephrosis _____ leukocytosis _____ *This condition, a slight increase in normal white blood cells, occurs as white blood cells multiply to fight an infection.*
-pathy	disease condition	enteropathy _____ *(ĕn-tĕ-RŎP-ă-thē)* adenopathy _____ *(ă-dĕ-NŎP-ă-thē)*
-scope	instrument to visually examine	endoscope _____ *Endo- means within. A cystoscope is an endoscope.*
-scopy	process of visually examining	endoscopy _____ *(ĕn-DŎS-kō-pē)*
-sis	state of	prognosis _____
-tomy	process of cutting, incision	osteotomy _____ *(ŏs-tē-ŎT-tō-mē)*
-y	process, condition	gastroenterology _____

Prefixes			
Prefix	**Meaning**	**Terminology**	**Meaning**
a-, an-	no, not, without	anemia _____ *Anemia means a decreased number of erythrocytes or an abnormality of the hemoglobin (a chemical) within the red blood cells. The result is decreased delivery of oxygen to cells of the body. Anemic patients looked so pale that they were thought to be "without blood."*	
auto-	self	autopsy _____ *Actually, an autopsy is the examination of a dead body (with one's own eyes) to determine the cause of death and nature of disease.*	
dia-	through, complete	diagnosis _____	

endo-	within	endocrinologist _____
epi-	above, upon	epigastric _____
		epidermis _____

The outermost layer of skin, lying above the middle layer of skin (called the dermis).

ex-	out	excision _____
exo-	out	exocrine glands _____
hyper-	excessive, above, more than normal	hyperglycemia _____

The term glyc/o means sugar.

| hypo- | deficient, below, less than normal | hypogastric _____ |

When hypo- is used with a part of the body, it means below.

hypoglycemia _____

In this term, hypo- means deficient.

| in- | into, in | incision _____ |
| peri- | surrounding, around | pericardium _____ |

The suffix -um means a structure. The pericardium is a membrane surrounding the heart.

| pro- | before | prognosis _____ |
| re- | back, backward, again | resection _____ |

An operation in which an organ is "cut back" or removed.

retro-	behind	retrocardiac _____
sub-	below, under	subhepatic _____
trans-	across, through	transhepatic _____

IV. Practical Applications

This is an opportunity for you to use your skill in understanding medical terms and to increase your knowledge of new terms. Be sure to check your answers with the Answers to Practical Applications on page 24. You should find helpful explanations there.

Specialists

Match the **abnormal condition** in COLUMN I with the **physician (specialist) who treats** it in COLUMN II.

Column I		Column II
1. heart attack	_____	A. gastroenterologist
2. ovarian cysts	_____	B. hematologist
		C. nephrologist
3. bipolar (manic-depressive) disorder	_____	D. cardiologist
		E. oncologist
4. breast adenocarcinoma	_____	F. gynecologist
		G. urologist
5. iron-deficiency anemia	_____	H. ophthalmologist
		I. neurologist
6. retinopathy	_____	J. psychiatrist
7. cerebrovascular accident	_____	
8. renal failure	_____	
9. inflammatory bowel disease	_____	
10. cystitis	_____	

V. Exercises

The exercises that follow are designed to help you learn the terms that are presented in the chapter. Writing terms over and over again is a good way to remember this new language. Answers are presented in Section VI so that they are easy to refer to as you work. *Check your answers carefully* to gain additional information from the correct answers. Each exercise is designed not as a test, but rather as an opportunity for you to learn the material.

A. Complete the following sentences.

1. Word beginnings are called _____.

2. Word endings are called _____.

3. The foundation of a word is known as the _____.

4. A letter linking a suffix and a root, or linking two roots, in a term is called

   the _____.

5. The combination of a root and a combining vowel is known as the _____.

B. Give the meanings of the following combining forms.

1. cardi/o _____   7. carcin/o _____

2. aden/o _____   8. cyst/o _____

3. bi/o _____   9. cyt/o _____

4. cerebr/o _____   10. derm/o or dermat/o _____

5. cephal/o _____   11. encephal/o _____

6. arthr/o _____   12. electr/o _____

C. Give the meanings of the following suffixes.

1. -oma _____   5. -scopy _____

2. -al _____   6. -ic _____

3. -itis _____   7. -gram _____

4. -logy _____   8. -opsy _____

D. Using slashes, divide the following terms into parts and give the meaning of the entire term.

1. cerebral _____

2. biopsy _____

3. adenitis _____

4. cephalic _____

5. carcinoma _____

6. cystoscopy _____

7. electrocardiogram _____

8. cardiology _____

9. electroencephalogram _____

10. dermatitis _____

11. arthroscopy _____

12. cytology _____

E. Give the meanings of the following combining forms.

1. erythr/o _____   7. nephr/o _____

2. enter/o _____   8. leuk/o _____

3. gastr/o _____   9. iatr/o _____

4. gnos/o _____   10. hepat/o _____

5. hemat/o _____   11. neur/o _____

6. cis/o _____   12. gynec/o _____

F. Complete the medical term based on its meaning, as provided.

1. white blood cell: _____ cyte

2. inflammation of the stomach: gastr _____

3. pertaining to being produced by treatment: _____ genic

4. study of kidneys: _____ logy

5. red blood cell: _____ cyte

6. mass of blood: _____ oma

7. view of living tissue: bi _____

8. pain of nerves: neur _____

9. process of viewing the eye: _____ scopy

10. inflammation of the small intestine: _____ itis

G. Match the English term in column I with its combining form in column II.

Column I
English Term

Column II
Combining Form

1. kidney _____

2. disease _____

3. eye _____

4. to cut _____

5. nose _____

6. flesh _____

7. mind _____

8. urinary tract _____

9. bone _____

10. x-rays _____

11. clotting _____

12. tumor _____

psych/o
ophthalm/o
oste/o
path/o
ren/o
rhin/o
radi/o
onc/o
sarc/o
thromb/o
ur/o
sect/o

H. Underline the suffix in each term and give the meaning of the entire term.

1. ophthalmoscopy _____

2. ophthalmoscope _____

3. oncology _____

4. osteitis _____

5. psychosis _____

6. thrombocyte _____

7. renal _____

8. nephrectomy _____

9. osteotomy _____

10. resection _____

11. carcinogenic _____

12. sarcoma _____

I. Match the suffix in column I with its meaning in column II. Write the meaning in the space provided.

Column I
Suffix

Column II
Meaning

1. -algia _____

2. -ion _____

3. -emia _____

4. -gram _____

5. -scope _____

6. -osis _____

7. -ectomy _____

8. -genic _____

9. -pathy _____

10. -tomy _____

11. -itis _____

12. -cyte _____

abnormal condition
record
pertaining to producing, produced by, or produced in
instrument to visually examine
pain
blood condition
removal, excision, resection
process
inflammation
cell
disease condition
incision, process of cutting into

J. Select from the following terms to complete the sentences below.

leukocytosis	leukemia	endocrine glands
arthralgia	hematoma	exocrine glands
enteropathy	carcinogenic	iatrogenic
cystitis	neuralgia	hepatoma

1. Cigarette smoke is an example of a (an) _____ substance.

2. When there is the abnormal condition of a slight increase in white blood cells due to infection in the body, the condition is called _____.

3. A tumor of the liver is a (an) _____.

4. The medical term for pain in joints is _____.

5. Organs that secrete chemical (hormones) directly into the blood are called

   _____.
   Examples are the thyroid gland (in the neck), the pituitary gland (at the base of the brain), and the adrenal glands (on top of the kidneys).

6. Organs that secrete chemicals out of the body through tubes (ducts) are

   called _____. Examples are sweat, tear, and salivary glands.

7. The medical term for nerve pain is _____.

8. Ms. Walsh went to her doctor with complaints of pain when urinating. The doctor's diagnosis of her condition was inflammation of the urinary bladder, also known as _____.

9. A collection (mass) of blood (under the skin) is a (an) _____.

10. Mr. Bell's white blood cell count is 10 times higher than normal. Examination of his blood shows cancerous white blood cells. His diagnosis is _____.

11. Mr. Kay was resuscitated (revived from potential or apparent death) in the emergency room (ER) after experiencing a heart attack. Unfortunately, he suffered a broken rib as a result of the physician's chest compressions. This is an example of a (an) _____ fracture.

12. After coming back from a trip during which he had eaten strange foods, Mr. Cameron had a disease (condition) in his intestines, called _____.

K. Give the meanings of the following prefixes.

1. dia- _____ 8. endo- _____

2. pro- _____ 9. retro- _____

3. auto- _____ 10. trans- _____

4. a-, an- _____ 11. peri- _____

5. hyper- _____ 12. ex- _____

6. hypo- _____ 13. sub- _____

7. epi- _____ 14. re- _____

L. Underline the prefix in the following terms and give the meaning of the entire term.

1. diagnosis _____

2. prognosis _____

3. subhepatic _____

4. pericardium _____

5. hyperglycemia _____

6. hypodermic _____

7. epigastric _____

8. resection _____

9. hypoglycemia _____

10. anemia _____

M. Complete the following terms (describing areas of medicine) based on their meanings as given below.

1. study of urinary tract: _____ logy

2. study of women and women's diseases: _____ logy

3. study of blood: _____ logy

4. study of tumors: _____ logy

5. study of the kidneys: _____ logy

6. study of nerves: _____ logy

7. treatment of children: _____ iatrics

8. study of x-rays: _____ logy

9. study of the eyes: _____ logy

10. study of the stomach and intestines: _____ logy

11. study of glands that secrete hormones: _____ logy

12. treatment of the mind: _____ iatry

13. study of disease: _____ logy

14. study of the heart: _____ logy

N. Give the meaning of the underlined word part and then define the term.

1. <u>cerebro</u>vascular accident _____

2. <u>encephal</u>itis _____

3. <u>cysto</u>scope _____

4. <u>trans</u>hepatic _____

5. <u>iatro</u>genic _____

6. <u>hypo</u>gastric _____

7. <u>endo</u>crine glands _____

8. neur<u>ectomy</u> _____

O. Select from the following terms to complete the sentences below.

anemia	nephrologist	neuropathy
biopsy	psychiatrist	psychologist
oncologist	urologist	oncogenic
pathogenic	thrombocyte	leukemia
prognosis	thrombosis	diagnosis
osteoarthritis		

1. Seventy-two-year-old Ms. Crick suffers from a degenerative joint disease that is caused by the wearing away of tissue around her joints. This condition, which literally means inflammation of

   bones and joints, is called _____.

2. The _____ sample was removed during surgery and sent to a pathologist to be examined under a microscope for a proper diagnosis.

3. A (an) _____ performed surgery to remove Mr. Simon's cancerous kidney.

4. Ms. Rose has suffered from hyperglycemia (diabetes) for many years. This condition can lead to

   long-term complications such as the disease of nerves called diabetic _____.

5. A virus or a bacterium produces disease and is therefore a (an) _____ organism.

6. Mr. Jordan has a disease caused by abnormal hemoglobin in his erythrocytes. The erythrocytes change shape, collapsing to form sickle-shaped cells that can become clots and stop the flow of

   blood. He has a condition called sickle-cell _____.

7. A (an) _____ is a doctor who treats carcinomas and sarcomas.

8. A cell that helps blood to clot is called a platelet or _____.

9. Dr. Susan Parker told Mr. Jones that his condition would improve with treatment in a few weeks.

   She said his _____ is excellent and he can expect total recovery.

10. A (an) _____ is a medical doctor who treats mental illness and can prescribe medications.

P. Select the correct term to complete each sentence.

1. Ms. Brody had a cough and fever. Her doctor instructed her to go to the **(pathology, radiology, hematology)** department for a chest x-ray.

2. Ms. Thompson had problems holding her urine (a condition known as urinary incontinence). She made an appointment with a **(gastroenterologist, gynecologist, urologist)**.

3. Dr. Monroe told a new mother she had lost much blood during delivery of her child. She had **(anemia, leukocytosis, adenitis)** and needed a blood transfusion immediately.

4. Mr. Preston was having chest pain during his morning walks. He made an appointment to discuss his new symptom with a **(nephrologist, neurologist, cardiologist)**.

5. After the skiing accident, Dr. Curtin suggested **(cystoscopy, biopsy, arthroscopy)** to visually examine my swollen, painful knee.

VI. Answers to Exercises

A

1. prefixes
2. suffixes
3. root
4. combining vowel
5. combining form

B

1. heart
2. gland
3. life
4. cerebrum, largest part of the brain
5. head
6. joint
7. cancer, cancerous
8. urinary bladder
9. cell
10. skin
11. brain
12. electricity

C

1. tumor, mass, swelling
2. pertaining to
3. inflammation
4. process of study
5. process of visual examination
6. pertaining to
7. record
8. process of viewing

D

1. cerebr/al—pertaining to the cerebrum or largest part of the brain
2. bi/opsy—process of viewing life (removal of living tissue and viewing it under the microscope)
3. aden/itis—inflammation of a gland
4. cephal/ic—pertaining to the head
5. carcin/oma—tumor that is cancerous (cancerous tumor)
6. cyst/o/scopy—process of visually examining the urinary bladder
7. electr/o/cardi/o/gram—record of the electricity in the heart
8. cardi/o/logy—process of study of the heart
9. electr/o/encephal/o/gram—record of the electricity in the brain
10. dermat/itis—inflammation of the skin
11. arthr/o/scopy—process of visual examination of a joint
12. cyt/o/logy—process of study of cells

E

1. red
2. intestines (usually small intestine)
3. stomach
4. knowledge
5. blood
6. to cut
7. kidney
8. white
9. treatment
10. liver
11. nerve
12. woman, female

F

1. leukocyte
2. gastritis
3. iatrogenic
4. nephrology

5. erythrocyte
6. hematoma
7. biopsy
8. neuralgia

9. ophthalmoscopy
10. enteritis

G

1. ren/o
2. path/o
3. ophthalm/o
4. sect/o

5. rhin/o
6. sarc/o
7. psych/o
8. ur/o

9. oste/o
10. radi/o
11. thromb/o
12. onc/o

H

1. ophthalmoscopy—process of visual examination of the eye
2. ophthalmoscope—instrument to visually examine the eye
3. oncology—study of tumors
4. osteitis—inflammation of bone
5. psychosis—abnormal condition of the mind

6. thrombocyte—clotting cell (platelet)
7. renal—pertaining to the kidney
8. nephrectomy—removal (excision) of the kidney
9. osteotomy—incision of (to cut into) a bone
10. resection—process of cutting back (in the sense of "out" or removal)

11. carcinogenic—pertaining to producing cancer
12. sarcoma—tumor of flesh (cancerous tumor of flesh tissue, such as bone, fat, and muscle)

I

1. pain
2. process
3. blood condition
4. record
5. instrument to visually examine

6. abnormal condition
7. removal, excision, resection
8. pertaining to producing, produced by, or produced in
9. disease condition

10. incision, process of cutting into
11. inflammation
12. cell

J

1. carcinogenic
2. leukocytosis
3. hepatoma
4. arthralgia

5. endocrine glands
6. exocrine glands
7. neuralgia
8. cystitis

9. hematoma
10. leukemia
11. iatrogenic
12. enteropathy

K

1. complete, through
2. before
3. self
4. no, not, without
5. excessive, above, more than normal

6. deficient, below, less than normal
7. above, upon
8. within
9. behind
10. across, through

11. surrounding
12. out
13. below, under
14. back

L

1. diagnosis—complete knowledge; a decision about the nature of the patient's condition after the appropriate tests are done
2. prognosis—before knowledge; a prediction about the outcome of treatment, and given after the diagnosis
3. subhepatic—pertaining to below the liver. A combining vowel is not needed between the prefix and the root.

4. pericardium—the membrane surrounding the heart
5. hyperglycemia—condition of excessive sugar in the blood
6. hypodermic—pertaining to under the skin
7. epigastric—pertaining to above the stomach
8. resection—process of cutting back (in the sense of cutting out)

9. hypoglycemia—condition of deficient (low) sugar in the blood
10. anemia—blood condition of low numbers of erythrocytes or deficient hemoglobin in the red blood cells

M

1. urology
2. gynecology
3. hematology
4. oncology
5. nephrology

6. neurology
7. pediatrics (combining vowel o has been dropped between ped and iatr)
8. radiology
9. ophthalmology

10. gastroenterology
11. endocrinology
12. psychiatry
13. pathology
14. cardiology

N

1. cerebrum (largest part of the brain). A cerebrovascular accident is damage to the blood vessels of the cerebrum leading to death of brain cells; also called a stroke.
2. brain. Encephalitis is inflammation of the brain.
3. urinary bladder. A cystoscope is an instrument used to visually examine the urinary bladder. The cystoscope is placed through the urethra into the bladder.
4. across, through. Transhepatic means pertaining to across or through the liver.
5. treatment. Iatrogenic means pertaining to an adverse side effect produced by treatment.
6. under, below, deficient. Hypogastric means pertaining to below the stomach.
7. within. Endocrine glands secrete hormones within the body. Examples of these are the pituitary, thyroid, and adrenal glands.
8. excision. Neurectomy is the removal of a nerve.

O

1. osteoarthritis
2. biopsy
3. urologist (a nephrologist is a medical doctor who treats kidney disorders but does not operate on patients)
4. neuropathy
5. pathogenic
6. anemia
7. oncologist
8. thrombocyte
9. prognosis
10. psychiatrist (a psychologist can treat mentally ill patients but is not a medical doctor and cannot prescribe medications)

P

1. radiology
2. urologist
3. anemia
4. cardiologist
5. arthroscopy

Answers to Practical Applications

1. **D** A **cardiologist** is an internal medicine specialist who takes additional (fellowship) training in the diagnosis and treatment of heart disease.
2. **F** A **gynecologist** trains in both surgery and internal medicine in order to diagnose and treat disorders of the female reproductive system. Ovarian cysts are sacs of fluid that form on and in the ovaries (female organs that produce eggs and hormones).
3. **J** A **psychiatrist** is a specialist in diagnosing and treating mental illness. In bipolar disorder (manic-depressive illness), the mood switches periodically from excessive mania (excitability) to deep depression (sadness, despair, and discouragement).
4. **E** An **oncologist** is an internal medicine specialist who takes fellowship training in the diagnosis and medical (drug) treatment of cancer.
5. **B** A **hematologist** is an internal medicine specialist who takes fellowship training in the diagnosis and treatment of blood disorders such as anemia and clotting diseases.
6. **H** An **ophthalmologist** trains in both surgery and internal medicine to diagnose and treat disorders of the eye. The retina is a sensitive layer of light-receptor cells in the back of the eye. Retinopathy can occur as a secondary complication of chronic diabetes (hyperglycemia).
7. **I** A **neurologist** is an internal medicine specialist who takes fellowship training in the diagnosis and treatment of disorders of nervous tissue (brain, spinal cord, and nerves). A CVA causes damage to areas of the brain and results in loss of function.
8. **C** A **nephrologist** is an internal medicine specialist who takes fellowship training in the diagnosis and medical treatment of kidney disease. A nephrologist does not perform surgery on the urinary tract, but treats kidney disease with drugs.
9. **A** A **gastroenterologist** is an internal medicine specialist who takes fellowship training in the diagnosis and treatment of disorders of the gastrointestinal tract. Examples of inflammatory bowel disease are ulcerative colitis (inflammation of the large intestine) and Crohn disease (inflammation of the last part of the small intestine).
10. **G** A **urologist** is a surgical specialist who treats and operates on organs of the urinary tract (such as the urinary bladder) and the male reproductive system.

VII. Pronunciation of Terms

The markings ¯ and ˘ above the vowels (a, e, i, o, and u) indicate the proper sounds of the vowels. When ¯ is above a vowel its sound is long, that is, exactly like its name; for example:

> ā as in āpe
> ē as in ēven
> ī as in īce
> ō as in ōpen
> ū as in ūnit

The ˘ marking indicates a short vowel sound, as in the following examples:

> ă as in ăpple
> ĕ as in ĕvery
> ĭ as in ĭnterest
> ŏ as in pŏt
> ŭ as in ŭnder

To test your understanding of the terminology in this chapter, write the meaning of each term in the space provided. In addition, you may wish to cover the terms and write them by looking at your definitions. Make sure your spelling is correct. The page number after each term indicates where it is defined or used in the text so you can easily check your responses.

Term	Pronunciation	Meaning
adenitis (6)	ăd-ĕ-NĪ-tĭs	_____
adenoma (6)	ăd-ĕ-NŌ-mă	_____
adenopathy (11)	ăd-ĕ-NŎP-ă-thē	_____
anemia (11)	ă-NĒ-mē-ă	_____
arthralgia (10)	ăr-THRĂL-jă	_____
arthritis (6)	ăr-THRĪ-tĭs	_____
autopsy (11)	ĂW-tŏp-sē	_____
biology (6)	bī-ŎL-ō-jē	_____
biopsy (6)	BĪ-ŏp-sē	_____
carcinogenic (10)	kăr-sĭ-nō-JĔN-ĭk	_____
carcinoma (6)	kăr-sĭ-NŌ-mă	_____
cardiac (10)	KĂR-dē-ăk	_____
cardiology (6)	kăr-dē-ŎL-ō-jē	_____
cephalic (6)	sĕ-FĂL-ĭk	_____

cerebral (6)   sĕ-RĒ-brăl or SĔR-ĕ-brăl   _____

cystitis (10)   sĭs-TĪ-tĭs   _____

cystoscopy (7)   sĭs-TŎS-kō-pē   _____

cytology (7)   sī-TŎL-ō-jē   _____

dermatitis (7)   dĕr-mă-TĪ-tĭs   _____

dermatology (7)   dĕr-mă-TŎL-ō-jē   _____

diagnosis (7)   dī-ăg-NŌ-sĭs   _____

electrocardiogram (7)   ē-lĕk-trō-KĂR-dē-ō-grăm   _____

electroencephalogram (7) ē-lĕk-trō-ĕn-SĔF-ă-lō-grăm   _____

endocrine glands (7)   ĔN-dō-krĭn glăndz   _____

endocrinologist (12)   ĕn-dō-krĭ-NŎL-ō-jĭst   _____

endocrinology (10)   ĕn-dō-krĭ-NŎL-ō-jē   _____

endoscope (11)   ĔN-dō-skōp   _____

endoscopy (11)   ĕn-DŎS-kō-pē   _____

enteritis (7)   ĕn-tĕ-RĪ-tĭs   _____

enteropathy (11)   ĕn-tĕ-RŎP-ă-thē   _____

epidermis (12)   ĕp-ĭ-DĔR-mĭs   _____

epigastric (12)   ĕp-ĭ-GĂS-trĭk   _____

erythrocyte (7)   ĕ-RĬTH-rō-sīt   _____

excision (7)   ĕk-SĬZH-ŭn   _____

exocrine glands (12)   ĔK-sō-krĭn glăndz   _____

gastrectomy (7)   găs-TRĔK-tō-mē   _____

gastric (10)   GĂS-trĭk   _____

gastroenterology (11)   găs-trō-ĕn-tĕr-ŎL-ō-jē   _____

gastrotomy (7)   găs-TRŎT-ō-mē   _____

gynecologist (10)   gī-nĕ-KŎL-ō-jĭst   _____

gynecology (8)   gī-nĕ-KŎL-ō-jē   _____

hematology (8)	hē-mă-TŎL-ō-jē	_____
hematoma (8)	hē-mă-TŌ-mă	_____
hepatitis (8)	hĕp-ă-TĪ-tĭs	_____
hepatoma (10)	hĕp-ă-TŌ-mă	_____
hyperglycemia (12)	hī-pĕr-glī-SĒ-mē-ă	_____
hypodermic (7)	hī-pō-DĔR-mĭk	_____
hypogastric (12)	hī-pō-GĂS-trĭk	_____
hypoglycemia (12)	hī-pō-glī-SĒ-mē-ă	_____
iatrogenic (8)	ī-ăt-rō-JĔN-ĭk	_____
incision (6)	ĭn-SĬZH-ŭn	_____
leukemia (10)	lū-KĒ-mē-ă	_____
leukocyte (8)	LŪ-kō-sīt	_____
leukocytosis (11)	lū-kō-sī-TŌ-sĭs	_____
nephrectomy (10)	nĕ-FRĔK-tō-mē	_____
nephritis (8)	nĕ-FRĪ-tĭs	_____
nephrology (8)	nĕ-FRŎL-ō-jē	_____
nephrosis (11)	nĕ-FRŌ-sĭs	_____
nephrotomy (8)	nĕ-FRŎT-ō-mē	_____
neural (10)	NŪ-răl	_____
neuralgia (10)	nū-RĂL-jă	_____
neurological (10)	nū-rō-LŎJ-ĭk-ăl	_____
neurology (8)	nū-RŎL-ō-jē	_____
oncologist (8)	ŏn-KŎL-ō-jĭst	_____
oncology (8)	ŏn-KŎL-ō-jē	_____
ophthalmologist (24)	ŏf-thăl-MŎL-ō-jĭst	_____
ophthalmoscope (8)	ŏf-THĂL-mō-skōp	_____
osteitis (8)	ŏs-tē-Ī-tĭs	_____

osteoarthritis (8)	ŏs-tē-ō-ăr-THRĪ-tĭs	_____
osteotomy (11)	ŏs-tē-ŎT-ō-mē	_____
pathogenic (10)	păth-ō-JĔN-ĭk	_____
pathologist (9)	pă-THŎL-ŏ-jĭst	_____
pathology (9)	pă-THŎL-ō-jē	_____
pediatric (9)	pē-dē-ĂT-rĭk	_____
pericardium (12)	pĕr-ĭ-KĂR-dē-ŭm	_____
prognosis (8)	prŏg-NŌ-sĭs	_____
psychiatrist (9)	sī-KĪ-ă-trĭst	_____
psychiatry (20)	sī-KĪ-ă-trē	_____
psychology (9)	sī-KŎL-ō-jē	_____
radiology (9)	rā-dē-ŎL-ō-jē	_____
renal (9)	RĒ-năl	_____
resection (9)	rē-SĔK-shŭn	_____
retrocardiac (12)	rĕt-rō-KĂR-dē-ăc	_____
rhinitis (9)	rī-NĪ-tĭs	_____
sarcoma (9)	săr-KŌ-mă	_____
subhepatic (12)	sŭb-hĕ-PĂT-ĭk	_____
thrombocyte (9)	THRŎM-bō-sīt	_____
transhepatic (12)	trănz-hĕ-PĂT-ĭk	_____
urology (9)	ū-RŎL-ō-jē	_____

VIII. Review Sheet

This review sheet and the others that follow each chapter are complete lists of the word elements contained in that chapter. The review sheets are designed to pull together the terminology and to reinforce your learning by giving you the opportunity to write the meanings of each word part in the spaces provided and test yourself. Check your answers with the information in the chapter or in the Glossary (Medical Terms—English) at the end of the book.

COMBINING FORMS

Combining Form	Meaning	Combining Form	Meaning
aden/o		hem/o, hemat/o	
arthr/o		hepat/o	
bi/o		iatr/o	
carcin/o		leuk/o	
cardi/o		log/o	
cephal/o		nephr/o	
cerebr/o		neur/o	
cis/o		onc/o	
crin/o		ophthalm/o	
cyst/o		oste/o	
cyt/o		path/o	
derm/o, dermat/o		ped/o	
electr/o		psych/o	
encephal/o		radi/o	
enter/o		ren/o	
erythr/o		rhin/o	
gastr/o		sarc/o	
glyc/o		sect/o	
gnos/o		thromb/o	
gynec/o		ur/o	

Continued on following page

SUFFIXES

Suffix	Meaning	Suffix	Meaning
-ac	_____	-itis	_____
-al	_____	-logy	_____
-algia	_____	-oma	_____
-cyte	_____	-opsy	_____
-ectomy	_____	-osis	_____
-emia	_____	-pathy	_____
-genic	_____	-scope	_____
-gram	_____	-scopy	_____
-ic, ical	_____	-sis	_____
-ion	_____	-tomy	_____
-ist	_____	-y	_____

PREFIXES

Prefix	Meaning	Prefix	Meaning
a-, an-	_____	hypo-	_____
auto-	_____	in-	_____
dia-	_____	peri-	_____
endo-	_____	pro-	_____
epi-	_____	re-	_____
ex-	_____	retro-	_____
exo-	_____	sub-	_____
hyper-	_____	trans-	_____

CHAPTER 2

Terms Pertaining to the Body as a Whole

This chapter is divided into the following sections

In this chapter you will

- Define terms that apply to the structural organization of the body;
- Identify the body cavities and recognize the organs contained within those cavities;
- Locate and identify the anatomical and clinical divisions of the abdomen;
- Locate and name the anatomical divisions of the back;
- Become acquainted with terms that describe positions, directions, and planes of the body; and
- Identify the meanings for new word elements and use them to understand new medical terms.

I. Structural Organization of the Body

Cells

The cell is the fundamental unit of all living things (animal or plant). Cells are everywhere in the human body—every tissue, every organ is made up of these individual units.

Similarity in Cells. All cells are similar in that they contain a gelatinous substance composed of water, protein, sugar, acids, fats, and various minerals. Several parts of a cell are described below and pictured in Figure 2–1 as they might look when photographed with an electron microscope. Label the structures on Figure 2–1. Throughout the book, numbers in brackets indicate that the boldfaced term preceding it is to be used in labeling.

The **cell membrane** [1] not only surrounds and protects the cell, but also regulates what passes into and out of the cell.

The **nucleus** [2] is the controlling structure of the cell. It directs the reproduction of the cell and determines the structure and function of the cell.

Chromosomes [3] are rod-like structures within the nucleus. All human body cells (except for the sex cells, the egg and sperm) contain 23 pairs of chromosomes. Each sperm and egg cell has only 23 unpaired chromosomes. After the egg and sperm cells unite to form the embryo, each cell of the embryo then has 46 chromosomes (23 pairs) (Fig. 2–2).

Chromosomes contain regions called **genes.** There are several thousand genes, in an orderly sequence, on each chromosome. Each gene is composed of a chemical called **DNA** (deoxyribonucleic acid). DNA regulates the activities of the cell by its sequence (arrangement into genes) on each chromosome. The DNA sequence is like a series of recipes in code. When the code is carried out of the nucleus to the rest of the cell, it directs the activities of the cell, such as cellular reproduction and the manufacture of proteins.

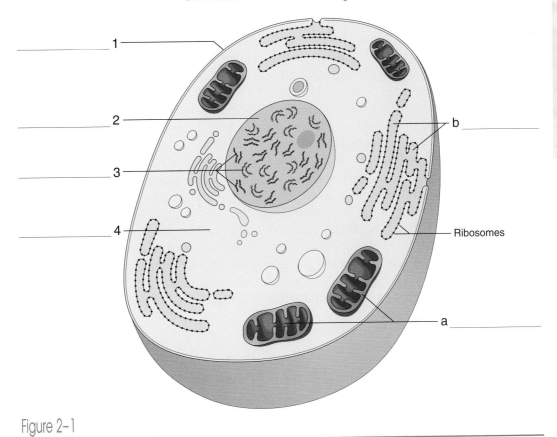

Figure 2-1

Major parts of a cell. Ribosomes (RĪ-bō-sōmz) are small granules that help the cell make proteins.

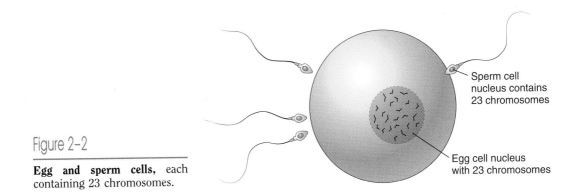

Figure 2-2

Egg and sperm cells, each containing 23 chromosomes.

Chromosomes within the nucleus can be analyzed in terms of their size, arrangement, and number by performing a **karyotype.** Karyotyping of chromosomes is useful to determine whether the chromosomes are normal in number and structure. For example, obstetricians often recommend an amniocentesis (puncture of the sac around the fetus for removal of fluid and cells) for a pregnant woman so that the karyotype of the baby can be examined. Figure 2–3 shows a karyotype, or chromosome "map," of a normal male. The chromosomes have been treated with chemicals so that bands (light and dark areas) can be seen.

If a baby is born with an abnormal number of chromosomes, serious problems can result. In Down syndrome, the karyotype shows 47 chromosomes instead of the normal number, which is 46. There is an extra number 21 chromosome. Thus, Down syndrome is also called trisomy-21 syndrome. Its incidence is about 1 in every 750 live births. The infant is born with physical malformations that may include a small, flattened skull; a short, flat-bridged nose; wide-set, slanted eyes; and short, broad hands and feet with a wide gap between the first and the second toes. Reproductive organs are often underdeveloped, congenital heart defects are not uncommon, and some degree of mental retardation is evident (Fig. 2–4).

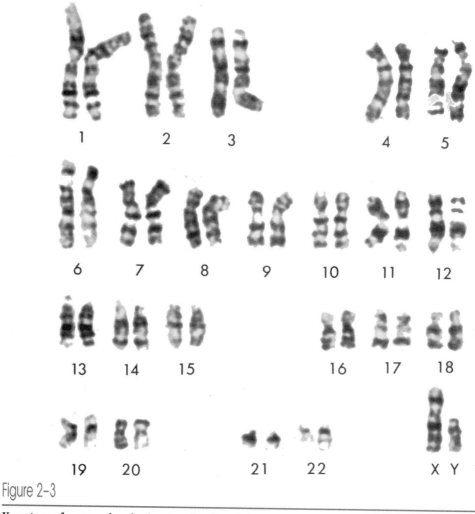

Figure 2-3

Karyotype of a normal male showing 23 pairs of chromosomes. The 23rd pair is the XY pair. In a normal female karyotype, the 23rd pair is XX. (From Behrman RE, Vaughn VC III [eds]: Nelson Textbook of Pediatrics, 13th ed. Philadelphia, WB Saunders, 1987, p 28.)

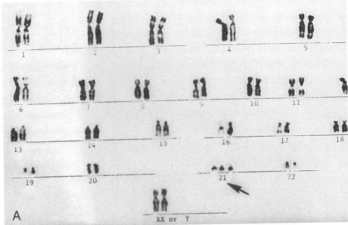

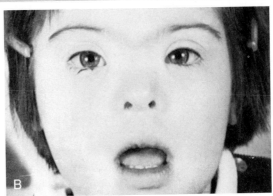

Figure 2–4

(A) Karyotype of a Down syndrome female patient showing trisomy 21. **(B) Photograph of a 3½-year-old girl with the typical facial appearance that occurs in Down syndrome.** This includes a flat nasal bridge, an upward slant of the eyes, and a protruding tongue. Other characteristics of Down syndrome patients are mental deficiency and heart defects. **(A,** From Zitelli BJ, Davis HW [eds]: Atlas of Pediatric Physical Diagnosis, 3rd ed. St. Louis, Mosby-Wolfe, 1997, p 10; **B,** From Jarvis C: Physical Examination and Health Assessment, 2nd ed. Philadelphia, WB Saunders, 1996, p 342.)

Continue labeling Figure 2–1.

Cytoplasm [4] (cyt/o = cell, -plasm = formation) is all the material outside the nucleus and enclosed by the cell membrane. It carries on the work of the cell (in a muscle cell, it does the contracting; in a nerve cell, it transmits impulses). The cytoplasm contains:

Mitochondria [a] are small, sausage-shaped bodies that, like miniature power plants, produce energy by burning food in the presence of oxygen. This chemical process is called **catabolism** (cata = down, bol = to cast, -ism = process). During catabolism, complex foods (sugar and fat) are broken down into simpler substances, and energy is released to do the work of the cell.

Endoplasmic reticulum [b] is a network (reticulum) of canals within the cell. These canals (containing small structures called ribosomes) are like a cellular tunnel system in which proteins are manufactured for use in the cell. This process of building up complex materials, such as proteins, from simpler parts is called **anabolism** (ana = up, bol = to cast, -ism = process). During anabolism, small pieces of protein are fitted together like links in a chain to make larger proteins.

The two processes, anabolism and catabolism, are known as **metabolism** (meta = change, bol = to cast, -ism = process). Metabolism is the total of the chemical processes occurring in a cell. If a person has a "fast metabolism," then foods, such as sugar and fat, are thought to be used up very quickly, and energy is released. If a person has a "slow metabolism," foods are thought to be burned slowly, and fat accumulates in cells.

STUDY SECTION 1

Practice spelling each term, and know its meaning.

anabolism
Process of building up complex materials (proteins) from simple materials.

catabolism
Process of breaking down complex materials (foods) to form simpler substances and release energy.

cell membrane
Structure surrounding and protecting the cell. It determines what enters and leaves the cell.

chromosomes
Rod-shaped structures in the nucleus that contain regions of DNA called genes. There are 46 chromosomes (23 pairs) in every cell except for the egg and sperm cells, which contain only 23 individual, unpaired chromosomes.

cytoplasm
All the material that is outside the nucleus and yet contained within the cell membrane.

DNA
Chemical found within each chromosome. Arranged like a sequence of recipes in code, it directs the activities of the cell.

endoplasmic reticulum
Structure (canals) within the cytoplasm. Site in which large proteins are made from smaller protein pieces.

genes
Regions of DNA within each chromosome.

karyotype
Picture of chromosomes in the nucleus of a cell. The chromosomes are arranged in a numerical order to determine their number and structure.

metabolism
The total of the chemical processes in a cell. It includes both catabolism and anabolism.

mitochondria
Structures in the cytoplasm in which foods are burned to release energy.

nucleus
Control center of the cell. It contains chromosomes and directs the activities of the cell.

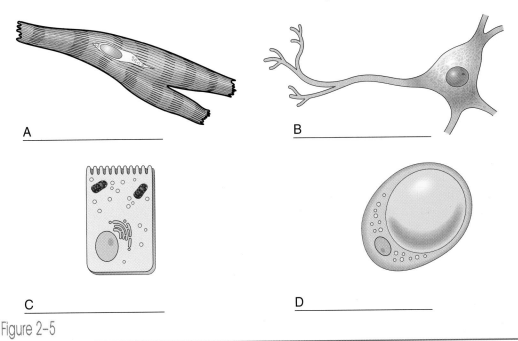

A _____

B _____

C _____

D _____

Figure 2–5

Types of cells. Label **(A)** muscle cell, **(B)** nerve cell, **(C)** epithelial cell, and **(D)** fat cell.

Differences in Cells. Cells are different, or specialized, throughout the body to carry out their individual functions. For instance, a **muscle cell** is long and slender and contains fibers that aid in contracting and relaxing; an **epithelial cell** (a lining and skin cell) may be square and flat to provide protection; a **nerve cell** may be quite long and have various fibrous extensions that aid in its job of carrying impulses; a **fat cell** contains large, empty spaces for fat storage. These are only a few of the many types of cells in the body. Different types of cells are pictured in Figure 2–5. Label the nerve cell, epithelial cell, fat cell, and muscle cell.

Tissues

A tissue is a group of similar cells working together to do a specific job. A **histologist** (hist/o = tissue) is a scientist who specializes in the study of tissues. Some types of tissues are:

Epithelial Tissue. Epithelial tissue is located all over the body and forms the linings of internal organs, makes up exocrine and endocrine glands, and forms the outer surface of the skin covering the body. The term **epithelial** was originally used to describe the tissue above (epi-) the breast nipple (thel/o). Now it describes tissue that covers the outside of the body and lines the inner surface of internal organs.

Muscle Tissue. Voluntary muscle is found in arms and legs and parts of the body where movement is voluntary, whereas involuntary muscle is found in the heart and digestive system, as well as in other places where movement is not under conscious control. Cardiac muscle is a specialized type of muscle found only in the heart and can be seen beating in a 6-week-old fetus.

Connective Tissue. Examples are **fat** (adipose tissue), **cartilage** (elastic, fibrous tissue attached to bones), bone, and blood.

Nerve Tissue. Nerve tissue conducts impulses all over the body.

Organs

Organs are structures composed of several kinds of tissue. For example, an organ like the stomach is composed of muscle tissue, nerve tissue, and glandular epithelial tissue. The medical term for internal organs is **viscera** (singular: **viscus**). Examples of abdominal viscera (organs located in the abdomen) are the liver, stomach, intestines, pancreas, spleen, and gallbladder.

Systems

Systems are groups of organs working together to perform complex functions. For example, the mouth, esophagus, stomach, and small and large intestines are organs that do the work of the digestive system to digest food and absorb it into the bloodstream.

Ten body systems are listed below with their organs. The organs in boldface are ones that you should learn to spell and identify.

System	Organs
Digestive	mouth, **pharynx** (throat), esophagus, stomach, intestines (small and large), liver, gallbladder, pancreas
Urinary or excretory	kidneys, **ureters** (tubes from the kidneys to the urinary bladder), urinary bladder, **urethra** (tube from the bladder to the outside of the body)
Respiratory	nose, pharynx, **larynx** (voice box), **trachea** (windpipe), bronchial tubes, lungs (where the exchange of gases takes place)
Reproductive	female: ovaries, fallopian tubes, **uterus** (womb), vagina, mammary glands; male: testes and associated tubes, urethra, penis, prostate gland
Endocrine	**thyroid gland** (in the neck), **pituitary gland** (at the base of the brain), sex glands (ovaries and testes), adrenal glands, pancreas (islets of Langerhans), parathyroid glands
Nervous	brain, spinal cord, nerves, and collections of nerves
Circulatory	heart, blood vessels (arteries, veins, and capillaries), lymphatic vessels and nodes, spleen, thymus gland
Muscular	muscles
Skeletal	bones and joints
Skin and sense organs	skin, hair, nails, sweat glands, and sebaceous (oil) glands; eye, ear, nose, and tongue

Practice spelling each term, and know its meaning.

adipose tissue	Collection of fat cells.
cartilage	Flexible connective tissue attached to bones at joints. For example, it surrounds the trachea, and forms part of the external ear and nose.
epithelial cell	Skin cells that cover the external body surface and line the internal surfaces of organs.
histologist	Specialist in the study of tissues.
larynx (LĂR-ĭnks)	Voice box; located at the upper part of the trachea.
pharynx (FĂR-ĭnks)	Throat. The pharynx is the common passageway for food (from the mouth going to the esophagus) and air (from the nose to the trachea).
pituitary gland	Endocrine gland at the base of the brain.
thyroid gland	Endocrine gland that surrounds the trachea in the neck.
trachea	Windpipe (tube leading from the throat to the bronchial tubes).
ureter	One of two tubes, each leading from a single kidney to the urinary bladder. Spelling clue: ureter has two e's and there are two of them.
urethra	Tube from the urinary bladder to the outside of the body. Spelling clue: urethra has one e and there is only one urethra.
uterus	The womb. The organ that holds the embryo and fetus as it develops.
viscera	Internal organs.

II. Body Cavities

A body cavity is a space within the body that contains internal organs (viscera). Label Figure 2–6 as you learn the names of the body cavities. Some of the important viscera contained within those cavities are listed as well.

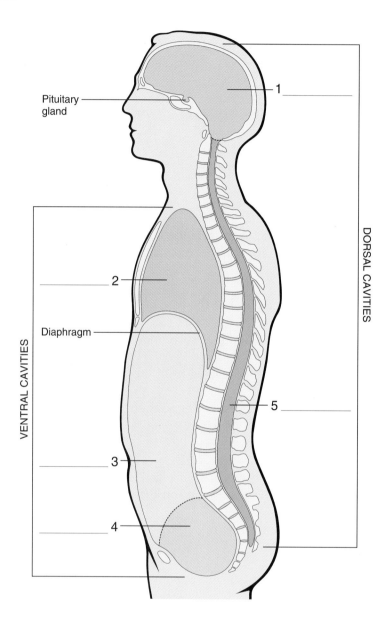

Pituitary gland

Diaphragm

VENTRAL CAVITIES

DORSAL CAVITIES

1

2

3

4

5

Figure 2-6

Body cavities. Ventral (anterior) cavities are in the front of the body. Dorsal (posterior) cavities are in the back.

Cavity	Organs
Cranial [1]	Brain, pituitary gland.
Thoracic [2]	Lungs, heart, esophagus, trachea, bronchial tubes, thymus gland, aorta (large artery).
	The thoracic cavity can be divided into two smaller cavities (Fig. 2–7):
	a. **Pleural cavity**—space between the membranes that surround each lung. Each pleural cavity is lined with a double-folded membrane called **pleura.** If the pleura becomes inflamed (as in pleuritis or pleurisy), the pleural cavity can fill with fluid.
	b. **Mediastinum**—centrally located area outside of and between the lungs. It contains the heart, aorta, trachea, esophagus, thymus gland, bronchial tubes, and many lymph nodes.
Abdominal [3]	Stomach, small and large intestines, spleen, pancreas, liver, and gallbladder.
	The **peritoneum** is the double-folded membrane surrounding the abdominal cavity (Fig. 2–8). The kidneys are two bean-shaped organs situated behind (retroperitoneal area) the abdominal cavity on either side of the backbone (see Fig. 2–10).
Pelvic [4]	Portions of the small and large intestines, rectum, urinary bladder, urethra, and ureters; uterus and vagina in the female.
Spinal [5]	Nerves of the spinal cord.

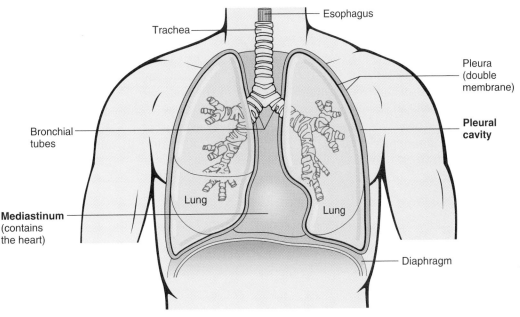

Figure 2–7

Divisions of the thoracic cavity.

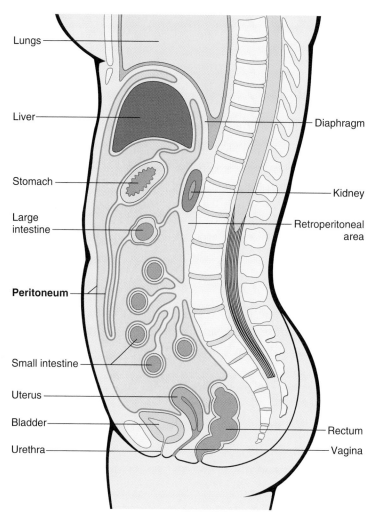

Lungs

Liver

Stomach

Large
intestine

Peritoneum

Small intestine

Uterus

Bladder

Urethra

Diaphragm

Kidney

Retroperitoneal
area

Rectum

Vagina

Figure 2-8

Abdominal cavity (side view).
Notice the **peritoneum,** which
is a membrane surrounding
the organs in the abdominal
cavity. The retroperitoneal area
is behind the peritoneum and
contains the kidneys.

The cranial and spinal cavities are **dorsal** body cavities because of their location on the back (posterior) portion of the body. The thoracic, abdominal, and pelvic cavities are **ventral** body cavities because they are on the front (anterior) portion of the body. See Figure 2–6.

The thoracic and abdominal cavities are separated by a muscular wall called the **diaphragm.** The abdominal and pelvic cavities are not separated by a muscular wall, and together they are frequently called the **abdominopelvic cavity.** Figures 2–9 and 2–10 show the abdominal and thoracic viscera from anterior (ventral) and posterior (dorsal) views.

▬ STUDY SECTION 3

Practice spelling each term, and know its meaning.

abdominal cavity	Space below the chest containing organs such as the liver, stomach, gallbladder, and intestines; also called the **abdomen.**
cranial cavity	Space in the head containing the brain and surrounded by the skull. **Cranial** means **pertaining to the skull.**
diaphragm	Muscle separating the abdominal and thoracic cavities.
dorsal (posterior)	Pertaining to the back.
mediastinum	Centrally located space between the lungs.
pelvic cavity	Space below the abdomen containing portions of the intestines, rectum, urinary bladder, and reproductive organs. **Pelvic** means **pertaining to the hip bone,** which surrounds the pelvic cavity.
peritoneum	Membrane surrounding the organs in the abdomen.
pleura	A double-layered membrane surrounding each lung.
pleural cavity	Space between the pleural membranes and surrounding each lung.
spinal cavity	Space within the spinal column (backbones) and containing the spinal cord. Also called the **spinal canal.**
thoracic cavity	Space in the chest containing the heart, lungs, bronchial tubes, trachea, esophagus, and other organs.
ventral (anterior)	Pertaining to the front.

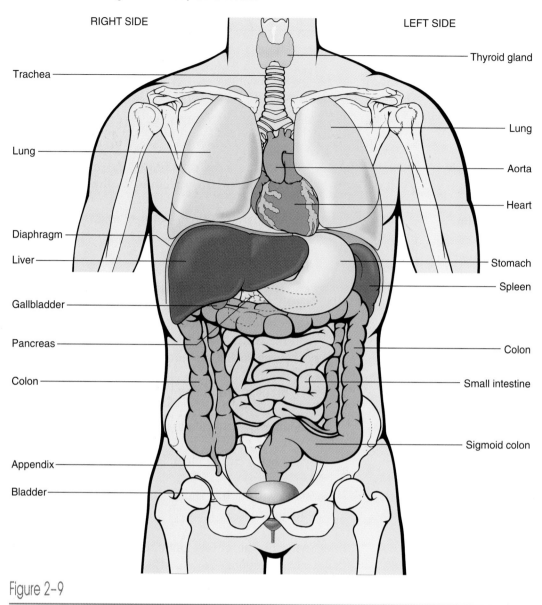

RIGHT SIDE   LEFT SIDE

Thyroid gland

Trachea

Lung

Lung

Aorta

Heart

Diaphragm

Liver

Stomach

Spleen

Gallbladder

Pancreas

Colon

Colon

Small intestine

Sigmoid colon

Appendix

Bladder

Figure 2-9

Organs of the abdominopelvic and thoracic cavities, anterior view.

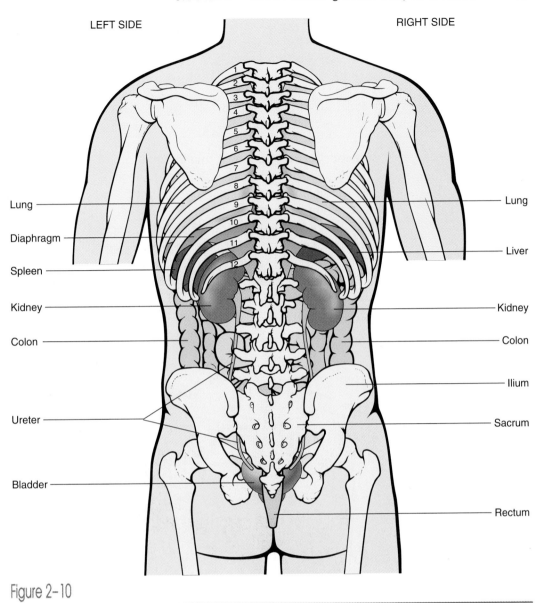

LEFT SIDE   RIGHT SIDE

Lung
Diaphragm
Spleen
Kidney
Colon
Ureter
Bladder

Lung
Liver
Kidney
Colon
Ilium
Sacrum
Rectum

Figure 2-10

Organs of the abdominopelvic and thoracic cavities, posterior view.

III. Abdominopelvic Regions and Quadrants

Regions

Figure 2–11 shows the division of the abdominal and pelvic cavities (abdomino-pelvic cavity) into nine regions, which are used by doctors to describe the regions in which internal organs are found. These regions are:

Hypochondriac regions: two upper right and left regions below the cartilage (chondr/o) of the ribs that extend over the abdomen.

Epigastric region: region above the stomach.

Lumbar regions: two middle right and left regions near the waist.

Umbilical region: region of the navel or umbilicus.

Inguinal regions: two lower right and left regions near the groin (inguin/o = groin), which is the area where the legs join the trunk of the body. These regions are also known as **iliac** regions because they are near the ilium, which is the upper portion of the hip bone on each side of the body.

Hypogastric region: lower middle region below the umbilical region.

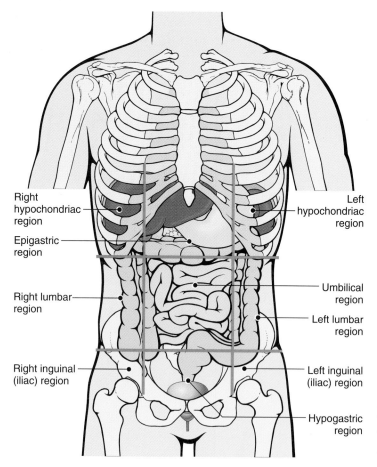

Right hypochondriac region

Epigastric region

Right lumbar region

Right inguinal (iliac) region

Left hypochondriac region

Umbilical region

Left lumbar region

Left inguinal (iliac) region

Hypogastric region

Figure 2-11

Abdominopelvic regions. These regions can be used clinically to locate internal organs.

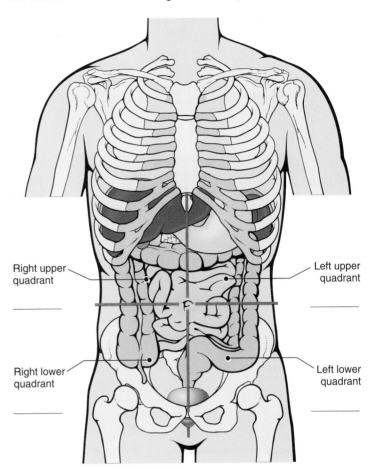

Right upper quadrant

Left upper quadrant

Right lower quadrant

Left lower quadrant

Figure 2-12

Abdominopelvic quadrants. Give the abbreviation for each quadrant on the line provided.

Quadrants

The abdominopelvic area can be divided into four quadrants by drawing two imaginary lines—one horizontally and one vertically through the body. Figure 2–12 shows these quadrants. You add the proper abbreviation on the line under each label on the diagram.

Right upper quadrant (RUQ) contains the liver (right lobe), gallbladder, part of the pancreas, parts of the small and large intestines.

Left upper quadrant (LUQ) contains the liver (left lobe), stomach, spleen, part of the pancreas, parts of the small and large intestines.

Right lower quadrant (RLQ) contains parts of the small and large intestines, right ovary, right fallopian tube, appendix, right ureter.

Left lower quadrant (LLQ) contains parts of the small and large intestines, left ovary, left fallopian tube, left ureter.

IV. Divisions of the Back (Spinal Column)

The back is separated into divisions that correspond to the regions of the spinal column. The spinal column is composed of a series of bones that extend from the neck to the tailbone. Each bone is called a **vertebra** (plural: **vertebrae**).

Label the divisions of the back on Figure 2–13 as you study the following:

Division of the Back	Abbreviation	Location
Cervical [1]	C	Neck region. There are 7 cervical vertebrae (C1–C7).
Thoracic [2]	T	Chest region. There are 12 thoracic vertebrae (T1–T12). Each bone is joined to a rib.
Lumbar [3]	L	Loin (waist) or flank region (between the ribs and the hip bone). There are 5 lumbar vertebrae (L1–L5).
Sacral [4]	S	Five bones (S1–S5) are fused to form one bone, the **sacrum.**
Coccygeal [5]		The **coccyx** (tailbone) is a small bone composed of 4 fused pieces.

An important distinction should be made between the **spinal column** (back bones or vertebrae) and the **spinal cord** (nerves surrounded by the column). The column is bone tissue, whereas the cord is composed of nerve tissue.

The spaces between the vertebrae (intervertebral spaces) are identified according to the two vertebrae between which they lie; for example, L5–S1 lies between the 5th lumbar and the 1st sacral vertebrae. Within the space and between vertebrae there is a small pad of cartilage called a **disc** or **disk.** The disc acts as a shock absorber. Occasionally, it moves out of place (ruptures) and puts pressure on a nerve. This is called a **slipped disc,** and it can be very painful.

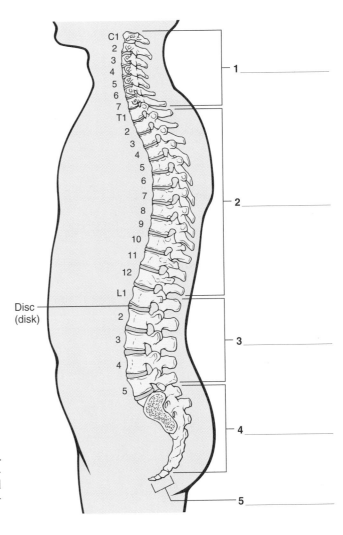

Figure 2–13

Anatomical divisions of the back (spinal column). A disc (disk) is a small pad of cartilage between each backbone (vertebra).

Practice spelling each term, and know its meaning.

ABDOMINOPELVIC REGIONS

hypochondriac	Upper right and left regions beneath the ribs.
epigastric	Upper middle region above the stomach.
lumbar	Middle right and left regions near the waist.
umbilical	Central region near the navel.
inguinal	Lower right and left regions near the groin. Also called **iliac regions.**
hypogastric	Lower middle region below the umbilical region.

Continued on following page

ABDOMINOPELVIC QUADRANTS

RUQ	Right upper quadrant
LUQ	Left upper quadrant
RLQ	Right lower quadrant
LLQ	Left lower quadrant

DIVISIONS OF THE BACK

cervical	Neck region (C1–C7)
thoracic	Chest region (T1–T12)
lumbar	Loin (waist) region (L1–L5)
sacral	Region of the sacrum (S1–S5)
coccygeal	Region of the coccyx (tailbone)

RELATED TERMS

vertebra	A single back bone.
vertebrae	Back bones.
spinal column	Bone tissue surrounding the spinal cavity.
spinal cord	Nervous tissue within the spinal cavity.
disc (disk)	A pad of cartilage between vertebrae.

V. Positional and Directional Terms

The following terms are used to describe the locations of organs in relationship to one another throughout the body.

Location	Relationship
Anterior (ventral)	Front side of the body. *Example:* The abdomen is anterior to the spinal cord. Ventral and anterior are the same position in a human; but in an animal (on four legs), ventral refers to the belly side and anterior to the front near the head.
Posterior (dorsal)	The back side of the body. *Example:* The spinal cord is posterior, or dorsal, to the stomach.
Deep	Away from the surface. *Example:* The stab wound penetrated deep into the abdomen.
Superficial	On the surface. *Example:* Superficial veins can be viewed through the skin.
Proximal	Near the point of attachment to the trunk or near the beginning of a structure. *Examples:* The proximal end of the upper armbone (humerus) joins with the shoulder bone. The proximal end of the stomach is at the esophagus.
Distal	Far from the point of attachment to the trunk or far from the beginning of a structure. *Examples:* At its distal end, the humerus joins with the lower armbones at the elbow. The distal end of the stomach is at the small intestine.
Inferior	Below another structure. *Example:* The urinary bladder lies inferior to the kidney. The term **caudal** (pertaining to the tail) means inferior in humans.
Superior	Above another structure. *Example:* The uterus is located superior to the vagina. The term **cephalic** (pertaining to the head) is also used to mean superior.
Medial	Pertaining to the middle or nearer the medial plane of the body. *Example:* In the anatomical position (see Fig. 2–14), the palms of the hands are facing outward and the fifth finger lies medial to the other fingers.
Lateral	Pertaining to the side. *Example:* The little toes are lateral to the big toes.
Supine	Lying on the back. *Example:* The patient is supine during an examination of the abdomen. The face is **up** in the **sup**ine position.
Prone	Lying on the belly. *Example:* The backbones can be examined with the patient in a prone position. The patient is lying **on** his or her face in the **prone** position.

VI. Planes of the Body

A plane is an imaginary flat surface. Label Figure 2–14 as you study the terms for the planes of the body:

Plane	Location
Frontal (coronal) [1]	Vertical plane that divides the body or structure into anterior and posterior portions. Also called a **coronal** plane. An AP (anterior-posterior) chest x-ray is taken in the frontal plane.
Sagittal (lateral) [2]	Lengthwise vertical plane that divides the body or structure into right and left sides. The **midsagittal** plane divides the body into right and left halves. A **lateral** chest x-ray is taken in the sagittal plane.
Transverse (cross-sectional) [3]	Plane running across the body parallel to the ground (horizontal). It divides the body or structure into upper and lower portions and is also called a **cross-sectional** plane. A CT (computed tomography; also known as computerized axial tomography or CAT) scan is a series of x-ray pictures taken in the transverse plane.

▪ STUDY SECTION 5

Practice spelling each term, and know its meaning.

anterior (ventral)	Pertaining to the front (belly side) of the body. (A fish's ventral fin is on its belly side.)
deep	Away from the surface.
distal	Far from the point of attachment to the trunk or far from the beginning of a structure.
frontal (coronal) plane	Vertical plane dividing the body into an anterior and a posterior portion.
inferior (caudal)	Below another structure.
lateral	Pertaining to the side.
medial	Pertaining to the middle or near the medial plane of the body.

Continued on page 54

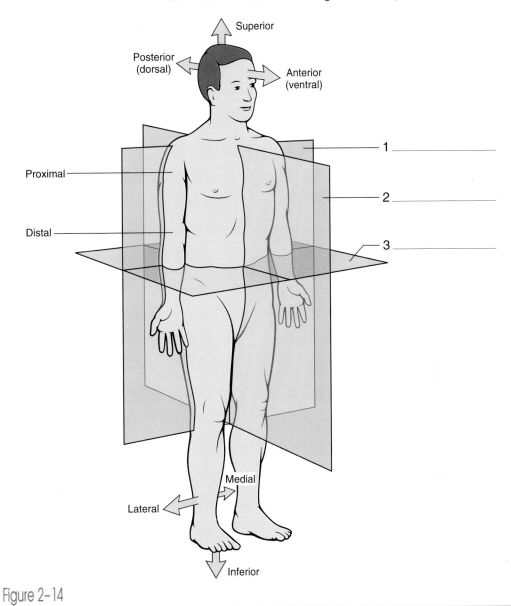

Figure 2-14

Planes of the body. The figure is standing in the anatomical position with the palms of the hands facing outward and the fifth finger lying medial to the other fingers.

posterior (dorsal)	Pertaining to the back of the body. (The dorsal fin of a fish is on its back side.)
prone	Lying on the belly (face down, palm down).
proximal	Near the point of attachment to the trunk or near the beginning of a structure.
sagittal plane	Vertical, lateral plane dividing the body into right and left sides. From the Latin *sagitta*, meaning arrow. As an arrow is shot from a bow it enters the body in the sagittal plane, dividing right from left. The **midsagittal plane** divides the body into right and left halves.
superficial	On the surface.
superior (cephalic)	Above another structure.
supine	Lying on the back (face up, palm up).
transverse plane	Horizontal plane dividing the body into upper and lower portions (cross-section).

VII. Combining Forms, Prefixes, and Suffixes

Write the meaning of the medical terms that follow in the spaces provided.

Combining Forms

Combining Form	Meaning	Terminology	Meaning
abdomin/o	abdomen	abdominal _____	
		The abdomen is the region below the chest containing internal organs (liver, intestines, stomach, gallbladder, etc.).	
adip/o	fat	adipose _____	
		The suffix -ose means pertaining to or full of.	
anter/o	front	anterior _____	
		The suffix -ior means pertaining to.	

bol/o	to cast (throw)	anabolism _____

The prefix ana- means up. The suffix -ism means process. In this cellular process, proteins are built up (protein synthesis).

cervic/o	neck (of the body or of the uterus)	cervical _____

The cervix is the neck of the uterus. The term cervical can mean pertaining to the neck of the body or the neck (lower part) of the uterus.

chondr/o	cartilage (type of connective tissue)	chondroma _____

This is a benign tumor.

chondrosarcoma _____

This is a malignant tumor. The term sarc indicates that the malignant tumor is a type of flesh or connective tissue.

chrom/o	color	chromosomes _____

These nuclear structures absorb the color of dyes used to stain the cell. The suffix -somes means bodies. Literally, this term means bodies of color, which is how they first appeared to doctors who saw them under the microscope.

coccyg/o	coccyx (tailbone)	coccygeal _____
crani/o	skull	craniotomy _____
cyt/o	cell	cytoplasm _____

The suffix -plasm means formation.

dist/o	far, distant	distal _____
dors/o	back portion of the body	dorsal _____
hist/o	tissue	histology _____
ili/o	ilium (part of the pelvic bone)	iliac _____

See Figure 2–10 for a picture of the ilium.

inguin/o	groin	inguinal _____
kary/o	nucleus	karyotype _____

The suffix -type means classification or picture.

later/o	side	lateral _____
lumb/o	lower back (side and back between the ribs and the pelvis)	lumbosacral _____
medi/o	middle	medial _____
nucle/o	nucleus	nucleic _____
pelv/o	hip, pelvic cavity	pelvic _____
poster/o	back, behind	posterior _____
proxim/o	nearest	proximal _____
sacr/o	sacrum	sacral _____
sarc/o	flesh	sarcoma _____
spin/o	spine, backbone	spinal _____
thel/o	nipple	epithelial cell _____

This cell, originally identified as covering nipples, is found covering body surfaces, externally (outside the body) and internally (lining cavities and organs).

thorac/o	chest	thoracic _____
		thoracotomy _____
trache/o	trachea, windpipe	tracheal _____
umbilic/o	navel, umbilicus	umbilical _____
ventr/o	belly side of the body	ventral _____
vertebr/o	vertebrae, back-bones	vertebral _____
viscer/o	internal organs	visceral _____

Prefixes

Prefix	Meaning	Terminology	Meaning
ana-	up	anabolic _____	
cata-	down	catabolism _____	
		The cellular process of breaking down foods to release energy.	
epi-	above	epigastric _____	
hypo-	below	hypochondriac regions _____	
		The Greeks thought organs (liver and spleen) in the hypochondriac region of the abdomen were the origin of imaginary illnesses. Hence the term hypochondriac, a person with unusual anxiety about his or her health and with symptoms not attributable to any disease process.	
inter-	between	intervertebral _____	
		A disc is an intervertebral structure.	
meta-	change	metabolism _____	
		Literally, to cast (bol/o) a change (meta-), meaning the chemical changes (processes) that occur in a cell.	

Suffixes

The following are some new suffixes introduced in this chapter.

Suffix	Meaning	Suffix	Meaning
-eal	pertaining to	**-ose**	pertaining to, full of
-iac	pertaining to	**-plasm**	formation
-ior	pertaining to	**-somes**	bodies
-ism	process	**-type**	picture, classification

VIII. Practical Applications

Be sure to check your answers with the Answers to Practical Applications on page 65.

Surgical Procedures

Match the **surgical procedure** in COLUMN I with a **reason** for performing it in COLUMN II:

Column I

1. Craniotomy _____

2. Thoracotomy _____

3. Discectomy _____

4. Mediastinoscopy _____

5. Tracheotomy _____

6. Laryngectomy _____

7. Arthroscopy _____

8. Peritoneoscopy _____

Column II

A. Emergency effort to remove foreign material from the windpipe

B. Inspection and repair of torn cartilage in the knee

C. Removal of a diseased or injured portion of the brain

D. Inspection of lymph nodes* in the region between the lungs

E. Removal of a squamous cell** carcinoma in the voicebox

F. Open-heart surgery; or removal of lung tissue

G. Inspection of abdominal organs and removal of diseased tissue

H. Relieving of symptoms of a bulging intervertebral pad of cartilage

*Lymph nodes are collections of tissue containing white blood cells called lymphocytes.
**A squamous cell is a type of epithelial cell.

IX. Exercises

Remember to check your answers carefully with those given in Section X, Answers to Exercises.

A. *The following terms are parts of a cell. Match each term with its meaning below.*

cell membrane   chromosomes   genes
nucleus   cytoplasm   DNA
mitochondria   endoplasmic reticulum

1. the material of the cell that is outside the nucleus and yet enclosed by the cell membrane

_____

2. regions of DNA within each chromosome _____

3. small, sausage-shaped structures; the place where food is burned to release energy

_____

4. canal-like structure in the cytoplasm; the place where proteins are made _____

5. the structure that surrounds and protects the cell _____

6. the control center of the cell, containing chromosomes _____

7. a chemical found within each chromosome _____

8. rod-shaped structures in the nucleus that contain regions called genes _____

B. *Use medical terms or numbers to complete the following sentences.*

1. A picture of chromosomes in the nucleus of a cell is called a (an) _____

2. The number of chromosomes in a normal male's muscle cell is _____

3. The number of chromosomes in a female's egg cell is _____

4. The process of building up proteins in a cell is called _____

5. The process of chemically burning or breaking down foods to release energy in cells is known as

_____

6. The total of the chemical processes in a cell is known as _____

7. A scientist who studies tissues is called a (an) _____

8. The medical term for internal organs is _____

C. Match the part of the body listed with its description below.

ureter	larynx	urethra
thyroid gland	cartilage	epithelial tissue
pharynx	trachea	adipose tissue
pituitary gland	uterus	pleura

1. the voice box _____

2. membrane surrounding the lungs _____

3. the throat _____

4. tube from the kidney to the urinary bladder _____

5. collection of fat cells _____

6. an endocrine organ located at the base of the brain _____

7. windpipe _____

8. flexible connective tissue attached to bones at joints _____

9. surface cells covering the outside of the body and lining internal organs _____

10. an endocrine gland surrounding the windpipe in the neck _____

11. the womb _____

12. a tube leading from the urinary bladder to the outside of the body _____

D. Name the five cavities of the body.

1. the cavity surrounded by the skull _____

2. the cavity in the chest surrounded by the ribs _____

3. the cavity below the chest containing the stomach, liver, and gallbladder _____

4. the cavity surrounded by the hip bone _____

5. the cavity surrounded by the bones of the back _____

E. Select from the following definitions to complete the sentences below (1–11).

space surrounding each lung
space between the lungs
muscle separating the abdominal and thoracic cavities
membrane surrounding the abdominal organs
area below the umbilicus (as well as below the stomach)
area above the stomach
area of the navel
areas near the groin
nervous tissue within the spinal cavity
bone tissue surrounding the spinal cavity
a pad of cartilage between each vertebra

1. The hypogastric region is the _____

2. The mediastinum is the _____

3. The spinal cord is _____

4. The diaphragm is a (an) _____

5. An intervertebral disc is _____

6. The pleural cavity is _____

7. The spinal column is _____

8. Inguinal areas are the _____

9. The peritoneum is the _____

10. The umbilical region is the _____

11. The epigastric region is the _____

F. Name the five divisions of the back.

1. region of the neck _____

2. region of the chest _____

3. region of the waist _____

4. region of the sacrum _____

5. region of the tailbone _____

G. Give the meanings of the following abbreviations.

1. LLQ _____

2. L5–S1 _____

3. RUQ _____

4. C3–C4 _____

5. RLQ _____

H. Give the opposites of the following terms.

1. deep _____   4. medial _____

2. proximal _____   5. dorsal _____

3. supine _____   6. superior _____

I. Select from the following medical terms to complete the sentences below.

vertebra	proximal	frontal
lateral	superior	inferior (caudal)
vertebrae	transverse	
distal	sagittal	

1. The kidney lies _____ to the spinal cord.

2. The _____ end of the thigh bone joins with the knee cap (patella).

3. The _____ plane is a vertical plane that divides the body into an anterior and a posterior portion.

4. A backbone is called a (an) _____ .

5. Several backbones are called _____ .

6. The diaphragm lies _____ to the organs in the thoracic cavity.

7. The _____ plane is a vertical plane that divides the body into right and left portions.

8. The _____ end of the upper armbone is at the shoulder.

9. The _____ plane is a horizontal plane that divides the body into upper and lower portions, like a cross section.

10. The pharynx is located _____ to the esophagus.

J. Give the meanings of the following medical terms.

1. craniotomy _____

2. cervical _____

3. chondroma _____

4. chondrosarcoma _____

5. nucleic _____

K. Give the medical term for the following definitions. Pay attention to spelling!

1. space below the chest containing the liver, stomach, gallbladder, and intestines:

_____

2. flexible connective tissue attached to bones at joints: _____

3. rod-shaped structures in the cell nucleus, containing regions of DNA: _____

4. muscle separating the abdominal and thoracic cavities: _____

5. the voice box: _____

6. vertical plane dividing the body into right and left sides: _____

7. pertaining to the neck: _____

8. tumor (benign) of cartilage: _____

9. control center of the cell; directs the activities of the cell: _____

10. pertaining to the windpipe: _____

L. Complete each term based on the meaning provided.

1. pertaining to internal organs: _____ al

2. tumor of flesh tissue (malignant): _____ oma

3. pertaining to the chest: _____ ic

4. picture of the chromosomes in the cell nucleus: _____ type

5. sausage-shaped cellular structures in which catabolism takes place: mito _____

6. space between the lungs: media _____

7. endocrine gland at the base of the brain: _____ ary gland

8. pertaining to skin (surface) cells: epi _____

M. Select the correct term to complete each sentence.

1. Dr. Curnen said the **(inguinal, superior, superficial)** wound barely scratched the surface.

2. The liver and spleen are on opposite sides of the body. The liver is in the **(RUQ, LUQ, LLQ)** of the abdominopelvic cavity and the spleen is in the **(RUQ, LUQ, RLQ)**.

3. When a gynecologist examines a patient's pelvis, the patient lies on her back in the **(ventral, dorsal, medial)** lithotomy position. (Lithotomy = incision of an organ to remove a stone—the position also used for removal of ureteral or kidney stones.)

4. Sally's pain was around her navel. The doctor described it as **(periumbilical, epigastric, hypogastric)**.

5. After sampling the fluid surrounding her 16-week-old fetus, the doctor told Mrs. Jones she was carrying a baby with trisomy-21. The diagnosis was made by analysis of an abnormal **(urine sample, thoracotomy, karyotype)**.

6. The **(spinal, sagittal, abdominal)** cavity contains digestive organs.

X. Answers to Exercises

A

1. cytoplasm
2. genes
3. mitochondria
4. endoplasmic reticulum
5. cell membrane
6. nucleus
7. DNA
8. chromosomes

B

1. karyotype
2. 46 (23 pairs)
3. 23
4. anabolism
5. catabolism
6. metabolism
7. histologist
8. viscera

C

1. larynx
2. pleura
3. pharynx
4. ureter
5. adipose tissue
6. pituitary gland
7. trachea
8. cartilage
9. epithelial tissue
10. thyroid gland
11. uterus
12. urethra

D

1. cranial
2. thoracic
3. abdominal
4. pelvic
5. spinal

E

1. area below the umbilicus
2. space between the lungs
3. nervous tissue within the spinal cavity
4. muscle separating the abdominal and thoracic cavities
5. a pad of cartilage between each vertebra
6. space surrounding each lung
7. bone tissue surrounding the spinal cavity
8. areas near the groin
9. membrane surrounding the abdominal organs
10. area of the navel
11. area above the stomach

F

1. cervical
2. thoracic
3. lumbar
4. sacral
5. coccygeal

G

1. left lower quadrant (of the abdominopelvic cavity)
2. between the 5th lumbar vertebra and the 1st sacral vertebra (a common place for a slipped disc)
3. right upper quadrant (of the abdominopelvic cavity)
4. between the 3rd cervical vertebra and the 4th cervical vertebra
5. right lower quadrant (of the abdominopelvic cavity)

H

1. superficial
2. distal
3. prone
4. lateral
5. ventral (anterior)
6. inferior (caudal)

I

1. lateral
2. distal
3. frontal (coronal)
4. vertebra
5. vertebrae
6. inferior (caudal)
7. sagittal
8. proximal
9. transverse
10. superior (cephalic)

J

1. incision of the skull
2. pertaining to the neck (of the body or the cervix of the uterus)
3. tumor of cartilage (benign or noncancerous tumor)
4. flesh tumor of cartilage (cancerous, malignant tumor)
5. pertaining to the nucleus

K

1. abdomen or abdominal cavity
2. cartilage
3. chromosomes
4. diaphragm
5. larynx
6. sagittal—note spelling with two t's
7. cervical
8. chondroma
9. nucleus
10. tracheal

L

1. visceral
2. sarcoma
3. thoracic
4. karyotype
5. mitochondria—memory tip: catabolism and mitochondria and cat and mouse!
6. mediastinum
7. pituitary gland
8. epithelial

M

1. superficial
2. RUQ; LUQ
3. dorsal; often called the dorsolithotomy position
4. periumbilical
5. karyotype
6. abdominal

Answers to Practical Applications

1. **C** A trephine is a type of circular saw used for craniotomy.
2. **F**
3. **H** Endoscopic discectomy is performed through a small incision on the back, lateral to the spine. All or a portion of the disc is removed.
4. **D** A small incision is made above the breastbone and an endoscope is inserted to inspect the lymph nodes around the trachea.
5. **A**
6. **E**
7. **B**
8. **G** A small incision is made near the navel, and a laparoscope is inserted. The procedure, also called laparoscopy (lapar/o means abdomen) or minimally invasive surgery, is used to examine organs and perform surgical operations, such as the removal of the gallbladder or appendix or the tying off of the fallopian tubes.

XI. Pronunciation of Terms

Pronunciation Guide

ā as in āpe   ă as in ăpple
ē as in ēven   ĕ as in ĕvery
ī as in īce   ĭ as in ĭnterest
ō as in ōpen   ŏ as in pŏt
ū as in ūnit   ŭ as in ŭnder

To test your understanding of the terminology in this chapter, write the meaning of each term in the space provided. In addition, you may wish to cover the terms and write them by looking at your definitions. Make sure your spelling is correct. The page number after each term indicates where it is defined or used in the text so you can easily check your responses.

Term	Pronunciation	Meaning
abdomen (43)	ĂB-dō-mĕn or ăb-DŌ-mĕn	
abdominal cavity (43)	ăb-DŎM-ĭ-năl KĂ-vĭ-tē	
adipose (54)	ĂD-ĭ-pōs	
anabolism (36)	ă-NĂB-ō-lĭzm	
anterior (51)	an-TĒ-rē-ŏr	
cartilage (39)	KĂR-tĭ-lĭj	
catabolism (36)	kă-TĂB-ō-lĭsm	
cell membrane (36)	sĕl MĔM-brān	
cephalic (54)	sĕ-FĂL-ĭk	
cervical (55)	SĔR-vĭ-kăl	
chondroma (55)	kŏn-DRŌ-mă	
chondrosarcoma (55)	kŏn-drō-săr-KŌ-mă	
chromosome (36)	KRŌ-mō-sōm	
coccygeal (55)	kŏk-sĭ-JĒ-ăl	
coccyx (48)	KŎK-sĭks	
cranial cavity (43)	KRĀ-nē-ăl KĂ-vĭ-tē	
craniotomy (55)	krā-nē-ŎT-ō-mē	
cytoplasm (36)	SĪ-tō-plăzm	
diaphragm (43)	DĪ-ă-frăm	
disc (disk) (50)	dĭsk	
distal (51)	DĬS-tăl	
dorsal (43)	DŎR-săl	

endoplasmic reticulum (36)	ĕn-dō-PLĂZ-mĭk rē-TĬK-ū-lŭm	
epigastric (46)	ĕp-ĭ-GĂS-trĭk	
epithelial cell (39)	ĕp-ĭ-THĒ-lē-ăl sĕl	
frontal plane (52)	FRŬN-tăl plān	
genes (36)	jēnz	
histology (55)	hĭs-TŎL-ō-jē	
hypochondriac (57)	hī-pō-KŎN-drē-ăk	
hypogastric (46)	hĭ-pō-GĂS-trĭk	
iliac (55)	ĬL-ē-ăk	
inguinal (55)	ĬNG-gwĭ-năl	
intervertebral (57)	ĭn-tĕr-VĔR-tĕ-brăl or ĭn-tĕr-vĕr-TĒ-brăl	
karyotype (36)	KĂR-ē-ō-tīp	
larynx (39)	LĂR-ĭnks	
lateral (51)	LĂT-ĕr-al	
lumbar (50)	LŬM-băr	
lumbosacral (56)	lŭm-bō-SĀ-krăl	
medial (51)	MĒ-dē-ăl	
mediastinum (43)	mē-dē-ă-STĪ-nŭm	
metabolism (36)	mĕ-TĂB-ō-lĭzm	
mitochondria (36)	mī-tō-KŎN-drē-ă	
nucleic (56)	nū-KLĒ-ĭk	
nucleus (36)	NŪ-klē-ŭs	
pelvic cavity (43)	PĔL-vĭk KĂ-vĭ-tē	
peritoneum (43)	pĕ-rĭ-tō-NĒ-um	
pharynx (39)	FĂR-ĭnks	
pituitary gland (39)	pĭ-TŪ-ĭ-tăr-ē glănd	
pleura (43)	PLOO-ră	
pleural cavity (43)	PLOOR-ăl KĂ-vĭ-tē	

posterior (51)	pōs-TĒR-ē-ŏr	_____
prone (51)	prōn	_____
proximal (51)	PRŎK-sĭ-măl	_____
sacral (56)	SĀ-krăl	_____
sacrum (48)	SĀ-krŭm	_____
sagittal plane (54)	SĂJ-ĭ-tăl plān	_____
sarcoma (56)	săr-KŌ-mă	_____
spinal cavity (43)	SPĪ-năl KĂ-vĭ-tē	_____
spinal column (50)	SPĪ-năl KŎL-ŭm	_____
spinal cord (50)	SPĪ-năl kŏrd	_____
superficial (54)	sū-pĕr-FĬSH-ăl	_____
supine (54)	SŪ-pīn	_____
thoracic cavity (43)	thō-RĂS-ĭk KĂ-vĭ-tē	_____
thoracotomy (56)	thō-ră-KŎT-ō-mē	_____
thyroid gland (39)	THĪ-royd glănd	_____
trachea (39)	TRĀ-kē-ă	_____
tracheal (56)	TRĀ-kē-ăl	_____
transverse plane (54)	trănz-VĔRS plān	_____
umbilical (56)	ŭm-BĬL-ĭ-kăl	_____
ureter (39)	Ū-rĕ-tĕr or ū-RĒ-tĕr	_____
urethra (39)	ū-RĒ-thră	_____
uterus (39)	Ū-tĕ-rŭs	_____
ventral (56)	VĔN-trăl	_____
vertebra (50)	VĔR-tĕ-bră	_____
vertebrae (50)	VĔR-tĕ-brā	_____
vertebral (56)	VĔR-tĕ-brăl or vĕr-TĒ-brăl	_____
viscera (39)	VĬS-ĕr-ă	_____
visceral (56)	VĬS-ĕr-ăl	_____

XII. Review Sheet

Write the meaning of each combining form in the space provided and test yourself. Check your answers with the information in the chapter or in the Glossary (Medical Terms—English) at the end of the book.

COMBINING FORMS

Combining Form	Meaning	Combining Form	Meaning
abdomin/o	_____	lumb/o	_____
adip/o	_____	medi/o	_____
anter/o	_____	nucle/o	_____
bol/o	_____	pelv/o	_____
cervic/o	_____	poster/o	_____
chondr/o	_____	proxim/o	_____
chrom/o	_____	sacr/o	_____
coccyg/o	_____	sarc/o	_____
crani/o	_____	spin/o	_____
cyt/o	_____	thel/o	_____
dist/o	_____	thorac/o	_____
dors/o	_____	trache/o	_____
hist/o	_____	umbilic/o	_____
ili/o	_____	vertebr/o	_____
inguin/o	_____	ventr/o	_____
kary/o	_____	viscer/o	_____
later/o	_____		

Continued on following page

PREFIXES

Prefix	Meaning	Prefix	Meaning
ana-	_____	hypo-	_____
cata-	_____	inter-	_____
epi-	_____	meta-	_____

SUFFIXES

Suffix	Meaning	Suffix	Meaning
-eal	_____	-ose	_____
-ectomy	_____	-plasm	_____
-iac	_____	-somes	_____
-ior	_____	-tomy	_____
-ism	_____	-type	_____
-oma	_____		

Label the regions and quadrants of the abdominopelvic cavity.

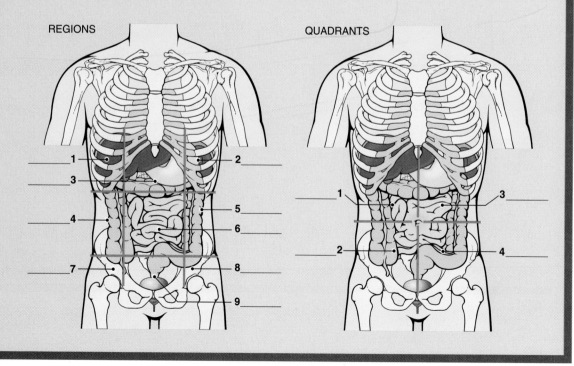

REGIONS   QUADRANTS

Name the divisions of the spinal column.

neck region (C1–C7) _____

chest region (T1–T12) _____

lower back (loin) region (L1–L5) _____

region of the sacrum (S1–S5) _____

tailbone region _____

Name the planes of the head as pictured below:

Brain   vertical plane that divides the body into anterior and posterior portions

_____

Brain   horizontal plane that divides the body into upper and lower portions

_____

Brain   vertical plane that divides the body into right and left portions

_____

Name the positional and directional terms.

front of the body _____

back of the body _____

away from the surface of the body _____

on the surface of the body _____

far from the point of attachment to the trunk or far from the beginning of a structure

_____

Continued on following page

near the point of attachment to the trunk or near the beginning of a structure

_____

below another structure _____

above another structure _____

pertaining to the side _____

pertaining to the middle _____

lying on the belly _____

lying on the back _____

Give the meanings of the following terms that pertain to the cell.

chromosomes _____

mitochondria _____

nucleus _____

DNA _____

endoplasmic reticulum _____

cell membrane _____

catabolism _____

anabolism _____

metabolism _____

Give the term that suits the meaning provided.

membrane surrounding the lungs _____

membrane surrounding the abdominal viscera _____

muscular wall separating the thoracic and abdominal cavities _____

space between the lungs, containing the heart, windpipe, aorta _____

a backbone _____

a pad of cartilage between each backbone and the next _____

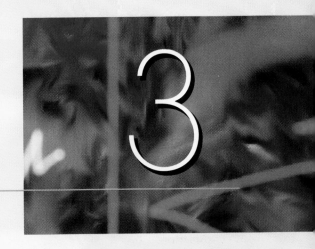

CHAPTER 3

Suffixes

This chapter is divided into the following sections

In this chapter you will
- Define new suffixes and review those presented in previous chapters;
- Gain practice in word analysis by using these suffixes with combining forms to build and understand terms; and
- Name and know the functions of the different types of blood cells in the body.

I. Introduction

This chapter has three purposes. The first is to teach many of the most common suffixes in the medical language. As you work through the entire book, the suffixes mastered in this chapter will appear often. An additional group of basic suffixes is presented in Chapter 6.

The second purpose is to teach new combining forms and use them to make words with suffixes. Your analysis of the terminology in Section III of this chapter will increase your medical language vocabulary.

The third purpose is to expand your understanding of terminology beyond basic word analysis. The appendices in Section IV give additional explanations of many terms listed. In particular, emphasis is placed on learning the names and functions of different types of blood cells. These terms are basic to the vocabulary of a person working in the allied health field.

II. Combining Forms

Read this list and underline those combining forms that are unfamiliar.

Combining Form	Meaning	Combining Form	Meaning
abdomin/o	abdomen	**encephal/o**	brain
acr/o	extremities, top, extreme point	**hydr/o**	water, fluid
acu/o	sharp, severe, sudden	**inguin/o**	groin
aden/o	gland	**isch/o**	to hold back
agor/a	marketplace	**lapar/o**	abdomen, abdominal wall
amni/o	amnion (sac surrounding the embryo in the uterus)	**laryng/o**	larynx (voice box)
angi/o	vessel	**lymph/o**	lymph
arteri/o	artery		*Lymph is clear fluid that bathes tissue spaces and is contained in special lymph vessels and nodes throughout the body.*
arthr/o	joint		
axill/o	armpit		
blephar/o	eyelid	**mamm/o**	breast
bronch/o	bronchial tubes (two tubes, one right and one left, that branch from the trachea to enter the lungs)	**mast/o**	breast
		morph/o	shape, form
		muc/o	mucus
carcin/o	cancer	**myel/o**	spinal cord, bone marrow
chem/o	drug, chemical		*Context of usage indicates which meaning is intended.*
chondr/o	cartilage	**my/o**	muscle
chron/o	time	**necr/o**	death (of cells or whole body)
col/o	colon (large intestine)	**nephr/o**	kidney
cyst/o	urinary bladder	**neur/o**	nerve

neutr/o	neutrophil (a white blood cell)	**pulmon/o**	lungs
ophthalm/o	eye	**rect/o**	rectum
oste/o	bone	**ren/o**	kidney
ot/o	ear	**sarc/o**	flesh
path/o	disease	**splen/o**	spleen
peritone/o	peritoneum	**staphyl/o**	clusters
phag/o	to eat, swallow	**strept/o**	twisted chains
phleb/o	vein	**thorac/o**	chest
plas/o	formation, development	**thromb/o**	clot
pleur/o	pleura (membranes surrounding lungs and adjacent to chest wall muscles)	**tonsill/o**	tonsils
		trache/o	trachea (windpipe)
pneumon/o	lungs	**ven/o**	vein

III. Suffixes and Terminology

Noun Suffixes

The following is a list of the most common noun suffixes. A medical term is given to illustrate the use of the suffix. The basic rule for building a medical word is that the combining vowel, such as **o**, is used to connect the root to the suffix, with the exception that the combining vowel is *not* used before suffixes that begin with a vowel. For example: **gastr/itis,** *not* **gastr/o/itis.**

Numbers above certain terms direct you to an Appendix that follows this list. The Appendix contains additional information that will help you understand the terminology.

Suffix	Meaning	Terminology	Meaning
-algia	pain	arthralgia _____	
		otalgia _____	
		neuralgia _____	
		myalgia _____	

-cele	hernia[1]	rectocele _____
		cystocele _____
-centesis	surgical puncture to remove fluid	thoracocentesis _____

This term is often shortened to thoracentesis.

amniocentesis[2] _____

abdominocentesis _____

This procedure is also known as a paracentesis.

-coccus (plural: **-cocci**)[3]	berry-shaped bacterium (plural: bacteria)	streptococcus[4] _____
		staphylococci _____
-cyte	cell	erythrocyte[5] _____
		leukocyte _____
		thrombocyte _____
-dynia	pain	pleurodynia _____

Pain in the chest wall muscles that is aggravated by breathing.

-ectomy	excision, removal, resection	laryngectomy[6] _____
		mastectomy _____
-emia	blood condition	anemia[7] _____
		ischemia[8] _____
-genesis	condition of producing, forming	carcinogenesis _____
		pathogenesis _____
		angiogenesis _____

---

[1] See Appendix A.
[2] See Appendix B.
[3] See Appendix C.
[4] See Appendix D.
[5] See Appendix E.
[6] See Appendix F.
[7] See Appendix G.
[8] See Appendix H.

| **-genic** | pertaining to producing, produced by, or in | carcinogenic _____ |
| | | osteogenic _____ |

An osteogenic sarcoma is a tumor produced by bone tissue.

| **-gram** | record | electroencephalogram _____ |
| | | myelogram _____ |

Myel/o means spinal cord in this term. This is an x-ray record taken after contrast material is injected into membranes around the spinal cord.

		mammogram _____
-graph	instrument for recording	electroencephalograph _____
-graphy	process of recording	electroencephalography _____
		angiography _____
-itis	inflammation	bronchitis _____
		tonsillitis[9] _____
		phlebitis _____
-logy	study of	ophthalmology _____
		morphology _____
-lysis	breakdown, destruction, separation	hemolysis _____

Breakdown of red blood cells with release of hemoglobin.

-malacia	softening	osteomalacia _____
		chondromalacia _____
-megaly	enlargement	acromegaly[10] _____
		splenomegaly[11] _____

---

[9] See Appendix I.
[10] See Appendix J.
[11] See Appendix K.

-oma   tumor, mass, collection of fluid

myoma _____

This is a benign tumor.

myosarcoma _____

This is a malignant tumor. Muscle is a type of flesh (sarc/o) tissue.

multiple myeloma _____

Myel/o means bone marrow in this term. This is a malignant tumor that occurs in bone marrow throughout the body.

hematoma _____

-opsy   to view

biopsy _____

necropsy _____

Autopsy or post mortem examination.

-osis   condition, usually abnormal

necrosis _____

hydronephrosis _____

leukocytosis[12] _____

-pathy   disease condition

cardiomyopathy _____

Primary disease of the heart muscle in the absence of a known underlying etiology (cause).

-penia   deficiency

erythropenia _____

neutropenia _____

In this term, neutr/o means neutrophil (a type of white blood cell).

thrombocytopenia _____

-phobia   fear

acrophobia _____

Fear of heights.

agoraphobia _____

An anxiety disorder marked by fear of venturing out into a crowded place.

---

[12] See Appendix L.

-plasia	development, formation, growth	achondroplasia[13] _____
-plasty	surgical repair	angioplasty _____

A narrowed blood vessel is opened using a balloon that is inflated after it is inserted into the blood vessel.

-ptosis[14]	drooping, sagging, prolapse	blepharoptosis _____

*The term **ptosis** (Tō-sĭs) is used alone to indicate prolapse of the upper eyelid.*

-sclerosis	hardening	arteriosclerosis _____

Atherosclerosis is a form of arteriosclerosis in which the artery becomes clogged with deposits of fat (ather/o means fatty material).

-scope	instrument for visual examination	laparoscope _____
-scopy	process of visual examination	laparoscopy[15] _____
-stasis	stopping, controlling	metastasis _____

Meta- means beyond. A metastasis is the spreading of a malignant tumor beyond its original site to a secondary organ or location.

hemostasis _____

Blood flow is stopped naturally by clotting or artificially by compression.

-stomy	opening to form a mouth (stoma)	colostomy _____
		tracheostomy _____
-therapy	treatment	hydrotherapy _____
		chemotherapy _____
		radiotherapy _____

---

[13] See Appendix M.
[14] See Appendix N.
[15] See Appendix O.

-tomy	incision, to cut into	laparotomy _____	

This is called exploratory surgery.

phlebotomy _____

-trophy	nourishment, development	hypertrophy _____	

Cells increase in size, not number. Muscles of weight lifters often hypertrophy.

atrophy _____

Cells decrease in size. Muscles atrophy when they are immobilized in a cast and not in use.

The following are shorter noun suffixes that are usually attached to roots in words.

Suffix	Meaning	Terminology	Meaning
-er	one who	radiographer _____	

A technologist who assists in the making of diagnostic x-ray pictures.

Suffix	Meaning	Terminology	Meaning
-ia	condition	leukemia _____	
		pneumonia _____	
-ist	one who specializes in	nephrologist _____	
-ole	little, small	arteriole[16] _____	
-ule	little, small	venule _____	
-um, ium	structure, tissue, thing	pericardium _____	

The pericardium is a membrane around the heart.

Suffix	Meaning	Terminology	Meaning
-y	condition, process	nephropathy _____	

---

[16] See Appendix P.

Adjective Suffixes

The following are adjective suffixes. There is no simple rule indicating which suffix meaning *pertaining to* is used with a specific combining form. Your job is to recognize the types of adjectival suffixes in each term.

Suffix	Meaning	Terminology	Meaning
-ac, iac	pertaining to	cardiac _____	
-al	pertaining to	peritoneal _____	
		inguinal _____	
		pleural _____	
-ar	pertaining to	tonsillar _____	
-ary	pertaining to	pulmonary _____	
		axillary _____	
-eal	pertaining to	laryngeal _____	
-ic, ical	pertaining to	chronic _____	

Acute is the opposite of chronic. It describes a disease that is of rapid onset and has severe symptoms and brief duration.

		pathological _____	
-oid	resembling	adenoids[17] _____	
-ose	pertaining to, full of	adipose _____	
-ous	pertaining to	mucous _____	

Mucus (a noun) is the sticky secretion produced by mucous membranes.

-tic	pertaining to	necrotic _____	

---

[17] See Appendix Q.

IV. Appendices

Appendix A: Hernia

A **hernia** is a bulging forth, or protrusion, of an organ or the muscular wall of an organ through the cavity that normally contains it. Some examples of hernias are a hiatal hernia (the stomach protrudes upward into the mediastinum through the esophageal opening in the diaphragm; see Fig. 5–21, page 160) and an inguinal hernia (part of the intestine protrudes downward into the groin region and commonly into the scrotal sac in the male; see Fig. 5–21). A **rectocele** is the protrusion of a portion of the rectum toward the vagina through a weak part of the vaginal wall muscles. An **omphalocele** (omphal/o = umbilicus, navel) is a hernia of the navel that occurs in infants at birth. A **cystocele** is the protrusion of part of the urinary bladder through the vaginal wall due to weakened pelvic muscles (Fig. 3–1).

Appendix B: Amniocentesis

The amnion is the sac (membrane) that surrounds the embryo (called the fetus after the 8th week) in the uterus. Fluid accumulates within the sac and can be withdrawn **(amniocentesis)** for analysis during the 12th to 18th week of pregnancy. Cells of the fetus are in the fluid and are grown (cultured) for microscopic analysis. A karyotype is made to analyze chromosomes, and the fluid can be examined for high levels of chemicals that indicate defects in the developing spinal cord and spinal column of the fetus (Fig. 3–2).

Appendix C: Plurals

Words ending in **-us** commonly form their plural by dropping the **-us** and adding **-i**. Thus, nucleus becomes nuclei and coccus becomes cocci (KŎK-sī). A guide to formation of plurals is found in Appendix 1, page 903, at the end of the book.

Appendix D: Streptococcus and Staphylococcus

A **streptococcus** is a berry-shaped bacterium that grows in twisted chains. One group of streptococci is responsible for such conditions as "strep" throat, tonsillitis, rheumatic fever, and certain kidney ailments, whereas another group causes infections in teeth, in the sinuses (cavities) of the nose and face, and sometimes in the valves of the heart.

Staphylococci are bacteria that grow in small clusters, like grapes. Staphylococcal lesions may be external (skin abscesses, boils, styes) or internal (abscesses in bone and kidney). (An abscess is a collection of pus, white blood cells, and protein that is present at the site of infection.)

Diplococci (organized in pairs) are **pneumococci** (pneum/o = lungs), which are the most common cause of bacterial pneumonia in adults, and **gonococci** (gon/o = seed), which invade the reproductive organs and cause gonorrhea. Figure 3–3 illustrates the pattern of growth of streptococci, staphylococci, and diplococci.

CYSTOCELE

RECTOCELE

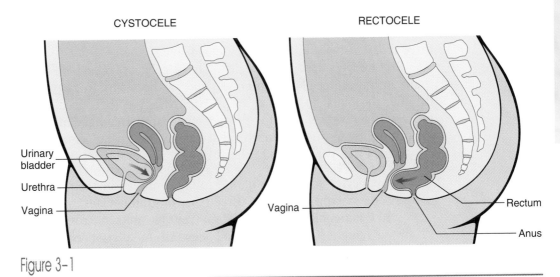

Urinary bladder

Urethra

Vagina

Vagina

Rectum

Anus

Figure 3–1

Cystocele and **rectocele**.

Figure 3–2

Amniocentesis. Under ultrasound (sound wave images) guidance, a needle is inserted through the uterine wall and amnion (the membrane surrounding the fetus) into the amniotic cavity. Amniotic fluid, containing fetal cells, is withdrawn for analysis. The physician uses continuous ultrasound pictures to locate the fetus and other structures within the uterus, and to ensure the proper placement of the needle.

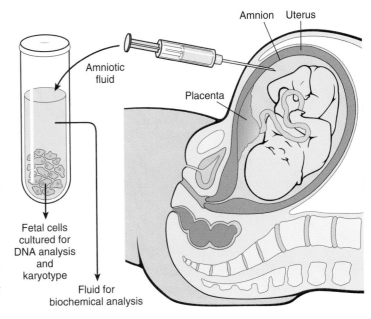

Amnion Uterus

Amniotic fluid

Placenta

Fetal cells cultured for DNA analysis and karyotype

Fluid for biochemical analysis

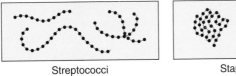

Streptococci

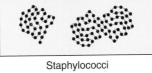

Staphylococci

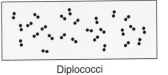

Diplococci

Figure 3–3

Types of coccal bacteria.

Appendix E: Blood Cells

Study Figure 3–4 as you read the following to note the differences among the three different types of cells in the blood.

Erythrocytes (red blood cells). These cells are made in the bone marrow (soft tissue in the center of certain bones) and are necessary to carry oxygen from the lungs through the blood to all body cells. The oxygen is then used up by body cells in the process of converting food to energy (catabolism). **Hemoglobin** (globin = protein) is an important protein in erythrocytes that carries the oxygen through the bloodstream.

Leukocytes (white blood cells). There are several types of leukocytes:

Granulocytes (cells with dark-staining granules in their cytoplasm) are formed in bone marrow. There are three types of granulocytes:

1. **Eosinophils** (granules stain red [eosin/o = rosy] with acidic stain) are thought to be active and elevated in allergic conditions such as asthma. About 3 per cent of leukocytes are eosinophils.

2. **Basophils** (granules stain blue with basic [bas/o = basic] stain). The function

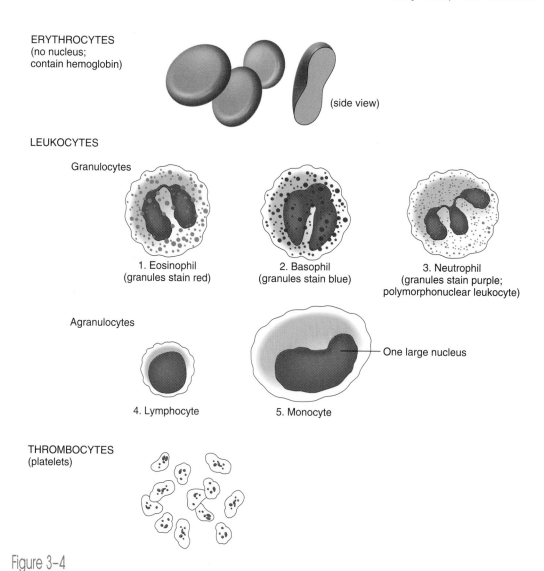

ERYTHROCYTES
(no nucleus;
contain hemoglobin)

(side view)

LEUKOCYTES

Granulocytes

1. Eosinophil
(granules stain red)

2. Basophil
(granules stain blue)

3. Neutrophil
(granules stain purple;
polymorphonuclear leukocyte)

Agranulocytes

4. Lymphocyte

5. Monocyte

One large nucleus

THROMBOCYTES
(platelets)

Figure 3–4

Types of blood cells.

of basophils is not clear, but they play a role in inflammation. Less than 1 per cent of leukocytes are basophils.

3. **Neutrophils** (granules stain blue and red [purple] with neutral stain) are important disease-fighting cells. They are called **phagocytes** (phag/o = eating, swallowing) because they engulf and digest bacteria. They are the most numerous disease-fighting "soldiers" and are often called **polymorphonuclear leukocytes** (poly = many, morph/o = shape) because of their nucleus, which is multilobed. Almost 60 per cent of leukocytes are neutrophils.

Agranulocytes (cells without dark-staining granules in the cytoplasm) are produced by lymph nodes and the spleen. There are two types of agranulocytes:

1. **Lymphocytes** (lymph cells) fight disease by producing antibodies and thus destroying foreign cells. They may also attach directly to foreign cells and destroy them. Two types of lymphocytes are T cells and B cells. About 32 per cent of leukocytes are lymphocytes.

2. **Monocytes** (cells with one [mon/o = one] very large nucleus) engulf and destroy cellular debris after neutrophils have attacked foreign cells. Monocytes leave the bloodstream and enter tissues (such as lung and liver) to become **macrophages,** which are large phagocytes. Monocytes make up about 4 per cent of all leukocytes.

Thrombocytes or **platelets** (clotting cells). These tiny fragments of blood cells are formed in the bone marrow and are necessary for blood clotting.

Appendix F: Pronunciation Clue

Pronunciation clue: The letters **g** and **c** are soft (as in ginger and cent) when followed by an **i** or **e,** and are hard (as in good and can) when followed by an **o** or **a.**

For example: laryngitis (lăr-ĭn-JĪ-tĭs)
laryngotomy (lă-rĭn-GŎT-ō-mē)

Appendix G: Anemia

Anemia literally means no blood. In medical language and usage, anemia refers to a medical condition in which there is a *reduction* in the number of erythrocytes or amount of hemoglobin in the circulating blood. There are many different kinds of anemias, classified on the basis of the many different problems that can arise with red blood cells and their circulation and content. **Aplastic** (a- = no, plas/o = formation) **anemia** is a severe type in which the bone marrow fails to produce not only erythrocytes but leukocytes and thrombocytes as well.

Appendix H: Ischemia

Ischemia literally means to hold back (isch/o) blood (-emia) from a part of the body. Tissue that becomes **ischemic** loses its normal flow of blood and becomes deprived of oxygen. The ischemia can be caused by mechanical injury to a blood vessel, by blood clots lodging in a vessel, or by the gradual closing off (occlusion) of a vessel owing to collection of fatty material.

Appendix I: Tonsillitis

Tonsils (notice the spelling with one letter l, whereas the combining form has a double letter l) are lymphatic tissue in the throat. They contain white blood cells (lymphocytes) and function to filter and fight bacteria, but they can also become infected and inflamed. Streptococcal infection of the throat can cause **tonsillitis,** which may lead to **tonsillectomy.**

Appendix J: Acromegaly

Acromegaly is an example of an endocrine disorder. The **pituitary gland** attached to the base of the brain produces an excessive amount of growth hormone after the completion of puberty. Hence, a person with acromegaly is of normal height, because the long bones have stopped growth after puberty, but has an abnormally large growth of bones and tissue in the hands, feet, and face. High levels of growth hormone before completion of puberty produce excessive growth of long bones (gigantism) as well as acromegaly.

Appendix K: Splenomegaly

The spleen is an organ in the left upper quadrant of the abdomen (below the diaphragm and to the side of the stomach). It is composed of lymph tissue and blood vessels. Its job is to dispose of dying red blood cells and manufacture white blood cells (lymphocytes) to fight disease. If the spleen must be removed (splenectomy), other organs carry out these functions.

Appendix L: Leukocytosis

When **-osis** is used as a suffix with blood cells, it means an abnormal condition in which there is a slight increase in number of normal circulating blood cells. Thus, in leukocytosis a slight elevation in numbers of *normal* white blood cells occurs in response to the presence of infection in the body. When **-emia** is used as a suffix with blood cells (**-cyte** is usually dropped, as in leukemia), the condition is an *abnormally* high or excessive increase in number of abnormal or cancerous blood cells.

Appendix M: Achondroplasia

Achondroplasia is an inherited disorder in which the bones of the arms and legs fail to grow to normal size owing to a defect in both cartilage and bone. It results in a type of dwarfism characterized by short limbs, a normal-sized head and body, and normal intelligence (Fig. 3–5).

Appendix N: -ptosis

The suffix **-ptosis** is pronounced TŌ-sĭs. When two consonants begin a word, the first is silent. If the two consonants are found in the middle of a word, both are pronounced—for example, blepharoptosis (blĕ-făr-ŏp-TŌ-sĭs). This condition occurs when eyelid muscles weaken, and a person has difficulty lifting the eyelid to keep it open (Fig. 3–6).

Appendix O: Laparoscopy

Laparoscopy (also known as **peritoneoscopy** or **minimally invasive surgery**) is visual examination of the abdominal (peritoneal) cavity using a laparoscope. The laparoscope, a lighted telescopic instrument, is inserted through an incision in the abdomen near the navel, and gas (carbon dioxide) is infused into the peritoneal cavity to prevent injury to abdominal structures during surgery. Laparoscopy is used to examine abdominal viscera for evidence of disease (performing biopsies) or for surgical procedures such as removal of the appendix or gallbladder and repair of hernias. It is also used to clip and collapse the fallopian tubes, thus preventing sperm cells from reaching eggs that are released from the ovary (Fig. 3–7).

Figure 3-5

A boy with achondroplasia showing short stature, short limbs and fingers, normal length of the trunk, bowed legs, a relatively large head, a prominent forehead, and a depressed nasal bridge. (Courtesy of Dr. A.E. Chudley, Professor of Pediatrics and Child Health, Children's Hospital and University of Manitoba, Winnipeg, Manitoba, Canada.)

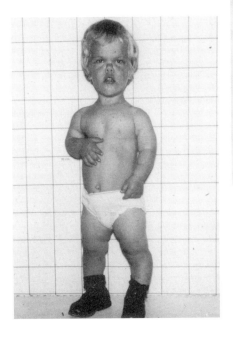

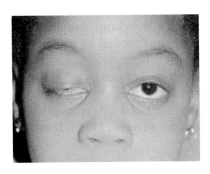

Figure 3-6

Ptosis of the upper eyelid (blepharoptosis) can occur with aging or may be associated with cerebrovascular accidents, cranial nerve damage, and other neurological disorders. (From Seidel HM, et al: Mosby's Guide to Physical Examination, 4th ed. St. Louis, Mosby, 1998, p 281.)

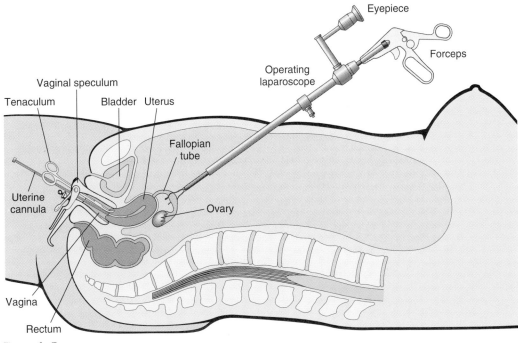

Figure 3-7

Laparoscopy for tubal ligation (interruption of the continuity of the fallopian tubes) as a means of preventing future pregnancy. The **tenaculum** is an instrument used to grasp the cervix. The **vaginal speculum** keeps the vaginal cavity open. The **uterine cannula** is a tube placed into the uterus to move the uterus during the procedure. **Forceps,** placed through the laparoscope, are used for grasping or manipulating tissue.

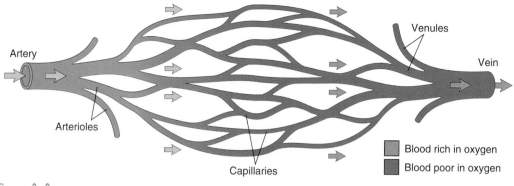

Figure 3-8

Relationship of blood vessels. An artery carries blood rich in oxygen from the heart to the organs of the body. In the organs, the artery narrows to form **arterioles** (small arteries), which branch into **capillaries** (the smallest blood vessels). Through the thin walls of capillaries, oxygen leaves the blood and enters cells. Thus, the capillaries branching into **venules** (small veins) carry blood poor in oxygen. Venules lead to a **vein** that brings oxygen-poor blood back to the heart.

Appendix P: Arteriole

The relationship among an artery, **arterioles,** capillaries (the tiniest of blood vessels), **venules** (small veins), and a vein is illustrated in Figure 3–8.

Appendix Q: Adenoids

The **adenoids** (the literal meaning is resembling glands, for they are neither endocrine nor exocrine glands) are lymphatic tissue in the part of the pharynx (throat) near the nose and nasal passages. Enlargement of this tissue may cause blockage of the airway from the nose to the pharynx, and adenoidectomy may be advised. The tonsils are also lymphatic tissue and their location as well as that of the adenoids is indicated in Figure 3–9.

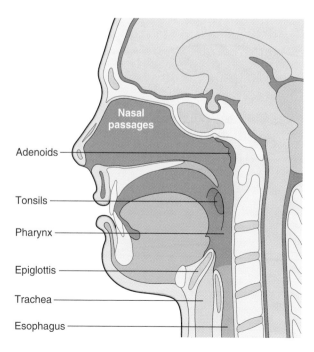

Figure 3-9

Adenoids and tonsils.

V. Practical Applications

Check your answers with the Answers to Practical Applications on page 98.

Procedures

Select from the diagnostic or treatment procedures that follow to complete the sentences below.

amniocentesis	angiography	angioplasty	mastectomy
paracentesis	laparoscopy	laparotomy	tonsillectomy
thoracentesis	tracheotomy	colostomy	

1. _____ is needed to remove abdominal fluid in the peritoneal space.

2. _____ is a large abdominal incision to remove an ovarian adenocarcinoma.

3. _____ is a treatment procedure to remove an adenocarcinoma of the breast.

4. _____ is a method used to determine the karyotype of a fetus.

5. _____ is used to establish an emergency airway path.

6. _____ is a surgical procedure to remove pharyngeal lymphatic tissue.

7. _____ is a surgical procedure to open clogged coronary arteries.

8. _____ is a method of removing fluid from the chest (pleural effusion).

9. _____ is used to drain feces from the body after bowel resection.

10. _____ is an x-ray procedure used to examine blood vessels before surgery.

11. _____ is a type of minimally invasive surgery within the abdomen.

VI. Exercises

Remember to check your answers carefully with those given in Section VII, Answers to Exercises.

A. Give the meanings for the following suffixes.

1. -cele _____

2. -emia _____

3. -coccus _____

4. -gram _____

5. -cyte _____

6. -algia _____

7. -ectomy _____

8. -centesis _____

9. -genesis _____

10. -graph _____

11. -itis _____

12. -graphy _____

B. Using the following combining forms and your knowledge of suffixes, build the following medical terms.

strept/o	cyst/o	arthr/o
staphyl/o	angi/o	carcino/o
mast/o	laryng/o	myel/o
thorac/o	isch/o	bronch/o
amni/o	ot/o	my/o
rect/o		

1. hernia of the urinary bladder _____

2. pain of muscle _____

3. process of producing cancer _____

4. record (x-ray) of the spinal cord _____

5. berry-shaped bacteria in twisted chains _____

6. surgical puncture to remove fluid from the chest _____

7. removal of the breast _____

8. inflammation of the tubes leading from the windpipe to the lungs _____

9. to hold back blood from cells _____

10. process of recording (x-ray) blood vessels _____

11. visual examination of joints _____

12. berry-shaped bacteria in clusters _____

13. resection of the voice box _____

14. surgical procedure to remove fluid from the sac around the fetus _____

C. Match the following terms, which describe blood cells, with their meanings below.

eosinophil   monocyte   erythrocyte
thrombocyte   neutrophil   lymphocyte
basophil

1. a granulocytic white blood cell that destroys foreign cells by engulfing and digesting them; also

   called a polymorphonuclear leukocyte _____

2. an agranular white blood cell that destroys foreign cells by making antibodies

   _____

3. a clotting cell; also called a platelet _____

4. a leukocyte whose granules turn red with stain and whose numbers are elevated in allergic

   reactions _____

5. a red blood cell _____

6. an agranular white blood cell that engulfs and digests cellular debris and contains one large

   nucleus _____

7. a white blood cell that contains granules in its cytoplasm and is prominent in causing an

   inflammatory reaction _____

D. Give the meanings of the following suffixes.

1. -logy _____   8. -megaly _____

2. -lysis _____   9. -oma _____

3. -pathy _____   10. -opsy _____

4. -penia _____   11. -plasia _____

5. -malacia _____   12. -plasty _____

6. -osis _____   13. -sclerosis _____

7. -phobia _____   14. -stasis _____

E. Using the following combining forms and your knowledge of suffixes, build the following medical terms.

hydr/o	splen/o	cardi/o
blephar/o	hem/o	acr/o
my/o	myel/o	rhin/o
nephr/o	bi/o	arteri/o
chondr/o	morph/o	agor/a
sarc/o	phleb/o	

1. fear of the marketplace (crowds) _____

2. enlargement of the spleen _____

3. study of the shape (of cells) _____

4. softening of cartilage _____

5. abnormal condition of water (fluid) in the kidney _____

6. disease condition of heart muscle _____

7. hardening of arteries _____

8. tumor (benign) of muscle _____

9. flesh tumor (malignant) of muscle _____

10. surgical repair of the nose _____

11. tumor of bone marrow _____

12. fear of heights _____

13. view of living tissue under the microscope _____

14. stoppage of the flow of blood (by mechanical or natural means) _____

15. inflammation of the eyelid _____

16. incision of a vein _____

F. Match the following terms with their meanings below.

acromegaly   achondroplasia   chemotherapy
laparoscopy   metastasis   hydrotherapy
osteomalacia   laparoscope   hypertrophy
necrosis   colostomy   atrophy

1. treatment using drugs _____

2. condition of death (of cells) _____

3. softening of bone _____

4. opening of the large intestine to the outside of the body _____

5. no development; shrinkage of cells _____

6. beyond control; spread of a cancerous tumor to another organ _____

7. instrument to visually examine the abdomen _____

8. enlargement of extremities; an endocrine disorder that causes excess growth hormone to be

    produced by the pituitary gland after puberty _____

9. condition of improper formation of cartilage in the embryo that leads to short bones and dwarf-

    like deformities _____

10. process of viewing the peritoneal (abdominal) cavity _____

11. treatment using water _____

12. excessive development of cells (increase in size of individual cells) _____

G. Give the meanings of the following suffixes.

1. -ia _____   7. -um _____

2. -trophy _____   8. -ule _____

3. -stasis _____   9. -y _____

4. -stomy _____   10. -oid _____

5. -tomy _____   11. -genic _____

6. -ole _____   12. -ptosis _____

H. Using the following combining forms and suffixes, build the following medical terms.

Combining Forms   *Suffixes*

pneumon/o	pleur/o	-gram	-ia	-pathy
nephr/o	mamm/o	-tomy	-ule	-plasty
arteri/o	lapar/o	-scopy	-dynia	-ectomy
ven/o	radi/o	-therapy	-ole	

1. incision of the abdomen _____

2. process of visual examination of the abdomen _____

3. a small artery _____

4. condition of the lungs _____

5. treatment using x-rays _____

6. record (x-ray) of the breast _____

7. pain of the chest wall and the membranes surrounding the lungs _____

8. a small vein _____

9. disease condition of the kidney _____

10. surgical repair of the breast _____

I. Underline the suffix in the following terms and give the meaning of the entire term.

1. laryngeal _____

2. inguinal _____

3. chronic _____

4. pulmonary _____

5. adipose _____

6. peritoneal _____

7. axillary _____

8. necrotic _____

9. mucoid _____

10. mucous _____

J. *Select from the following terms relating to blood and blood vessels to complete the sentences below.*

ischemia	leukemia	hematoma
anemia	multiple myeloma	arterioles
hemostasis	leukocytosis	venules
thrombocytopenia	angioplasty	hemolysis

1. Billy was diagnosed as having excessively high numbers of cancerous white blood cells, a disease

    known as _____. Chemotherapy was prescribed by his doctor, and his
    prognosis is excellent.

2. Mr. Clark's angiogram showed that he had serious atherosclerosis of one of the arteries supplying

    blood to his heart. His doctor recommended that _____ would be helpful to
    open up his clogged artery by threading a catheter (tube) through his artery and opening a
    balloon at the end of the catheter to widen the artery.

3. Mrs. Jackson's blood count showed a greatly reduced number of red blood cells, a condition called

    _____. The cause of this condition was destruction of her (red) blood cells,

    known as _____.

4. Doctors were unable to operate on Joe Hite because his platelet count was so low. His condition

    is called _____.

5. Blockage of an artery leading to Mr. Stein's brain led to the holding back of blood flow to nerve

    tissue in his brain. This condition, called _____, could lead to necrosis of
    tissue and a cerebrovascular accident.

6. Small arteries, called _____, were broken under Ms. Bein's scalp when
    she was struck on the head with a rock. She soon developed a mass of blood, called a (an)

    _____, under the skin in that region of her head.

7. Sarah Jones had a staphylococcal infection that caused her white blood cell count to be elevated.

    This slight elevation of white blood cells is called _____.

8. Within the body, the bone marrow (soft tissue within bones) is the "factory" for making blood
    cells. Mr. Scott developed a malignant condition of the bone marrow cells in his hip, upper arm,

    and thigh bones, a condition known as _____.

9. During surgery, clamps are used to close off blood vessels and prevent blood loss. Therefore,

    _____ is maintained and there is no need for blood transfusions.

10. Small vessels that carry blood back toward the heart from the capillaries and tissues of the body

    are known as _____.

K. Complete the medical term for the following definitions.

Definition	Medical Term
1. The membrane surrounding the heart	peri _____
2. Hardening of arteries	arterio _____
3. Enlargement of the liver	hepato _____
4. New opening of the windpipe to the outside of the body	tracheo _____
5. Inflammation of the tonsils	_____ itis
6. Surgical puncture to remove fluid from the abdomen	abdomino _____
7. Muscle pain	my _____
8. Pertaining to the membranes surrounding the lungs	_____ al
9. Study of the eye	_____ logy
10. Berry-shaped bacteria in clusters	_____ cocci
11. Beyond control (spread of a cancerous tumor)	meta _____
12. Pertaining to the voice box	_____ eal

L. Select the correct term to complete the following sentences.

1. Ms. Daley has nine children and presents to her doctor complaining of problems urinating. After examining her, the doctor finds her bladder protruding into her vagina and tells her she has a **(rectocele, cystocele, hiatal)** hernia.

2. Suzy coughed constantly for a week. Her doctor told her that her chest x-ray showed pneumonia. Her sputum (material coughed up from her chest) demonstrated **(ischemic, pleuritic, pneumococcal)** bacteria.

3. Mr. Manion went to the doctor complaining that he couldn't keep his left upper eyelid from sagging. His doctor told him that he had a neurological problem called Horner syndrome, characterized by **(necrosis, hydronephrosis, ptosis)** of his eyelid.

4. After 6 weeks in a cast to set her broken arm, Jill's arm muscles were smaller and weaker. They had **(atrophied, hypertrophied, metastasized)** and she was advised to have physical therapy to strengthen them.

5. Ms. Brody was diagnosed with breast cancer. The first phase of her treatment included a **(nephrectomy, mastectomy, pulmonary resection)** to remove her breast and the tumor. Following the surgery her doctors recommended **(chemotherapy, radiotherapy, hydrotherapy)** using drugs such as methotrexate and 5-fluorouracil.

6. As she grew older, Miriam's facial features became coarser and her hands and tongue became bigger; doctors told her she had a slowly progressive endocrine condition called **(thyromegaly, splenomegaly, acromegaly)**.

VII. Answers to Exercises

A

1. hernia
2. blood condition
3. berry-shaped bacterium
4. record
5. cell
6. pain
7. removal, excision, resection
8. surgical puncture to remove fluid
9. process of producing, forming
10. instrument to record
11. inflammation
12. process of recording

B

1. cystocele
2. myalgia (myodynia is not used)
3. carcinogenesis
4. myelogram
5. streptococci (bacteria is a plural term)
6. thoracocentesis or thoracentesis
7. mastectomy
8. bronchitis
9. ischemia
10. angiography
11. arthroscopy
12. staphylococci
13. laryngectomy
14. amniocentesis

C

1. neutrophil
2. lymphocyte
3. thrombocyte
4. eosinophil
5. erythrocyte
6. monocyte
7. basophil

D

1. process of study
2. breakdown, separation, destruction
3. process of disease
4. deficiency, less than normal
5. softening
6. condition, abnormal condition
7. fear of
8. enlargement
9. tumor, mass
10. process of viewing
11. condition of formation, growth
12. surgical repair
13. hardening, to harden
14. to stop, control

E

1. agoraphobia
2. splenomegaly
3. morphology
4. chondromalacia
5. hydronephrosis
6. cardiomyopathy
7. arteriosclerosis
8. myoma
9. myosarcoma
10. rhinoplasty
11. myeloma (called multiple myeloma)
12. acrophobia
13. biopsy
14. hemostasis
15. blepharitis
16. phlebotomy

F

1. chemotherapy
2. necrosis
3. osteomalacia
4. colostomy
5. atrophy
6. metastasis
7. laparoscope
8. acromegaly
9. achondroplasia
10. laparoscopy
11. hydrotherapy
12. hypertrophy

G

1. condition
2. development, nourishment
3. to stop, control
4. new opening
5. incision, cut into
6. small, little
7. structure
8. small, little
9. condition, process
10. resembling
11. pertaining to producing, produced by or in
12. prolapse, drooping, sagging

H

1. laparotomy
2. laparoscopy
3. arteriole
4. pneumonia (this condition is actually pneumonitis)
5. radiotherapy
6. mammogram
7. pleurodynia
8. venule
9. nephropathy
10. mammoplasty

I

1. laryngeal—pertaining to the voice box
2. inguinal—pertaining to the groin
3. chronic—pertaining to time (over a long period of time)
4. pulmonary—pertaining to the lung
5. adipose—pertaining to (or full of) fat
6. peritoneal—pertaining to the peritoneum (membrane around the abdominal organs)
7. axillary—pertaining to the armpit, under arm
8. necrotic—pertaining to death
9. mucoid—resembling mucus
10. mucous—pertaining to mucus

J

1. leukemia
2. angioplasty
3. anemia; hemolysis
4. thrombocytopenia

5. ischemia
6. arterioles; hematoma
7. leukocytosis
8. multiple myeloma

9. hemostasis
10. venules

K

1. pericardium
2. arteriosclerosis
3. hepatomegaly
4. tracheostomy
5. tonsillitis

6. abdominocentesis (this procedure is also known as a paracentesis)
7. myalgia
8. pleural
9. ophthalmology

10. staphylococci
11. metastasis
12. laryngeal

L

1. cystocele
2. pneumococcal
3. ptosis

4. atrophied
5. mastectomy; chemotherapy
6. acromegaly

Answers to Practical Applications

1. paracentesis (abdominocentesis)
2. laparotomy
3. mastectomy
4. amniocentesis

5. tracheotomy
6. tonsillectomy
7. angioplasty
8. thoracentesis

9. colostomy
10. angiography
11. laparoscopy

VIII. Pronunciation of Terms

Pronunciation Guide

To test your understanding of the terminology in this chapter, write the meaning of each term in the space provided. In addition, you may wish to cover the terms and write them by looking at your definitions. Make sure your spelling is correct. The page number after each term indicates where it is defined or used in the text so you can easily check your responses.

ā as in āpe   ă as in ăpple
ē as in ēven   ĕ as in ĕvery
ī as in īce   ĭ as in ĭnterest
ō as in ōpen   ŏ as in pŏt
ū as in ūnit   ŭ as in ŭnder

Term	Pronunciation	Meaning
abdominocentesis (76)	ăb-dŏm-ĭ-nō-sĕn-TĒ-sĭs	_____
achondroplasia (79)	ā-kŏn-drō-PLĀ-zē-ă	_____
acromegaly (77)	ăk-rō-MĔG-ă-lē	_____
acrophobia (78)	ăk-rō-FŌ-bē-ă	_____
acute (81)	ă-KŪT	_____
adenoids (81)	ĂD-ĕ-noydz	_____
adipose (81)	Ă-dĭ-pōs	_____
agoraphobia (76)	ă-gŏr-ă-FŌ-bē-ă	_____

amniocentesis (76)	ăm-nē-ō-sĕn-TĒ-sĭs	_____
anemia (76)	ă-NĒ-mē-ă	_____
angiogenesis (76)	ăn-jē-ō-JĔN-ĕ-sĭs	_____
angiography (77)	ăn-jē-ŎG-ră-fē	_____
angioplasty (79)	ăn-jē-ō-PLĂS-tē	_____
arteriole (80)	ăr-TĒR-ē-ōl	_____
arteriosclerosis (79)	ăr-tē-rē-ō-sklĕ-RŌ-sĭs	_____
arthralgia (75)	ăr-THRĂL-jă	_____
atrophy (80)	ĂT-rō-fē	_____
axillary (81)	ĂK-sĭ-lār-ē	_____
basophil (84)	BĀ-sō-fĭl	_____
biopsy (78)	BĪ-ŏp-sē	_____
blepharoptosis (79)	blĕ-fă-rŏp-TŌ-sĭs	_____
bronchitis (77)	brŏng-KĪ-tĭs	_____
carcinogenesis (76)	kăr-sĭ-nō-JĔN-ĕ-sĭs	_____
cardiomyopathy (78)	kăr-dē-ō-mī-ŎP-ă-thē	_____
chemotherapy (79)	kē-mō-THĔR-ĕ-pē	_____
chondromalacia (77)	kŏn-drō-mă-LĀ-shă	_____
chronic (81)	KRŎN-ĭk	_____
colostomy (79)	kō-LŎS-tō-mē	_____
cystocele (76)	SĬS-tō-sēl	_____
electroencephalogram (77)	ē-lĕk-trō-ĕn-SĔF-ă-lō-grăm	_____
electroencephalograph (77)	ē-lĕk-trō-ĕn-SĔF-ă-lō-grăf	_____
electroencephalography (77)	ē-lĕk-trō-ĕn-sĕf-ă-LŎG-ră-fē	_____
eosinophil (84)	ē-ō-SĬN-ō-fĭl	_____
erythrocyte (76)	ĕ-RĬTH-rō-sīt	_____
erythropenia (78)	ĕ-rĭth-rō-PĒ-nē-ă	_____
hematoma (78)	hē-mă-TŌ-mă	_____
hemolysis (77)	hē-MŎL-ĭ-sĭs	_____

hemostasis (79)	hē-mō-STĀ-sĭs	_____
hydronephrosis (78)	hī-drō-nĕ-FRŌ-sĭs	_____
hydrotherapy (79)	hī-drō-THĔR-ă-pē	_____
hypertrophy (80)	hī-PĔR-trō-fē	_____
inguinal (81)	ĬNG-wă-năl	_____
ischemia (76)	ĭs-KĒ-mē-ă	_____
laparoscope (79)	LĂP-ă-rō-skōp	_____
laparoscopy (79)	lă-pă-RŎS-kō-pē	_____
laparotomy (80)	lăp-ă-RŎT-ō-mē	_____
laryngeal (81)	lă-RĬN-jē-ăl or lăr-ĭn-JĒ-ăl	_____
laryngectomy (76)	lăr-ĭn-JĔK-tō-mē	_____
leukemia (80)	lū-KĒ-mē-ă	_____
leukocytosis (78)	lū-kō-sī-TŌ-sĭs	_____
lymphocyte (85)	LĬM-fō-sīt	_____
mammogram (77)	MĂM-mō-grăm	_____
mastectomy (76)	măs-TĔK-tō-mē	_____
metastasis (79)	mĕ-TĂS-tă-sĭs	_____
monocyte (89)	MŎN-ō-sīt	_____
morphology (77)	mŏr-FŎL-ō-jē	_____
mucous (81)	MŪ-kŭs	_____
myalgia (75)	mī-ĂL-jă	_____
myelogram (77)	MĪ-ĕ-lō-grăm	_____
myeloma (78)	mī-ĕ-LŌ-mă	_____
myoma (78)	mī-Ō-mă	_____
myosarcoma (78)	mī-ō-săr-KŌ-mă	_____
necrosis (78)	nĕ-KRŌ-sĭs	_____
necrotic (81)	nĕ-KRŎT-ĭk	_____
nephrologist (80)	nĕ-FRŎL-ō-jĭst	_____
nephropathy (80)	nĕ-FRŎP-ă-thē	_____

neuralgia (75)	nū-RĂL-jă	_____
neutropenia (78)	nū-trō-PĒ-nē-ă	_____
neutrophil (85)	NŪ-trō-fĭl	_____
ophthalmology (77)	ŏf-thăl-MŎL-ō-jē	_____
osteogenic (77)	ŏs-tē-ō-JĔN-ĭk	_____
osteomalacia (77)	ŏs-tē-ō-mă-LĀ-shă	_____
otalgia (75)	ō-TĂL-jă	_____
paracentesis (76)	pă-ră-cĕn-TĒ-sĭs	_____
pathogenesis (76)	păth-ŏ-JĔN-ĕ-sĭs	_____
pericardium (80)	pĕr-ē-KĂR-dē-ŭm	_____
peritoneal (81)	pĕr-ĭ-tō-NĒ-ăl	_____
phlebitis (77)	flĕ-BĪ-tis	_____
phlebotomy (80)	flĕ-BŎT-ō-mē	_____
platelet (85)	PLĀT-lĕt	_____
pleurodynia (76)	plŭr-ō-DĬN-ē-ă	_____
pneumonia (80)	nū-MŌN-yă	_____
polymorphonuclear leukocyte (85)	pŏl-ē-mŏr-fō-NŪ-klē-ăr LŪ-kō-sīt	_____
ptosis (79)	Tō-sĭs	_____
pulmonary (81)	PŬL-mō-nă-rē	_____
radiotherapy (79)	rā-dē-ō-THĔ-ră-pē	_____
rectocele (76)	RĔK-tō-sēl	_____
splenomegaly (77)	splē-nō-MĔG-ă-lē	_____
staphylococci (76)	stăf-ĭ-lō-KŎK-sī	_____
streptococcus (76)	strĕp-tō-KŎK-ŭs	_____
thoracentesis (76)	thō-ră-sĕn-TĒ-sĭs	_____
thrombocytopenia (78)	thrŏm-bō-sī-tō-PĒ-nē-ă	_____
tonsillitis (77)	tŏn-sĭ-LĪ-tĭs	_____
tracheostomy (79)	trā-kē-ŎS-tō-mē	_____
venule (80)	VĔN-ūl	_____

IX. Review Sheet

Write the meanings of each word part in the space provided and test yourself. Check your answers with the information in the chapter or in the glossary (Medical Terms—English) at the end of the book.

NOUN SUFFIXES

Suffix	Meaning	Suffix	Meaning
-algia	_____	-ole	_____
-cele	_____	-oma	_____
-centesis	_____	-opsy	_____
-coccus	_____	-osis	_____
-cyte	_____	-pathy	_____
-dynia	_____	-penia	_____
-ectomy	_____	-phobia	_____
-emia	_____	-plasia	_____
-er	_____	-plasty	_____
-genesis	_____	-ptosis	_____
-genic	_____	-sclerosis	_____
-gram	_____	-scope	_____
-graph	_____	-scopy	_____
-graphy	_____	-stasis	_____
-ia	_____	-stomy	_____
-ist	_____	-therapy	_____
-itis	_____	-tomy	_____
-logy	_____	-trophy	_____
-lysis	_____	-ule	_____
-malacia	_____	-um, -ium	_____
-megaly	_____	-y	_____

ADJECTIVE SUFFIXES

Suffix	Meaning	Suffix	Meaning
-ac	_____	-oid	_____
-al	_____	-ose	_____
-ary	_____	-ous	_____
-eal	_____	-tic	_____
-ic, -ical	_____		

COMBINING FORMS

Combining Form	Meaning	Combining Form	Meaning
abdomin/o	_____	chondr/o	_____
acr/o	_____	chron/o	_____
aden/o	_____	col/o	_____
adip/o	_____	cyst/o	_____
agor/a	_____	encephal/o	_____
amni/o	_____	erythr/o	_____
angi/o	_____	hem/o	_____
arteri/o	_____	hepat/o	_____
arthr/o	_____	hydr/o	_____
axill/o	_____	inguin/o	_____
bi/o	_____	lapar/o	_____
blephar/o	_____	laryng/o	_____
bronch/o	_____	leuk/o	_____
carcin/o	_____	lymph/o	_____
cardi/o	_____	mamm/o	_____
chem/o	_____	mast/o	_____

Continued on following page

morph/o	_____	pleur/o	_____
muc/o	_____	pneumon/o	_____
my/o	_____	pulmon/o	_____
myel/o	_____	radi/o	_____
necr/o	_____	rect/o	_____
nephr/o	_____	rhin/o	_____
neur/o	_____	sarc/o	_____
neutr/o	_____	splen/o	_____
nucle/o	_____	staphyl/o	_____
ophthalm/o	_____	strept/o	_____
oste/o	_____	thorac/o	_____
ot/o	_____	thromb/o	_____
peritone/o	_____	tonsill/o	_____
phleb/o	_____	ven/o	_____
plas/o	_____		

Do you remember the following combining forms from previous chapters?

Combining Form	Meaning	Combining Form	Meaning
anter/o	_____	later/o	_____
cephal/o	_____	onc/o	_____
cervic/o	_____	poster/o	_____
crani/o	_____	ren/o	_____
dist/o	_____	trache/o	_____
dors/o	_____	vertebr/o	_____
gynec/o	_____	viscer/o	_____

CHAPTER

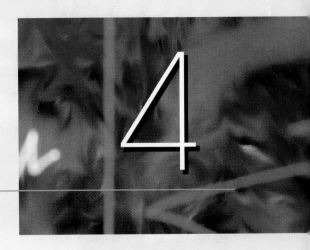

4

Prefixes

This chapter is divided into the following sections
- I. Introduction
- II. Combining Forms and Suffixes
- III. Prefixes and Terminology
- IV. Appendices
- V. Practical Applications
- VI. Exercises
- VII. Answers to Exercises
- VIII. Pronunciation of Terms
- IX. Review Sheet

In this chapter you will
- Define basic prefixes used in the medical language;
- Analyze medical terms that combine prefixes and other word elements; and
- Learn about the Rh condition as an example of an antigen-antibody reaction.

1. Introduction

This chapter on prefixes, like the preceding chapter on suffixes, is designed to give you practice in word analysis and provide a foundation for the study of the terminology of body systems that follows.

The list of combining forms, suffixes, and their meanings in Section II will help you analyze the terminology in the rest of the chapter. The appendices (Section IV) are included to provide more complete understanding of the terms and to explain the words with reference to the anatomy, physiology, and diseases of the body.

II. Combining Forms and Suffixes

Combining Forms

Combining Form	Meaning	Combining Form	Meaning
carp/o	wrist bones	nect/o	to bind, tie, connect
cib/o	meals	norm/o	rule, order
cis/o	to cut	ox/o	oxygen
cost/o	rib	seps/o	infection
cutane/o	skin	somn/o	sleep
dactyl/o	fingers, toes	son/o	sound
duct/o	to lead, carry	the/o	to put, place
flex/o	to bend	thel/o	nipple
furc/o	forking, branching	thyr/o	shield; the shape of the thyroid gland resembled (-oid) a shield to those who named it.
gloss/o	tongue		
glyc/o	sugar	top/o	place, position, location
immun/o	protection	tox/o	poison
morph/o	shape, form	trache/o	windpipe, trachea
mort/o	death	urethr/o	urethra
nat/i	birth		

Suffixes

Suffix	Meaning	Suffix	Meaning
-blast	embryonic, immature	-gen	producing, forming
-cyesis	pregnancy	-lapse	to slide, fall, sag
-drome	to run	-lysis	breakdown, separation, loosening
-fusion	to pour	-meter	to measure

-mission	to send	**-plasm**	development, formation
-or	one who	**-pnea**	breathing
-partum	birth, labor	**-ptosis**	droop, sag, prolapse
-phoria	to bear, carry; feeling (mental state)	**-rrhea**	flow, discharge
		-stasis	stop, control; place
-physis	to grow	**-trophy**	nourishment, development
-plasia	development, formation		

III. Prefixes and Terminology

Write the meaning of the medical term in the space provided.

Prefix	Meaning	Terminology	Meaning
a-, an-	no, not, without	apnea _____	
		anoxia _____	
ab-	away from	abnormal _____	
		abductor _____	
		A muscle that draws a limb away from the body.	
ad-	toward	adductor _____	
		adrenal glands[1] _____	
ana-	up, apart	anabolism _____	
		analysis _____	
		Urinalysis (urin/o + [an]alysis) is laboratory examination of urine to aid in diagnosis.	
ante-	before, forward	ante cibum _____	
		a. c. is a notation on prescription orders. It means prior to (before) meals.	
		anteflexion _____	
		ante partum _____	

---

[1]See Appendix A.

anti-	against	antisepsis _____

An antiseptic (-sis changes to -tic to form an adjective) substance is used against infections. Anti- is pronounced ăn-tŭh.

antibiotic[2] _____

antigen[3] _____

In this word, anti- stands for antibody.

antibody _____

antitoxin _____

auto-	self, own	autoimmune[4] _____
bi-	two	bifurcation _____
		bilateral _____
brady-	slow	bradycardia _____
cata-	down	catabolism _____
con-	with, together	congenital anomaly[5] _____
		connective _____
contra-	against, opposite	contraindication _____

Contra- means against in this term.

contralateral[6] _____

Contra- means opposite in this term.

de-	down, lack of	dehydration _____
dia-	through, complete	diameter _____
		diarrhea _____
		dialysis[7] _____
dys-	bad, painful, difficult, abnormal	dyspnea _____
		dysplasia _____
ec-, ecto-	out, outside	ectopic pregnancy[8] _____

---

[2]See Appendix B.
[3]See Appendix C.
[4]See Appendix D.
[5]See Appendix E.
[6]See Appendix F.
[7]See Appendix G.
[8]See Appendix H.

en-, endo-	in, within	endotracheal _____
		endoscope _____
		endocardium _____
epi-	upon, on, above	epithelium _____
eu-	good, normal	euthyroid _____

Normal thyroid function.

euphoria _____

Exaggerated feeling of well-being.

| **ex-** | out, away from | exophthalmos _____ |

Protrusion of the eyeball associated with enlargement and overactivity of the thyroid gland; also called proptosis (pro = forward, -ptosis = prolapse).

| **hemi-** | half | hemiglossectomy _____ |
| **hyper-** | excessive, above, | hyperplasia _____ |

Increase in cell numbers.

hypertrophy _____

Increase in size of individual cells.

hyperglycemia _____

hypo-	deficient, under	hypodermic _____
		hypoglycemia _____
in-	not	insomniac _____
in-	into	incision _____
infra-	beneath	infracostal _____
inter-	between	intercostal _____
intra-	into, within	intravenous _____
macro-	large	macrocephalic _____
mal-	bad	malignant _____

From the Latin ignis *meaning fire.* **Benign** *(ben- = good) tumors are noncancerous, whereas malignant tumors are cancerous.*

malaise _____

From the French malaise *meaning a vague feeling of bodily discomfort.*

meta-   change, beyond   metamorphosis _____

Meta- means change in this term.

metastasis _____

Meta = beyond and -stasis = control, or meta = change and -stasis = place.
A metastasis is the spread of a cancerous tumor to a secondary location.

metacarpal bones _____

These are five hand bones. They lie beyond the wrist bones, but before the
finger bones (phalanges).

micro-   small   microscope _____

neo-   new   neoplasm _____

neonatal _____

pan-   all   pancytopenia _____

Deficiency of erythrocytes, leukocytes, and thrombocytes.

para-   near, beside,   parathyroid glands[9] _____
abnormal

paralysis _____

Abnormal disruption of the connection between nerve and muscle.
Originally from the Greek paralusis *meaning to separate, loosen on one*
side, describing the loss of movement on one side of the body (occurring in
stroke patients).

per-   through   percutaneous _____

peri-   surrounding   pericardium _____

periosteum _____

poly-   many, much   polymorphonuclear _____

polyneuritis _____

post-   after, behind   post mortem _____

postnatal _____

pre-   before, in front of   precancerous _____

prenatal _____

pro-   before, forward   prodrome _____

Prodromal symptoms (rash, fever) appear before the actual illness and
signal its onset.

[9]See Appendix I.
[10]See Appendix J.

prolapse[10] _____

pseudo-	false	pseudocyesis _____
		Development of signs of pregnancy but without the presence of an embryo.
re-	back, again	relapse _____
		A disease or its symptoms return after an apparent recovery.
		remission _____
		Symptoms lessen and the patient feels better.
		recombinant DNA[11] _____
retro-	behind, backward	retroperitoneal _____
		retroflexion _____
sub-	under	subcutaneous _____
supra-	above, upper	suprathoracic _____
		suprarenal glands _____
syn-, sym-	together, with	syndactyly _____
		synthesis _____
		syndrome[12] _____
		Before the letters b, p, and m, syn becomes sym.
		symbiosis[13] _____
		symmetry _____
		What is asymmetry?
		symphysis[14] _____
tachy-	fast	tachypnea _____
trans-	across, through	transfusion _____
		transurethral[15] _____
ultra-	beyond, excess	ultrasonography[16] _____
uni-	one	unilateral _____

---

[11] See Appendix K.
[12] See Appendix L.
[13] See Appendix M.
[14] See Appendix N.
[15] See Appendix O.
[16] See Appendix P.

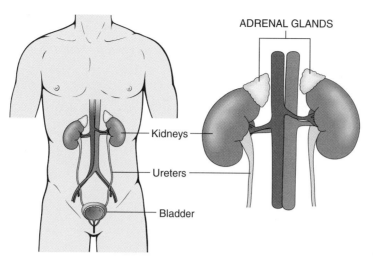

ADRENAL GLANDS

Kidneys

Ureters

Bladder

Figure 4-1

Adrenal glands.

IV. Appendices

Appendix A: Adrenal Glands

The **adrenal glands** (also called suprarenal glands) are endocrine glands located above each kidney. They secrete chemicals called hormones that affect the functioning of the body. One of these hormones is called adrenaline (epinephrine). It causes the bronchial tubes to widen, the heart to beat more rapidly, and blood pressure to rise (Fig. 4–1).

Appendix B: Antibiotic

An **antibiotic** is a chemical that destroys or inhibits the growth of microorganisms (small living things) such as bacteria. The first antibiotic, penicillin, was produced from immature plants called molds or fungi.

Appendix C: Antigens and Antibodies; the Rh Condition

An **antigen** is a substance, usually foreign to the body (such as a poison, virus, or bacterium), that stimulates the production of antibodies. **Antibodies** are protein substances made by white blood cells in response to the presence of foreign antigens. For example, the flu virus (antigen) enters the body, causing the production of antibodies in the bloodstream. These antibodies will then attach to and destroy the antigens (viruses) that produced them. The reaction between an antigen and an antibody is called an immune reaction (immun/o means protection).

Another example of an antigen-antibody is the **Rh condition.** A person who is Rh$^+$ has a protein coating (antigen) on his or her red blood cells (RBCs). This antigen factor is something that the person is born with and is normal for him or her. A person who is Rh$^-$ has normal RBCs as well, but they do not carry the Rh factor antigen.

If an Rh$^-$ woman and an Rh$^+$ man conceive an embryo, the embryo may be Rh$^-$ or Rh$^+$. A dangerous condition arises only when the embryo is Rh$^+$. During delivery of the first Rh$^+$ baby, some of the baby's blood cells containing antigens may escape into the mother's bloodstream. This sensitizes the mother so that she produces a low level of antibodies to the Rh$^+$ antigen. Because this occurs at delivery, the first baby is generally not affected and is normal at birth. Sensitization can also occur after a miscarriage or an abortion.

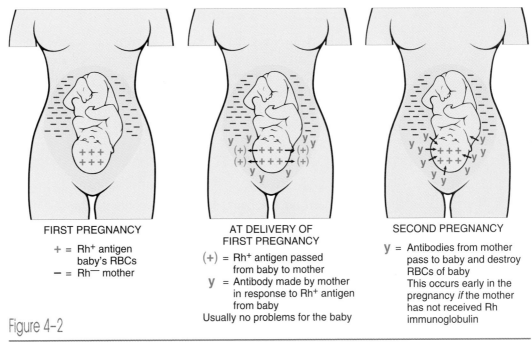

FIRST PREGNANCY

+ = Rh⁺ antigen
       baby's RBCs
− = Rh⁻ mother

AT DELIVERY OF
FIRST PREGNANCY

(+) = Rh⁺ antigen passed
        from baby to mother
y = Antibody made by mother
     in response to Rh⁺ antigen
     from baby
Usually no problems for the baby

SECOND PREGNANCY

y = Antibodies from mother
     pass to baby and destroy
     RBCs of baby
     This occurs early in the
     pregnancy *if* the mother
     has not received Rh
     immunoglobulin

Figure 4-2

Rh condition as an example of an antigen-antibody reaction.

Difficulties arise with the second Rh⁺ pregnancy. If the embryo is Rh⁺ again, during pregnancy the mother's acquired antibodies will enter the infant's bloodstream and attack the infant's RBCs (Rh⁺). The infant's RBCs are destroyed, and the infant attempts to compensate for this loss of cells by making many new immature RBCs (erythroblasts). The infant is born with a condition known as **erythroblastosis fetalis, or hemolytic disease of the newborn (HDN).**

One of the clinical symptoms of erythroblastosis fetalis is jaundice, or yellow skin pigmentation. The jaundice results from the excessive destruction of RBCs, which causes a substance called **bilirubin** (chemical pigment produced when hemoglobin from dying RBCs is broken down) to accumulate in the blood. To prevent bilirubin from affecting the brain cells of the infant, newborns are often treated by exposure to bright lights (phototherapy). The light changes the bilirubin so that it can be easily excreted from the body in feces.

To prevent hemolytic disease of the newborn, Rh immune globulin is given to the mother at 28 weeks of pregnancy and within 72 hours after each Rh⁺ delivery or after every abortion and miscarriage if the father is Rh⁺. The globulin binds to Rh⁺ cells that have escaped into the mother's circulation, and thus prevents the mother from making Rh⁺ antibodies. This ensures that future babies will not develop HDN. Figure 4–2 reviews the antigen-antibody reaction in the Rh condition in a diagrammatic fashion.

Appendix D: Autoimmune

Part of the normal immune reaction (protecting the body against foreign invaders) involves making antibodies to fight against viruses and bacteria. However, in an **auto-immune** reaction, the body makes antibodies against its own good cells and tissues, causing inflammation and injury. Examples of autoimmune disorders are rheumatoid arthritis (joints are affected), systemic lupus erythematosus (connective tissues, skin, and internal organs are affected), and Graves disease (hyperthyroidism—the thyroid gland is affected).

Appendix E: Congenital Anomaly

An anomaly is an irregularity in a structure or organ. Examples of **congenital anomalies** (those that an infant is born with) are webbed fingers or toes (syndactyly) and heart defects. Some congenital anomalies are recognized as hereditary (passed to the infant through chromosomes from the father or mother, or both), whereas others are produced by factors present during pregnancy. For example, cocaine addiction in the mother produces addiction and brain damage in the infant at birth.

Appendix F: Contralateral

Often, after a stroke involving the motor (movement) area of the brain, the effect on the body is seen on the **contralateral** side. This means that if the brain damage is located on the right side of the brain, the patient will have paralysis on the left side of the body. The muscles on one side of the body are controlled by nerves on the opposite (contralateral) side of the brain. **Ipsilateral (ipsi-** means same) means the same side.

Appendix G: Dialysis

Dialysis literally means complete separation. A dialysis machine (artificial kidney) can completely separate out from the blood the harmful waste products of the body that are normally removed by the urine.

Appendix H: Ectopic Pregnancy

In a normal pregnancy, the embryo develops within the uterus. In an **ectopic pregnancy,** the embryo is implanted outside the uterus—most often it is found in the fallopian tubes and sometimes in the ovary or abdominal cavity (Fig. 4–3).

Appendix I: Parathyroid Glands

There are four **parathyroid glands** located on the dorsal side of the thyroid gland. The parathyroids are endocrine glands that produce a hormone and function entirely

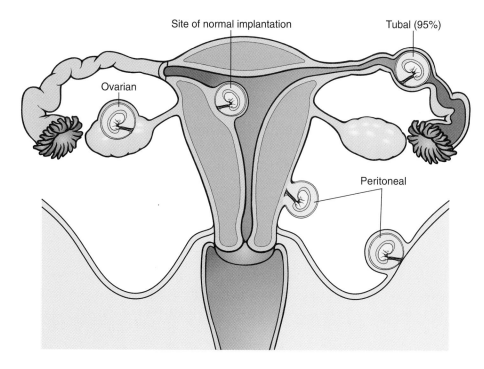

Figure 4-3

Sites of ectopic pregnancies. Normal pregnancy implantation is in the upper portion of the uterus. (Modified from Damjanov I: Pathology for the Health-Related Professions, Philadelphia, WB Saunders, 1996, p 393.)

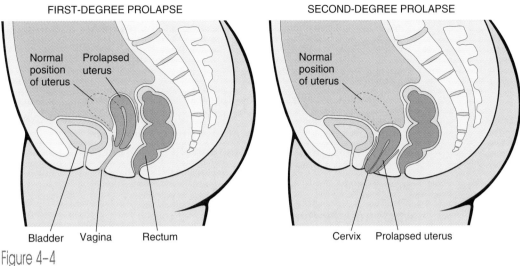

FIRST-DEGREE PROLAPSE   SECOND-DEGREE PROLAPSE

Normal position of uterus   Prolapsed uterus

Normal position of uterus

Bladder   Vagina   Rectum

Cervix   Prolapsed uterus

Figure 4-4

First- and second-degree prolapse of the uterus. In **first-degree** prolapse, the uterus descends into the vaginal canal. In **second-degree** prolapse, the body of the uterus is still within the vagina, but the cervix protrudes from the vaginal orifice (opening). In **third-degree** prolapse (not pictured), the entire uterus projects permanently outside the orifice. As treatment, the uterus may be held in position by a plastic pessary (oval supporting object) that is inserted into the vagina. Some patients may require hysterectomy (removal of the uterus).

separately from the thyroid gland. The **parathyroid hormone** increases blood calcium and maintains it at a normal level.

Appendix J: Prolapse

-Lapse means to slide, sag, or fall. If an organ or tissue **prolapses,** it slides forward or downward. Prolapse of the uterus is a common example. If the muscles that hold the uterus in place become weak, the uterus may slide downward toward the vagina (Fig. 4–4).

Appendix K: Recombinant DNA

This is the process of taking a gene (a region of DNA) from one organism and inserting it (recombining it) into the DNA of another organism. An example is the **recombinant DNA** technique used to manufacture insulin outside the body. The gene that codes for insulin (i.e., contains the recipe for making insulin) is cut out of a human chromosome (using special enzymes) and transferred into a bacterium, such as *Escherichia coli.* The bacterium then contains the gene for making human insulin and, because it divides very rapidly, can produce insulin in large quantities. The insulin is given to diabetic patients who are unable to make their own insulin. Polymerase chain reaction (PCR) is a method of producing multiple copies of a single gene, and it is an important tool for making recombinant DNA.

Appendix L: Syndrome

A **syndrome** is a group of signs or symptoms that commonly occur together and indicate a particular disease or abnormal condition. An example of a syndrome is Reye syndrome, characterized by vomiting, swelling of the brain, increased intracranial pressure, hypoglycemia, and dysfunction of the liver. It can occur in children following a viral infection that has been treated with aspirin.

Fetal alcohol syndrome is a group of symptoms (pre- and postnatal growth deficiency and craniofacial anomalies such as microcephaly and limb and heart defects) in an infant caused by the mother's intake of alcohol during pregnancy.

Appendix M: Symbiosis

Symbiosis refers to the living together in close association of two organisms, either for mutual benefit or not. The bacteria that normally live in the digestive tract of humans are an example of symbiosis. **Parasitism** is an example of symbiosis in which one organism benefits and the other does not.

In psychiatry, symbiosis is a relationship between two persons who are emotionally dependent on each other.

Appendix N: Symphysis

A **symphysis** is a type of joint in which the bony surfaces are covered by a layer of cartilage. The surfaces act as shock absorbers. Examples are the pubic symphysis where the pubic bones of the pelvis have grown together and the symphysis of the two halves of the lower jaw bone (mandible) that unite before birth.

Appendix O: Transurethral

A **transurethral** resection of the prostate gland (TURP) is a removal of a portion of the prostate gland by means of an instrument that is passed through **(trans-)** the urethra. The procedure is necessary when the prostatic tissue enlarges (hypertrophies) and interferes with urination. Figure 4–5 shows the location of the prostate gland at the base of the urinary bladder.

Appendix P: Ultrasonography

Ultrasonography is a diagnostic technique using ultrasound waves (inaudible sound waves) to produce an image or photograph of an organ or tissue. The ultrasonic echoes are recorded as they pass through different types of tissue. **Echocardiograms** are ultrasound images of the heart. Figure 4–6 shows an ultrasound image **(sonogram)** of a fetus.

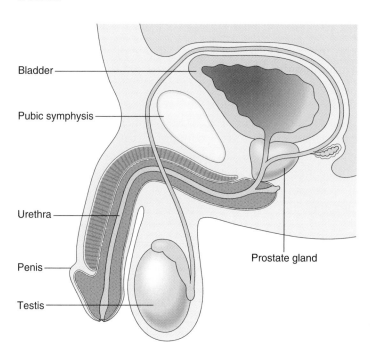

Figure 4–5

Location of the prostate gland.

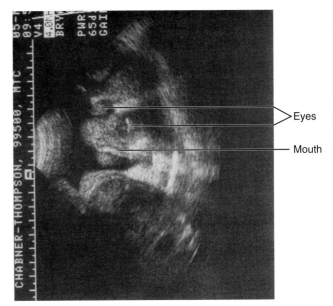

Eyes

Mouth

Figure 4-6

Ultrasonography. Notice the facial features of this beautiful 30-week-old fetus (my granddaughter, Beatrix Bess Thompson)! (Courtesy of Dr. Elizabeth Chabner Thompson.)

V. Practical Applications

Check your answers with the Answers to Practical Applications on page 125.

Procedures

Match the **procedure** or **treatment** in COLUMN I with the best **reason for using it** in COLUMN II:

Column I

1. Ultrasonography _____
2. Hemiglossectomy _____
3. Percutaneous liver biopsy _____
4. Transfusion of blood cells _____
5. Gastric endoscopy _____
6. Autopsy _____
7. Endotracheal intubation _____
8. Dialysis _____
9. Antibiotics _____
10. Transurethral resection of a gland below the bladder in a male _____

Column II

A. Diagnosis hepatopathy
B. Treat renal failure
C. Obtain prenatal images
D. Determine the post mortem status of organs
E. Treat carcinoma of the tongue
F. Treat benign prostatic hyperplasia
G. Diagnose disease in the stomach
H. Establish an airway during surgery
I. Treat pancytopenia
J. Treat staphylococcemia

VI. Exercises

Remember to check your answers carefully with those given in Section VII, Answers to Exercises.

A. Give the meanings of the following prefixes.

1. ante- _____
2. ab- _____
3. ana- _____
4. anti- _____
5. a-, an- _____
6. ad- _____

7. auto- _____
8. cata- _____
9. brady- _____
10. contra- _____
11. bi- _____
12. con- _____

B. Match the following terms with their meanings below.

bilateral
congenital anomaly
contralateral
ante partum

adductor
antisepsis
analysis
anteflexion

bradycardia
apnea
anoxia
adrenal

1. bending forward _____
2. a muscle that carries the limb toward the body _____
3. before birth _____
4. slow heartbeat _____
5. a gland located near (above) each kidney _____
6. not breathing _____
7. pertaining to the opposite side _____
8. against infection _____
9. to separate apart _____
10. pertaining to two (both) sides _____
11. condition of no oxygen in tissues _____
12. an irregularity that is present at birth _____

C. Select from the following terms to complete the sentences below.

autoimmune   antibody   catabolism
antitoxin   antibiotic   contraindication
antigen   anabolism

1. A chemical substance, such as erythromycin (-mycin = mold), that is made from molds and used

   against bacterial life is a (an) _____ .

2. The process of burning food (breaking it down) and releasing the energy stored in the food is

   _____ .

3. A reason that a doctor would advise against taking a specific medication would be a (an)

   _____ .

4. A disorder in which the body's own leukocytes make antibodies that damage its own good tissue is

   a (an) _____ disorder.

5. A foreign agent (virus or bacterium) is known as a (an) _____
   because it causes the production of antibodies by white blood cells.

6. A protein made by lymphocytes in response to the presence in the blood of a specific antigen is a

   (an) _____ .

7. A type of antibody that acts against poisons that enter the body is a (an) _____ .

8. The process of building up proteins in cells by putting together small pieces of proteins, called

   amino acids, is called _____ .

D. Give the meanings of the following prefixes.

1. ec- _____   9. en- _____

2. dys- _____   10. eu- _____

3. de- _____   11. in- _____

4. dia- _____   12. inter- _____

5. hemi- _____   13. intra- _____

6. hypo- _____   14. infra- _____

7. epi- _____   15. macro- _____

8. hyper- _____

E. Complete the following terms based on their meanings as given below.

1. normal thyroid function: _____ thyroid

2. painful breathing: _____ pnea

3. pregnancy that is out of place (outside the uterus): _____ topic

4. instrument to visually examine within the body: endo _____

5. removal of half of the tongue: _____ glossectomy

6. good (exaggerated) feeling (of well-being): _____ phoria

7. pertaining to within the windpipe: endo _____

8. a blood condition of less than normal sugar: _____ glycemia

9. pertaining to (having) a large head: _____ cephalic

10. pertaining to between the ribs: _____ costal

11. pertaining to within a vein: intra _____

12. condition of bad (abnormal) formation (of cells): dys _____

13. condition of excessive formation (numbers of cells): _____ plasia

14. the structure (membrane) that forms the inner lining of the heart: endo _____

15. pertaining to below the ribs: infra _____

16. a blood condition of excessive amount of sugar: hyper _____

F. Match the following terms with their meanings below.

dialysis	incision	metastasis
dehydration	malignant	pancytopenia
diarrhea	metamorphosis	microscope
insomnia	malaise	exophthalmos

1. a vague feeling of bodily discomfort _____

2. not able to sleep _____

3. lack of water _____

4. spread of a cancerous tumor to a secondary organ or tissue _____

5. instrument used to see small objects _____

6. to cut into an organ or tissue _____

7. eyeballs that bulge outward (proptosis) _____

8. condition of change in shape or form _____

9. watery discharge (of wastes from the colon) _____

10. deficiency of all (blood) cells _____

11. separation of wastes from the blood by using a machine that does the job of the kidney

_____

12. harmful, cancerous _____

G. *Give the meanings of the following prefixes.*

1. mal- _____   11. sub- _____

2. pan- _____   12. supra- _____

3. per- _____   13. re- _____

4. meta- _____   14. retro- _____

5. para- _____   15. tachy- _____

6. peri- _____   16. syn- _____

7. poly- _____   17. uni- _____

8. post- _____   18. trans- _____

9. pro- _____   19. neo- _____

10. pre- _____   20. epi- _____

H. *Underline the prefix in the following terms and give the meaning of the entire term.*

1. periosteum _____

2. percutaneous _____

3. retroperitoneal _____

4. postnatal _____

5. polyneuritis _____

6. retroflexion _____

7. transurethral _____

8. subcutaneous _____

9. tachypnea _____

10. unilateral _____

11. pseudocyesis _____

I. Match the following terms with their meanings below.

syndrome	parathyroid	relapse	recombinant DNA
prodrome	suprarenal	prolapse	syndactyly
paralysis	remission	neoplasm	ultrasonography

1. the return of a disease or its symptoms _____

2. loss of movement in muscles _____

3. a congenital anomaly in which fingers or toes are webbed (formed together)

_____

4. four endocrine glands that are located near (behind) another endocrine gland in the neck

_____

5. glands that are located above the kidneys _____

6. symptoms that come before the actual illness _____

7. the technique of transferring genetic material from one organism into another _____

8. sliding, sagging downward or forward _____

9. new growth or tumor _____

10. process of using sound waves to create an image of organs and structures in the body

_____

11. group of symptoms that occur together and indicate a particular disorder

_____

12. symptoms lessen and a patient feels better _____

J. Complete the following terms based on their meanings as given below.

1. pertaining to new birth: neo _____

2. after death: post _____

3. spread of a cancerous tumor: meta _____

4. branching into two: bi _____

5. increase in development (size of cells): hyper _____

6. pertaining to a chemical that works against bacterial life: _____ biotic

7. hand bones (beyond the wrist): _____ carpals

8. protein produced by leukocytes to fight foreign organisms: anti _____

9. group of symptoms that occur together: _____ drome

10. surface or skin tissue of the body: _____ thelium

K. Select the correct term to complete each sentence.

1. Dr. Tate felt that Mrs. Snow's condition of thrombocytopenia was a clear **(analysis, contraindication, synthesis)** to performing elective surgery.

2. Medical science was revolutionized by the introduction of **(antigens, antibiotics, antibodies)** in the 1940s. Now we occasionally treat an infection with only one dose.

3. The elderly gentleman was having **(malaise, dialysis, insomnia)** despite taking the sleeping medication that his doctor prescribed.

4. During her pregnancy, Ms. Payne described pressure on her **(pituitary gland, parathyroid gland, pubic symphysis)**, making it difficult for her to find a comfortable position, even when seated.

5. Many times, people with diabetes accidentally take too much insulin. This results in the lowering of their blood sugar so much that they may be admitted to the emergency room (ER) with **(hyperplasia, hypoglycemia, hyperglycemia)**.

6. Before his migraine headaches would begin, John noticed changes in his eyesight, such as bright spots, zigzag lines, and double vision. His physician told him that these were **(symbiotic, exophthalmos, prodromal)** symptoms.

VII. Answers to Exercises

A

1. before, forward
2. away from
3. up, apart
4. against
5. no, not, without
6. toward
7. self, own
8. down
9. slow
10. against, opposite
11. two
12. together, with

B

1. anteflexion
2. adductor
3. ante partum
4. bradycardia
5. adrenal
6. apnea
7. contralateral
8. antisepsis
9. analysis
10. bilateral
11. anoxia
12. congenital anomaly

C

1. antibiotic
2. catabolism
3. contraindication
4. autoimmune
5. antigen
6. antibody
7. antitoxin
8. anabolism

D

1. out, outside
2. bad, painful, difficult
3. down, lack of
4. through, complete
5. half
6. deficient, under
7. upon, on, above
8. excessive, above, beyond
9. in, within
10. good, well
11. in, not
12. between
13. within
14. below, inferior
15. large

E

1. euthyroid
2. dyspnea
3. ectopic
4. endoscope
5. hemiglossectomy
6. euphoria
7. endotracheal
8. hypoglycemia
9. macrocephalic
10. intercostal
11. intravenous
12. dysplasia
13. hyperplasia
14. endocardium
15. infracostal
16. hyperglycemia

F

1. malaise
2. insomnia
3. dehydration
4. metastasis
5. microscope
6. incision
7. exophthalmos (proptosis)
8. metamorphosis
9. diarrhea
10. pancytopenia
11. dialysis
12. malignant

G

1. bad
2. all
3. through
4. change, beyond
5. near, beside, abnormal
6. surrounding
7. many, much
8. after, behind
9. before, forward
10. before, in front of
11. under
12. above
13. back, again
14. behind, backward
15. fast
16. together, with
17. one
18. across, through
19. new
20. above, upon, on

H

1. periosteum—membrane (structure) surrounding bone
2. percutaneous—pertaining to through the skin
3. retroperitoneal—pertaining to behind the peritoneum
4. postnatal—pertaining to after birth
5. polyneuritis—inflammation of many nerves
6. retroflexion—bending backward
7. transurethral—pertaining to through the urethra
8. subcutaneous—pertaining to below the skin
9. tachypnea—rapid, fast breathing
10. unilateral—pertaining to one side
11. pseudocyesis—false pregnancy (no pregnancy actually occurs)

I

1. relapse
2. paralysis
3. syndactyly
4. parathyroid
5. suprarenal (adrenal glands)
6. prodrome
7. recombinant DNA
8. prolapse
9. neoplasm
10. ultrasonography
11. syndrome
12. remission

J

1. neonatal
2. post mortem
3. metastasis
4. bifurcation
5. hypertrophy
6. antibiotic
7. metacarpals
8. antibody
9. syndrome
10. epithelium

K

1. contraindication
2. antibiotics
3. insomnia
4. pubic symphysis
5. hypoglycemia
6. prodromal

Answers to Practical Applications

1. **C** Ultrasonography is especially useful to detect fetal structures because no x-rays are used.
2. **E** Malignancies of the oral (mouth) cavity are often treated with surgery to remove the cancerous growth.
3. **A** Diseases such as hepatitis or hepatoma are diagnosed by performing a liver biopsy.
4. **I** Transfusion of leukocytes, erythrocytes, and platelets will increase numbers of these cells in the bloodstream.
5. **G** Placement of an endoscope through the mouth and esophagus and into the stomach is used to diagnose gastric (stomach) disease.
6. **D** A veterinarian performs a post mortem examination of an animal, which is called a necropsy.
7. **H** Endotracheal intubation is necessary during surgery in which general anesthesia is used.
8. **B** Patients experiencing loss of kidney function need dialysis to remove waste materials from the blood.
9. **J** Examples of antibiotics are penicillin, erythromycin, and amoxicillin.
10. **F** A TURP is a transurethral resection of the prostate gland.

VIII. Pronunciation of Terms

Pronunciation Guide

To test your understanding of the terminology in this chapter, write the meaning of each term in the space provided. In addition, you may wish to cover the terms and write them by looking at your definitions. Make sure your spelling is correct. The page number after each term indicates where it is defined or used in the text so you can easily check your responses.

ā as in āpe   ă as in ăpple
ē as in ēven   ě as in ěvery
ī as in īce   ĭ as in ĭnterest
ō as in ōpen   ŏ as in pŏt
ū as in ūnit   ŭ as in ŭnder

Term	Pronunciation	Meaning
abductor (107)	ăb-DŬK-tŏr	_____
adductor (107)	ă-DŬK-tŏr	_____
adrenal glands (107)	ă-DRĒ-năl glăndz	_____

analysis (107)	ă-NĂL-ĭ-sĭs	_____
anoxia (107)	ă-NŎK-sē-ă	_____
ante cibum (107)	ăn-tē se-bum	_____
anteflexion (107)	ăn-tē-FLĔK-shŭn	_____
ante partum (107)	ĂN-tē PĂR-tŭm	_____
antibiotic (108)	ăn-tĭ-bī-ŎT-ĭk	_____
antibody (108)	ĂN-tĭ-bŏd-ē	_____
antigen (108)	ĂN-tĭ-jĕn	_____
antisepsis (108)	ăn-tĭ-SĔP-sĭs	_____
antitoxin (108)	ăn-tĭ-TŎK-sĭn	_____
apnea (107)	ĂP-nē-ă or ăp-NĒ-ă	_____
autoimmune (108)	ăw-tō-ĭ-MŪN	_____
benign (109)	bē-NĪN	_____
bifurcation (108)	bī-fŭr-KĀ-shŭn	_____
bilateral (108)	bī-LĂT-ĕr-ăl	_____
bradycardia (108)	brăd-ē-KĂR-dē-ă	_____
congenital anomaly (108)	kŏn-JĔN-ĭ-tăl ă-NŎM-ă-lē	_____
contraindication (108)	kŏn-tră-ĭn-dĭ-KĀ-shŭn	_____
contralateral (108)	kŏn-tră-LĂT-ĕr-ăl	_____
dehydration (108)	dē-hī-DRĀ-shŭn	_____
dialysis (108)	dī-ĂL-ĭ-sĭs	_____
diarrhea (108)	dī-ă-RĒ-ă	_____
dysplasia (108)	dĭs-PLĀ-zē-ă	_____
dyspnea (108)	DĬSP-nē-ă or dĭsp-NĒ-ă	_____
ectopic pregnancy (108)	ĕk-TŎP-ĭk PRĔG-năn-sē	_____
endocardium (109)	ĕn-dō-KĂR-dē-ŭm	_____
endoscope (109)	ĔN-dō-skōp	_____
endotracheal (109)	ĕn-dō-TRĀ-kē-ăl	_____

epithelium (109)   ĕp-ĭ-THĒ-lē-ŭm   _____

euphoria (109)   ū-FŎR-ē-ă   _____

euthyroid (109)   ū-THĪ-royd   _____

exophthalmos (109)   ĕk-sŏf-THĂL-mŏs   _____

hemiglossectomy (109)   hĕm-ē-glŏs-SĔK-tō-mē   _____

hyperglycemia (109)   hī-pĕr-glī-SĒ-mē-ă   _____

hyperplasia (109)   hī-pĕr-PLĀ-zē-ă   _____

hypertrophy (109)   hī-PĔR-trō-fē   _____

hypodermic (109)   hī-pō-DĔR-mĭk   _____

hypoglycemia (109)   hī-pō-glī-SĒ-mē-ă   _____

infracostal (109)   ĭn-fră-KŎS-tăl   _____

insomniac (109)   ĭn-SŎM-nē-ăk   _____

intercostal (109)   ĭn-tĕr-KŎS-tăl   _____

intravenous (109)   ĭn-tră-VĒ-nŭs   _____

macrocephalic (109)   măk-rŏ-sĕ-FĂL-ĭk   _____

malaise (109)   măl-ĀZ   _____

malignant (109)   mă-LĬG-nănt   _____

metacarpal bones (110)   mĕ-tă-KĂR-păl bōnz   _____

metamorphosis (110)   mĕt-ă-MŎR-fŏ-sĭs   _____

metastasis (110)   mĕ-TĂS-tă-sĭs   _____

microscope (110)   MĪ-krō-skōp   _____

neonatal (110)   nē-ō-NĀ-tăl   _____

neoplasm (110)   NĒ-ō-plăzm   _____

pancytopenia (110)   păn-sī-tō-PĒ-nē-ă   _____

paralysis (110)   pă-RĂL-ĭ-sĭs   _____

parathyroid (110)   păr-ă-THĪ-royd   _____

percutaneous (110)   pĕr-kū-TĀ-nē-ŭs   _____

periosteum (110)   pĕr-ē-ŎS-tē-ŭm   _____

polymorphonuclear (110)	pŏl-ĕ-mŏr-fō-NŪ-klē-ăr	
polyneuritis (110)	pŏl-ē-nū-RĪ-tĭs	
post mortem (110)	pōst MŎR-tĕm	
postnatal (110)	pōst-NĀ-tăl	
precancerous (110)	prē-KĂN-sĕr-ŭs	
prodrome (110)	PRŌ-drōm	
prolapse (110)	PRŌ-lăps	
pseudocyesis (111)	sū-dō-sī-Ē-sĭs	
recombinant DNA (111)	rē-KŎM-bĭ-nănt DNA	
relapse (111)	RĒ-lăps	
remission (111)	rē-MĬ-shŭn	
retroflexion (111)	rĕt-rō-FLĔK-shŭn	
retroperitoneal (111)	rĕt-rō-pĕr-ĭ-tō-NĒ-ăl	
subcutaneous (111)	sŭb-kū-TĀ-nē-ŭs	
suprarenal (111)	soo-pră-RĒ-năl	
suprathoracic (111)	soo-pră-thō-RĂ-sĭk	
symbiosis (111)	sĭm-bē-Ō-sĭs	
symmetry (111)	SĬM-mĕ-trē	
symphysis (111)	SĬM-fĭ-sĭs	
syndactyly (111)	sĭn-DĂK-tĭ-lē	
syndrome (111)	SĬN-drōm	
synthesis (111)	SĬN-thĕ-sĭs	
tachypnea (111)	tă-KĬP-nē-ă or tăk-ĭp-NĒ-ă	
transfusion (111)	trăns-FŪ-zhŭn	
transurethral (111)	trăns-ū-RĒ-thrăl	
ultrasonography (111)	ŭl-tră-sŏn-ŎG-ră-fē	
unilateral (111)	ū-nē-LĂT-ĕr-ăl	

IX. Review Sheet

Write out the meanings of each word part in the space provided and test yourself. Check your answers with the information in the chapter or in the Glossary (Medical Terms—English) at the end of the book.

PREFIXES

Prefix	Meaning	Prefix	Meaning
a-, an-	_____	ex-	_____
ab-	_____	hemi-	_____
ad-	_____	hyper-	_____
ana-	_____	hypo-	_____
ante-	_____	in-	_____
anti-	_____	infra-	_____
auto-	_____	inter-	_____
bi-	_____	intra-	_____
brady-	_____	macro-	_____
cata-	_____	mal-	_____
con-	_____	meta-	_____
contra-	_____	micro-	_____
de-	_____	neo-	_____
dia-	_____	pan-	_____
dys-	_____	para-	_____
ec-, ecto-	_____	per-	_____
en-, endo-	_____	peri-	_____
epi-	_____	poly-	_____
eu-	_____	post-	_____

Continued on following page

pre-	_____	supra-	_____
pro-	_____	syn-, sym-	_____
pseudo-	_____	tachy-	_____
re-	_____	trans-	_____
retro-	_____	ultra-	_____
sub-	_____	uni-	_____

COMBINING FORMS

Combining Form	Meaning	Combining Form	Meaning
carp/o	_____	nect/o	_____
cib/o	_____	norm/o	_____
cost/o	_____	ophthalm/o	_____
cutane/o	_____	ox/o	_____
dactyl/o	_____	ren/o	_____
duct/o	_____	seps/o	_____
flex/o	_____	somn/o	_____
furc/o	_____	son/o	_____
gloss/o	_____	the/o	_____
glyc/o	_____	thyr/o	_____
immun/o	_____	top/o	_____
later/o	_____	tox/o	_____
morph/o	_____	trache/o	_____
mort/o	_____	urethr/o	_____
nat/i	_____	ven/o	_____
necr/o	_____		

SUFFIXES

Combining Form	Meaning	Combining Form	Meaning
-blast		-phoria	
-crine		-physis	
-cyesis		-plasia	
-drome		-plasm	
-gen		-pnea	
-lapse		-ptosis	
-lysis		-rrhea	
-mission		-stasis	
-partum		-trophy	

PREFIXES WITH SIMILAR MEANINGS

Prefix	Meaning
a- (an-), in-	
ante-, pre-, pro-	
anti-, contra-	
con-, syn- (sym-)	
de-, cata-	
dia-, per-, trans-	
dys-, mal-	
ec- (ecto-), ex-	
en- (endo-), in-, intra-	
epi-, hyper-, supra-	
hypo-, infra-, sub-	
re-, retro-, post-	
ultra-, meta-	

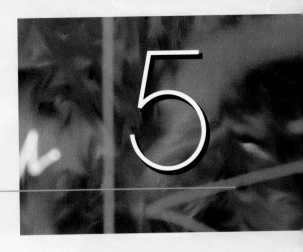

CHAPTER 5

Digestive System

This chapter is divided into the following sections

In this chapter you will

- Name the organs of the digestive system and describe their locations and functions;
- Describe disease processes and symptoms that affect these organs; and
- Define combining forms for organs and the meaning of related terminology using these word parts.

I. Introduction

The digestive system, also called the **alimentary canal** or **gastrointestinal tract,** begins with the mouth, where food enters the body, and ends with the anus, where solid waste material leaves the body. The primary functions of the organs of the digestive system are threefold.

First, complex food material taken into the mouth must be **digested,** or broken down, mechanically and chemically, as it travels through the gastrointestinal tract (passageway). Digestive **enzymes** speed up chemical reactions and help in the breakdown (digestion) of complex nutrients. Complex proteins are digested to simpler **amino acids;** complicated sugars are reduced to simple sugars, such as **glucose;** and large fat molecules **(triglycerides)** are broken down to **fatty acids** and glycerol.

133

Second, the digested food must be **absorbed** into the bloodstream by passing through the walls of the small intestine. In this way, valuable nutrients, such as sugar and amino acids, can travel to all the cells of the body. Cells then catabolize (burn) nutrients in the presence of oxygen to release energy stored within the food. Cells also use amino acid nutrients to anabolize (build) large protein molecules needed for growth and development. Although the walls of the small intestine also absorb fatty acids and glycerol, these nutrients enter lymphatic vessels rather than blood vessels. Digested fats eventually enter the bloodstream as lymph vessels join with blood vessels in the upper chest region.

The third function of the digestive system is the **elimination** of the solid waste materials that cannot be absorbed into the bloodstream. The large intestine concentrates these solid wastes, called **feces,** and the wastes finally pass out of the body through the anus.

II. Anatomy and Physiology

Oral Cavity

The alimentary canal begins with the oral cavity, or mouth. Label Figure 5–1 as you learn the major parts of the oral cavity.

The **cheeks** [1] form the walls of the oval-shaped oral cavity, and the **lips** [2] surround the opening to the cavity.

The **hard palate** [3] forms the anterior portion of the roof of the mouth, and the muscular **soft palate** [4] lies posterior to it. **Rugae** are irregular ridges in the mucous membrane covering the anterior portion of the hard palate. Hanging from the soft palate is a small, soft tissue called the **uvula** [5]. The word uvula means little grape. The structure functions to aid in producing sounds and speech.

The **tongue** [6] extends across the floor of the oral cavity, and muscles attach it to the lower jaw bone. It moves food around during **mastication** (chewing) and **deglutition** (swallowing). **Papillae,** small raised areas on the tongue, contain taste buds that are sensitive to the chemical nature of foods and allow discrimination of different tastes as food moves across the tongue.

The **tonsils** [7] are masses of lymphatic tissue located in depressions of the mucous membranes on both sides if the oropharynx (part of the throat near the mouth). They act as filters to protect the body from the invasion of microorganisms and produce lymphocytes, which are white blood cells able to fight disease.

The **gums** [8] are made of fleshy tissue and surround the sockets of the **teeth** [9]. Figure 5–2 shows a dental arch with 16 permanent teeth (there are 32 permanent teeth in the entire oral cavity). Label the figure with the following names of teeth:

Central incisor [1]	Second premolar [5]
Lateral incisor [2]	First molar [6]
Canine [3]	Second molar [7]
First premolar [4]	Third molar (wisdom tooth) [8]

Dentists use special terms to describe the surfaces of teeth (Fig. 5–2). The **labial** surface (labi/o means lip), for incisor and canine teeth, is nearest the lips. The **buccal** surface (bucc/o means cheek), for premolar and molar teeth, is adjacent to the cheek.

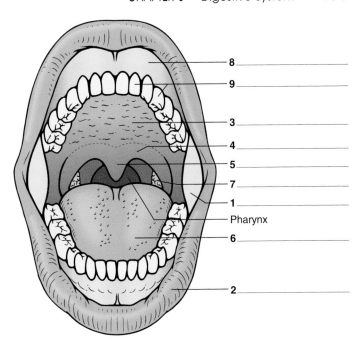

Figure 5–1

Oral cavity.

These are indicated on the left side of Figure 5–2. Some dentists refer to both the labial and the buccal surfaces as the **facial** surface (faci/o means face). Opposite to the facial surface, all teeth have a **lingual** surface (lingu/o means tongue). The **mesial** surface of a tooth lies nearest to the median line and the **distal** surface, farthest from the medial line. Premolars and molars have an additional **occlusal** surface (occlusion means to close) that comes in contact with a corresponding tooth in the opposing arch. The incisors and cuspids have a sharp **incisal** edge.

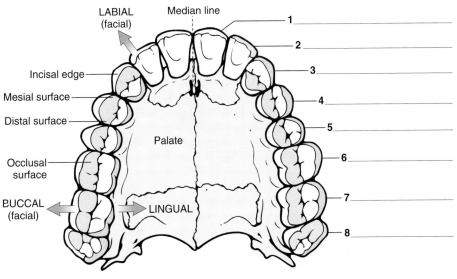

Figure 5–2

Upper permanent teeth within the dental arch.

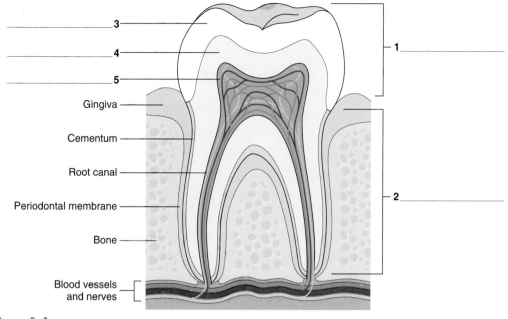

3

4

5

Gingiva

Cementum

Root canal

Periodontal membrane

Bone

Blood vessels
and nerves

1

2

Figure 5-3

Anatomy of a tooth.

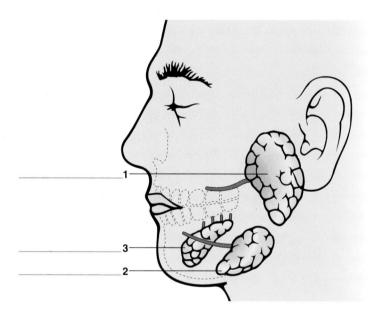

1

3

2

Figure 5-4

Salivary glands.

Figure 5–3 shows the inner anatomy of a tooth. Label it as you read the following description:

A tooth consists of a **crown** [1], which shows above the gumline and a **root** [2], which lies within the bony tooth socket. The outermost protective layer of the crown, the **enamel** [3], protects the tooth. Enamel is a dense, hard, white substance—the hardest substance in the body. **Dentin** [4], the main substance of the tooth, lies beneath the enamel and extends throughout the crown. Yellow in color, dentin is composed of bony tissue that is softer than enamel. The **cementum** covers, protects, and supports the dentin in the root. A **periodontal membrane** surrounds the cementum and holds the tooth in place in the tooth socket.

The **pulp** [5] lies underneath the dentin. It is soft and delicate tissue and fills the center of the tooth. Blood vessels, nerve endings, connective tissue, and lymphatic vessels are within the pulp canal (also called the **root canal**). Root canal therapy is often necessary when disease or abscess (pus collection) occurs in the pulp canal. A dentist opens the tooth from above and cleans the canal of infection, nerves, and blood vessels. The canal is then disinfected and filled with material to prevent the entrance of microorganisms and decay.

Three pairs of **salivary glands** (Fig. 5–4) surround the oral cavity. These exocrine glands produce a fluid called **saliva** that contains important digestive **enzymes.** Saliva is released from the **parotid gland** [1], **submandibular gland** [2], and **sublingual gland** [3] on each side of the mouth. Narrow ducts carry the saliva into the oral cavity.

Pharynx

Refer to Figure 5–5. The **pharynx** or **throat** is a muscular tube, about 5 inches long, lined with a mucous membrane. It serves as a common passageway for air traveling from the nose (nasal cavity) to the windpipe (trachea) and food traveling from the oral cavity to the **esophagus.** When swallowing **(deglutition)** occurs, a flap of tissue, the epiglottis, covers the trachea so that food cannot enter and become lodged there. See Figure 5–5 (A and B).

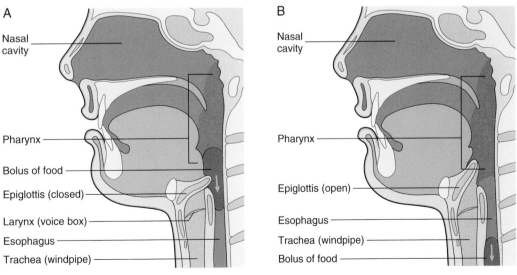

Figure 5–5

Deglutition (swallowing). **(A)** Epiglottis closes over the trachea as the bolus of food passes down the pharynx toward the esophagus. **(B)** Epiglottis opens as the bolus moves down the esophagus.

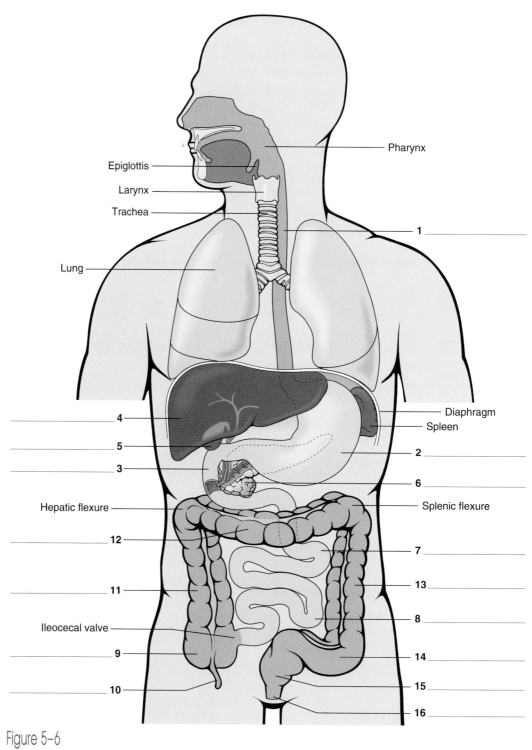

Epiglottis

Larynx

Trachea

Lung

Pharynx

1

Diaphragm

Spleen

4

5

3

2

6

Hepatic flexure

Splenic flexure

12

7

11

13

Ileocecal valve

8

9

14

10

15

16

Figure 5-6

The gastrointestinal tract.

Figure 5–6 traces the passage of food from the esophagus through the gastrointestinal tract. Label it as you read the following paragraphs.

Esophagus

The **esophagus** [1], meaning swallowing (phag/o) inward (eso-), is a 9- to 10-inch muscular tube extending from the pharynx to the stomach. Rhythmic contractions of muscles in the wall of the esophagus propel food toward the stomach. **Peristalsis,** meaning constriction (-stalsis) surrounding (peri-), is this involuntary, progressive, rhythm-like contraction of the esophagus and the other gastrointestinal tubes. The process is like squeezing a marble (the **bolus,** or semisolid mass of food) through a rubber tube.

Stomach

Food passes from the esophagus into the **stomach** [2]. The stomach is composed of an upper portion called the **fundus,** a middle section known as the **body,** and a lower portion, the **antrum** (Fig. 5–7). Rings of muscles called **sphincters** control the openings into and leading out of the stomach. The **lower esophageal sphincter (cardiac sphincter)** relaxes and contracts to move food from the esophagus into the stomach, whereas the **pyloric sphincter** allows food to leave the stomach when it is ready. Folds in the mucous membrane **(mucosa)** lining the stomach are called **rugae.** The rugae contain digestive glands that produce the enzyme **pepsin** (to begin digestion of proteins) and **hydrochloric acid.**

The role of the stomach is to prepare the food chemically and mechanically so that it can be received in the small intestine for digestion and absorption into the bloodstream. Food does not enter the bloodstream through the walls of the stomach. The stomach controls the passing of foods into the first part of the small intestine so that it proceeds only when it is chemically ready and in small amounts. Food leaves the stomach in 1–4 hours or longer, depending upon the amount and type of food eaten.

Figure 5-7

Parts of the stomach. The fundus and **body** (often referred to collectively as the fundus) are a reservoir for ingested food and an area for action by acid and pepsin (gastric enzyme). The **antrum** is a muscular grinding chamber that pulverizes food and feeds it gradually into the duodenum.

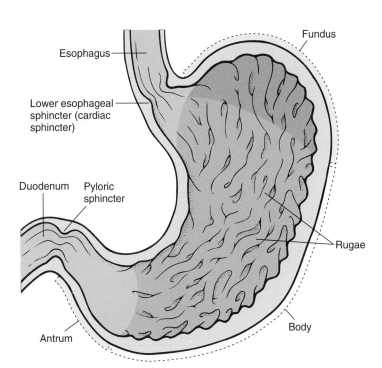

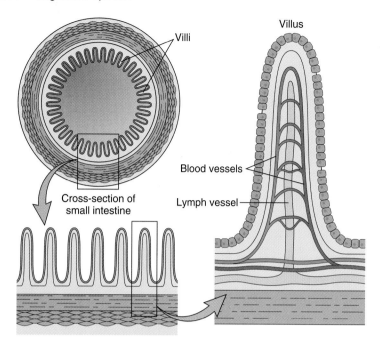

Villi

Villus

Blood vessels

Lymph vessel

Cross-section of
small intestine

Figure 5-8

**Villi in the lining of the small
intestine.**

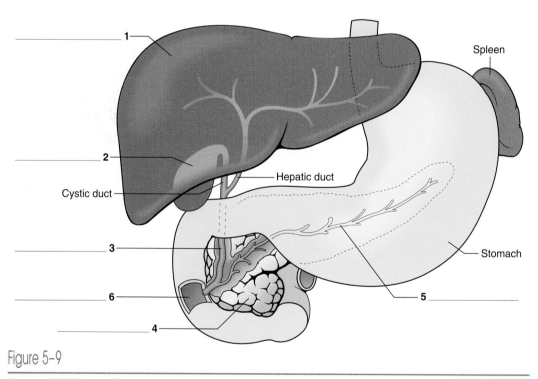

1

Spleen

2

Hepatic duct

Cystic duct

Stomach

3

6

5

4

Figure 5-9

Liver, gallbladder, and pancreas.

Small Intestine (Small Bowel)

(Continue labeling Fig. 5–6 on page 138.)

The **small intestine (small bowel)** extends for 20 feet from the pyloric sphincter to the first part of the large intestine. It has three parts. The first section is the **duodenum** [3], only 1 foot in length, which receives food from the stomach as well as **bile** from the **liver** [4] and **gallbladder** [5] and pancreatic juice from the **pancreas** [6]. Enzymes and bile help to digest food before it passes into the second part of the small intestine, the **jejunum** [7], about 8 feet long. The jejunum connects with the third section, the **ileum** [8], about 11 feet long. The ileum attaches to the first part of the large intestine.

Millions of tiny, microscopic projections called **villi** line the walls of the small intestine. The tiny capillaries (microscopic blood vessels) in the villi absorb the digested nutrients into the bloodstream and lymph vessels. Figure 5–8 shows several different views of villi in the lining of the small intestine.

Large Intestine (Large Bowel)

(Continue labeling Fig. 5–6.)

The large intestine extends from the end of the ileum to the anus. It is divided into six parts: cecum, ascending colon, transverse colon, descending colon, sigmoid colon, and rectum. The **cecum** [9] is a pouch on the right side that connects to the ileum at the ileocecal valve (sphincter). The **appendix** [10] hangs from the cecum. The appendix has no clear function and can become inflamed and infected when it is clogged or blocked. The **colon** (large intestine), about 5 feet long, has three divisions. The **ascending colon** [11] extends from the cecum to the undersurface of the liver, where it turns to the left (hepatic flexure or bend) to become the **transverse colon** [12]. The transverse colon passes horizontally to the left toward the spleen, and turns downward (splenic flexure) into the **descending colon** [13]. The **sigmoid colon** [14], shaped like an S (resembling the Greek letter sigma, which curves like an S), lies at the distal end of the descending colon and leads into the **rectum** [15]. The rectum terminates in the lower opening of the gastrointestinal tract, the **anus** [16].

The large intestine receives the fluid waste products of digestion (the material unable to pass into the bloodstream) and stores these wastes until they can be released from the body. Because the large intestine absorbs most of the water within the waste material, the body can expel solid **feces** (stools). Defecation is the expulsion or passage of feces from the body through the anus. Diarrhea, watery stools, can result from lack of absorption of the water through the walls of the large intestine.

Liver, Gallbladder, and Pancreas

Three important additional organs of the digestive system—the liver, gallbladder, and pancreas—play crucial roles in the proper digestion and absorption of nutrients. Label Figure 5–9 as you study the following:

The **liver** [1], located in the right upper quadrant (RUQ) of the abdomen, manufactures a thick, yellowish-brown, sometimes greenish, fluid called **bile.** Bile contains cholesterol (a fatty substance), bile acids, and several bile pigments. One of these pigments, **bilirubin,** is produced from the breakdown of hemoglobin during normal red blood cell destruction. Bilirubin then travels via the bloodstream to the liver where it is conjugated (combined) with another substance so that it can be added to bile. Thus, conjugated bilirubin enters the intestine with bile. In the colon, bilirubin is degraded by bacteria into a variety of pigments that give feces a brownish color. Bilirubin and bile leave the body in feces.

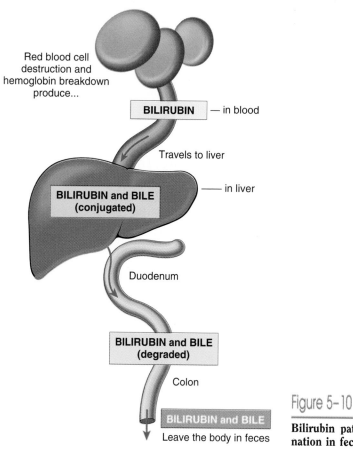

Red blood cell destruction and hemoglobin breakdown produce...

BILIRUBIN — in blood

Travels to liver

BILIRUBIN and BILE (conjugated) — in liver

Duodenum

BILIRUBIN and BILE (degraded)

Colon

BILIRUBIN and BILE

Leave the body in feces

Figure 5-10

Bilirubin pathway from bloodstream to elimination in feces.

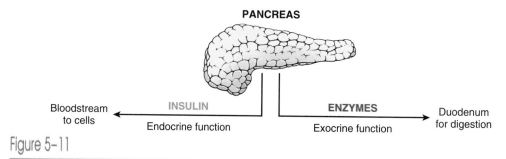

PANCREAS

Bloodstream to cells ← **INSULIN** Endocrine function | **ENZYMES** Exocrine function → Duodenum for digestion

Figure 5-11

The pancreas and its functions.

If bilirubin cannot leave the body, it remains in the bloodstream, causing **jaundice (hyperbilirubinemia),** which is yellow discoloration of the skin, whites of the eyes, and mucous membranes. Figure 5–10 reviews the path of bilirubin from red blood cell destruction (hemolysis) to elimination with bile in the feces.

(Continue labeling Figure 5–9.)

The liver continuously releases bile, which then travels through the **hepatic duct** to the **cystic duct.** The cystic duct leads to the **gallbladder** [2], a pear-shaped sac under the liver, which stores and concentrates the bile for later use. After meals, in response to the presence of food in the stomach and duodenum, the gallbladder contracts, forcing the bile out the cystic duct into the **common bile duct** [3]. Meanwhile, the **pancreas** [4] secretes pancreatic juices (enzymes) that travel via the **pancreatic duct** [5] to join with the common bile duct just as it enters the **duodenum** [6]. The duodenum thus receives a mixture of bile and pancreatic juices.

Bile has a detergent-like effect on fats in the duodenum. It breaks apart large fat globules, creating more surface area so that enzymes from the pancreas can digest the fats. This is called **emulsification.** Without bile, most of the fat taken into the body would remain undigested.

The liver, besides producing bile, has several other vital and important functions. Some of these are:

1. Keeping the amount of **glucose** (sugar) in the blood at a normal level. The liver removes excess glucose from the bloodstream and stores it as **glycogen** (starch) in liver cells. When the blood sugar level becomes dangerously low the liver can convert stored glycogen back into glucose via a process called glycogenolysis. In addition, the liver can also convert proteins and fats into glucose, when the body needs sugar, by a process called gluconeogenesis.
2. Manufacture of some blood proteins, particularly those necessary for blood clotting.
3. Release of bilirubin, a pigment in bile.
4. Removal of poisons (detoxification) from the blood.

The **portal vein** brings blood to the liver from the intestines. Digested foods pass into the portal vein directly after being absorbed into the bloodstream from the small intestine, thus giving the liver the first chance to use the nutrients.

The **pancreas** (Fig. 5–11) is both an exocrine and an endocrine organ. As an exocrine gland, it produces enzymes to digest starch, such as **amylase** (amyl/o = starch, -ase = enzyme), to digest fat, such as **lipase** (lip/o = fat), and to digest proteins, such as **protease** (prote/o = protein). These pass into the duodenum through the pancreatic duct.

As an endocrine gland (secreting into the bloodstream), the pancreas secretes **insulin.** This hormone, needed to help release sugar from the blood, acts as a carrier to bring glucose into cells of the body to be used for energy.

Figure 5–12 is a flow chart that traces the pathway of food through the gastrointestinal tract.

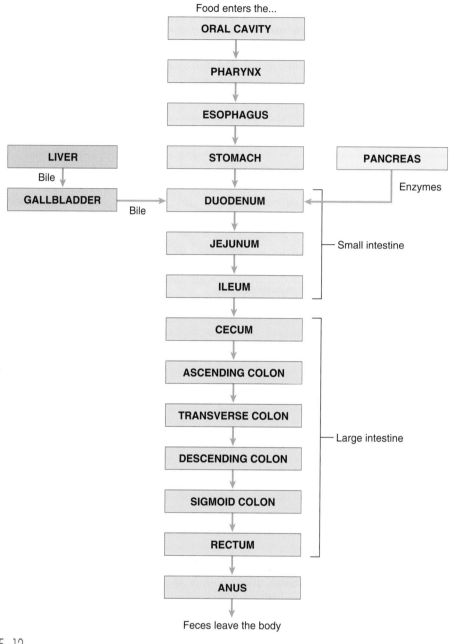

Figure 5-12

Pathway of food through the gastrointestinal tract.

III. Vocabulary

This list will help you review many of the new terms introduced in the text. Short definitions will reinforce your understanding of the terms. See Section VIII of this chapter for help in pronouncing the more difficult terms.

absorption	Passage of materials through the walls of the intestine into the bloodstream.
alimentary canal	The digestive tract (canal); aliment means food.
amino acids	Small substances that are the building blocks of proteins and are produced when proteins are digested.
amylase	Enzyme secreted by the pancreas to digest starch.
anus	Opening of the digestive tract to the outside of the body.
appendix	Blind pouch hanging from the first part of the colon (cecum). It literally means hanging (pend/o) on (ap-). Usually found in the RLQ.
bile	Digestive juice made in the liver and stored in the gallbladder. It physically breaks up (emulsifies) large fat globules. Bile was originally called gall (Latin *bilis* meaning gall or anger), probably because it has a bitter taste. It is composed of bile pigments, cholesterol, and bile salts.
bilirubin	Pigment released by the liver in bile; produced from the destruction of hemoglobin, a blood protein (-globin). In the intestine, bilirubin is degraded by bacteria to a variety of pigments that give stool (feces) its brown color.
bowel	Intestine.
canine teeth	Pointed, dog-like (canine) teeth, next to (distal to) the incisors. Also called cuspids or eyeteeth.
cecum	First part of the large intestine.
colon	Large intestine; cecum, ascending, transverse, and descending colon, and rectum.
common bile duct	Carries bile from the liver and gallbladder to the duodenum.
defecation	Expulsion or passage of feces from the body through the anus.
deglutition	Swallowing.
dentin	Major tissue composing teeth, covered by the enamel in the crown and a protective layer of cementum in the root.

digestion	Breakdown of complex foods to simpler forms.
duodenum	First part of the small intestine. Duo = 2, den = 10; the duodenum measures 12 inches in length.
emulsification	Physical process of breaking up large fat globules into smaller globules, thus increasing the surface area that enzymes can use to digest the fat.
enamel	Hard, outermost layer of a tooth.
enzyme	A chemical that speeds up a reaction between substances. Digestive enzymes help in the breakdown of complex foods to simpler foods.
esophagus	Tube connecting the throat to the stomach.
fatty acids	Substances produced when fats are digested.
feces	Solid wastes; stools.
gallbladder	Small sac under the liver; stores bile.
glucose	Simple sugar.
glycogen	Starch; glucose is stored in the form of glycogen in liver cells.
hydrochloric acid	Substance produced by the stomach; necessary for digestion of food.
ileum	Third part of the small intestine; from the Greek *eilos,* meaning twisted. When the abdomen was viewed at necropsy (autopsy), the intestine appeared twisted and the ileum was often an area of obstruction.
incisor	One of four front teeth in the dental arch.
insulin	Hormone produced by the endocrine cells of the pancreas. It transports sugar into cells from the blood and stimulates glycogen formation by the liver.
jejunum	Second part of the small intestine. The Latin *jejunus* means empty; this part of the intestine was always empty when a body was examined after death.
lipase	Pancreatic enzyme necessary to digest fats.
liver	A large organ located in the RUQ of the abdomen. The liver secretes bile; stores sugar, iron, and vitamins; produces blood proteins; and destroys worn-out red blood cells. The normal adult liver weighs about 2½–3 pounds.
lower esophageal sphincter	Ring of muscles between the esophagus and the stomach. Also called **cardiac sphincter.**

mastication

Chewing.

palate

Roof of the mouth. The hard palate is anterior to the soft palate.

pancreas

Organ under the stomach; produces insulin (for transport of sugar into cells) and enzymes (for digestion of foods).

papillae (singular: **papilla**)

Small elevations on the tongue. A papilla is any nipple-like elevation.

parotid gland

Salivary gland within the cheek, just anterior to the ear.

peristalsis

Rhythm-like contractions of the tubes of the gastrointestinal (GI) tract and other tubular structures. Peristalsis moves the contents through the GI tract at different rates; stomach (0.5 to 2 hours), small intestine (2–6 hours), and colon (6–72 hours).

pharynx

Throat, the common passageway for food from the mouth and air from the nose.

portal vein

Large vein bringing blood to the liver from the intestines.

proteases

Enzymes that digest protein.

pulp

Soft tissue within a tooth, containing nerves and blood vessels.

pyloric sphincter

Ring of muscle at the distal region of the stomach, where it joins the duodenum. From Greek *pyloros,* meaning gatekeeper.

rectum

Last section of the colon.

rugae

Ridges on the hard palate and the wall of the stomach.

saliva

Digestive juice produced by salivary glands.

salivary glands

Parotid, sublingual, and submandibular glands.

sigmoid colon

Lower part of the colon; shaped like an S.

sphincter

Ring of muscles within a tube.

stomach

Muscular organ that receives food from the esophagus. It is divided into the fundus, body, and antrum (distal portion).

triglycerides

Large fat molecules composed of three molecules of fatty acids with one molecule of glycerol.

uvula

Soft tissue hanging from the soft palate into the mouth.

villi (singular: **villus**)

Microscopic projections in the walls of the small intestine that absorb nutrients into the bloodstream.

IV. Combining Forms, Suffixes, and Terminology

Check Section VIII of this chapter for help with pronunciation of terms. Write the meaning of the medical term in the space provided.

Parts of the Body Combining Form	Meaning	Terminology	Meaning
an/o	anus	perianal _____	
append/o	appendix	appendectomy _____	
appendic/o	appendix	appendicitis _____	
		See Figure 5–13.	
bucc/o	cheek	buccal mucosa _____	
		The mucosa is composed of epithelial cells.	
cec/o	cecum	cecal _____	
celi/o	belly, abdomen	celiac _____	

Abdomin/o and lapar/o also mean abdomen. When there is more than one combining form with the same meaning there is no rule indicating when one or the other is used. Your job is to recognize each in its proper context.

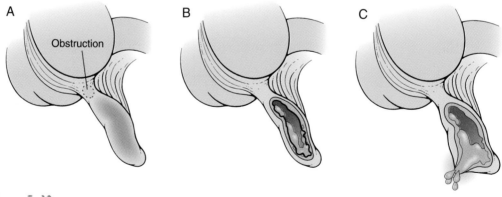

Figure 5-13

Stages of appendicitis. (A) Obstruction and bacterial infection cause red, swollen, and inflamed appendix. **(B)** Pus and bacteria invade the wall of the appendix. **(C)** Pus perforates (ruptures through) the wall of the appendix into the abdomen, leading to peritonitis (inflammation of the peritoneum). (Modified from Damjanov I: Pathology for the Health-Related Professions. Philadelphia, WB Saunders, 1966, page 274.)

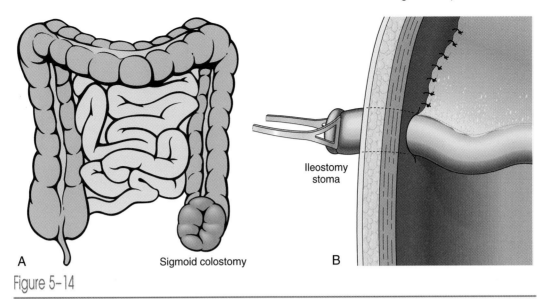

Figure 5-14

(A) **Sigmoid colostomy** after resection of the rectum and part of the sigmoid colon. (B) Ileostomy after resection of the entire colon. The ileum is drawn through the abdominal wall to form an ileostomy stoma.

cheil/o	lip	cheilosis _____

Labi/o also means lip.

cholecyst/o	gallbladder	cholecystectomy _____

choledoch/o	common bile duct	choledochotomy _____

col/o	colon, large intestine	colostomy _____

*-stomy, when used with a combining form for an organ, means an opening to the outside of the body. A **stoma** is an opening between an organ and the surface of the body (Fig. 5–14).*

colon/o	colon	colonic _____
		colonoscopy _____

dent/i	tooth	dentibuccal _____

Odont/o also means tooth.

duoden/o	duodenum	duodenal _____

enter/o	intestines, usually small intestine	enterocolitis _____

When two combining forms for gastrointestinal organs are in a term, the one closest to the mouth appears first.

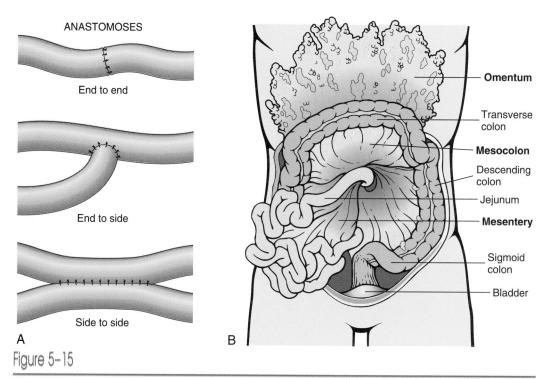

Figure 5-15

(A) Three types of anastomoses. (B) Mesentery. The **omentum** and **mesocolon** are parts of the mesentery. The omentum (raised in this figure) actually hangs down like an apron over the intestines.

enterocolostomy _____

*-stomy, when used with two or more combining forms for organs, means the surgical creation of an opening between those organs inside the body. This is also called an **anastomosis** (ana = up, stom = opening, -sis = state of) (Fig. 5–15A).*

mesentery _____

This membrane is a part of the double fold of peritoneum that stretches around the organs in the abdomen and holds them in place. It is literally in the middle (mes-) of the intestines, attaching the intestines to the muscle wall at the back of the abdomen (Fig. 5–15B).

parenteral _____

Par (from para-) means apart from in this term. Parenteral nutrition is food (glucose) given intravenously (IV) and not through the intestinal tract. Parenteral injections can be subcutaneous and intramuscular, as well.

esophag/o   esophagus   esophageal _____

Note that the final g is softened (ji) by changing the suffix from al to eal.

faci/o	face	facial _____
gastr/o	stomach	gastrostomy _____
gingiv/o	gums	gingivitis _____
gloss/o	tongue	hypoglossal _____

Lingu/o also means tongue.

hepat/o	liver	hepatoma _____
		hepatomegaly _____
ile/o	ileum	ileocecal sphincter _____

Also called the ileocecal valve.

ileitis _____

ileostomy _____

See Figure 5–14B.

jejun/o	jejunum	gastrojejunostomy _____

An anastomosis.

choledochojejunostomy _____

An anastomosis.

labi/o	lip	labial _____
lapar/o	abdomen	laparoscopy _____

Minimally invasive surgery. Laparoscopic cholecystectomy and appendectomy are examples.

lingu/o	tongue	sublingual _____
mandibul/o	lower jaw, mandible	submandibular _____
odont/o	tooth	orthodontist _____

Orth/o means straight.

periodontist _____

endodontist _____

Does root canal therapy.

or/o	mouth	oral _____

Stomat/o also means mouth.

palat/o	palate	palatoplasty _____
pancreat/o	pancreas	pancreatitis _____
pharyng/o	throat	pharyngeal _____
peritone/o	peritoneum	peritonitis _____

The e of the root has been dropped in this term.

proct/o	anus and rectum	proctologist _____
pylor/o	pyloric sphincter	pyloroplasty _____
rect/o	rectum	rectocele _____
sialaden/o	salivary gland	sialadenitis _____
sigmoid/o	sigmoid colon	sigmoidoscopy _____
stomat/o	mouth	stomatitis _____

Substances

Combining Form	Meaning	Terminology	Meaning
amyl/o	starch	amylase _____	

-ase means enzyme.

bil/i	gall, bile	biliary _____

The biliary tract includes the organs (liver and gallbladder) and ducts (hepatic, cystic, and common bile ducts) that secrete, store, and empty bile into the duodenum.

bilirubin/o	bilirubin (bile pigment)	hyperbilirubinemia _____
chol/e	gall, bile	cholelithiasis _____

lith/o means stone or calculus; -iasis means abnormal condition.

chlorhydr/o	hydrochloric acid	achlorhydria _____

Absence of gastric juice is associated with gastric carcinoma.

gluc/o	sugar	gluconeogenesis _____

New sugar is made by liver cells from fats and proteins.

glyc/o	sugar	hyperglycemia _____
glycogen/o	glycogen, animal starch	glycogenolysis _____

Liver cells can change glycogen back to glucose when blood sugar is low.

lip/o	fat, lipid	lipoma _____
lith/o	stone	cholecystolithiasis _____
prote/o	protein	protease _____
sial/o	saliva, salivary	sialolith _____
steat/o	fat	steatorrhea _____

Fats are improperly digested (malabsorbed) and appear in the feces.

Suffixes			
Suffix	**Meaning**	**Terminology**	**Meaning**
-ase	enzyme	lipase _____	
-chezia	defecation, elimination of wastes	hematochezia _____	
		(hem-ă-tō-KĒ-zē-ă). Bright red blood is found in the feces.	
-iasis	abnormal condition	choledocholithiasis _____	
-prandial	meal	postprandial _____	
		Post cibum also means after meals (cib/o means meal).	

V. Pathology of the Digestive System

This section is divided into terms that describe symptoms (signs of illness) and terms that describe pathological conditions. The sentences following the definitions use medical words that are familiar to you and often describe the **etiology** (eti/o = cause) of the illness and its treatment. If the etiology is neither known nor understood, it is called **idiopathic** (idi/o = unknown).

Symptoms

anorexia

Lack of appetite (-orexia = appetite).

Often a sign of malignancy or liver disease. Anorexia nervosa is loss of appetite owing to emotional problems such as anger, anxiety, and fear. It is an eating disorder and is discussed, along with a similar disorder, bulimia nervosa, in Chapter 22.

ascites

Abnormal accumulation of fluid in the abdomen.

This condition, previously called dropsy, occurs when fluid seeps out of the bloodstream and collects in the peritoneal cavity. It can be a symptom of neoplasm or inflammatory disorders in the abdomen, venous hypertension (high blood pressure) caused by liver disease (cirrhosis), and heart failure (Fig. 5–16).

borborygmus

Rumbling or gurgling noises produced by the movement of gas, fluid, or both in the gastrointestinal tract.

These noises are often audible from a distance.

constipation

Difficult, delayed elimination of feces.

Stools (feces) are dry and hard when peristalsis is slow. A medication that encourages movement of feces from the colon is called a **laxative.** A **cathartic** is a strong laxative.

diarrhea

Frequent, loose, watery stools.

Rapid onset of diarrhea soon after eating suggests an acute infection or toxin. However, certain infections may not cause diarrhea for several hours. Watery or bloody stools are a symptom of inflammation or disease in the GI tract.

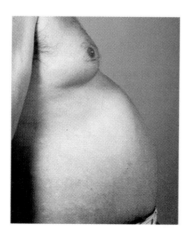

Figure 5–16

Ascites in a male patient. The photograph was taken after a paracentesis (puncture to remove fluid from the abdomen) was performed. Notice the gynecomastia (condition of female breasts) in this patient due to an excess of estrogen that can accompany cirrhosis, especially in alcoholics. (From Lewis SM, Collier IC, Heitkemper MM: Medical-Surgical Nursing, 4th edition, St. Louis, Mosby, 1996, page 1274.)

dysphagia

Difficulty in swallowing.

This sensation occurs when a swallowed bolus fails to progress, either because of a physical obstruction (obstructive dysphagia) or because of a motor disorder in which esophageal peristalsis is not properly coordinated (motor dysphagia). **Odynophagia** is painful swallowing.

flatus

Gas expelled through the anus.

Eructation (belching) is the expelling of gas from the stomach through the mouth. Flatulence is the presence of excessive gas in both the stomach and the intestines. Flatulent refers to a person experiencing flatulence.

hematochezia

Bright, fresh, red blood discharged from the rectum.

Hematochezia is associated with rapid bleeding, as from a duodenal ulcer, ulcerative colitis, or hemorrhoids.

jaundice

Yellow-orange coloration of the skin and other tissues due to high levels of bilirubin in the blood (hyperbilirubinemia).

Jaundice **(icterus)** can occur in three major ways: (1) excessive destruction of erythrocytes, as in **hemolysis,** causes excess bilirubin in the blood; (2) malfunction of liver cells (hepatocytes) because of **liver disease** prevents the liver from excreting bilirubin with bile; (3) **obstruction of bile flow,** such as from choledocholithiasis or tumor, prevents bilirubin in bile from being excreted into the duodenum.

melena

Black, tarry stools; feces containing blood.

This symptom usually reflects a condition in which blood has had time to be digested (acted on by intestinal juices).

nausea

Unpleasant sensation in the stomach and a tendency to vomit.

This term comes from a Greek word meaning seasickness. Irritation of nerve endings in the stomach or other parts of the body sends a message to the vomiting reflex center in the brain. Nausea and vomiting may be symptomatic of a perforation (hole in the wall) of an abdominal organ; obstruction of a bile duct, stomach, or intestine; or toxins (poisons).

steatorrhea

Fat in the feces.

Improper digestion or absorption of fat can cause fat to remain in the intestine. This may occur with disease of the pancreas (pancreatitis) when pancreatic enzymes are not excreted. It is also a symptom of disease of the small intestine that involves malabsorption of fat.

Pathological Conditions

Oral Cavity and Teeth

aphthous stomatitis

Inflammation of the mouth with small ulcers.

This idiopathic condition is also known as **canker** (KĂNK-ĕr) **sores.** Aphth/o means ulcer.

dental caries

Tooth decay (caries means decay).

Dental plaque is the accumulation of foods, proteins from saliva, and necrotic debris on the tooth enamel. Bacteria grow in the plaque and cause the production of acid that dissolves the tooth enamel, resulting in a cavity (area of decay). If the bacterial infection reaches the pulp of the tooth (causing pulpitis), root canal therapy may be necessary.

herpetic stomatitis

Inflammation of the mouth (gingiva, lips, palate, and tongue) **by infection with the herpesvirus.**

Commonly called **fever blisters** or **cold sores.**

oral leukoplakia

White plaques or patches (-plakia means plaque) **on the mucosa of the mouth.**

A precancerous condition; major etiological factors are chronic tobacco and alcohol use.

periodontal disease

Inflammation and degeneration of gums, teeth, and surrounding bone; also called **pyorrhea** (py/o means pus).

Chronic inflammation of gums (gingivitis) occurs as a result of accumulation of **dental plaque** (noncalcified collection of oral microorganisms and their products) and **dental calculus** or **tartar** (a white, brown, or yellow-brown calcified deposit at or below the gingival margin of teeth). Gingivectomy (a metal instrument is used to scrape away plaque and tartar from teeth) may be necessary to remove pockets of pus and allow new tissue to form. Infected areas are treated with targeted antibiotics.

Gastrointestinal Tract

achalasia

Failure of the lower esophagus sphincter (LES) muscle to relax (-chalasia means relaxation).

In achalasia there is also loss of peristalsis so that food cannot pass easily through the esophagus. Both failure of the LES to relax and the loss of peristalsis cause dilation and widening of the esophagus (Fig. 5–17A). Physicians often recommend a bland diet low in bulk, and dilation of the LES to relieve symptoms (Fig. 5–17B).

anal fistula

Abnormal tube-like passageway near the anus (Fig. 5–18A).

The fistula usually, but not always, opens into the rectum. An **anal fissure** is a narrow crack or slit in the mucous membrane of the anus.

colonic polyposis

Polyps (small benign growths) protrude from the mucous membrane of the colon.

Figure 5–18A illustrates two types of polyps: **pedunculated** (attached to the membrane by a stalk or peduncle) and **sessile** (sitting directly on the mucous membrane). Figure 5–18B shows multiple polyps of the colon. The polyps protrude into the lumen of the colon.

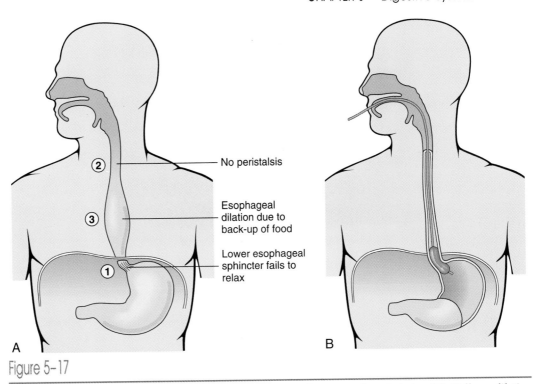

Figure 5-17

(A) **Achalasia.** Numbers refer to the sequence of events that occur in achalasia. (B) **Balloon dilation (dilatation)** of the lower esophageal sphincter (LES) as treatment for achalasia.

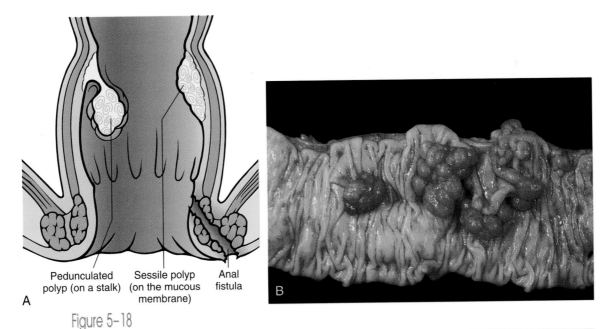

Figure 5-18

(A) **Anal fistula and two types of polyps.** (B) **Multiple polyps of the colon.** (Part B from Damjanov I: Pathology for the Health-Related Professions, Philadelphia, WB Saunders, 1996, page 281.)

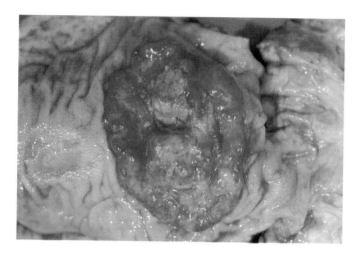

Figure 5-19

Adenocarcinoma of the colon. This tumor appears ulcerated (characterized by open, exposed surfaces). (From Damjanov I: Pathology for the Health-Related Professions, Philadelphia, WB Saunders, 1996, page 283.)

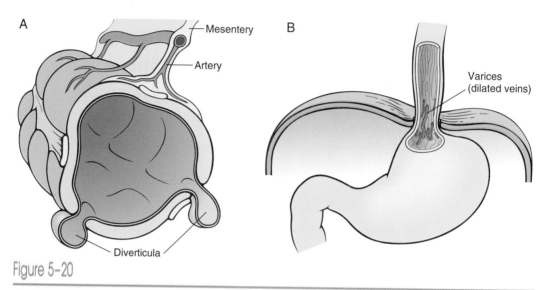

Figure 5-20

(A) Diverticula. The mucous lining of the colon bulges through the muscular wall to form diverticula. **(B) Esophageal varices.** (Part B from Damjanov I: Pathology for the Health-Related Professions. Philadelphia, WB Saunders, 1996, page 261.)

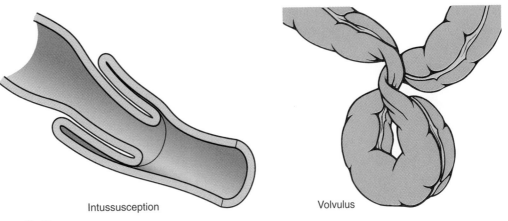

Intussusception   Volvulus

Figure 5-22

Intussusception and volvulus. (From Damjanov I: Pathology for the Health-Related Professions. Philadelphia, WB Saunders, 1996, page 276.)

irritable bowel syndrome

A group of GI symptoms (diarrhea and constipation, lower abdominal pain, and bloating) associated with stress and tension. Also called **spastic colon.**

No pathological lesions are found in the intestines. Treatment includes psychotherapy to manage stress and medications (antidiarrheals and bulk-forming laxatives) to relieve symptoms. A diet high in bran and fiber also helps soften stools and establish regular bowel movements.

ulcer

Open sore or lesion (wound) **of skin** (epithelial) **tissue.**

Gastric or duodenal ulcers (both are **peptic ulcers**) are examples. Duodenal ulcers are now thought to be caused by a bacterium, *Helicobacter pylori (H. pylori)*. The combination of bacteria, hyperacidity, and gastric juice (particularly pepsin) damages epithelial linings. Treatment includes drugs to reduce the production of hydrochloric acid and protect the lining of the stomach and intestine. Antibiotics are commonly used against *H. pylori*.

ulcerative colitis

Chronic inflammation of the colon with the presence of ulcers.

This is an idiopathic, chronic, recurrent diarrheal disease **(inflammatory bowel disease)** with rectal bleeding and pain. Often beginning in the rectum, the inflammation spreads proximally, involving the entire colon. Resection of diseased bowel with ileostomy may be necessary as treatment. Ulcerative colitis is associated with a higher risk of colon cancer.

volvulus

Twisting of the intestine upon itself.

A surgical emergency, the volvulus must be released immediately (see Fig. 5–22).

Liver, Gallbladder, and Pancreas

cirrhosis

Chronic disease of the liver with degeneration of liver cells.

Alcoholism combined with malnutrition is a common etiological factor, but infection and poisons can affect the liver cells as well. Alcohol has a toxic effect on hepatocytes, causing fat cells to accumulate, followed by necrosis and fibrous scarring, and discoloration (cirrh/o refers to the liver's orange-yellow

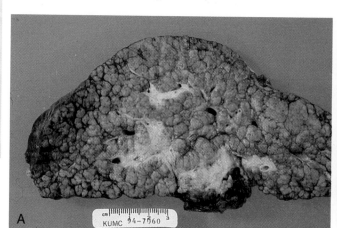
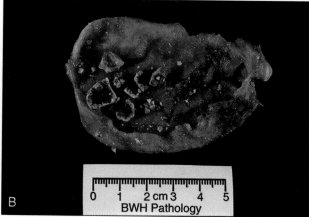

Figure 5–23

(A) Liver with alcoholic cirrhosis. The normal liver cells (hepatocytes) have been replaced by nodules that are yellow because of their high fat content. (B) Cholesterol gallstones. Mechanical manipulation during laparoscopic cholecystectomy has caused fragmentation of several cholesterol gallstones, revealing interiors that are pigmented because of entrapped bile pigments. The gallbladder mucosa is reddened and irregular as a result of coexistent acute and chronic cholecystitis. (Part A from Damjanov I: Pathology for the Health-Related Professions. WB Saunders, Philadelphia, 1996, page 301; Part B from Kumar V, Cotran RS, and Robbins S: Basic Pathology, 6th ed. Philadelphia, WB Saunders, 1997, page 551.)

color). As with other liver diseases, jaundice results when the liver cells fail to function and bilirubin is not eliminated from the body (Fig. 5–23A).

gallstones (cholelithiasis and choledocholithiasis)

Crystallization of cholesterol and other materials to form stones in the gallbladder or bile ducts (Fig. 5–23B).

Calculi (stones) can prevent bile from leaving the gallbladder and bile ducts to enter the duodenum (Fig. 5–24). The majority of patients with gallstones remain asymptomatic and do not require treatment. However, if a

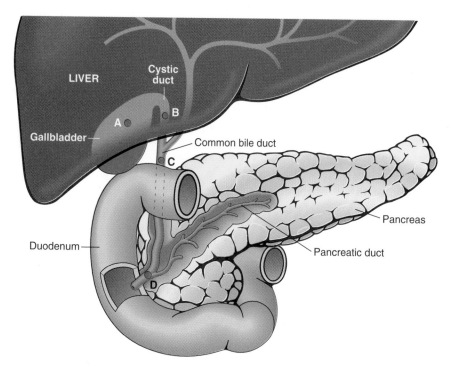

Figure 5–24

Gallstone positions. (A) Stone in the gallbladder causing mild or no symptoms. (B) Stone obstructing the cystic duct causing pain. (C) Stone obstructing the common bile duct causing pain and jaundice. (D) Stone at the lower end of the common bile duct and pancreatic duct causing pain, jaundice, and pancreatitis.

Figure 5-25

Trocars in place for laparoscopic cholecystectomy. Trocars are used to puncture and enter the abdomen. They are metal sleeves consisting of a hollow metal tube (cannula) into which fits an obturator (a solid, removable metal instrument with a sharp, three-cornered tip) used to puncture the wall of a body cavity. Once the obturator is removed, an endoscope and other instruments can be introduced through the trocar to perform laparoscopic surgery. **(1)** is an umbilical 10/11-mm trocar (the largest trocar diameter is 15). **(2)** is a 10/11-mm trocar at the midline. **(3)** and **(4)** are 5-mm trocars at the axillary line.

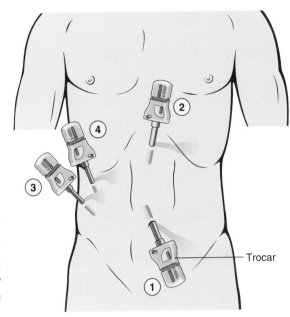

Trocar

patient experiences episodes of **biliary colic** (pain from blocked cystic or common bile duct), treatment is required. Conventional treatment has been cholecystectomy or choledocholithotomy. Currently, more cholecystectomies are performed using a laparoscopic technique **(laparoscopic cholecystectomy)** similar to that used to tie off the fallopian tubes (Fig. 5–25).

pancreatitis

Inflammation of the pancreas.

Digestive enzymes attack pancreatic tissue, leading to damage to the gland. Alcoholism and gallstones may be causative factors, but chronic or acute inflammation can develop from abdominal trauma or chemical injury. Acute pancreatitis (marked by massive swelling, bleeding, and necrosis of the pancreas) may be complicated by sacs of fluid called pseudocysts (in the pancreas) and systemic problems such as shock, renal failure, and respiratory collapse. Treatment includes medications to relieve epigastric pain, intravenous fluids, and, rarely, surgery to remove portions of the pancreas.

viral hepatitis

Inflammation of the liver caused by virus.

There are three major types of viral hepatitis: **Hepatitis A** (caused by type A virus and previously called infectious hepatitis) is a benign, acute, self-limited disorder transmitted by infected water and food (the virus is also excreted in feces). **Hepatitis B** (caused by type B virus and called serum hepatitis) is acquired parenterally, through blood (transfusions, hypodermic needles, and dental and surgical instruments) and via body fluids, such as tears, saliva, and semen. A vaccine that provides immunity to hepatitis B is recommended for hospital personnel, dentists, laboratory technicians, and persons requiring frequent transfusions. **Hepatitis C** is transmitted by blood or blood products; transmission through sexual contact and from mother to infant is rare. About 10 per cent of patients develop hepatic fibrosis and cirrhosis. In all types, liver enzymes may be elevated, indicating damage to liver tissue. Symptoms include malaise, anorexia, occasional joint pain, and in severe cases, nausea and jaundice.

VI. Exercises

Remember to check your answers carefully with those given in Section VII, Answers to Exercises.

A. Match the following digestive system structures with their meanings below.

anus	sigmoid colon	ileum
esophagus	pancreas	liver
jejunum	gallbladder	colon
pharynx	cecum	duodenum

1. large intestine _____

2. small sac under the liver; stores bile _____

3. first part of the large intestine _____

4. opening of the digestive tract to the outside of the body _____

5. second part of the small intestine _____

6. tube connecting the throat to the stomach _____

7. third part of the small intestine _____

8. large organ located in the RUQ; secretes bile, stores sugar, produces blood proteins

   _____

9. throat _____

10. lower part of the colon _____

11. first part of the small intestine _____

12. organ under the stomach; produces insulin and digestive enzymes _____

B. Circle the term that correctly fits the definition given. You should be able to define the other terms as well!

1. **microscopic projections in the walls of the small intestine:**
   papillae   villi   rugae

2. **salivary gland near the ear:**
   submandibular   sublingual   parotid

3. **ring of muscle at the distal end of the stomach:**
   pyloric sphincter   uvula   lower esophageal sphincter

4. **soft, inner section of a tooth:**
   dentin   enamel   pulp

5. **chemical that speeds up reactions and helps digest foods:**
   triglyceride   amino acid   enzyme

6. **pigment released with bile:**
   glycogen   bilirubin   melena

7. **hormone produced by endocrine cells of the pancreas:**
   insulin   amylase   lipase

8. **rhythm-like movement of the muscles in the walls of the gastrointestinal tract:**
   deglutition   mastication   peristalsis

9. **breakdown of large fat globules:**
   absorption   emulsification   anabolism

10. **pointed, dog-like tooth medial to premolars:**
    incisor   canine   molar

C. Complete the following.

1. labi/o and cheil/o both mean _____

2. gloss/o and lingu/o both mean _____

3. or/o and stomat/o both mean _____

4. dent/i and odont/o both mean _____

5. lapar/o and celi/o both mean _____

6. gluc/o and glyc/o both mean _____

7. lip/o, steat/o, and adip/o all mean _____

8. -iasis and -osis both mean _____

9. chol/e and bil/i both mean _____

10. -ectomy and resection both mean _____

D. Build medical terms.

1. removal of a salivary gland _____

2. pertaining to the throat _____

3. hernia of the rectum _____

4. enlargement of the liver _____

5. surgical repair of the roof of the mouth _____

6. after meals _____

7. visual examination of the anal and rectal region _____

8. study of the cause (of disease) _____

9. incision of the common bile duct _____

10. pertaining to tooth and cheek (the surface of tooth against the cheek) _____

11. disease condition of the small intestine _____

12. new opening between the common bile duct and the jejunum _____

13. pertaining to surrounding the anus _____

14. new opening from the colon to the outside of the body _____

15. pertaining to under the lower jaw _____

16. pertaining to the face _____

E. Match the following doctors or dentists with their specialties.

oral surgeon   endodontist   colorectal surgeon
orthodontist   proctologist   nephrologist
gastroenterologist   periodontist   urologist

1. diagnoses and treats disorders of the anus and rectum _____

2. operates on the organs of the urinary tract _____

3. straightens teeth _____

4. performs root canal therapy _____

5. operates on the mouth and teeth _____

6. diagnoses and uses drugs to treat kidney disorders _____

7. diagnoses and treats gastrointestinal tract disorders _____

8. treats gum disease _____

9. operates on the intestinal tract _____

F. Build medical terms to describe the following inflammations.

1. inflammation of the appendix _____

2. inflammation of the large intestine _____

3. inflammation of the tube from the throat to the stomach _____

4. inflammation of the membrane around the abdomen _____

5. inflammation of the gallbladder _____

6. inflammation of the third part of the small intestine _____

7. inflammation of the pancreas _____

8. inflammation of the gums _____

9. inflammation of the liver _____

10. inflammation of the mouth _____

11. inflammation of the salivary gland _____

12. inflammation of the small and large intestine _____

G. Match the following terms with their meanings below.

anastomosis	hyperglycemia	mesentery
mucosa	portal vein	parenteral
biliary	dysphagia	gluconeogenesis
defecation	hyperbilirubinemia	glycogenolysis

1. high level of blood sugar _____

2. difficulty in swallowing _____

3. pertaining to administration other than through the intestinal tract _____

4. a mucous membrane _____

5. expulsion of feces from the body through the anus _____

6. breakdown (conversion) of animal starch to sugar _____

7. membrane that connects the small intestine to the abdominal wall _____

8. large vessel that takes blood to the liver from the intestines _____

9. new surgical connection between two previously unconnected organs _____

10. pertaining to bile ducts and organs _____

11. process of forming new sugar from proteins and fats _____

12. high levels of a bile pigment in the bloodstream _____

H. Give the names of the following gastrointestinal symptoms based on their descriptions.

1. bright red blood discharged from the rectum _____

2. lack of appetite _____

3. discharge of fat in the feces _____

4. black, tarry stools; feces containing blood _____

5. abnormal accumulation of fluid in the abdomen _____

6. rumbling noises produced by gas in the GI tract _____

7. gas expelled through the anus _____

8. an unpleasant sensation in the stomach and a tendency to vomit _____

9. loose, watery stools _____

10. difficult, delayed elimination of feces with dry, hard stools _____

I. Give short answers for the following.

1. What is jaundice? _____

2. Give three ways in which a patient can become jaundiced:

   a. _____

   b. _____

   c. _____

3. What does it mean when a disease is described as *idiopathic?* _____

J. Using the pathological terminology listed below, complete the following sentences.

herpetic stomatitis	aphthous stomatitis	achalasia
dental caries	oral leukoplakia	periodontal disease
colorectal cancer	colonic polyposis	anal fistula
Crohn disease		

1. Ms. Jones' dysphagia was diagnosed by her doctor as being caused by a failure of the muscles in her lower esophagus to relax during swallowing. Her condition is also known as

_____.

2. Mr. Rosen's proctalgia was related to the abnormal tube-like passageway that formed near his anus. His doctor performed surgery to close off the _____.

3. When bacteria produce acid that eats away at tooth enamel, the result can be tooth decay, otherwise known as _____.

4. Nancy Cole's symptoms of chronic diarrhea, abdominal cramps, and fever led her doctor to suspect that she suffered from an inflammatory bowel disease that affected the distal portion of her ileum. The doctor prescribed steroid drugs to heal her condition, which is known as

_____.

5. The results of President Reagan's colonoscopy revealed the presence of small benign growths protruding from the mucous membrane of his large intestine. His diagnosis was

_____.

6. During a routine dental checkup, Dr. Payne discovered white plaques on Jim's buccal mucosa. A chronic smoker and alcoholic, Jim was advised that the lesions were precancerous and should be

removed. His diagnosis was _____.

7. Every time Bob had a stressful time at work he developed a fever blister (cold sore) on his lip, resulting from reactivation of a previous viral infection. His doctor told him his condition was

called _____.

8. After biopsy of the neoplasm in Mr. Greenberg's ascending colon, and determination that the

lesion was malignant, Dr. Jones' diagnosis was _____.
He advised radical (complete) colectomy followed by colostomy.

9. The small ulcers (canker sores) on Diane's gums and buccal mucosa were both painful and

annoying. Her dentist told her that the condition is known as _____,
and that its cause is unknown.

10. Failure to floss her teeth and remove dental plaque regularly led to Sharon's gingivitis and

pyorrhea. Her dentist called the condition _____
and advised consulting a specialist who could treat her condition.

K. Match the following pathological diagnoses with their definitions.

hepatitis	pancreatitis	cirrhosis
ileus	dysentery	irritable bowel syndrome
diverticula	cholecystolithiasis	hiatal hernia
peptic ulcer	intussusception	volvulus
esophageal varices	ulcerative colitis	hemorrhoids

1. protrusion of the upper part of the stomach through the esophageal opening in the diaphragm

   _____

2. painful, inflamed intestines caused by bacterial infection _____

3. swollen, twisted veins in the rectal region _____

4. a sore or lesion of the mucous membrane in the gastric or duodenal region

   _____

5. failure of peristalsis _____

6. twisting of the intestine upon itself _____

7. swollen, twisted veins around the distal end of the esophagus _____

8. abnormal side-pockets in the intestinal wall _____

9. chronic inflammation of the large bowel with ulcers _____

10. telescoping of the intestines _____

11. inflammation of the liver caused by type A, type B, or type C virus _____

12. inflammation of the pancreas _____

13. calculi in the sac that stores bile _____

14. chronic liver disease resulting from alcoholism and malnutrition _____

15. a group of symptoms (diarrhea and constipation, abdominal pain, bloating) associated with stress

    and tension, but without inflammation of the intestine _____

L. Complete the following terms from their meanings given below.

1. membrane (peritoneal fold) that holds the intestines together: mes _____

2. removal of the gallbladder: _____ ectomy

3. black or dark brown, tarry stools containing blood: mel _____

4. high levels of pigment in the blood (jaundice): hyper _____

5. pertaining to under the tongue: sub _____

6. twisting of the intestine upon itself: vol _____

7. organ under the stomach that produces insulin and digestive enzymes:

   pan _____

8. lack of appetite: an _____

9. swollen, twisted veins in the rectal region: _____ oids

10. new connection between two previously unconnected tubes: ana _____

11. absence of acid in the stomach: a _____

12. solid and fluids return to the mouth from the stomach: gastro _____

    re _____ disease

VII. Answers to Exercises

A

1. colon
2. gallbladder
3. cecum
4. anus
5. jejunum
6. esophagus
7. ileum
8. liver
9. pharynx
10. sigmoid colon
11. duodenum
12. pancreas

B

1. Villi. Papillae are nipple-like projections in the tongue where taste buds are located, and rugae are folds in the mucous membrane of the stomach and hard palate.
2. Parotid. The submandibular gland is under the lower jaw, and the sublingual gland is under the tongue.
3. Pyloric sphincter. The uvula is soft tissue hanging from the soft palate, and the lower esophageal sphincter is a ring of muscle between the esophagus and stomach.
4. Pulp. Dentin is the hard part of the tooth directly under the enamel and in the root, and enamel is the hard, outermost part of the tooth composing the crown.
5. Enzyme. A triglyceride is a large fat molecule, and an amino acid is substance produced when proteins are digested.
6. Bilirubin. Glycogen is animal starch that is produced in liver cells from sugar, and melena is dark, tarry stools.
7. Insulin. Amylase and lipase are digestive enzymes produced by the exocrine cells of the pancreas.
8. Peristalis. Deglutition is swallowing, and mastication is chewing.
9. Emulsification. Absorption is the passage of materials through the walls of the small intestine into the bloodstream, and anabolism is the process of building up proteins in a cell (protein synthesis).
10. Canine. An incisor is one of the four front teeth in the dental arch (not pointed or dog-like), and a molar is one of three large teeth just behind (distal to) the two premolar teeth.

C

1. lip
2. tongue
3. mouth
4. tooth
5. abdomen
6. sugar
7. fat
8. abnormal condition
9. gall, bile
10. removal, excision

D

1. sialadenectomy
2. pharyngeal
3. rectocele
4. hepatomegaly
5. palatoplasty
6. postprandial (post cibum—cib/o means meals)
7. proctoscopy
8. etiology
9. choledochotomy
10. dentibuccal
11. enteropathy
12. choledochojejunostomy
13. perianal
14. colostomy
15. submandibular
16. facial

E

1. proctologist
2. urologist
3. orthodontist
4. endodontist
5. oral surgeon
6. nephrologist
7. gastroenterologist
8. periodontist
9. colorectal surgeon

F

1. appendicitis
2. colitis
3. esophagitis
4. peritonitis (note that the e is dropped)
5. cholecystitis
6. ileitis
7. pancreatitis
8. gingivitis
9. hepatitis
10. stomatitis
11. sialadenitis
12. enterocolitis (when two combining forms for gastrointestinal organs are in a term, use the one that is closest to the mouth first)

G

1. hyperglycemia
2. dysphagia
3. parenteral
4. mucosa
5. defecation
6. glycogenolysis
7. mesentery
8. portal vein
9. anastomosis
10. biliary
11. gluconeogenesis
12. hyperbilirubinemia

H

1. hematochezia
2. anorexia
3. steatorrhea
4. melena
5. ascites
6. borborygmus
7. flatus
8. nausea
9. diarrhea
10. constipation

I

1. yellow-orange coloration of the skin and other tissues (hyperbilirubinemia)
2. **a** any liver disease (hepatopathy—such as cirrhosis, hepatoma, or hepatitis), so that bilirubin is not processed into bile and cannot be excreted in feces
b obstruction of bile flow, so that bile and bilirubin are not excreted and accumulate in the bloodstream
c excessive hemolysis leading to overproduction of bilirubin and high levels in the bloodstream
3. its cause is not known

J

1. achalasia
2. anal fistula
3. dental caries
4. Crohn disease
5. colonic polyposis
6. oral leukoplakia
7. herpetic stomatitis
8. colorectal cancer
9. aphthous stomatitis
10. periodontal disease

K

1. hiatal hernia
2. dysentery
3. hemorrhoids
4. peptic ulcer
5. ileus
6. volvulus
7. esophageal varices
8. diverticula (diverticulosis)
9. ulcerative colitis
10. intussusception
11. viral hepatitis
12. pancreatitis
13. cholecystolithiasis (gallstones)
14. cirrhosis
15. irritable bowel syndrome

L

1. mesentery
2. cholecystectomy
3. melena
4. hyperbilirubinemia
5. sublingual
6. volvulus
7. pancreas
8. anorexia
9. hemorrhoids
10. anastomosis
11. achlorhydria
12. gastroesophageal reflux disease

VIII. Pronunciation of Terms

Pronunciation Guide

ā as in āpe   ă as in ăpple
ē as in ēven   ĕ as in ĕvery
ī as in īce   ĭ as in ĭnterest
ō as in ōpen   ŏ as in pŏt
ū as in ūnit   ŭ as in ŭnder

To test your understanding of the terminology in this chapter, write the meaning of each term in the space provided. In addition, you may wish to cover the terms and write them by looking at your definitions. Make sure your spelling is correct. The page number after each term indicates where it is defined or used in the text so you can easily check your responses.

Vocabulary and Terminology Sections

Term	Pronunciation	Meaning
absorption (145)	ăb-SŎRP-shŭn	
achlorhydria (153)	ā-chlōr-HĪ-drē-ă	
alimentary canal (145)	ăl-ĕ-MĔN-tăr-ē kă-NĂL	
amino acids (145)	ă-MĒ-nō ĂS-ĭdz	
amylase (145)	ĂM-ĭ-lās	
anus (145)	Ā-nŭs	
appendectomy (148)	ăp-ĕn-DĔK-tō-mē	
appendicitis (148)	ă-pĕn-dĭ-SĪ-tĭs	
appendix (145)	ă-PĔN-dĭks	
bile (145)	BĪL	
biliary (152)	BĬL-ē-ăr-ē	
bilirubin (145)	bĭl-ĭ-ROO-bĭn	
bowel (145)	BŎW-ĕl	
buccal mucosa (148)	BŬK-ăl mū-KŌ-să	
canine teeth (145)	KĀ-nīn tēth	
cecal (148)	SĒ-kăl	
cecum (145)	SĒ-kŭm	
celiac (148)	SĒ-lē-ăk	
cheilosis (149)	kī-LŌ-sĭs	

cholecystectomy (149)	kō-lĕ-sĭs-TĔK-tō-mē	_____
choledocholithiasis (153)	kō-lĕd-ō-kō-lĭ-THĪ-ă-sĭs	_____
choledochojejunostomy (151)	kō-lĕd-ō-kō-jĭ-jū-NŎS-tō-mē	_____
choledochotomy (149)	kō-lĕd-ō-KŎT-ō-mē	_____
cholelithiasis (152)	kō-lē-lĭ-THĪ-ă-sĭs	_____
colon (145)	KŌ-lĕn	_____
colonic (149)	kō-LŎN-ĭk	_____
colonoscopy (149)	kō-lŏn-ŎS-kō-pē	_____
colostomy (149)	kŏ-LŎS-tō-mē	_____
common bile duct (145)	KŎM-ĭn bīl dŭkt	_____
defecation (145)	dĕf-ĕ-KĀ-shŭn	_____
deglutition (145)	dē-gloo-TĬSH-ŭn	_____
dentibuccal (149)	dĕn-tē-BŬK-ăl	_____
dentin (145)	DĔN-tĭn	_____
digestion (146)	dī-JĔST-yŭn	_____
duodenal (149)	dū-ō-DĒ-năl or dū-ŎD-dĕ-năl	_____
duodenum (146)	dū-ō-DĒ-nŭm or dū-ŎD-dĕ-ŭm	_____
emulsification (146)	ē-mŭl-sĭ-fĭ-KĀ-shŭn	_____
enamel (146)	ē-NĂM-ĕl	_____
endodontist (151)	ĕn-dō-DŎN-tĭst	_____
enterocolitis (149)	ĕn-tĕr-ō-kō-LĪ-tĭs	_____
enterocolostomy (150)	ĕn-tĕr-ō-kō-LŎS-tō-mē	_____
enzyme (146)	ĔN-zīm	_____
esophageal (150)	ĕ-sŏf-ă-JĒ-ăl	_____
esophagus (146)	ĕ-SŎF-ă-gŭs	_____
facial (146)	FĀ-shŭl	_____
feces (146)	FĒ-sēz	_____
gallbladder (146)	găl-BLĂ-dĕr	_____

gastrojejunostomy (151)	găs-trō-jĭ-jū-NŎS-tō-mē	_____
gastrostomy (151)	găs-TRŎS-tō-mē	_____
gluconeogenesis (153)	gloo-kō-nē-ō-JĔN-ĕ-sĭs	_____
glucose (146)	GLOO-kōs	_____
glycogen (146)	GLĪ-kō-jĕn	_____
glycogenolysis (153)	glī-kō-jĕ-NŎL-ĭ-sĭs	_____
hepatoma (151)	hĕ-pă-TŌ-mă	_____
hepatomegaly (151)	hĕ-pă-tō-MĔG-ă-lē	_____
hydrochloric acid (146)	hī-drō-KLŎR-ĭk Ă-sĭd	_____
hyperbilirubinemia (152)	hī-pĕr-bĭl-ĭ-roo-bĭ-NĒ-mē-ă	_____
hyperglycemia (153)	hī-pĕr-glī-SĒ-mē-ă	_____
hypoglossal (151)	hī-pō-GLŎ-săl	_____
ileitis (151)	ĭl-ē-Ī-tĭs	_____
ileocecal sphincter (151)	ĭl-ē-ō-SĒ-kăl SFĬNGK-tĕr	_____
ileostomy (151)	ĭl-ē-ŎS-tō-mē	_____
ileum (146)	ĬL-ē-ŭm	_____
incisor (146)	ĭn-SĪ-zŏr	_____
insulin (146)	ĬN-sŭ-lĭn	_____
jejunum (146)	jĕ-JOO-nŭm	_____
labial (151)	LĀ-bē-ăl	_____
laparoscopy (151)	lă-pă-RŎS-kō-pē	_____
lipase (146)	LĪ-pās	_____
liver (146)	LĬ-vĕr	_____
mastication (147)	măs-tĭ-KĀ-shŭn	_____
mesentery (150)	MĔS-ĕn-tĕr-ē	_____
molar teeth (134)	MŌ-lăr tēth	_____
oral (152)	ŎR-ăl	_____
orthodontist (151)	ŏr-thō-DŎN-tĭst	_____
palate (147)	PĂL-ăt	_____

palatoplasty (152)	PĂL-ă-tō-plăs-tē	_____
pancreas (147)	PĂN-krē-ăs	_____
pancreatitis (152)	păn-krē-ă-TĪ-tĭs	_____
papillae (147)	pă-PĬL-ē	_____
parenteral (150)	pă-RĔN-tĕr-ăl	_____
parotid gland (147)	pă-RŎT-ĭd gland	_____
perianal (148)	pĕ-rē-Ā-năl	_____
periodontist (151)	pĕr-ē-ō-DŎN-tĭst	_____
peristalsis (147)	pĕr-ĭ-STĂL-sĭs	_____
pharyngeal (152)	făr-ăn-JĒ-ăl or fă-RĬN-jē-ăl	_____
pharynx (147)	FĂR-ĭnks	_____
portal vein (147)	PŎR-tăl vān	_____
postprandial (153)	pōst-PRĂN-dē-ăl	_____
premolar teeth (134)	prē-MŌ-lăr tēth	_____
proctologist (152)	prŏk-TŎL-ō-jĭst	_____
proteases (147)	PRŌ-tē-ā-sĕz	_____
pulp (147)	pŭlp	_____
pyloric sphincter (147)	pī-LŎR-ĭk SFĬNGK-tĕr	_____
pyloroplasty (152)	pī-LŎR-ō-plăs-tē	_____
rectocele (152)	RĔK-tō-sēl	_____
rectum (147)	RĔK-tŭm	_____
rugae (147)	ROO-gē	_____
saliva (147)	să-LĪ-vă	_____
salivary glands (147)	SĂL-ĭ-vĕr-ē glăndz	_____
sialadenitis (152)	sī-ăl-ă-dĕ-NĪ-tĭs	_____
sialolith (153)	sī-ĂL-ō-lĭth	_____
sigmoid colon (147)	SĬG-moyd KŌ-lŏn	_____
sigmoidoscopy (152)	sĭg-moy-DŎS-kō-pē	_____

sphincter (147)	SFĬNGK-tĕr	_____
steatorrhea (153)	stē-ă-tō-RĒ-ă	_____
stomatitis (152)	stō-mă-TĪ-tĭs	_____
sublingual (151)	sŭb-LĬNG-wăl	_____
submandibular (151)	sŭb-măn-DĬB-ū-lăr	_____
triglycerides (147)	trī-GLĬ-sĕ-rīdz	_____
uvula (147)	Ū-vū-lă	_____
villi (147)	VĬL-ī	_____

Pathological Terminology

Term	Pronunciation	Meaning
achalasia (156)	ăk-ăh-LĀ-zē-ă	_____
anal fistula (156)	Ā-năl FĬS-tū-lă	_____
anorexia (154)	ăn-ō-RĔK-sē-ă	_____
aphthous stomatitis (155)	ĂF-thŭs stō-mă-TĪ-tĭs	_____
ascites (154)	ă-SĪ-tēz	_____
borborygmus (154)	bŏr-bō-RĬG-mŭs	_____
cholelithiasis (162)	kō-lĕ-lĭ-THĪ-ă-sĭs	_____
cirrhosis (161)	sĭr-RŌ-sĭs	_____
colonic polyposis (156)	kō-LŎN-ĭk pŏl-ĭ-PŌ-sĭs	_____
colorectal cancer (159)	kō-lō-RĔK-tăl KĂN-sĕr	_____
constipation (154)	cŏn-stĭ-PĀ-shŭn	_____
Crohn disease (159)	krōn dĭ-ZĒZ	_____
dental caries (156)	DĔN-tăl KĂR-ēz	_____
diarrhea (154)	dī-ăh-RĒ-ă	_____
diverticula (159)	dī-vĕr-TĬK-ū-lă	_____
dysentery (159)	DĬS-ĕn-tĕr-ē	_____
dysphagia (155)	dĭs-PHĀ-jē-ă	_____
esophageal varices (159)	ē-sŏf-ăh-JĒ-ăl VĂR-ĭ-sēz	_____

etiology (154)	ē-tē-ŎL-ō-jē	_____
flatus (155)	FLĀ-tŭs	_____
gastric carcinoma (159)	GĂS-trĭk kăr-sĭ-NŌ-mă	_____
gastroesophageal reflux disease (160)	găs-trō-ē-sŏf-ă-JĒ-ăl RĒ-flŭx dĭ-ZĒZ	_____
hematochezia (155)	hēm-ă-tō-KĒ-zē-ă	_____
hemorrhoids (160)	HĔM-ō-roydz	_____
herpetic stomatitis (156)	hĕr-PĔT-ĭk stō-măh-TĪ-tĭs	_____
hiatal hernia (160)	hī-Ā-tăl HĔR-nē-ă	_____
icterus (155)	ĬK-tĕr-ŭs	_____
idiopathic (154)	ĭd-ē-ō-PĂTH-ĭk	_____
ileus (160)	ĬL-ē-ŭs	_____
inflammatory bowel disease (161)	ĭn-FLĂ-mă-tō-rē BŎW-ĕl dĭ-ZĒZ	_____
inguinal hernia (160)	ĬNG-wă-năl HĔR-nē-ă	_____
intussusception (160)	ĭn-tŭs-sŭs-SĔP-shŭn	_____
irritable bowel syndrome (161)	ĬR-ĭh-tăl-bil BŎW-ĕl SĬN-drōm	_____
jaundice (155)	JĂWN-dĭs	_____
melena (155)	MĔl-ĕh-nă or mĕ-LĒ-nă	_____
nausea (155)	NĂW-zē-ă	_____
oral leukoplakia (156)	ŎR-ăl lū-kō-PLĀ-kē-ă	_____
pancreatitis (163)	păn-krē-ă-TĪ-tĭs	_____
periodontal disease (156)	pĕr-ē-ō-DŎN-tăl dĭ-ZĒZ	_____
ulcer (161)	ŬL-sĕr	_____
ulcerative colitis (161)	ŬL-sĕr-ă-tĭv kō-LĪ-tĭs	_____
viral hepatitis (163)	VĪ-răl hĕp-ă-TĪ-tĭs	_____
volvulus (161)	VŎL-vū-lŭs	_____

NOTE: The review sheet for this chapter is combined with the review sheet for Chapter 6 on page 200.

CHAPTER 6

Additional Suffixes and Digestive System Terminology

This chapter is divided into the following sections

In this chapter you will

- Define new suffixes and use them with digestive system combining forms;
- List and explain laboratory tests, clinical procedures, and abbreviations common to the digestive system;
- Apply your new knowledge to understanding medical terms in their proper context, such as in medical reports and records.

I. Introduction

This chapter will give you practice in word building, while not introducing a large number of new terms. It is designed to give you a breather after a long and difficult chapter.

Study the new suffixes in Section II first and complete the meanings of the terms in Sections II and III. Checking the meanings of the terms with a dictionary may prove helpful and add additional understanding.

The information included in Section IV (Laboratory Tests, Clinical Procedures, and Abbreviations) should be useful to those of you who work in laboratory or clinical areas and should also serve as a helpful reference.

Section V (Practical Applications) is designed to give you examples of medical language in context. Congratulate yourself as you decipher medical sentences, operation reports, case studies, and other material. You may also find this section useful in class as an oral reading exercise.

II. Suffixes

Write the meaning of the medical term in the space provided.

Suffix	Meaning	Terminology	Meaning
-ectasis, -ectasia	stretching, dilation, dilatation	bronchiectasis _____ *Bronchi/o means bronchial tubes.* lymphangiectasia _____	
-emesis	vomiting	hematemesis _____	
-lysis	destruction, breakdown, separation	hemolysis _____ *Red blood cells are destroyed.*	
-pepsia	digestion	dyspepsia _____	
-phagia	eating, swallowing	polyphagia _____ *Appetite is increased.* dysphagia _____ odynophagia _____ *Pain (odyn/o) caused by swallowing.*	

-plasty	surgical repair	rhinoplasty _____
		blepharoplasty _____
-ptosis	prolapse, fall, sag	proptosis _____

Pro- means before, forward. This term refers to the forward protrusion of the eye (exophthalmos).

| **-ptysis** | spitting | hemoptysis _____ |

From the respiratory tract and lungs.

| **-rrhagia, -rrhage** | bursting forth of blood | hemorrhage _____ |
| | | menorrhagia _____ |

Men/o means menstrual flow or menstruation. Menorrhagia is excessive bleeding at the time of menstruation.

| **-rrhaphy** | suture | herniorrhaphy _____ |

Herni/o means hernia. The hernia is repaired.

-rrhea	flow, discharge	dysmenorrhea _____
-spasm	sudden, involuntary contraction of muscles	pylorospasm _____
		bronchospasm _____
-stasis	stopping, controlling	cholestasis _____
		hemostasis _____
-stenosis	tightening, stricture, narrowing	pyloric stenosis _____

A narrowed lumen (space within a tubular structure).

| **-tresia** | opening | atresia _____ |

A structure that should be open is closed.

esophageal atresia _____

A congenital anomaly in which the esophagus does not connect with the stomach. It is commonly accompanied by a tracheoesophageal fistula.

biliary atresia _____

Congenital hypoplasia or nonformation of bile ducts resulting in jaundice.

Many of the suffixes that are listed above are also used alone as separate terms. They are listed below with examples of how the term would be used in a sentence.

ectasia	Mammary duct **ectasia** may cause mastitis.
lysis	The disease caused **lysis** of liver cells.
emesis (emetic)	If a child swallows poison, a drug to induce **emesis** is prescribed. A strong solution of salt or ipecac syrup is an example of an emetic.
ptosis	Mr. Smith's weakened eyelid muscles caused **ptosis** of his lids.
spasm	Eating spicy foods can lead to **spasm** of gastric sphincters.
stasis	Overgrowth of bacteria within the small intestine causes **stasis** of the intestinal contents.
stenosis	Projectile vomiting in an infant during feeding is a symptom of pyloric **stenosis.**

III. Combining Forms and Terminology

Write the meaning of the combining form and then the meaning of the term that includes that combining form in the spaces provided.

Combining Form	Meaning	Terminology	Meaning
bucc/o	_____	buccal _____	
cec/o	_____	cecal volvulus _____	
celi/o	_____	celiac artery _____	
		Carries blood from the aorta to the abdomen.	
cheil/o	_____	cheilosis _____	
chol/e	_____	cholelithiasis _____	
cholangi/o	_____	cholangiectasis _____	
cholecyst/o	_____	cholecystectomy _____	
choledoch/o	_____	choledochal _____	

col/o	_____	colectomy _____
colon/o	_____	colonoscopy _____
dent/i	_____	dentalgia _____
duoden/o	_____	gastroduodenal anastomosis _____
		_____
enter/o	_____	gastroenteritis _____
esophag/o	_____	esophageal atresia _____

A congenital anomaly that must be corrected surgically.

gastr/o	_____	gastrojejunostomy _____
gingiv/o	_____	gingivectomy _____
gloss/o	_____	glossopharyngeal _____
glyc/o	_____	glycolysis _____
hepat/o	_____	hepatomegaly _____
herni/o	_____	herniorrhaphy _____
ile/o	_____	ileostomy _____
jejun/o	_____	cholecystojejunostomy _____
labi/o	_____	labioglossopharyngeal _____
lingu/o	_____	sublingual _____
lip/o	_____	lipase _____
lith/o	_____	cholecystolithiasis _____
odont/o	_____	periodontal membrane _____
or/o	_____	oropharynx _____

The tonsils are in the oropharynx.

| palat/o | _____ | palatoplasty _____ |

This surgical procedure is performed to correct a congenital anomaly called cleft (split) palate.

pancreat/o _____   pancreatic _____

proct/o _____   proctosigmoidoscopy _____

pylor/o _____   pyloric stenosis _____

rect/o _____   rectosigmoidectomy _____

sialaden/o _____   sialadenectomy _____

splen/o _____   splenic flexure _____

The bend in the transverse colon downward near the spleen.

steat/o _____   steatorrhea _____

stomat/o _____   aphthous stomatitis _____

IV. Laboratory Tests, Clinical Procedures, and Abbreviations

Laboratory Tests

Liver Function Tests

ALT (alanine transaminase); called also **SGPT**
AST (aspartate transaminase); called also **SGOT**

Both tests reveal levels of enzymes (transaminases) in the blood serum. Serum is the clear fluid that remains after blood has clotted. These enzymes are normally present in many tissues, but levels are elevated when liver cells are damaged. A high **ALT** is especially indicative of acute damage to liver cells (as in hepatitis). High serum levels of **AST** may indicate damage to liver cells and also to muscle tissue, such as in a myocardial infarction, or heart attack.

alkaline phosphatase

This is another blood serum enzyme test. An increased level of alkaline phosphatase **(alk phos)** is found in liver disease, cancers, and other abnormal conditions.

serum bilirubin; called also **icterus index**

High levels of bilirubin in the blood are associated with jaundice in a patient. A **direct bilirubin** test measures conjugated bilirubin (combined with a substance in the liver). High levels indicate liver disease or obstruction of the biliary tract. An **indirect bilirubin** test measures unconjugated bilirubin (not yet combined in the liver). Increased levels are found in hepatic disease and with excessive hemolysis (as may occur in a newborn).

Stool Analyses

stool culture

Feces are placed in a growth medium to test for microorganisms that are abnormally present or are present in large numbers.

stool guaiac or **Hemoccult test**　　Test to determine the presence of blood in the feces and an important screening test for colon cancer. **Guaiac** (GWĪ-ăk) is a chemical from the wood of trees. It is added to a stool sample and reacts with occult (hidden) blood.

Clinical Procedures

X-Ray Tests

lower gastrointestinal series (barium enema)　　Radiologists inject barium sulfate, a contrast medium (substance that x-rays cannot penetrate) by enema into the rectum, and x-rays are taken of the rectum and colon. Figure 6–1A shows a barium enema of a colon with diverticulosis.

upper gastrointestinal series (barium swallow)　　Barium sulfate is swallowed and x-rays are taken of the esophagus, stomach, and small intestine. Often performed immediately after an upper gastrointestinal series, a **small-bowel follow-through** shows sequential x-ray pictures of the small intestine as barium passes through (Fig. 6–1B).

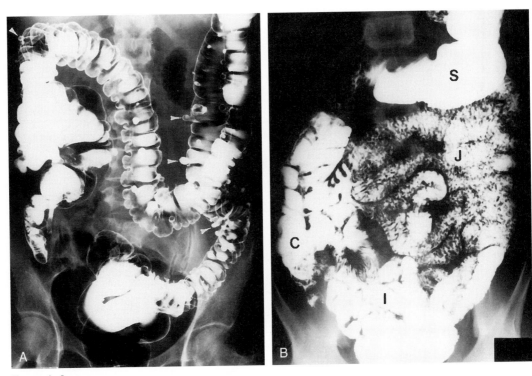

Figure 6-1

(A) Barium enema. This x-ray record of a barium enema with air contrast demonstrates diverticulosis. The arrowheads point to the diverticula throughout the colon. The majority of patients with diverticula are asymptomatic, but complications (diverticulitis, perforated diverticulum, obstruction, or hemorrhage) may occur. **(B)** An x-ray record of a **small-bowel follow-through** demonstrating the normal appearance of the jejunum (J) in the left upper abdomen and of the ileum (I) in the right lower abdomen. There is also contrast within the stomach (S) and cecum (C). (From Heuman DM, Mills AS, and McGuire HH: Gastroenterology. Philadelphia, WB Saunders, 1997, pages 120 and 110.)

cholangiography

X-ray images are taken after injecting contrast material into bile ducts. Contrast can be injected by putting a needle through the abdominal wall into the liver **(percutaneous transhepatic cholangiography)** or by endoscopically inserting a catheter (tube) retrograde (in a direction that is the reverse of the normal flow) into the biliary system **(endoscopic retrograde cholangiopancreatography, or ERCP)** (Fig. 6–2A and B). These invasive techniques also allow diagnostic or therapeutic measures such as sampling for cytology, dilatation of strictures (narrowed areas), and removal of stones.

computed tomography; also called **CT** or **CT scan**

A series of x-ray pictures is taken and processed by a computer to show a cross-sectional (transverse or axial) image of internal organs. A circular array of x-ray beams produces the cross-sectional image based upon differences in tissue densities. Contrast material also is introduced to visualize the GI tract, blood vessels, and organs (Fig. 6–3A, B, and C). **Tomography** (tom/o means to cut) is an x-ray procedure in which a *series* of x-ray pictures is taken to see multiple views of an organ.

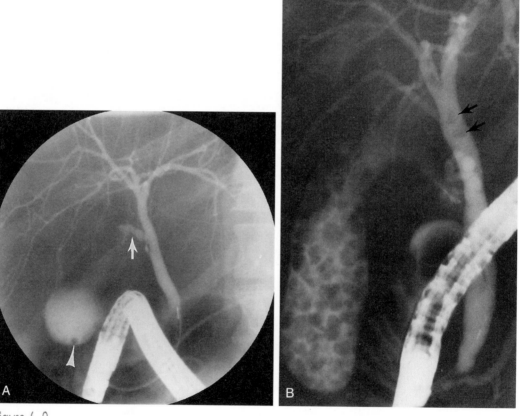

Figure 6–2

(A) Endoscopic retrograde cholangiopancreatography (ERCP) demonstrating normal bile ducts. Note the small stone (arrowhead) in the gallbladder, which is partially opacified through the cystic duct (arrow). **(B) ERCP showing choledocholithiasis** in a patient with biliary colic (pain). Multiple stones are visible in the gallbladder and common bile duct. The stones (arrows) are seen as filling defects in the contrast-opacified gallbladder and duct. (From Heuman DM, Mills AS, and McGuire HH: Gastroenterology. Philadelphia, WB Saunders, 1997, page 87.)

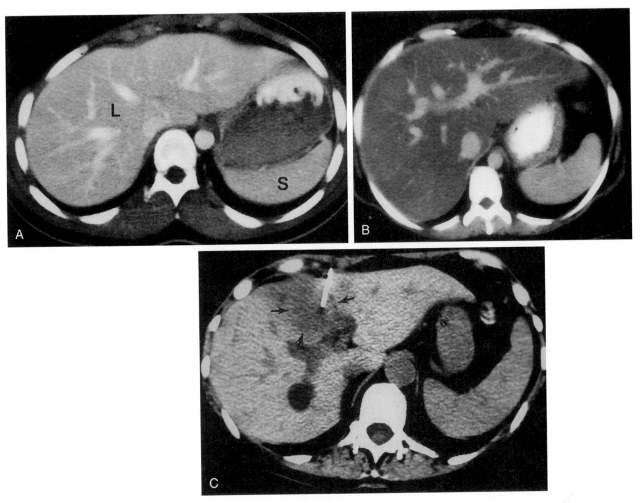

Figure 6-3

Computed tomographic images of normal and diseased liver. **(A) Normal liver.** Contrast material has been injected intravenously, making blood vessels appear bright. The liver (L) and spleen (S) are the same density. **(B) Fatty liver.** The radiodensity of the liver tissue is reduced because of the large volume of fat contained in the tissue, making it appear darker than normal. Compare to the spleen. **(C) CT-guided needle aspiration biopsy of a liver lesion.** The lesion (arrows) has a lower density than the surrounding liver. A needle has been placed into the liver tissue and its tip can be seen in the center of the lesion. Microscopic examination of material aspirated from the lesion revealed it to be a hepatocellular carcinoma. CT-guided needle placement can also be used to insert a catheter for drainage of a liver abscess (a collection of infection and pus). (From Heuman DM, Mills AS, and McGuire HH: Gastroenterology. Philadelphia, WB Saunders, 1997, page 166.)

Ultrasound

abdominal ultrasonography (ultrasound or sonography)

Sound waves are beamed into the abdomen, and a record is made of the echoes as they bounce off abdominal viscera. Ultrasonography is especially useful for examination of fluid-filled structures such as the gallbladder.

magnetic resonance imaging (MRI)

This is a noninvasive and non–x-ray diagnostic technique in which a patient is subjected to a strong magnetic field, and images are produced from subtle differences in tissue composition. Images in all three planes (3-dimensional) are possible and cross-sectional images are particularly helpful to show abdominal structures.

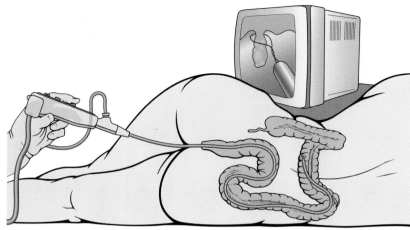

Figure 6-4

Colonoscopy and polypectomy. Prior to this procedure, agents are given to clean the bowel of feces. The patient is sedated and the gastroenterologist advances the instrument retrograde, guided by images from a video camera on the tip of the colonoscope. When a polyp is located, a wire snare is passed through the endoscope and looped around the stalk. After the loop is gently tightened, an electric current is applied to cut through the stalk. The polyp is removed for microscopic examination (biopsy).

Radioactive

liver scan   Radioactive material (radioisotope) is injected intravenously and taken up by the liver cells. An image of the liver (scintiscan) is made using a special scanner (gamma camera) that records the uptake of radioactive material by the liver cells.

Other Procedures

gastrointestinal endoscopy   A flexible fiberoptic tube is placed through the mouth or anus to visualize parts of the gastrointestinal tract. *Examples:* **esophagogastroduodenoscopy, colonoscopy** (Fig. 6–4), flexible **sigmoidoscopy,** rigid **proctoscopy,** and **anoscopy.** A patient with a family history of gastrointestinal cancer should relate this information to his or her gastroenterologist so that the appropriate type of endoscopy is performed.

liver biopsy   A needle is inserted percutaneously into the liver, and a sample of liver tissue is removed for microscopic examination. A local anesthetic is injected into the skin overlying the liver so that insertion of the needle is relatively painless. The average sample is less than 1 inch long. This procedure is useful in diagnosis of cirrhosis, chronic hepatitis, and tumors.

nasogastric intubation   A nasogastric tube (NG tube) is passed through the nose into the stomach and upper region of the small intestine. The procedure is used to remove fluid postoperatively and to obtain gastric or intestinal contents for analysis.

paracentesis (abdominocentesis)   Surgical puncture to remove fluid from the abdomen (peritoneal cavity). This procedure is performed to remove fluid from a patient with ascites and for diagnostic purposes.

ABBREVIATIONS

ALP	alkaline phosphatase	**IBD**	inflammatory bowel disease
ALT, AST	alanine transaminase, aspartate transaminase (enzyme tests of liver function)	**LFTs**	liver function tests; ALP, bilirubin, AST (SGOT), ALT (SGPT)
		MRI	magnetic resonance imaging
BE	barium enema	**NG tube**	nasogastric tube
BRBPR	bright red blood per (through) rectum; hematochezia	**NPO**	nothing by mouth (*nulla per os*)
BM	bowel movement	**PEG tube**	percutaneous endoscopic gastrostomy tube (feeding tube)
CT scan	computed tomography	**PEJ tube**	percutaneous endoscopic jejunostomy tube (feeding tube)
EGD	esophagogastroduodenoscopy		
ERCP	endoscopic retrograde cholangiopancreatography	**PUD**	peptic ulcer disease
		SGOT, SGPT	enzyme tests of liver function
GB	gallbladder	**TPN**	total parenteral nutrition
GERD	gastroesophageal reflux disease		This intravenous (IV) solution contains sugar (dextrose), proteins (amino acids), electrolytes (sodium, potassium, chloride), and vitamins.
GI	gastrointestinal		
HBV	hepatitis B virus		

V. Practical Applications

This section contains an actual medical report using terms that you have studied in this and previous chapters. Explanations of more difficult terms are added in brackets. Questions based on your reading of the report follow. Check your answers on page 197, Answers to Practical Applications.

Colonoscopy Report

The patient is a 73-year-old female who underwent colonoscopy and polypectomy on June 10, 1997. Biopsy revealed an invasive carcinoma, and on June 12, 1997, she underwent a low anterior resection and coloproctostomy. Sixteen months later, on August 2, 1998, she was seen in the office for flexible sigmoidoscopy, and a polyp was detected. Colonoscopy was scheduled.

Description of Procedure. The fiberoptic colonoscope was introduced, and I could pass it to about 15 cm, at which point there appeared to be an anastomosis. The colonoscope passed easily through a wide-open anastomosis to 30 cm, at which point a very friable [easily crumbled] polyp, irregular, on a short little stalk, was encountered. This was snared, the coagulating [blood clotting] current was applied, and the pedicle [stalk of the polyp] was severed and recovered and sent to pathology for histological identification. The colonoscope was then reintroduced and passed through the rectum to the sigmoid colon. Again the

Continued on following page

anastomosis was seen, and proximal to this, the fulgurated [destroyed by high-frequency electric current] base of the removed polyp could be seen. No bleeding was encountered, and I continued to advance the colonoscope through the descending colon. I proceeded to advance the colonoscope through the splenic flexure in the transverse colon. In spite of vigorous mechanical bowel preparation and the shortened colon from the previous resection, she had a considerable amount of stool, and it became progressively more difficult to visualize as I approached the hepatic flexure. Finally, at the hepatic flexure, I abandoned further evaluation and began to withdraw the colonoscope. The colonoscope passed through the transverse colon, splenic flexure, descending colon, sigmoid colon, rectum, and anus and was withdrawn. She tolerated the procedure well, but had some nausea. I will await the results of pathology, and in the event that it is not an invasive carcinoma, I would recommend a repeat colonoscopy in 6 months, at which time we will use a 48-hour, more vigorous mechanical bowel preparation.

Questions about the Colonoscopy Report

1. On June 10th, the initial procedure that the patient underwent was
   A. Anastomosis of two parts of the colon
   B. Visual examination of the rectum and anus
   C. Visual examination of the large bowel and removal of a growth
   D. Resection of a portion of the colon

2. On June 12th the patient had additional surgery to
   A. Remove a portion of the colon and reattach the cut end to the rectum
   B. Join two parts of the small intestine
   C. Reconnect the colon to the small intestine
   D. Remove a portion of the distal end of the small intestine

3. Which term in the report refers to an anastomosis?
   A. Sigmoidoscopy
   B. Colonoscopy
   C. Low anterior resection
   D. Coloproctostomy

4. Why was it impossible to visualize the entire colon?
   A. The patient experienced nausea
   B. Feces were blocking the colon
   C. Tumor was blocking the colon
   D. The hepatic flexure was twisted

VI. Exercises

Remember to check your answers carefully with those given in Section VII, Answers to Exercises.

A. Give the meanings of the following suffixes.

1. -pepsia _____

2. -ptysis _____

3. -emesis _____

4. -phagia _____

5. -ptosis _____

6. -rrhea _____

7. -rrhagia _____

8. -rrhaphy _____

9. -plasty _____

10. -lysis _____

11. -ectasis _____

12. -stenosis _____

13. -stasis _____

14. -spasm _____

15. -ectasia _____

B. *Using the suffixes listed in exercise A and the following combining forms, build medical terms.*

blephar/o
hemat/o
hem/o
pylor/o

chol/e
men/o
rhin/o

lymphangi/o
herni/o
bronch/o

1. painful menstrual flow _____

2. stoppage of bile (flow) _____

3. suture of a hernia _____

4. dilation of lymph vessels _____

5. spitting up blood (from the respiratory tract) _____

6. vomiting blood (from the digestive tract) _____

7. dilation of tubes leading from the windpipe into the lungs _____

8. surgical repair of eyelids _____

9. stopping blood flow _____

10. surgical repair of the nose _____

11. destruction of blood (red blood cells) _____

12. sudden involuntary contraction of muscles at the distal region of the stomach

_____

13. excessive bleeding (bursting forth of blood) during menstruation _____

14. sudden involuntary contraction of muscles within the bronchial tubes _____

C. Give the meanings of the following terms.

1. dysphagia _____

2. polyphagia _____

3. dyspepsia _____

4. biliary atresia _____

5. proptosis _____

6. cholestasis _____

7. esophageal atresia _____

8. odynophagia _____

9. emesis _____

10. stenosis _____

D. Match the following surgical procedures with their meanings below.

herniorrhaphy	blepharoplasty	rectosigmoidectomy
cecostomy	gastroduodenal anastomosis	cholecystectomy
sphincterotomy	colectomy	cholecystojejunostomy
gingivectomy	paracentesis	ileostomy

1. removal of the gallbladder _____

2. large bowel resection _____

3. suture of a weakened muscular wall (hernia) _____

4. new opening of the first part of the colon to the outside of the body _____

5. surgical repair of the eyelid _____

6. incision of a ring of muscles _____

7. new surgical connection between the stomach and the first part of the small intestine

_____

8. opening of the third part of the small intestine to the outside of the body _____

9. removal of gum tissue _____

10. new surgical connection between the gallbladder and the second part of the small intestine

_____

11. surgical puncture of the abdomen for withdrawal of fluid _____

12. removal of the rectum and sigmoid colon _____

E. Complete the following terms based on their meanings.

1. discharge of fat: steat _____

2. difficulty in swallowing: dys _____

3. abnormal condition of gallstones: chole _____

4. pertaining to the cheek: _____ al

5. pain in a tooth: dent _____

6. prolapse of an eyelid: blepharo _____

7. enlargement of the liver: hepato _____

8. pertaining to under the tongue: sub _____

9. removal of the gallbladder: _____ ectomy

10. pertaining to the common bile duct: chole _____

F. Give the meanings of the following terms.

1. cecal volvulus _____

2. aphthous stomatitis _____

3. celiac artery _____

4. lipase _____

5. cheilosis _____

6. oropharynx _____

7. glycolysis _____

8. glossopharyngeal _____

9. sialadenectomy _____

10. periodontal membrane _____

G. Match the name of the laboratory test or clinical procedure with its description.

CT of the abdomen
liver scan
percutaneous transhepatic
    cholangiography
stool guaiac (Hemoccult)

endoscopic retrograde
    cholangiopancreatography
abdominal ultrasonography
serum bilirubin
barium swallow

stool culture
barium enema
nasogastric intubation
liver biopsy

1. measurement of bile pigment in the blood _____

2. feces are placed in a growth medium for bacterial analysis _____

3. x-ray examination of the lower gastrointestinal tract _____

4. sound waves are used to image abdominal organs _____

5. test to reveal hidden blood in feces _____

6. upper gastrointestinal x-rays _____

7. contrast material is injected through the liver and x-rays are taken of bile vessels

    _____

8. tube is inserted through the nose into the stomach _____

9. transverse x-ray pictures of the abdominal organs _____

10. contrast material is injected through an endoscope, and x-ray images of the pancreas and bile

    ducts are taken _____

11. percutaneous removal of liver tissue followed by microscopic examination

    _____

12. radioactive material is injected intravenously, and an image is produced as the material is taken

    up by liver cells _____

H. Give the meanings of the following abbreviations and then select the letter from the sentences that follow that is the best association for each.

Column I

1. TPN _____ ____

2. PUD _____ ____

3. EGD _____ ____

4. IBD _____ ____

5. BE _____ ____

6. BRBPR _____ ____

7. LFTs _____ ____

8. GERD _____ ____

9. HBV _____ ____

10. CT _____ ____

Column II

A. ALT, AST, ALP, and serum bilirubin are examples of these tests.
B. Heartburn is a symptom of this condition.
C. Crohn disease and ulcerative colitis are examples of this general condition.
D. *H. pylori* is an etiological agent of this condition.
E. Intravenous feeding is allowed, but nothing is permitted by mouth (NPO).
F. This is also called a lower gastrointestinal series.
G. In this x-ray procedure, a series of cross-sectional images are taken.
H. This infectious agent causes chronic inflammation of the liver.
I. Hematochezia describes this gastrointestinal symptom.
J. This is an endoscopic visualization of the upper gastrointestinal tract.

I. Give the suffixes for the following terms.

1. hemorrhage _____

2. flow, discharge _____

3. suture _____

4. dilation _____

5. narrowing, stricture _____

6. vomiting _____

7. spitting _____

8. prolapse _____

9. excision _____

10. digestion _____

11. eating, swallowing _____

12. hardening _____

13. stopping, controlling _____

14. surgical repair _____

15. opening _____

16. surgical puncture _____

17. involuntary contraction _____

18. new opening _____

19. incision _____

20. destruction, breakdown _____

J. Circle the correct term in parentheses to complete each sentence.

1. When Mrs. Smith developed diarrhea and crampy abdominal pain, she consulted a **(urologist, nephrologist, gastroenterologist)** and worried that she might have **(inflammatory bowel disease, esophageal varices, achalasia).**

2. After taking a careful history and physical, Dr. Blakemore diagnosed Mr. Bean, a long-time drinker, with **(hemorrhoids, pancreatitis, appendicitis).** Mr. Bean had complained of sharp mid-epigastric pain and a change in bowel habits.

3. Many pregnant women cannot lie flat after eating because of a burning sensation in their chest and throat. Doctors call this condition **(volvulus, dysentery, gastroesophageal reflux).**

4. Pediatric surgeons must be wary of **(inguinal hernia, intussusception, oral leukoplakia)** in young infants who have not had a bowel movement in many days and have projectile vomiting.

5. Boris had terrible problems with his teeth. Not only did he need a periodontist for his **(anorexia, ascites, gingivitis),** but also an **(endodontist, oral surgeon, orthodontist)** to straighten his teeth.

6. After six weeks of radiation therapy to her throat, Betty experienced severe esophageal irritation and inflammation. She complained to her doctor about her **(dyspepsia, odynophagia, hematemesis).**

VII. Answers to Exercises

A

1. digestion
2. spitting (from the respiratory tract)
3. vomiting
4. eating, swallowing
5. prolapse, falling, sagging

6. flow, discharge
7. bursting forth of blood
8. suture
9. surgical repair
10. destruction, breakdown, separation

11. stretching, dilation, dilatation
12. tightening, narrowed lumen, stricture
13. stopping, controlling
14. sudden, involuntary contraction of muscles
15. dilation, stretching, dilatation

B

1. dysmenorrhea
2. cholestasis
3. herniorrhaphy
4. lymphangiectasis
5. hemoptysis

6. hematemesis
7. bronchiectasis
8. blepharoplasty
9. hemostasis
10. rhinoplasty

11. hemolysis
12. pylorospasm
13. menorrhagia
14. bronchospasm

C

1. difficulty in swallowing
2. excessive (much) eating
3. difficult digestion
4. biliary ducts are not open (congenital anomaly)

5. forward prolapse (bulging) of the eyes (exophthalmos)
6. stoppage of flow of bile
7. esophagus is not open (closed off) at birth (congenital anomaly)

8. pain caused by swallowing
9. vomiting
10. tightening, stricture, narrowing

D

1. cholecystectomy
2. colectomy
3. herniorrhaphy
4. cecostomy
5. blepharoplasty

6. sphincterotomy
7. gastroduodenal anastomosis (gastroduodenostomy)—both are acceptable
8. ileostomy

9. gingivectomy
10. cholecystojejunostomy (cholecystojejunal anastomosis)
11. paracentesis (abdominocentesis)
12. rectosigmoidectomy

E

1. steatorrhea
2. dysphagia
3. cholelithiasis
4. buccal

5. dentalgia
6. ptosis
7. hepatomegaly
8. sublingual

9. cholecystectomy
10. choledochal

F

1. twisted intestine in the area of the cecum
2. inflammation of the mouth with small ulcers
3. blood vessel bringing blood to the abdomen
4. enzyme to digest fat
5. abnormal condition of lips
6. the part of the throat near the mouth
7. breakdown of sugar
8. pertaining to the tongue and the throat
9. removal of a salivary gland
10. membrane surrounding a tooth

G

1. serum bilirubin
2. stool culture
3. barium enema
4. abdominal ultrasonography
5. stool guaiac (Hemoccult)
6. barium swallow
7. percutaneous transhepatic cholangiography
8. nasogastric intubation
9. CT scan of the abdomen
10. endoscopic retrograde cholangiopancreatography (ERCP)
11. liver biopsy
12. liver scan

H

1. total parenteral nutrition. E
2. peptic ulcer disease. D
3. esophagoduodenoscopy. J
4. inflammatory bowel disease. C
5. barium enema. F
6. bright red blood per rectum. I
7. liver function tests. A
8. gastroesophageal reflux disease. B
9. hepatitis B virus. H
10. computed tomography. G

I

1. -rrhagia, -rrhage
2. -rrhea
3. -rrhaphy
4. -ectasis, -ectasia
5. -stenosis
6. -emesis
7. -ptysis
8. -ptosis
9. -ectomy
10. -pepsia
11. -phagia
12. -sclerosis
13. -stasis
14. -plasty
15. -tresia
16. -centesis
17. -spasm
18. -stomy
19. -tomy
20. -lysis

J

1. gastroenterologist; inflammatory bowel disease
2. pancreatitis
3. gastroesophageal reflux
4. intussusception
5. gingivitis; orthodontist
6. odynophagia

Answers to Practical Applications

1. C
2. A
3. D
4. B

VIII. Pronunciation of Terms

Pronunciation Guide

ā as in āpe   ă as in ăpple
ē as in ēven   ĕ as in ĕvery
ī as in īce   ĭ as in ĭnterest
ō as in ōpen   ŏ as in pŏt
ū as in ūnit   ŭ as in ŭnder

To test your understanding of the terminology in this chapter, write the meaning of each term in the space provided. In addition, you may wish to cover the terms and write them by looking at your definitions. Make sure your spelling is correct. The page number after each term indicates where it is defined or used in the text so you can easily check your responses.

Term	Pronunciation	Meaning
abdominal ultrasonography (187)	ăb-DŎM-ĭn-ăl ŭl-tră-sō-NŎG-ră-fē	_____
aphthous stomatitis (184)	ĂF-thŭs stō-mă-TĪ-tĭs	_____

atresia (181)	ā-TRĒ-zē-ă	_____
biliary atresia (181)	BĬL-ē-ăr-ē ā-TRĒ-zē-ă	_____
bronchiectasis (180)	brŏng-kē-ĔK-tă-sĭs	_____
buccal (182)	BŬK-ăl	_____
cecal volvulus (182)	SĒ-kăl VŎL-vū-lŭs	_____
celiac artery (182)	SĒ-lē-ăk ĂR-tĕr-ē	_____
cheilosis (182)	kī-LŌ-sis	_____
cholangiectasis (182)	kōl-ăn-jē-ĔK-tă-sĭs	_____
cholangiography (186)	kōl-ăn-jē-ŎG-ră-fē	_____
cholangiopancreatography (186)	kŏl-ăn-jē-ō-păn-krē-ă-TŎG-ră-fē	_____
cholecystectomy (182)	kō-lē-sĭs-TĔK-tō-mē	_____
cholecystojejunostomy (183)	kō-lē-sĭs-tō-jĕ-jŭ-NŎS-tō-mē	_____
cholecystolithiasis (183)	kō-lē-sĭs-tō-lĭ-THĬ-ă-sĭs	_____
choledochal (182)	kō-lē-DŎK-ăl	_____
cholelithiasis (182)	kō-lē-lĭ-THĬ-ă-sĭs	_____
cholestasis (181)	kō-lē-STĀ-sĭs	_____
colectomy (183)	kō-LĔK-tō-mē	_____
colonoscopy (183)	kō-lŏn-ŎS-kō-pē	_____
dentalgia (183)	dĕn-TĂL-jă	_____
dysmenorrhea (181)	dĭs-mĕn-ŏr-RĒ-ă	_____
dyspepsia (180)	dĭs-PĔP-sē-ă	_____
dysphagia (180)	dĭs-FĀ-jē-ă	_____
esophageal atresia (181)	ĕ-sŏf-ă-JĒ-ăl ā-TRĒ-zē-ă	_____
gastroduodenal anastomosis (183)	găs-trō-dū-ō-DĒ-năl ă-nă-stō-MŌ-sĭs	_____
gastroenteritis (183)	găs-trō-ĕn-tĕ-RĪ-tĭs	_____
gastrointestinal endoscopy (188)	găs-trō-ĭn-TĔS-tĭn-ăl ĕn-DŎS-kō-pē	_____
gastrojejunostomy (183)	găs-trō-jĕ-jŭ-NŎS-tō-mē	_____

gingivectomy (183)	gĭn-gĭ-VĔK-tō-mē	_____
glossopharyngeal (183)	glŏs-ō-fă-rĭn-GĒ-al	_____
glycolysis (183)	glī-KŎL-ĭ-sis	_____
hematemesis (180)	hē-mă-TĔM-ĕh-sĭs	_____
hemolysis (180)	hē-MŎL-ĭ-sĭs	_____
hemoptysis (181)	hē-MŎP-tĭ-sĭs	_____
hemorrhage (181)	HĔM-ŏr-ĭj	_____
hemostasis (181)	hē-mō-STĀ-sĭs	_____
hepatomegaly (183)	hĕp-ă-tō-MĔG-ă-lē	_____
herniorrhaphy (181)	hĕr-nē-ŎR-ă-fē	_____
ileostomy (183)	ĭl-ē-ŎS-tō-mē	_____
labioglossopharyngeal (183)	lā-bē-ō-glŏs-ō-fă-RĬN-jē-ăl	_____
lipase (183)	LĪ-pās	_____
lymphangiectasia (180)	lĭm-făn-jē-ĕk-TĀ-zē-ă	_____
menorrhagia (181)	mĕn-ŏr-RĀ-jă	_____
odynophagia (180)	ō-dĭn-ō-FĀ-jē-ă	_____
oropharynx (183)	ŏr-ō-FĂR-ĭnks	_____
palatoplasty (183)	PĂL-ă-tō-plăs-tē	_____
pancreatic (184)	păn-krē-ĂH-tĭk	_____
periodontal membrane (183)	pĕr-ē-ō-DŎN-tăl MĔM-brān	_____
polyphagia (180)	pŏl-ē-FĀ-jē-ă	_____
proctosigmoidoscopy (184)	prŏk-tō-sĭg-mŏyd-ŎS-kō-pē	_____
proptosis (181)	prŏp-TŌ-sĭs	_____
pyloric stenosis (184)	pī-LŎR-ĭk stĕ-NŌ-sĭs	_____
pylorospasm (181)	pī-LŎR-ō-spăsm	_____
rectosigmoidectomy (184)	rĕk-tō-sĭg-mŏy-DĔK-tō-mē	_____
rhinoplasty (181)	rī-nō-PLĂS-tē	_____
splenic flexure (184)	SPLĔ-nĭk FLĔK-shŭr	_____

IX. Review Sheet

Write meanings for combining forms and suffixes in the space provided. Check your answers with information in Chapters 5 and 6 or in the Glossary (Medical Terms—English) at the end of the book.

COMBINING FORMS

Combining Form	Meaning	Combining Form	Meaning
amyl/o		col/o	
an/o		colon/o	
append/o		dent/i	
appendic/o		duoden/o	
bil/i		enter/o	
bilirubin/o		esophag/o	
bronch/o		eti/o	
bucc/o		gastr/o	
cec/o		gingiv/o	
celi/o		gloss/o	
cervic/o		gluc/o	
cheil/o		glyc/o	
chlorhydr/o		glycogen/o	
cholangi/o		hem/o	
chol/e		hemat/o	
cholecyst/o		hepat/o	
choledoch/o		herni/o	
cib/o		idi/o	
cirrh/o		ile/o	

jejun/o	_____	pancreat/o	_____
labi/o	_____	peritone/o	_____
lapar/o	_____	pharyng/o	_____
lingu/o	_____	proct/o	_____
lip/o	_____	prote/o	_____
lith/o	_____	pylor/o	_____
lymphangi/o	_____	rect/o	_____
mandibul/o	_____	sialaden/o	_____
men/o	_____	sigmoid/o	_____
necr/o	_____	splen/o	_____
odont/o	_____	steat/o	_____
odyn/o	_____	stomat/o	_____
or/o	_____	tonsill/o	_____
palat/o	_____		

SUFFIXES

Suffix	Meaning	Suffix	Meaning
-ase	_____	-emia	_____
-centesis	_____	-genesis	_____
-chezia	_____	-graphy	_____
-ectasia	_____	-iasis	_____
-ectasis	_____	-lysis	_____
-ectomy	_____	-megaly	_____
-emesis	_____	-orexia	_____

Continued on following page

-pathy _____

-pepsia _____

-phagia _____

-plasty _____

-prandial _____

-ptosis _____

-ptysis _____

-rrhage _____

-rrhagia _____

-rrhaphy _____

-rrhea _____

-scopy _____

-spasm _____

-stasis _____

-stenosis _____

-stomy _____

-tomy _____

-tresia _____

CHAPTER 7

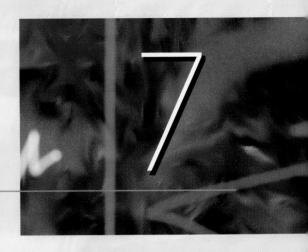

Urinary System

This chapter is divided into the following sections

In this chapter you will
- Name the organs of the urinary system and describe their locations and functions;
- Give the meaning of various pathological conditions affecting the system;
- Recognize the use and interpretation of urinalysis as a diagnostic test;
- Detail the meanings of combining forms, prefixes, and suffixes of the system's terminology;
- List and explain some clinical procedures, laboratory tests, and abbreviations that pertain to the urinary system; and
- Apply your new knowledge to understanding medical terms in their proper contexts, such as medical reports and records.

I. Introduction

You have just learned how food is brought into the bloodstream by the digestive system. In a future chapter you will learn how oxygen is brought into the bloodstream by the respiratory system. Food and oxygen are combined in the cells of the body to produce energy (catabolism). In the process, however, the substance of the food and oxygen is not destroyed. Instead, the small particles of which the food and oxygen are made are actually rearranged into new combinations. These are waste products. When foods like sugars and fats, which contain particles of carbon, hydrogen, and oxygen, combine with oxygen in cells, the wastes produced are gases called carbon dioxide (carbon and oxygen) and water (hydrogen and oxygen) in the form of vapor. These gases are removed from the body by exhalation through the lungs.

Foods composed of protein are more complicated than sugars and fats. They contain carbon, hydrogen, and oxygen **plus** nitrogen and other elements. The waste that is produced when proteins combine with oxygen is called **nitrogenous waste,** and it is more difficult to excrete (to separate out) from the body than are gases like carbon dioxide and water vapor.

The body cannot efficiently put the nitrogenous waste into a gaseous form and exhale it, so it excretes it in the form of a soluble (dissolved in water) waste substance called **urea.** The major function of the urinary system is to remove urea from the bloodstream so that it does not accumulate in the body and become toxic.

Urea is formed in the liver from ammonia, which in turn is derived from the breakdown of simple proteins (amino acids) in the body cells. The urea is carried in the bloodstream to the kidneys, where it passes with water, salts, and acids out of the bloodstream and into the kidney tubules as **urine.** Urine then travels down the ureters into the bladder and out of the body.

Besides removing urea from the blood, another important function of the kidneys is to maintain the proper balance of water, salts, and acids in the body fluids. Salts, such as **sodium** and **potassium,** and some acids are known as **electrolytes** (small molecules that conduct an electrical charge). Electrolytes are necessary for the proper functioning of muscle and nerve cells. The kidney adjusts the amounts of water and electrolytes by secreting some substances into the urine and holding back others in the bloodstream for use in the body.

In addition to forming urine and eliminating it from the body, the kidneys also act as endocrine organs, secreting into the bloodstream substances that act at some distant site in the body. Examples of the kidneys' endocrine function include the secretion of **renin** (RĒ-nĭn), a substance important in the control of blood pressure, and **erythropoietin** (erythr/o = red, -poietin = substance that forms), a hormone that regulates the production of red blood cells. The kidneys also secrete an active form of vitamin D, necessary for the absorption of calcium from the intestine. In addition, hormones such as insulin and parathyroid hormone are degraded and extracted from the bloodstream by the kidney.

II. Anatomy of the Major Organs

The organs of the urinary system are (label Figure 7–1 as you read these paragraphs):

Two **kidneys** [1]—bean-shaped organs situated behind the abdominal cavity (retroperitoneal) on either side of the vertebral column in the lumbar region of the spine. The kidneys are embedded in a cushion of adipose tissue and surrounded by fibrous connective tissue for protection. They are fist-sized and weigh about 4 to 6 ounces each.

The kidneys consist of an outer **cortex** region (cortex means outer portion or bark, as the bark of a tree) and an inner **medulla** region (medulla means marrow or inner portion). The depression on the medial border of the kidney, through which blood vessels and nerves pass, is called the **hilum.**

Two **ureters** [2]—muscular tubes (16 to 18 inches long) lined with mucous membranes. They convey urine in peristaltic waves from the kidneys to the urinary bladder.

The **urinary bladder** [3]—a hollow, muscular, distensible sac in the pelvic cavity. It serves as a temporary reservoir for urine. The **trigone** is a triangular space at the base of the bladder where the ureters enter and the urethra exits.

The **urethra** [4]—a membranous tube through which urine is discharged from the urinary bladder. The process of expelling **(voiding)** urine through the urethra is called

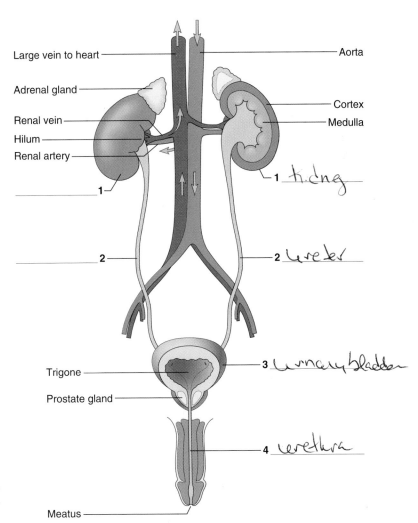

Large vein to heart

Aorta

Adrenal gland

Cortex

Renal vein

Medulla

Hilum

Renal artery

1— kidney

2— ureter

3— urinary bladder

Trigone

Prostate gland

4— urethra

Meatus

Figure 7–1

Organs of the urinary system in a male.

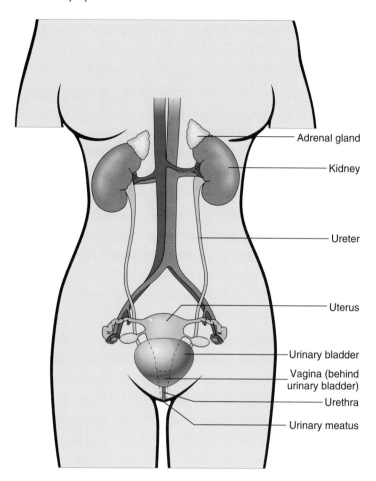

Figure 7–2

Female urinary system.

micturition. The external opening of the urethra is called the urethral or urinary **meatus.** The female urethra is about 1½ inches long, lying anterior to the vagina and vaginal meatus. The male urethra is about 8 inches long and extends downward through the prostate gland to the meatus at the tip of the penis. Figure 7–2 illustrates the female urinary system. Compare it with Figure 7–1, which shows the male urinary system.

III. How the Kidneys Produce Urine

Blood enters each kidney from the aorta by way of the right and left **renal arteries.** After the renal artery enters the kidney (at the hilum), the artery branches into smaller and smaller arteries. The smallest arteries are called **arterioles,** and these are located throughout the cortex of the kidney (Fig. 7–3A).

Because the arterioles are small, blood passes through them slowly, but constantly. Blood flow through the kidney is so essential that the kidneys have their own special device for maintaining blood flow. If blood pressure falls in the vessels of the kidney, so that blood flow is diminished, the kidney produces **renin** and discharges it into the blood. Renin leads to the formation of a substance that stimulates the contraction of arterioles so that blood pressure is increased and blood flow in the kidneys is restored to normal.

Each arteriole in the cortex of the kidney leads into a mass of very tiny, coiled and intertwined smaller blood vessels called **capillaries.** The collection of capillaries, shaped in the form of a tiny ball, is called a **glomerulus.** There are about 1 million glomeruli in the cortex region of each kidney.

The kidneys produce urine by a process of **filtration.** As blood passes through the many glomeruli, the walls of each glomerulus (the filter) are thin enough to permit water, salts, sugar, and **urea** (with other nitrogenous wastes such as **creatinine** and **uric acid**) to leave the bloodstream. These materials are collected in a tiny, cup-like structure called a **Bowman capsule,** which surrounds each glomerulus (Fig. 7–3B). The walls of the glomeruli prevent large substances such as proteins and blood cells from filtering into the Bowman capsule. These substances remain in the blood and normally do not appear in urine.

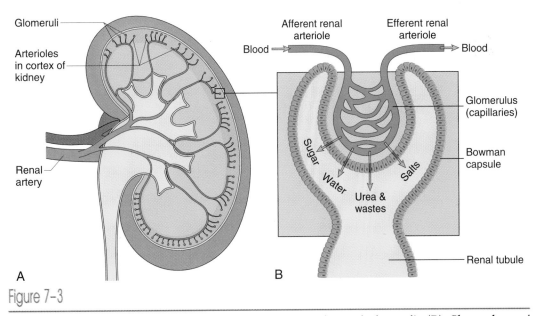

Figure 7-3

(A) Renal artery branching to form smaller arteries, arterioles, and glomeruli. **(B) Glomerulus** and **Bowman capsule**. Afferent arteriole carries blood toward (af-) the glomerulus. Efferent arteriole carries blood away (ef-) from the glomerulus.

Attached to each Bowman capsule is a long, twisted tube called a **renal tubule** (Figs. 7–3B and 7–4). As water, sugar, salts, urea, and other wastes pass through the renal tubule, most of the water, all of the sugar, and some salts (such as sodium) return to the bloodstream through tiny capillaries surrounding each tubule. This **reabsorption** ensures that the body retains essential substances such as sugar, water, and salts. The final process in the formation of urine is the **secretion** of some substances from the bloodstream into the renal tubule. Most are waste products of metabolism that become toxic if allowed to accumulate in the body. This is the method by which acids, drugs (such as penicillin), and potassium (a salt) are eliminated in urine.

Thus, only wastes, water, salts, acids, and some drugs remain in the renal tubule. Each renal tubule, now containing urine (95 per cent water, 5 per cent urea, creatinine, salts, acids, and drugs), ends in a larger collecting tubule. See Figure 7–4, which reviews the steps involved in urine formation.

Thousands of collecting tubules lead to the **renal pelvis,** a basin-like area in the central part of the kidney. Small, cup-like regions of the renal pelvis are called **calices** or **calyces** (singular: **calix** or **calyx**). Figure 7–5 illustrates a section of the kidney and shows the renal pelvis and calices.

The renal pelvis narrows into the **ureter,** which carries the urine to the **urinary bladder** where the urine is temporarily stored. The exit area of the bladder to the **urethra** is closed by sphincters that do not permit urine to leave the bladder. As the bladder fills up, pressure is placed on the base of the bladder, which causes the desire to urinate.

Study the flow diagram in Figure 7–6 to trace the process of forming urine and expelling it from the body.

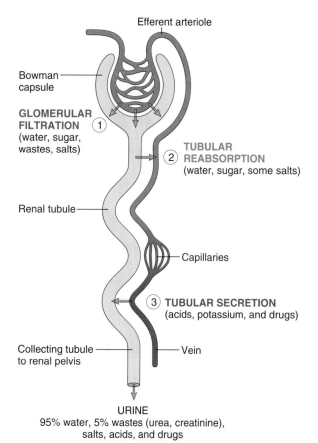

Efferent arteriole

Bowman capsule

GLOMERULAR FILTRATION ① (water, sugar, wastes, salts)

Renal tubule

TUBULAR REABSORPTION ② (water, sugar, some salts)

Capillaries

③ TUBULAR SECRETION (acids, potassium, and drugs)

Collecting tubule to renal pelvis — Vein

URINE
95% water, 5% wastes (urea, creatinine), salts, acids, and drugs

Figure 7-4

Three steps in the formation of urine. (1) Glomerular filtration of water, sugar, wastes (urea and creatinine), and salts. **(2) Tubular reabsorption** of water, sugar, and some salts. **(3) Tubular secretion** of acids, potassium, and drugs.

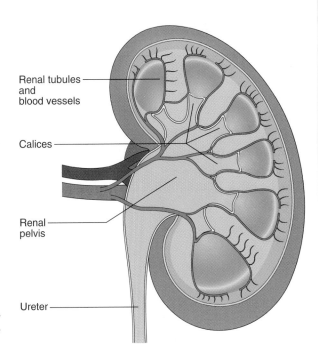

Renal tubules and blood vessels

Calices

Renal pelvis

Ureter

Figure 7-5

Section of the kidney showing renal pelvis, calices, and ureter.

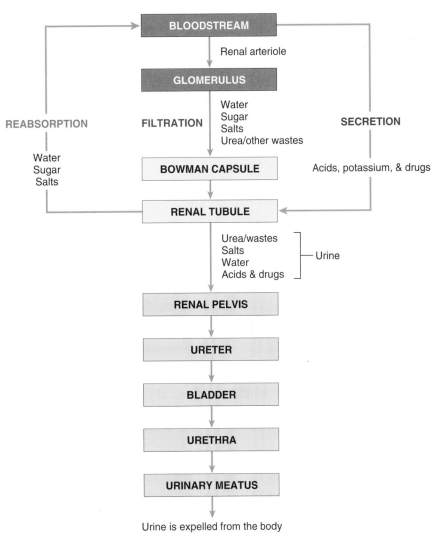

BLOODSTREAM

Renal arteriole

GLOMERULUS

REABSORPTION   FILTRATION   Water   SECRETION
                             Sugar
                             Salts
                             Urea/other wastes

Water   Acids, potassium, & drugs
Sugar   BOWMAN CAPSULE
Salts

                 RENAL TUBULE

                 Urea/wastes
                 Salts   ⎤
                 Water   ⎬ Urine
                 Acids & drugs ⎦

                 RENAL PELVIS

                 URETER

                 BLADDER

                 URETHRA

                 URINARY MEATUS

Urine is expelled from the body

Figure 7-6

Flow diagram illustrating the process of forming and expelling urine.

IV. Vocabulary

arteriole	A small artery.
Bowman capsule	A cup-shaped capsule surrounding each glomerulus.
calix or **calyx** (plural: **calices** or **calyces**)	Cup-like collecting region of the renal pelvis.
catheter	A tube for injecting or removing fluids.
cortex	Outer region; the renal cortex is the outer region of the kidney (**cortical** means pertaining to the cortex).
creatinine	A waste product of muscle metabolism; nitrogenous waste excreted in urine.
electrolyte	A chemical that carries an electrical charge in a solution.
erythropoietin	A hormone secreted by the kidney to stimulate the production of red blood cells.
filtration	Process whereby some substances, but not all, pass through a filter or other material. Blood pressure forces materials through the filter. About 180 quarts of fluid are filtered from the blood daily, but the kidney returns 98–99 per cent of the water and salts. Only about 1½ quarts (1500 mL) of urine are excreted daily.
glomerulus (plural: **glomeruli**)	Tiny ball of capillaries (microscopic blood vessels) in cortex of kidney.
hilum	Depression or pit in that part of an organ where blood vessels and nerves enter and leave. Also called a hilus.
kidney	One of two bean-shaped organs located behind the abdominal cavity on either side of the backbone in the lumbar region.
meatus	Opening or canal.
medulla	Inner region; the renal medulla is the inner region of the kidney (**medullary** means pertaining to the medulla).
micturition	Urination; the act of voiding.
nitrogenous wastes	Substances containing nitrogen and excreted in urine.
potassium (K$^+$)	A salt (electrolyte) secreted from the bloodstream into the renal tubules to leave the body in urine.

reabsorption	The process of accepting again or taking back. Materials necessary to the body are reabsorbed into the blood from the renal tubules as urine is formed.
renal artery	Carries blood to the kidney.
renal pelvis	Central collecting region in the kidney.
renal tubules	Microscopic tubes in the kidney where urine is formed and where water, sugar, and salts are reabsorbed (secreted back) into the bloodstream.
renal vein	Carries blood away from the kidney.
renin	A hormone synthesized, stored, and secreted by the kidney; it raises blood pressure by influencing vasoconstriction (narrowing of blood vessels).
sodium (Na⁺)	A salt (electrolyte) regulated in the blood and urine by the kidneys.
trigone	Triangular area in the bladder where the ureters enter and the urethra exits.
urea	Major nitrogenous waste product excreted in urine.
ureter	Tube leading from each kidney to the bladder.
urethra	Tube leading from the bladder to the outside of the body.
uric acid	Nitrogenous waste excreted in the urine.
urinary bladder	Sac that holds urine.
voiding	Expelling urine (micturition).

V. Terminology: Structures, Substances, and Urinary Symptoms

Write the meanings of the medical terms in the spaces provided.

Structures			
Combining Form	**Meaning**	**Terminology**	**Meaning**
cali/o **calic/o**	calix (calyx)	caliectasis _____	
		caliceal _____	

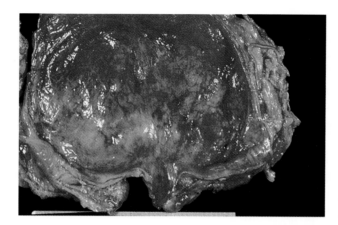

Figure 7–7

Acute cystitis. Notice that the mucosa of the bladder is red and swollen. Bacterial infections may be acquired during sexual intercourse ("honeymoon cystitis") or following surgical procedures and urinary catheterization. A UTI (urinary tract infection) such as cystitis is more common in women than in men because of the shorter urethra in women, which allows easier bacterial colonization of the urinary bladder. (From Damjanov I: Pathology for the Health-Related Professions. Philadelphia, WB Saunders, 1996, p 345.)

cyst/o	urinary bladder	cystitis _____

Acute or chronic cystitis often is caused by bacterial infection. In acute cystitis, the bladder is congested (contains blood) as a result of mucosal hemorrhages (Fig. 7–7).

cystectomy _____

cystostomy _____

An opening is made into the urinary bladder from the outside of the body. A catheter is placed into the bladder for drainage.

glomerul/o	glomerulus (collection of capillaries)	glomerular _____

meat/o	meatus	meatal stenosis _____

meatotomy _____

nephr/o	kidney	paranephric _____

nephropathy _____
(ně-FRŎ-pă-thē)

nephroptosis _____

nephrolithotomy _____

Incision (percutaneous) into the kidney to remove a stone.

nephrosclerosis _____

Arterioles in the kidney are affected.

hydronephrosis _____

Obstruction of urine flow may be caused by renal calculi (Fig. 7–8), stricture (narrowing) of the ureter, or hyperplasia of the prostate gland at the base of the bladder in males.

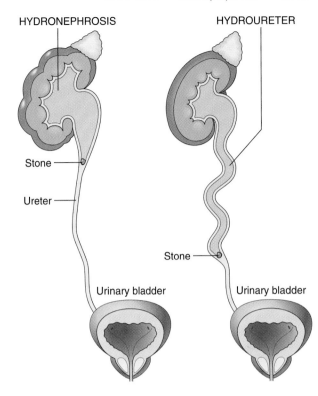

HYDRONEPHROSIS   HYDROURETER

Stone

Ureter

Stone

Urinary bladder   Urinary bladder

Figure 7–8

Hydronephrosis caused by a stone (obstruction) in the upper part of a ureter and **hydroureter** with hydronephrosis caused by a stone in the lower part of the ureter.

nephrostomy _____

Temporary opening to the outside of the body (from the renal pelvis). This is necessary when a ureter becomes obstructed and the renal pelvis becomes distended with urine (hydronephrosis).

pyel/o   renal pelvis   pyelolithotomy _____

Removal of a large calculus (stone) that contributes to blockage of urine flow and development of infection.

pyelogram _____

Intravenous (IVP) and retrograde pyelograms are discussed on pages 220 and 221, Section VIII, under Clinical Procedures.

ren/o   kidney   renal ischemia _____

renal transplantation _____

See page 224, Section VIII, under Clinical Procedures.

renal colic _____

Colic is intermittent spasms of pain caused by inflammation and distention of a hollow organ. In renal colic, pain results from calculi in the kidney or ureter.

trigon/o   trigone (region
of the bladder)   trigonitis _____

ureter/o	ureter	ureteroplasty _____	
		ureterolithotomy _____	
		ureteroileostomy _____	
		After cystectomy, a segment of the ileum is used in place of the bladder to carry urine from the ureters out of the body. Also called an ileal conduit.	
urethr/o	urethra	urethritis _____	
		urethroplasty _____	
		urethral stricture _____	
		A stricture is an abnormal narrowing of an opening or passageway.	
vesic/o	urinary bladder	perivesical _____	
		Do not confuse the term vesical with the term vesicle, which is a small blister on the skin.	
		vesicoureteral reflux _____	

Substances and Symptoms			
Combining Form or Suffix	**Meaning**	**Terminology**	**Meaning**
albumin/o	albumin (a protein in the blood)	albuminuria _____ *-uria means urine condition. This finding can indicate malfunction of the kidney as protein leaks out of damaged glomeruli.*	
azot/o	nitrogen	azotemia _____ *This is reflected in an elevated BUN (blood urea nitrogen) test.*	
bacteri/o	bacteria	bacteriuria _____ *Usually a sign of infection.*	
dips/o	thirst	polydipsia _____ *A sign of diabetes insipidus or diabetes mellitus (see pages 219 and 220, Section VII, Pathological Terminology).*	
ket/o **keton/o**	ketone bodies (ketoacids and acetone)	ketosis _____ *Often called ketoacidosis because acids accumulate in the blood and tissues. See page 216, Ketone bodies, Section VI, Urinalysis.*	
		ketonuria _____	

lith/o	stone	nephrolithiasis _____

noct/i	night	nocturia _____

Noctiphobia is an irrational fear of night or darkness.

olig/o	scanty	oliguria _____

-poietin	substance that forms	erythropoietin _____

py/o	pus	pyuria _____

-tripsy	to crush	lithotripsy _____

See page 222, Section VIII, Clinical Procedures.

ur/o	urine (urea)	uremia _____

This toxic state results when nitrogenous waste products accumulate greatly in the blood.

enuresis _____

Literally, a condition of being "in urine," and also called bedwetting.

diuresis _____

di- (from dia-) means complete. Caffeine and alcohol can produce diuresis, acting as diuretics to produce a diluted urine.

antidiuretic hormone _____

This substance (a hormone from the pituitary gland, and literally meaning against diuresis) normally acts on the renal tubules to cause water to be reabsorbed into the bloodstream. Also called ADH.

urin/o	urine	urinary incontinence _____

Incontinence literally means not (in-) able to hold (tin) together (con-). This is loss of control of the passage of urine from the bladder. Stress incontinence is due to strain on the bladder opening when coughing or sneezing, and urgency incontinence is the inability to hold back urination when feeling the urge to void.

urinary retention _____

This symptom results when there is blockage to the outflow of urine from the bladder.

-uria	urination, urine condition	dysuria _____

anuria _____

hematuria _____

glycosuria _____

A symptom of diabetes mellitus.

polyuria _____

A symptom of both diabetes insipidus and diabetes mellitus. See pages 219 and 220, Section VII, Pathological Terminology.

VI. Urinalysis

Urinalysis is an examination of urine to determine the presence of abnormal elements that may indicate various pathological conditions.

The following are some of the tests made in a urinalysis:

1. **Color**—Normal urine color is yellow (amber) or straw-colored. A colorless, pale urine indicates a large amount of water in the urine, whereas a smoky-red or brown color of urine is usually due to the presence of large amounts of blood. Foods such as beets and certain drugs can also produce red hues in urine.

2. **pH**—This is a test of the chemical nature of urine. The pH test indicates to what degree a solution (such as urine or blood) is **acidic** or **alkaline (basic).** The pH range is between 0 (very acid) and 14 (very alkaline). Normal urine is slightly acidic (6.5). However, in infections of the bladder, the urine pH may be alkaline, owing to the actions of bacteria in the urine that break down the urea and release an alkaline substance called ammonia.

3. **Protein**—Small amounts of protein are normally found in the urine but not in sufficient quantity to produce a positive result by ordinary methods of testing. When urinary tests for protein become positive, **albumin** is usually responsible. Albumin is the major protein in blood plasma. If it is detected in urine **(albuminuria),** it may indicate a leak in the glomerular membrane, which allows albumin to enter the renal tubule and pass into the urine.

   Through more sensitive testing, abnormal amounts of albumin may be detected **(microalbuminuria)** when ordinary tests are negative. Microalbuminuria is recognized as the earliest sign of renal involvement in diabetes mellitus (see page 219) and essential hypertension (see page 219).

4. **Glucose**—Sugar is not normally found in the urine. In most cases, when it does appear **(glycosuria),** it indicates **diabetes mellitus.** In diabetes mellitus, there is an excess of sugar in the bloodstream (hyperglycemia), which leads to the "spilling over" of sugar into the urine. The renal tubules are unable to reabsorb all the sugar that filters out through the glomerular membrane.

5. **Specific gravity**—The specific gravity of urine reflects the amounts of wastes, minerals, and solids in the urine. It is a comparison of the density of urine with that of water. The urine of patients with diabetes mellitus has a higher-than-normal specific gravity because of the presence of sugar.

6. **Ketone bodies**—Ketones (sometimes referred to as **acetones,** which are a type of ketone body) are breakdown products resulting from fat catabolism in cells. Ketones accumulate in large quantities in blood and urine when fat, instead of sugar,

is used as fuel for energy in cells. This happens, for example, in diabetes mellitus when cells that are deprived of sugar must use up their available fat for energy. In starvation, when sugar is not available, ketonuria and ketosis (ketones in the blood) occur as fat is abnormally catabolized.

The presence of ketones in the blood is quite dangerous because ketones increase the acidity of the blood **(acidosis).** This can lead to coma (unconsciousness) and death.

7. **Sediment**—Abnormal particles are present in the urine as a sign of a pathological condition. Included are cells (epithelial cells, white blood cells, or red blood cells), bacteria, crystals, or **casts** (cylindrical structures of protein often containing cellular elements).

8. **Pus—Pyuria** gives a **turbid** (cloudy) appearance to urine. Large numbers of leukocytes (polymorphonuclears) are present because of infection or inflammation in the kidney or bladder.

9. **Phenylketonuria (PKU)**—Phenylketones are substances that accumulate in the urine of infants born lacking an important enzyme. The enzyme (phenylalanine hydroxylase) is necessary in cells to change one amino acid (phenylalanine) to another amino acid (tyrosine). Lack of the enzyme causes phenylalanine to reach high levels in the infant's bloodstream, and this will eventually lead to mental retardation. The PKU test, done just after birth, can detect the phenylketonuria or phenylalanine in the blood. When it is detected, the infant is fed a low-protein diet that excludes phenylalanine so that mental retardation is prevented. This strict diet is necessary until the child is an adult.

10. **Bilirubin**—This pigment substance, which results from hemoglobin breakdown may appear in the urine, darkening it, as an indication of liver or gallbladder disease. The diseased liver has difficulty removing bilirubin from the blood **(hyperbilirubinemia),** which causes excessive bilirubin to appear in the urine **(bilirubinuria).**

VII. Pathological Terminology: Kidney, Bladder, and Associated Conditions

Your expanding knowledge of medical terminology should help you understand the terminology in the following paragraphs.

Kidney

glomerulonephritis   **Inflammation of the kidney glomerulus** (Bright disease).

Acute glomerulonephritis may develop as part of a systemic disorder (a condition that affects many organs in the body) or may be idiopathic. It can also occur after an acute infection, as in poststreptococcal glomerulonephritis. In this condition, which appears 10–14 days after a streptococcal infection, no bacteria are actually found in the kidney, but inflammation results from an immune (antigen and antibody) reaction in the glomerulus. Most patients recover spontaneously, but in some cases the disease becomes chronic. Chronic glomerulonephritis can result in hypertension (high blood pressure), albuminuria (protein seeps through damaged glomerular walls), renal failure, and uremia. Drugs may be useful to control inflammation, and dialysis or transplant may be necessary if uremia occurs.

interstitial nephritis	**Inflammation of the renal interstitium (connective tissue that lies between the renal tubules).**

Acute interstitial nephritis is an increasingly common disorder that may develop after the administration of drugs. It is characterized by fever, skin rash, eosinophils in the blood and urine, and poor renal function. Recovery may be anticipated when the offending agent is discontinued and may be hastened by the use of *corticosteroids* (anti-inflammatory agents).

nephrolithiasis — **Kidney stones (renal calculi).**

Kidney stones are usually composed of uric acid or calcium salts. Although the etiology is often unknown, conditions associated with an increase in the concentration of calcium (parathyroid gland tumors) or high levels of uric acid in the blood (**hyperuricemia**—associated with gouty arthritis) may contribute to the formation of calculi. Stones often lodge in the ureter or bladder as well as in the renal pelvis and may require removal by extracorporeal shock wave **lithotripsy** (see page 222, Section VIII, under Clinical Procedures) or surgery.

nephrotic syndrome — **A group of symptoms caused by excessive protein loss in the urine (also called nephrosis).**

In addition to marked proteinuria, symptoms include **edema** (swelling due to fluid in tissue spaces), hypoalbuminemia, hypercholesterolemia, and susceptibility to infections. Nephrotic syndrome may follow glomerulonephritis, exposure to toxins or drugs, and other pathological conditions, such as diabetes mellitus and malignant disease. Drugs may be useful to heal the leaky glomerulus.

polycystic kidneys — **Multiple fluid-filled sacs (cysts) within and upon the kidney.**

This is a hereditary condition that usually remains **asymptomatic** (without symptoms) until adult life. Cysts progressively develop in both kidneys, leading to nephromegaly, hematuria, urinary tract infection, hypertension, and uremia. Figure 7–9A shows polycystic kidney disease.

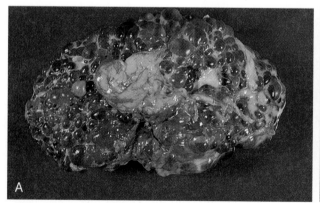 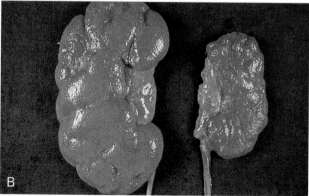

Figure 7-9

(A) Polycystic kidney disease. The kidneys contain masses of cysts. Typically, polycystic kidneys weigh 20 times more than their usual weight (150–200 grams). **(B) Chronic pyelonephritis.** Notice that one kidney is small, shrunken, and irregularly scarred. The other kidney is of normal size but also shows scarring. (From Damjanov I: Pathology for the Health-Related Professions. Philadelphia, WB Saunders, 1996, pp 337 and 345.)

pyelonephritis

Inflammation of the renal pelvis and renal medulla.

This common type of kidney disease is caused by bacterial infection. In acute pyelonephritis, many small **abscesses** (collections of pus) form in the renal pelvis and adjacent medulla. Pyuria is found on urinalysis. Treatment consists of antibiotics and surgical correction of any obstruction to urine flow. Chronic pyelonephritis may evolve from acute pyelonephritis. Recurrent infections lead to destruction of renal tissue and to scar formation (Fig. 7–9B).

renal cell carcinoma

Cancerous tumor of the kidney in adulthood.

This tumor accounts for 2 per cent of all cancers in adults. Its primary symptom is hematuria, and the tumor often metastasizes to the bones and lungs. Likelihood of survival depends on the extent of spread of the tumor. Nephrectomy is the treatment of choice.

renal failure

Failure of the kidney to excrete urine.

The kidney stops excreting nitrogenous waste products and acids derived from diet and body metabolism. Renal failure may be acute or chronic, reversible or progressive, mild or severe. The final phase of chronic renal failure is **end-stage renal disease (ESRD).** If untreated, the condition is fatal. Erythropoietin is used to treat patients with ESRD. It increases red blood cells and results in marked improvement in energy levels.

renal hypertension

High blood pressure resulting from kidney disease.

Renal hypertension is the most common type of **secondary hypertension** (high blood pressure caused by an abnormal condition, such as glomerulonephritis or renal artery stenosis). If the cause of high blood pressure is not known, it is called **essential hypertension.** Chronic essential hypertension can cause arteriole walls in the kidney to become narrowed and thickened (nephrosclerosis), and this can produce glomerular ischemia, atrophy, and scarring of kidney tissue.

Wilms tumor

Malignant tumor of the kidney occurring in childhood.

This tumor may be treated with surgery, radiation, and chemotherapy.

Urinary Bladder

bladder cancer

Malignant tumor of the urinary bladder.

The bladder is the most common site of malignancy of the urinary system. It occurs more frequently in men (often smokers) and in persons over the age of 50, especially industrial workers exposed to dyes and leather. Symptoms include gross (visible to the naked eye) or microscopic hematuria and dysuria and increased urinary frequency. Cystoscopy with biopsy is the most common diagnostic procedure. Staging of the tumor is based on the depth to which the bladder wall (urothelium) has been penetrated and the extent of metastasis. Superficial tumors are removed by electrocauterization (burning). Cystectomy, chemotherapy, and radiation therapy are helpful for more invasive disease.

Associated Conditions

diabetes insipidus

Inadequate secretion or resistance of the kidney to the action of antidiuretic hormone (ADH).

Two major symptoms of this condition are polydipsia and polyuria. Lack of ADH prevents water from being reabsorbed into the blood through the renal tubules. Insipidus means tasteless, reflecting that the urine is very dilute and watery, not sweet as in diabetes mellitus. The term **diabetes** is taken from a Greek word meaning siphon. It leads to an inability of the kidneys to hold water in the body, which instead runs through the body as through a siphon (a tube for carrying fluid).

diabetes mellitus

Inadequate secretion or improper utilization of insulin.

Major symptoms of diabetes mellitus are glycosuria, hyperglycemia, polyuria, and polydipsia. Without insulin, sugar is prevented from leaving the bloodstream and cannot be used by body cells for energy. Sugar thus remains in the blood (hyperglycemia) and spills over into the urine (glycosuria) when the kidney cannot reabsorb it through the renal tubules. Mellitus means sweet, reflecting the content of the urine. The term diabetes, when used by itself, usually refers to the more common condition, diabetes mellitus, rather than diabetes insipidus.

VIII. Laboratory Tests, Clinical Procedures, and Abbreviations

Laboratory Tests

blood urea nitrogen (BUN)

This test measures the amount of urea in the blood. Normally, the urea level is low because urea is excreted in the urine continuously. When the kidney is diseased or fails, however, urea accumulates in the blood (a condition known as uremia), and this can lead to unconsciousness and death.

creatinine clearance test

This test measures the ability of the kidney to remove creatinine from the blood. A blood sample is drawn and the amount of creatinine concentration is compared with the amount of creatinine excreted in the urine during a 24-hour period. If the kidney is not functioning well in its job of clearing creatinine from the blood, there will be a disproportionate amount of creatinine in the blood compared with the amount in the urine.

Clinical Procedures

X-Rays

CT scans

Transverse x-ray views of the kidney are taken with or without contrast material and are useful in the diagnosis of tumors, cysts, abscesses, and hydronephrosis. Studies may be obtained in renal failure, when contrast material should not be given.

intravenous pyelogram (IVP)

Contrast material is injected into a vein and travels to the kidney where it is filtered into the urine. X-rays are then taken showing the contrast material filling the kidneys, ureters, bladder, and urethra. These x-rays provide a test of renal function as well as show cysts, tumors, infections, hydronephrosis, and calculi. Also called an **excretory urogram.** IVP **tomograms** show a series of images of the kidney and may be required to see details.

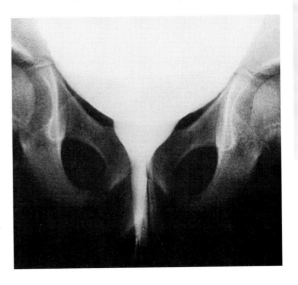

Figure 7-10

Voiding cystourethrogram showing a normal female urethra. (Courtesy of William H. Bush, Jr., M.D., University of Washington, Seattle.)

kidneys, ureters, and bladder (KUB)	This x-ray record (no contrast material is used) demonstrates the size and location of the kidneys in relation to other organs in the abdominopelvic region.
renal angiography	Contrast material is injected into the bloodstream and x-rays are taken of the blood vessels (vascular system) of the kidney. This procedure is helpful for the diagnosis of kidney tumors and to outline renal vessels in hypertensive patients.
retrograde pyelogram	Contrast material is introduced directly into the bladder and ureters through a cystoscope, and x-rays are taken to determine the presence of stones or obstructions. This technique may be indicated when poor renal function makes it impossible to visualize the kidneys, ureters, and bladder by use of intravenous dye as in an IVP. It may also be used as a substitute for an IVP when a patient is allergic to intravenous contrast material.
voiding cystourethrogram (VCUG)	The bladder is filled with contrast material, as in a retrograde pyelogram, and x-rays are taken of the bladder and urethra as a patient is expelling urine (Fig. 7-10).

Ultrasound

ultrasonography	Kidney size, tumors, hydronephrosis, polycystic kidney, and ureteral and bladder obstruction are some of the many conditions that can be diagnosed using sound waves, but no information about renal function is obtained.

Radioactive

radioisotope studies	A radioactive substance (isotope) is injected into the bloodstream in small amounts and is taken up by the kidneys. Pictures show the size and shape of the kidney **(renal scan)** and its function **(renogram).** These studies can indicate size of blood vessels, diagnose obstruction, and determine the individual functioning of each kidney.

Magnetic Imaging

magnetic resonance imaging (MRI)

The patient lies surrounded by a cylindrical magnetic resonance machine, and images are made of the pelvic and retroperitoneal regions using magnetic waves. This high-technology machine produces an image of internal organs based upon the movement of small particles called protons. The images can be taken in all three planes of the body—frontal, sagittal, and transverse—and are useful in showing pelvic, retroperitoneal, and vascular anatomy.

Other Procedures

cystoscopy

Cystoscopy is the visual examination of the urinary bladder by means of a cystoscope. A hollow metal tube is introduced into the urinary meatus and passed through the urethra into the bladder. By means of a light source, special lenses, and mirrors, the bladder mucosa is examined for tumors, calculi, or inflammation. By placing a catheter through the cystoscope, urine samples can be withdrawn and contrast material can be injected into the bladder. Cystoscopy is shown in Figure 7–11. A **panendoscope** is a cystoscope that gives a wide-angle view of the bladder.

dialysis

Waste materials such as urea are separated from the bloodstream when the kidneys can no longer function. There are two kinds of dialysis:

> **hemodialysis (HD)**—uses an artificial kidney machine that receives waste-filled blood from the patient's bloodstream, filters it, and returns the dialysed blood to the patient's body.
> **peritoneal dialysis (PD)**—using a peritoneal **catheter** (tube), fluid is introduced into the peritoneal (abdominal) cavity. The fluid causes wastes in the capillaries of the peritoneum to pass out of the bloodstream and into the fluid. Fluid (with wastes) is then removed by catheter. When used to treat patients with end-stage renal disease, PD may be performed continuously by the patient without artificial support (CAPD, continuous ambulatory PD) or with the aid of a mechanical apparatus at night during sleep (CCPD, continuous cycling PD). Figure 7–12 illustrates CAPD.

extracorporeal shock wave lithotripsy (ESWL)

Shock waves are used to crush urinary tract stones into tiny fragments that can then be passed out with urine. After receiving anesthesia, the patient is immersed in a tank of water and shock waves are generated electrically. Using an x-ray picture screen (fluoroscopy) the physician can position the patient so that the stone will receive the shock waves properly.

renal biopsy

Biopsy of the kidney may be performed at the time of surgery (open) or through the skin (percutaneous, or closed). When the latter technique is used, the patient lies in the prone position and, following administration of local anesthesia to the overlying skin and muscles of the back, a biopsy needle is inserted with the aid of fluoroscopy (x-rays on a screen) or ultrasonography, and tissue is obtained for microscopic examination by a pathologist.

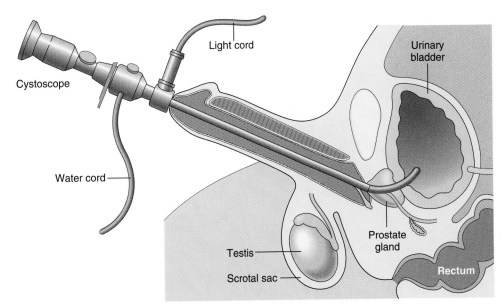

Figure 7-11

Cystoscopy.

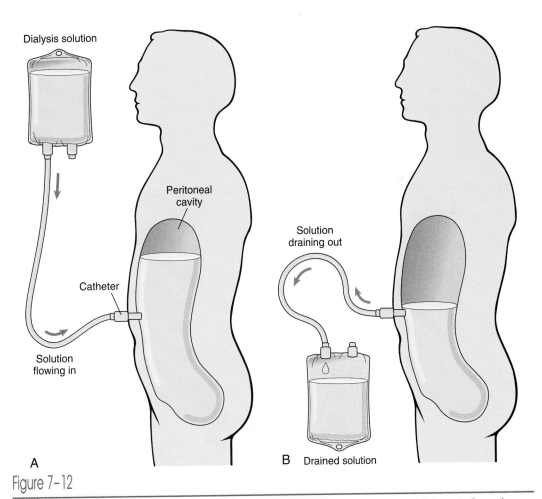

A

B   Drained solution

Figure 7-12

Continuous ambulatory peritoneal dialysis (CAPD). (A) The dialysis solution (dialysate) flows from a collapsible plastic bag through a catheter (a Tenckhoff peritoneal catheter) into the patient's peritoneal cavity. The empty bag is folded and inserted into undergarments. **(B)** After 4–8 hours, the bag is unfolded, and the fluid is allowed to drain into it by gravity. The full bag is discarded, and a new bag of fresh dialysate is attached.

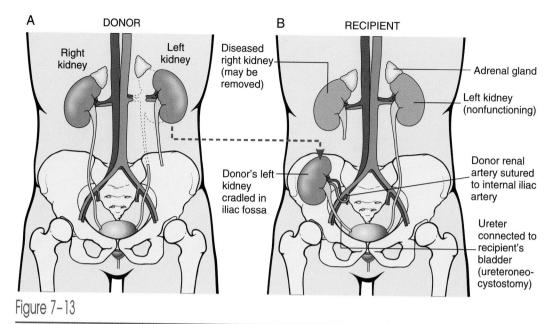

Figure 7-13

Renal (kidney) transplantation. (A) Left kidney of donor is removed for transplant. **(B)** Kidney is transplanted to right pelvis of the recipient. The renal artery and vein of the donor kidney are joined to the recipient's artery and vein, and the lower end of the donor ureter is connected to the recipient's bladder (**ureteroneocystostomy**). The health of the donor is not affected by losing one kidney. In fact, the remaining kidney enlarges (hypertrophies) to take over full function.

renal transplantation

A kidney is transplanted into a patient with renal failure from an identical twin (isograft) or other individual (allograft). Best results occur when the donor is closely related to the recipient, and better than 90 per cent of the kidneys survive for 1 year or longer (Fig. 7-13).

urinary catheterization

A flexible, tubular instrument is passed through the urethra into the urinary bladder. Catheters are used primarily for short- or long-term drainage of urine. A **Foley catheter** is an indwelling (left in the bladder) catheter held in place by a balloon inflated with air or liquid (Fig. 7-14).

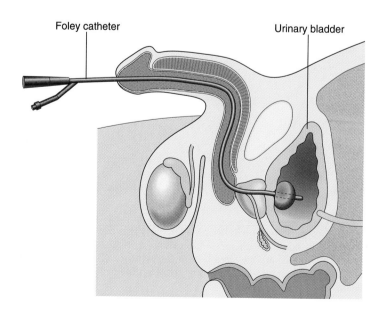

Figure 7-14

A **Foley catheter** in place in the urinary bladder.

ABBREVIATIONS

ADH	antidiuretic hormone; vasopressin	**HD**	hemodialysis
ARF	acute renal failure	**IC**	interstitial cystitis; chronic inflammation of the bladder wall; not caused by bacterial infection and not responsive to conventional antibiotic therapy.
BILI	bilirubin		
BUN	blood urea nitrogen	**IVP**	intravenous pyelogram
CAPD	continuous ambulatory peritoneal dialysis	**K+**	potassium; an electrolyte
Cath	catheter, catheterization	**KUB**	kidney, ureter, and bladder
CCPD	continuous cycling peritoneal dialysis	**Na+**	sodium; an electrolyte
Cl−	chloride; an electrolyte excreted by the kidney	**PD**	peritoneal dialysis
		pH	symbol for degree of acidity or alkalinity
CRF	chronic renal failure; progressive loss of kidney function	**PKU**	phenylketonuria
cysto	cystoscopic examination	**sp gr**	specific gravity
ESRD	end-stage renal disease; A period during which serum creatinine and BUN levels continue to rise and there is impairment of all body systems.	**UA**	urinalysis
		UTI	urinary tract infection
		VCUG	voiding cystourethrogram
ESWL	extracorporeal shock wave lithotripsy		
HCO3−	bicarbonate; an electrolyte conserved by the kidney		

IX. Practical Applications

This section contains an actual medical report using terms that you have studied in this and previous chapters. Questions are included to test your understanding. Answers to the questions are on page 234 after Answers to Exercises.

Case Report

The patient, a 50-year-old woman, presented herself at the clinic complaining of dysuria. This symptom was followed by sudden onset of hematuria and clots. There had been no history of urolithiasis, pyuria, or previous hematuria. Nocturia had been present about 5 years earlier. Panendoscopy revealed a carcinoma located about 2 cm from the left ureteral orifice. A partial cystectomy was carried out and the lesion cleared. No ileal conduit was necessary. A metastatic workup was negative. Bilateral pelvic lymphadenectomy revealed no positive nodes.

Continued on following page

Questions on the Case Report

1. Urological refers to which system of the body?
   (A) digestive
   (B) reproductive
   (C) excretory

2. What was the patient's reason for appearing at the clinic?
   (A) scanty urination
   (B) inability to urinate
   (C) painful urination

3. What acute symptom followed?
   (A) blood in the feces
   (B) blood in the urine
   (C) excessive urea in the blood

4. Which of the following was a previous symptom?
   (A) pus in the urine
   (B) blood in the urine
   (C) excessive urination at night

5. What diagnostic procedure was carried out?
   (A) lithotripsy
   (B) cystoscopy using a wide-angle view of the bladder
   (C) urinalysis

6. The patient's diagnosis was
   (A) malignant tumor of the bladder
   (B) tumor in the proximal ureter
   (C) lymph nodes were affected by tumor

7. Treatment was
   (A) ureteroileostomy
   (B) removal of tumor and subtotal removal of the bladder
   (C) not necessary because of negative lymph nodes

X. Exercises

Remember to check your answers carefully with those given in Section XI, Answers to Exercises.

A. *Using the following terms, trace the path of urine formation from afferent renal arterioles to the point at which urine leaves the body.*

renal pelvis   renal tubule   urinary meatus   Bowman capsule
glomerulus   ureter   urinary bladder   urethra

1. _____   5. _____

2. _____   6. _____

3. _____   7. _____

4. _____   8. _____

B. *Match the term in column I with the letter of a definition or term of similar meaning in column II.*

Column I

1. voiding _____ C

2. trigone _____ I

3. renal cortex _____ J

4. renal medulla _____ G

5. urea _____ D

6. erythropoietin _____ A

7. renin _____ H

8. electrolyte _____ F

9. hilum _____ B

10. calix (calyx) _____ E

Column II

A. a hormone secreted by the kidney that stimulates formation of red blood cells
B. notch on the surface of the kidney where blood vessels and nerve enter
C. micturition
D. nitrogenous waste
E. cup-like collecting region of the renal pelvis
F. a small molecule that carries an electric charge in solution
G. inner region of the kidney
H. hormone made by the kidney that causes blood pressure to rise
I. triangular area in the bladder
J. outer section of the kidney

C. *Give the meanings of the following medical terms.*

1. caliceal _____

2. uric acid _____

3. urinary meatal stenosis _____

4. cystocele _____

5. pyelolithotomy _____

6. trigonitis _____

7. ureteroileostomy _____

8. urethral stricture _____

9. vesicoureteral reflux _____

10. creatinine _____

11. medullary _____

12. cortical _____

D. Select the correct term to complete the sentences below.

1. After diagnosis of renal cell carcinoma (made by renal biopsy), Dr. Davis advised Donna that **(nephrostomy, meatotomy, nephrectomy)** would be necessary.

2. Ever since Bill's condition of gout was diagnosed, he has been warned that uric acid crystals could accumulate in his blood and tissues, leading to **(pyuria, renal calculi, cystocele).**

3. The voiding cystourethrogram demonstrated blockage of urine flow from Jim's bladder and **(hydronephrosis, renal ischemia, azotemia).**

4. Narrowed arterioles in the kidney increase blood pressure, and thus **(urinary incontinence, urinary retention, nephrosclerosis)** is often associated with hypertension.

5. Eight-year-old Willy was wetting his bed at night while sleeping. His mother limited Willy's intake of fluids in the evening to discourage his **(nocturia, oliguria, enuresis).**

6. David's chronic juvenile diabetes eventually resulted in **(nephropathy, meatal stenosis, urolithiasis),** which led to renal failure.

7. After Sue's bilateral renal failure, her doctor advised **(cystostomy, nephrolithotomy, renal transplantation)** to save her life.

8. When Betty's left kidney stopped functioning, her contralateral kidney overdeveloped or **(metastasized, atrophied, hypertrophied)** to meet the increased workload.

E. Give the meanings of the following terms that relate to urinary symptoms.

1. azotemia _____

2. polydipsia _____

3. nocturia _____

4. urinary incontinence _____

5. oliguria _____

6. bacteriuria _____

7. albuminuria _____

8. enuresis _____

9. urinary retention _____

10. dysuria _____

11. polyuria _____

12. glycosuria _____

13. ketosis _____

14. anuria _____

F. Give short answers for the following.

1. What is the difference between hematuria and uremia? _____

2. What is diuresis? _____

3. What is a diuretic? _____

4. What is antidiuretic hormone? _____

G. Match the following terms that pertain to urinalysis with their meanings below.

specific gravity	pH	glycosuria	ketonuria
bilirubinuria	sediment	albuminuria	phenylketonuria
hematuria	pyuria		

1. Abnormal particles present in the urine—cells, bacteria, casts, and crystals.

_____

2. High levels of a substance appear in urine when a baby is born with a deficiency of an enzyme. The infant can become mentally retarded if she or he is not put on a strict diet that prevents the substance from accumulating in the blood and urine. _____

3. Color of the urine is smoky-red owing to the presence of blood. _____

4. Urine is turbid (cloudy) owing to the presence of polymorphonuclear leukocytes and pus.

_____

5. Sugar in the urine; a symptom of diabetes mellitus and a result of hyperglycemia.

_____

6. This urine test reflects the acidity or alkalinity of the urine. _____

7. High levels of acids and acetones accumulate in the urine as a result of abnormal fat catabolism.

_____

8. Dark pigment accumulates in urine as a result of liver or gallbladder disease.

_____

9. This urine test reflects the concentration of the urine. _____

10. Leaky glomeruli can produce accumulation of protein in the urine. _____

H. Describe the following abnormal conditions that affect the kidney.

1. renal failure _____

2. polycystic kidney _____

3. interstitial nephritis _____

4. glomerulonephritis _____

5. nephrolithiasis _____

6. renal cell carcinoma _____

7. pyelonephritis _____

8. Wilms tumor _____

9. nephrotic syndrome _____

10. renal hypertension _____

I. Match the following terms with their meanings below.

edema   nephroptosis   diabetes mellitus
abscess   stricture   secondary hypertension
catheter   essential hypertension   diabetes insipidus
renal colic

1. high blood pressure that is idiopathic _____

2. swelling, fluid in tissues _____

3. a narrowed area in a tube _____

4. collection of pus _____

5. inadequate secretion of insulin or improper utilization of insulin leads to this condition

   _____

6. high blood pressure caused by kidney disease or another disease _____

7. a tube for withdrawing or giving fluid _____

8. inadequate secretion or resistance of the kidney to the action of antidiuretic hormone

   _____

9. prolapse of a kidney _____

10. severe pain resulting from a stone that is blocking a ureter or a kidney

_____

J. Give the meanings of the following abbreviations and then select the letter of the sentence that is the best association for each.

Column I

1. CAPD _____ ____

2. BUN _____ ____

3. IVP _____ ____

4. cysto _____ ____

5. UA _____ ____

6. UTI _____ ____

7. ESRD _____ ____

8. K⁺ _____ ____

9. VCU _____ ____

10. HD _____ ____

Column II

A. Bacterial invasion leads to this condition; acute cystitis is an example.

B. This electrolyte is secreted by renal tubules into the urine.

C. A patient's blood is filtered through a machine to remove nitrogenous wastes.

D. When levels of this test are high, renal disease is suspected.

E. This endoscopic procedure is used to examine the interior of the urinary bladder.

F. Dialysate (fluid) is injected into the peritoneal cavity and then drained out.

G. Contrast is injected into veins and x-rays are taken of the kidneys and urinary tract.

H. X-rays are taken of the urinary bladder and urethra while a patient is urinating.

I. Specific gravity, color, protein, glucose, and pH are all parts of this test.

J. This condition involves severe kidney failure, with impairment of body systems.

K. Match the following procedures with their meanings below.

cystectomy
cystostomy
extracorporeal shock wave
   lithotripsy

meatotomy
nephrectomy
nephrostomy
nephrolithotomy

ureteroileostomy (ileal
   conduit)
ureterolithotomy
urethroplasty

1. Excision of a kidney _____

2. Surgical incision into the kidney to remove a stone _____

3. Incision of the urinary meatus for enlargement _____

4. Crushing of stones (with sound waves generated outside the body) _____

5. New opening of the ureters to a segment of ileum (in place of the bladder)

_____

6. Surgical repair of the urethra _____

7. Creation of an artificial opening into the kidney (via catheter) from the outside of the body

_____

8. Surgical formation of an opening from the bladder to the outside of the body

_____

9. Removal of the urinary bladder _____

10. Incision of a ureter to remove a stone _____

XI. Answers to Exercises

A

1. glomerulus
2. Bowman capsule
3. renal tubule

4. renal pelvis
5. ureter
6. urinary bladder

7. urethra
8. urinary meatus

B

1. C
2. I
3. J
4. G

5. D
6. A
7. H
8. F

9. B
10. E

C

1. pertaining to a calix (collecting cup of renal pelvis)
2. a nitrogenous waste excreted in urine; high levels of uric acid in the blood are associated with gouty arthritis

3. narrowing of the urinary meatus
4. hernia of the urinary bladder
5. incision to remove a stone from the renal pelvis
6. inflammation of the trigone (triangular

area in the bladder where the ureters enter and urethra exits)
7. new opening between the ureter and the ileum (an anastomosis); urine then leaves the body through an ileostomy;

this surgery is performed when the bladder has been resected
8. narrowing (narrowed portion) of the urethra
9. backflow of urine from the bladder into the ureter

10. a nitrogenous waste produced as a result of muscle metabolism and excreted in the urine
11. pertaining to the inner, middle section (of the kidney)

12. pertaining to the outer section (of the kidney)

D

1. nephrectomy
2. renal calculi
3. hydronephrosis

4. nephrosclerosis
5. enuresis
6. nephropathy

7. renal transplantation
8. hypertrophied

E

1. excess nitrogenous waste in the bloodstream
2. condition of much thirst
3. excessive urination at night
4. inability to hold urine in the bladder
5. scanty urination

6. bacteria in the urine (sign of infection)
7. protein in the urine
8. bedwetting
9. inability to release urine from the bladder
10. painful urination

11. excessive urination
12. sugar in the urine
13. abnormal condition of ketone bodies (acids and acetones) in the blood and body tissues
14. no urination

F

1. Hematuria is the presence of blood in the urine and uremia is a toxic condition of excess urea (nitrogenous waste) in the bloodstream. Hematuria is a symptomatic condition of the urine (-uria), and uremia is an abnormal condition of the blood (-emia).

2. Diuresis is the excessive production of urine (polyuria).
3. A diuretic is a drug or chemical (caffeine or alcohol) that causes diuresis to occur.
4. Antidiuretic hormone is a hormone produced by the pituitary gland that

normally helps the renal tubules to reabsorb water back into the bloodstream. It works against diuresis to help retain water in the blood.

G

1. sediment
2. phenylketonuria (phenylketones in the urine)
3. hematuria (blood in the urine)

4. pyuria (pus in the urine)
5. glycosuria (sugar in the urine)
6. pH
7. ketonuria (ketone bodies in the urine)

8. bilirubinuria (high levels of bilirubin in the urine)
9. specific gravity
10. albuminuria

H

1. kidney does not produce urine
2. multiple fluid-filled sacs form in and on the kidney
3. inflammation of the connective tissue (interstitium) lying between the renal tubules
4. inflammation of the glomerulus of the kidney (may be a complication following a streptococcal infection)

5. condition of kidney stones (renal calculi)
6. malignant tumor of the kidney in adults
7. inflammation of the kidney and renal pelvis (caused by a bacterial infection, such as *Escherichia coli,* that enters the urinary tract from the gastrointestinal tract)

8. malignant tumor of the kidney in children
9. group of symptoms (proteinuria, edema, hypoalbuminemia) that appears when the kidney is damaged by disease; also called nephrosis
10. high blood pressure caused by kidney disease

I

1. essential hypertension
2. edema
3. stricture
4. abscess

5. diabetes mellitus
6. secondary hypertension
7. catheter
8. diabetes insipidus

9. nephroptosis
10. renal colic

J

1. continuous ambulatory peritoneal dialysis. F
2. blood, urea, nitrogen. D
3. intravenous pyelogram. G

4. cystoscopy. E
5. urinalysis. I
6. urinary tract infection. A
7. end-stage renal disease. J
8. potassium. B

9. voiding cystourethrogram. H
10. hemodialysis. C

K

1. nephrectomy
2. pyelolithotomy
3. meatotomy
4. extracorporeal shock wave lithotripsy

5. ureteroileostomy
6. urethroplasty
7. nephrostomy
8. cystostomy

9. cystectomy
10. ureterolithotomy

Answers to Practical Applications

1. C	4. C	6. A
2. C	5. B	7. B
3. B		

XII. Pronunciation of Terms

Pronunciation Guide

ā as in āpe   ă as in ăpple
ē as in ēven   ĕ as in ĕvery
ī as in īce   ĭ as in ĭnterest
ō as in ōpen   ŏ as in pŏt
ū as in ūnit   ŭ as in ŭnder

To test your understanding of the terminology in this chapter, write the meaning of each term in the space provided. In addition, you may wish to cover the terms and write them by looking at your definitions. Make sure your spelling is correct. The page number after each term indicates where it is defined or used in the text so you can easily check your responses.

Term	Pronunciation	Meaning
abscess (219)	ĂB-sĕs	_____
acetone (216)	ĂS-ĕ-tōn	_____
albuminuria (214)	ăl-bū-mĭ-NŪ-rē-ă	_____
antidiuretic hormone (215)	ăn-tĭ-dī-ū-RĔ-tĭk HŎR-mōn	_____
azotemia (214)	ă-zō-TĒ-mē-ă	_____
bacteriuria (214)	băk-tē-rē-Ū-rē-ă	_____
caliceal (211)	kā-lĭ-SĒ-ăl	_____
caliectasis (211)	kā-lē-ĔK-tă-sĭs	_____
calix (calyx); calices (210)	KĀ-lĭks; KĀ-lĭ-sēz	_____
catheter (210)	KĂ-thĕ-tĕr	_____
cortex (210)	KŎR-tĕks	_____
cortical (210)	KŎR-tĭ-kăl	_____
creatinine (210)	krē-ĂT-ĭ-nēn	_____
cystectomy (212)	sĭs-TĔK-tō-mē	_____
cystitis (212)	sĭs-TĪ-tĭs	_____
cystoscopy (222)	sĭs-TŎS-kō-pē	_____
cystostomy (212)	sĭs-TŎS-tō-mē	_____

diabetes insipidus (219)	dī-ă-BĒ-tēz ĭn-SĬP-ĭ-dŭs	_____
diabetes mellitus (220)	dī-ă-BĒ-tēz MĔL-ĭ-tŭs	_____
diuresis (215)	dī-ūr-RĒ-sĭs	_____
dysuria (215)	dĭs-Ū-rē-ă	_____
edema (218)	ĕ-DĒ-mă	_____
electrolyte (210)	ē-LĔK-trō-līt	_____
enuresis (215)	ĕn-ū-RĒ-sĭs	_____
erythropoietin (210)	ĕ-rĭth-rō-PŌ-ĭ-tĭn	_____
essential hypertension (219)	ĕ-SĔN-shŭl hī-pĕr-TĒN-shŭn	_____
glomerular (212)	glō-MĔR-ū-lăr	_____
glomerulonephritis (217)	glō-mĕr-ū-lō-nĕ-FRĪ-tĭs	_____
glomerulus; glomeruli (210)	glō-MĔR-ū-lŭs; glō-MĔR-ū-lī	_____
glycosuria (216)	glī-kōs-Ū-rē-ă	_____
hematuria (215)	hēm-ă-TŪ-rē-ă	_____
hemodialysis (222)	hē-mō-dī-ĂL-ĭ-sĭs	_____
hilum (210)	HĪ-lŭm	_____
hydronephrosis (212)	hī-drō-nĕ-FRŌ-sĭs	_____
interstitial nephritis (218)	ĭn-tĕr-STĬ-shŭl nĕ-FRĪ-tĭs	_____
intravenous pyelogram (220)	ĭn-tră-VĒ-nŭs PĪ-ĕl-ō-grăm	_____
ketonuria (214)	kē-tōn-Ū-rē-ă	_____
ketosis (214)	kē-TŌ-sĭs	_____
lithotripsy (222)	LĬTH-ō-trĭp-sē	_____
meatal stenosis (212)	mē-Ā-tăl stĕ-NŌ-sĭs	_____
meatotomy (212)	mē-ā-TŎT-ō-mē	_____
meatus (210)	mē-Ā-tŭs	_____
medulla (210)	mĕ-DŪL-ă or mĕ-DŬL-ă	_____
medullary (210)	MĔD-ū-lăr-ē	_____

micturition (210)	mĭk-tū-RĬSH-ŭn	_____
nephrolithiasis (218)	nĕf-rō-lĭ-THĪ-ă-sĭs	_____
nephrolithotomy (212)	nĕf-rō-lĭ-THŎT-ō-mē	_____
nephropathy (212)	nĕf-RŎP-ă-thē	_____
nephroptosis (212)	nĕf-rŏp-TŌ-sĭs	_____
nephrosclerosis (212)	nĕf-rō-sklĕ-RŌ-sĭs	_____
nephrostomy (213)	nĕ-FRŎS-tō-mē	_____
nephrotic syndrome (218)	nĕ-FRŎT-ĭk SĬN-drōm	_____
nitrogenous waste (210)	nĭ-TRŎJ-ĕ-nŭs wāst	_____
nocturia (215)	nŏk-TŪ-rē-ă	_____
oliguria (215)	ŏl-ĭ-GŪ-rē-ă	_____
paranephric (212)	pă-ră-NĚF-rĭk	_____
peritoneal dialysis (222)	pĕr-ĭ-tō-NĒ-ăl dī-ĂL-ĭ-sĭs	_____
perivesical (214)	pĕ-rē-VĚS-ĭ-kăl	_____
phenylketonuria (217)	fē-nĭl-kē-tō-NŪ-rē-ă or fĕn-ĭl-kē-tō-NŪ-rē-ă	_____
polycystic kidneys (218)	pŏl-ē-SĬS-tĭk KĬD-nēz	_____
polydipsia (214)	pŏl-ē-DĬP-sē-ă	_____
polyuria (216)	pŏl-ē-Ū-rē-ă	_____
potassium (210)	pō-TĂ-sē-ŭm	_____
pyelogram (213)	PĪ-ĕ-lo-grăm	_____
pyelolithotomy (213)	pī-ĕ-lō-lĭ-THŎT-ō-mē	_____
pyelonephritis (219)	pī-ĕ-lō-nĕf-RĪ-tĭs	_____
pyuria (215)	pī-Ū-rē-ă	_____
renal angiography (221)	RĒ-nal ăn-jē-ŎG-ră-fē	_____
renal calculi (218)	RĒ-năl KĂL-kū-lī	_____
renal cell carcinoma (219)	RĒ-năl sĕl kăr-sĭ-NŌ-mă	_____
renal colic (213)	RĒ-năl KŎL-ĭk	_____
renal failure (219)	RĒ-năl FĀL-ŭr	_____

renal hypertension (219)	RĒ-năl hī-pĕr-TĔN-shŭn	_____
renal ischemia (213)	RĒ-năl ĭs-KĒ-mē-ă	_____
renal pelvis (211)	RĒ-năl PĔL-vĭs	_____
renal transplantation (224)	RĒ-năl trăns-plăn-TĀ-shŭn	_____
renin (211)	RĒ-nĭn	_____
retrograde pyelogram (221)	RĔ-trō-grād PĪ-ĕ-lō-grăm	_____
secondary hypertension (219)	SĔ-kŏn-dă-rē hī-pĕr-TĔN-shŭn	_____
sodium (211)	SŌ-dē-ŭm	_____
stricture (212)	STRĬK-shŭr	_____
trigone (211)	TRĪ-gōn	_____
trigonitis (213)	trī-gō-NĪ-tĭs	_____
urea (211)	ū-RĒ-ă	_____
uremia (215)	ū-RĒ-mē-ă	_____
ureter (211)	ū-RĒ-tĕr or ŪR-ĕ-tĕr	_____
ureteroileostomy (214)	ū-rē-tĕr-ō-ĭl-ē-ŌS-tō-mē	_____
ureterolithotomy (214)	ū-rē-tĕr-ō-lĭ-THŎT-ō-mē	_____
ureteroneocystostomy (224)	ū-rē-tĕr-ō-nē-ō-sĭs-TŎS-tō-mē	_____
ureteroplasty (214)	ū-rē-tĕr-ō-PLĂS-tē	_____
urethra (211)	ū-RĒ-thră	_____
urethritis (214)	ū-rē-THRĬ-tĭs	_____
urethroplasty (214)	ū-rē-thrō-PLĂS-tē	_____
uric acid (211)	Ū-rĭk ĀS-ĭd	_____
urinalysis (216)	ū-rĭn-ĂL-ĭ-sĭs	_____
urinary incontinence (215)	ŬR-ĭ-năr-ē ĭn-KŎN-tĭ-nĕns	_____
urinary retention (215)	ŬR-ī-năr-ē rē-TĔN-shŭn	_____
vesicoureteral reflux (214)	vĕs-ĭ-kō-ū-RĒ-tĕr-ăl RĒ-flŭks	_____
voiding (211)	VOY-dĭng	_____
Wilms tumor (219)	wĭlmz TŪ-mŭr	_____

XIII. Review Sheet

Write the meanings of the combining forms, suffixes, and prefixes in the spaces provided. Check your answers with the information in the chapter or in the glossary (Medical Terms—English) at the end of the book.

COMBINING FORMS

Combining Form	Meaning	Combining Form	Meaning
albumin/o		meat/o	
angi/o		necr/o	
arteri/o		nephr/o	
azot/o		noct/i	
bacteri/o		olig/o	
cali/o		py/o	
calic/o		pyel/o	
cyst/o		ren/o	
dips/o		tom/o	
glomerul/o		tox/o	
glyc/o		trigon/o	
glycos/o		ur/o	
hydr/o		ureter/o	
isch/o		urethr/o	
ket/o		urin/o	
keton/o		vesic/o	
lith/o			

SUFFIXES

Suffix	Meaning	Suffix	Meaning
-ectasis	_____	-rrhea	_____
-emia	_____	-sclerosis	_____
-lithiasis	_____	-spasm	_____
-lithotomy	_____	-stenosis	_____
-lysis	_____	-stomy	_____
-megaly	_____	-tomy	_____
-ole	_____	-tripsy	_____
-plasty	_____	-trophy	_____
-poietin	_____	-ule	_____
-ptosis	_____	-uria	_____
-rrhaphy	_____		

PREFIXES

Prefix	Meaning	Prefix	Meaning
a-, an-	_____	en-	_____
anti-	_____	peri-	_____
dia-	_____	poly-	_____
dys-	_____	retro-	_____

Continued on following page

REVIEW OF ANATOMICAL TERMS

Match the number of the urinary system structure in column I with its location or function in column II.

Column I

Tiny structure surrounding each glomerulus; receives filtered materials from blood. _____

Tubes carrying urine from kidney to urinary bladder. _____

Tubules leading from the Bowman capsule. Urine is formed there as water, sugar, and salts are reabsorbed into the bloodstream. _____

Inner (middle) region of the kidney. _____

Muscular sac that serves as a reservoir for urine. _____

Cup-like divisions of the renal pelvis that receive urine from the renal tubules. _____

Tube carrying urine from the bladder to the outside of the body. _____

Central urine-collecting basin in the kidney that narrows into the ureter. _____

Collection of capillaries through which materials from the blood are filtered into the Bowman capsule. _____

Outer region of the kidney. _____

Column II

1. urethra
2. cortex
3. Bowman capsule
4. calices
5. renal pelvis
6. glomerulus
7. medulla
8. renal tubules
9. urinary bladder
10. ureters

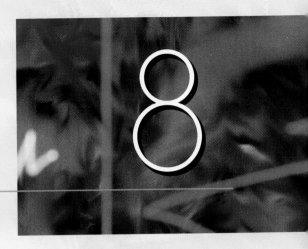

CHAPTER 8

Female Reproductive System

This chapter is divided into the following sections

In this chapter you will

- Name the organs of the female reproductive system, their locations, and combining forms;
- Explain how these organs and their hormones function in the processes of menstruation and pregnancy;
- Identify abnormal conditions of the female reproductive system and of the newborn child;
- Explain important laboratory tests, clinical procedures, and abbreviations related to gynecology and obstetrics; and
- Apply your new knowledge to understanding medical terms in their proper contexts, such as medical reports and records.

I. Introduction

Sexual reproduction is the union of the nuclei of the female sex cell **(ovum)** and the male sex cell **(sperm)** that results in the creation of a new individual. The ovum and sperm cell are specialized cells differing primarily from normal body cells in one important way. Each sex cell (also called a **gamete**) contains exactly half the number of chromosomes that a normal body cell contains. When the nuclei of ovum and sperm cell unite, the cell produced receives half of its genetic material from its female parent and half from its male parent; thus it contains a full, normal complement of hereditary material.

Gametes are produced in special organs called **gonads** in both males and females. The female gonads are the **ovaries,** and the male gonads are the **testes.** An ovum, after leaving the ovary, travels down a duct **(fallopian tube)** leading to the **uterus** (womb). If **coitus** (copulation, sexual intercourse) has occurred, and sperm cells are present in the fallopian tube, union of the ovum and sperm may take place. The union is called **fertilization.** The **embryo** (called the **fetus** after the 2nd month) then begins a 40-week (approximately 9-month) period of development **(gestation, pregnancy)** within the uterus.

The female reproductive system consists of organs that produce **ova** and provide a place for the growth of the embryo. In addition, the female reproductive organs supply important hormones that contribute to the development of female secondary sex characteristics (body hair, breast development, structural changes in bones and fat).

Ova mature and are released from the ovary from the onset of **puberty** (beginning of the fertile period when secondary sex characteristics develop) to **menopause** (cessation of fertility and diminishing of hormone production). Women are born with all the eggs that they will possibly release. However, it is not until the onset of puberty that the eggs mature and leave the ovary. If fertilization occurs at any time during the years between puberty and menopause, the fertilized egg may grow and develop within the uterus. Various hormones are secreted from the ovary and from a blood-vessel–filled organ **(placenta)** that grows in the wall of the uterus during pregnancy. If fertilization does not occur, hormone changes result in the shedding of the uterine lining, and bleeding, or **menstruation,** occurs.

The names of the hormones of the ovaries that play important roles in the processes of menstruation and pregnancy, and in the development of secondary sex characteristics, are **estrogen** and **progesterone.** Other hormones that govern the functions of the ovaries, breasts, and uterus are secreted by the **pituitary gland,** which is located behind the bridge of the nose at the base of the brain.

Gynecology is the study of the female reproductive system (organs, hormones, and diseases); **obstetrics** (obstetrix means midwife) is a specialty concerned with pregnancy and the delivery of the fetus; and **neonatology** is the study and treatment of the newborn child.

II. Organs of the Female Reproductive System

Uterus, Ovaries, and Associated Organs

Figures 8–1 and 8–3 should be labeled as you read and study the following paragraphs.

Figure 8–1 is a lateral view of the female reproductive organs and shows their relationship to the other organs in the pelvic cavity. The **ovaries** [1] (only one ovary is shown in this lateral view) are a pair of small, almond-shaped organs located in the lower abdomen. The **fallopian tubes** [2] (only one is shown in this view) lead from each ovary to the **uterus** [3], which is a muscular organ situated between the urinary bladder and the rectum. The uterus is normally in a bent-forward position and about 3 inches in length in a nonpregnant woman. Midway between the uterus and the rectum is a region in the abdominal cavity known as the **cul-de-sac** [4]. This region is often examined for the presence of cancerous growths.

The **vagina** [5] is a tube extending from the uterus to the exterior of the body. **Bartholin glands** [6] are two small, rounded glands on either side of the vaginal orifice. These glands produce a mucous secretion that lubricates the vagina. The **clitoris** [7] is an organ of sensitive, erectile tissue located anterior to the vaginal orifice and in front of the urethral meatus. The clitoris is similar in structure to the penis in the male.

The region between the vaginal orifice and the anus is called the **perineum** [8]. The perineum can be torn in childbirth and cause injury to the anus. To avoid a perineal tear, the obstetrician often cuts the perineum posteriorly before delivery. This incision is called an **episiotomy.** The perineum is then sewn together (repaired) after childbirth.

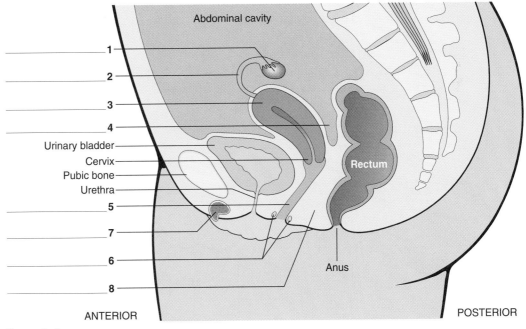

Figure 8–1

Organs of the female reproductive system, lateral view.

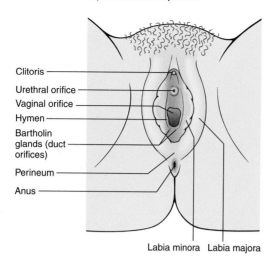

Clitoris
Urethral orifice
Vaginal orifice
Hymen
Bartholin glands (duct orifices)
Perineum
Anus

Labia minora   Labia majora

Figure 8-2

Female external genitalia (vulva).

The external genitalia (organs of reproduction) of the female are collectively called the **vulva.** Figure 8–2 shows the various structures that are part of the vulva. The **labia majora** are the outer lips of the vagina, and the **labia minora** are the smaller, inner lips. The **hymen** is a mucous membrane that normally partially covers the entrance to the vagina. The clitoris and Bartholin glands are also parts of the vulva.

Figure 8–3 is an anterior view of the female reproductive system. Each **ovary** [1] is held in place on either side of the uterus by a **utero-ovarian ligament** [2].

Within each ovary are thousands of small sacs called **graafian follicles** [3]. Each graafian follicle contains an **ovum** [4]. When an ovum is mature, the graafian follicle ruptures to the surface and the ovum leaves the ovary. The release of the ovum from the ovary is called **ovulation.** The ruptured follicle fills first with blood, and then with a yellow, fat-like material. It is then called the **corpus luteum** [5] (meaning yellow body).

Near each ovary is a duct, about 5½ inches long, called a **fallopian tube** [6]. Collectively, the fallopian tubes, ovaries, and supporting ligaments are called the **adnexa** (accessory structures) of the uterus. The egg, after its release from the ovary, is

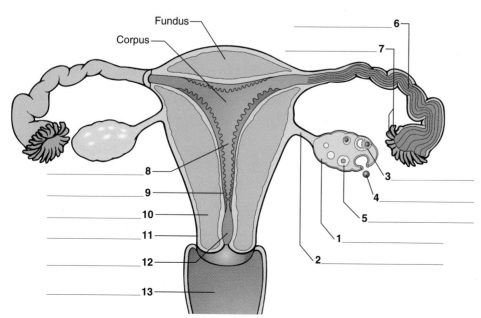

Fundus
Corpus

6
7
8
9
10
11
12
13
3
4
5
1
2

Figure 8-3

Organs of the female reproductive system, anterior view.

caught up by the finger-like ends of the fallopian tube. These ends are called **fimbriae** [7]. The tube itself is lined with small hairs that, through their motion, sweep the ovum along. It usually takes the ovum about 5 days to pass through the fallopian tube.

It is within the fallopian tube that fertilization takes place if any sperm cells are present. If coitus takes place near the time of ovulation and no contraception is used, there is a high likelihood that sperm cells will be in the fallopian tube when the egg cell is passing through it. If coitus has not taken place, the ovum remains unfertilized and, after a day or two, disintegrates.

The fallopian tubes, one on either side, lead into the **uterus** [8], a pear-shaped organ with muscular walls and a mucous membrane lining filled with a rich supply of blood vessels. The rounded upper portion of the uterus is the **fundus,** and the larger, central section is the **corpus** (body of the organ). The specialized epithelial mucosa of the uterus is the **endometrium** [9]; the middle, muscular layer is the **myometrium** [10], and the outer, membranous tissue layer is the **uterine serosa** [11]. A serosa is the outermost coat or layer of an organ that is in the abdomen or thorax.

The narrow, lower portion of the uterus is the **cervix** [12] (meaning neck). The cervical opening leads into a 3-inch-long tube called the **vagina** [13], which opens to the outside of the body.

The Breast (Accessory Organ of Reproduction)

Label Figure 8–4 as you read the following description of breast structures.

The breasts are two **mammary glands** located in the upper anterior region of the chest. They are composed of **glandular tissue** [1], containing milk glands, that develop in response to hormones from the ovaries during puberty. The breasts also contain **fibrous** and **fatty tissue** [2], special **lactiferous** (milk-carrying) **ducts** [3], and **sinuses** (cavities) [4] that carry milk to the opening, or nipple. The breast nipple is called the **mammary papilla** [5], and the dark-pigmented area around the mammary papilla is called the **areola** [6].

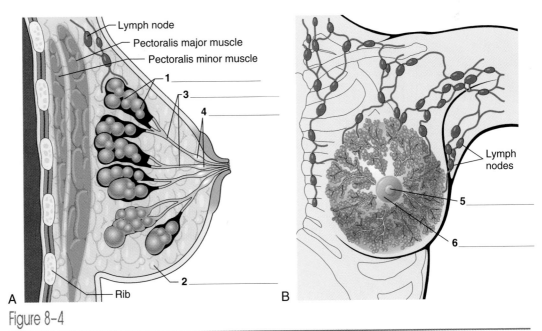

Figure 8–4

Views of the breast. (A) Sagittal. **(B)** Frontal. Notice the numerous lymph nodes.

During pregnancy, the hormones from the ovaries and the placenta stimulate glandular tissues in the breasts to their full development. After **parturition** (giving birth), hormones from the pituitary gland stimulate the production of milk **(lactation).**

III. Menstruation and Pregnancy

Menstrual Cycle (Fig. 8–5)

The beginning of menstruation at the time of puberty is called **menarche.** Each menstrual cycle is divided into 28 days. These days can be grouped into four time periods, which are useful in describing the events of the cycle. The approximate time periods are:

Days 1–5 (menstrual period) These are the days during which bloody fluid containing disintegrated endometrial cells, glandular secretions, and blood cells is discharged through the vagina.

Days 6–12 After the menstrual period ends, the endometrium begins to repair itself as the hormone **estrogen** is released by the maturing graafian follicle in the ovaries. This is also the period of the growth of the ovum in the graafian follicle.

Days 13–14 (ovulatory period) On about the 14th day of the cycle, the graafian follicle ruptures **(ovulation)** and the egg leaves the ovary to travel slowly down the fallopian tube.

Days 15–28 The empty graafian follicle fills with a yellow material and becomes known as the **corpus luteum.** The corpus

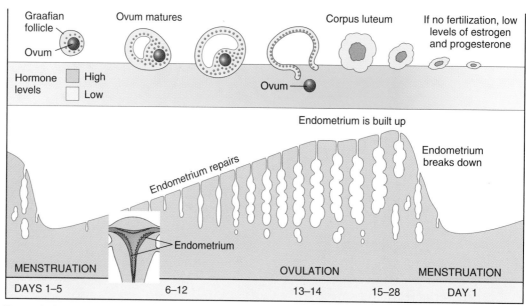

Figure 8-5

The menstrual cycle.

luteum functions as an endocrine organ and secretes two hormones, **estrogen** and **progesterone,** into the bloodstream. These hormones stimulate the building up of the lining of the uterus in anticipation of fertilization of the egg and pregnancy.

If fertilization does *not* occur, the corpus luteum in the ovary stops producing progesterone and estrogen and regresses. At this time, owing to the lowered levels of progesterone and estrogen, some women have symptoms of depression, breast tenderness, and irritability prior to menstruation. These symptoms are known as **premenstrual syndrome (PMS).** About 5 days after the fall in hormones, the uterine endometrium breaks down and the menstrual period begins (days 1–5).

Pregnancy

If fertilization does occur in the uterine tube, the fertilized egg travels to the uterus and implants in the uterine endometrium. The corpus luteum in the ovary continues to produce progesterone and estrogen, which support the vascular and muscular development of the uterine lining.

The **placenta,** a vascular organ, now forms within the uterine wall. The placenta is derived from maternal endometrium and from the **chorion,** the outermost membrane that surrounds the developing embryo. The **amnion** is the innermost of the embryonic membranes, and it holds the fetus suspended in an amniotic cavity surrounded by a fluid called the **amniotic fluid.** The amnion and fluid are sometimes known as the "bag of water," which usually ruptures (breaks) during labor.

The maternal blood and the fetal blood never mix during pregnancy, but important nutrients, oxygen, and wastes are exchanged as the blood vessels of the baby (coming from the umbilical cord) lie side by side with the mother's blood vessels in the placenta. Figure 8–6A and B shows the embryo's implantation in the uterus and its relationship to the placenta and enveloping membranes (the chorion and amnion).

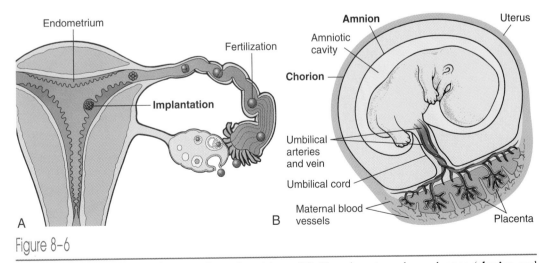

Figure 8–6

(A) Implantation of the embryo in the endometrium. (B) The placenta and membranes (**chorion** and **amnion**).

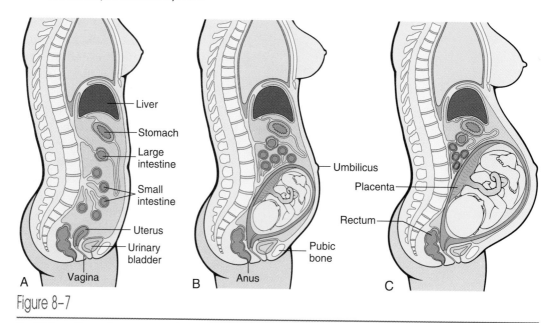

Figure 8-7

Sagittal sections of pregnancy. (A) Nonpregnant woman. **(B)** Woman 20 weeks pregnant. **(C)** Woman 30 weeks pregnant.

The placenta produces its own hormone as it develops in the uterus. This placental hormone is called **human chorionic gonadotropin (HCG).** HCG is the hormone tested for in the urine of women who suspect that they are pregnant. HCG stimulates the corpus luteum to continue producing hormones until about the 3rd month of pregnancy, when the placenta itself takes over the endocrine function and releases estrogen and progesterone. Progesterone maintains the development of the placenta. Low levels of progesterone can lead to spontaneous abortion in pregnant women and menstrual irregularities in nonpregnant women.

The uterus normally lies in the pelvis. During pregnancy, the uterus expands as the fetus grows, and the superior part rises out of the pelvic cavity. By about 28–30 weeks, it occupies a large part of the abdominopelvic cavity and reaches the epigastric region (Fig. 8–7).

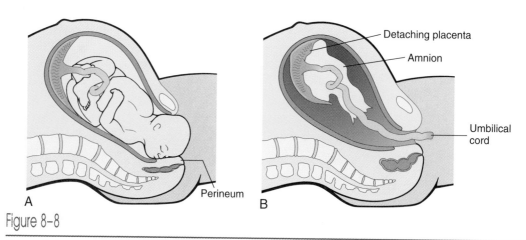

Figure 8-8

(A) Cephalic presentation of the fetus during delivery from the vaginal (birth) canal. **(B)** Between 10 and 15 minutes after parturition (birth), the placenta separates from the uterine wall. Forceful contractions expel the placenta and attached membranes, also called the afterbirth.

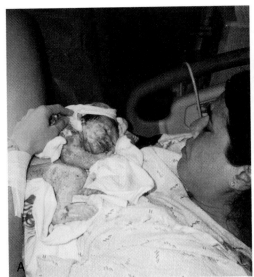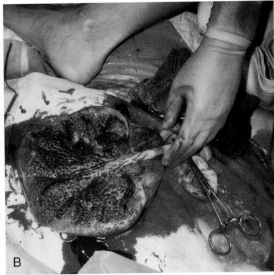

Figure 8-9

(A) My newborn granddaughter, Beatrix Bess (Bebe) Thompson, and her mother, Dr. Elizabeth Chabner Thompson, minutes after Bebe's birth. Notice that Bebe's skin is covered with vernix caseosa, a mixture of a fatty secretion from fetal sebaceous (oil) glands and dead skin. The vernix protects the fetus' delicate skin from abrasions, chapping, and hardening as a result of being bathed in amniotic fluid. **(B)** The placenta and umbilical cord just after expulsion from the uterus.

The onset of true labor is marked by rhythmic contractions, dilation of the cervix, and a discharge of bloody mucus from the cervix and vagina ("show"). In a normal delivery position, the head appears first (cephalic presentation) and helps to dilate the cervix. After the baby is delivered, the umbilical cord is expelled and cut (Fig. 8–8). Figure 8–9A and B shows photographs of a newborn and its placenta with attached cord, minutes after birth. The expelled placenta is known as the **afterbirth.**

IV. Hormonal Interactions

The events of menstruation and pregnancy are dependent not only upon hormones from the ovaries (estrogen and progesterone) but also on hormones from the **pituitary gland.** These pituitary gland hormones are **follicle-stimulating hormone (FSH)** and **luteinizing hormone (LH).** After the onset of menstruation, the pituitary gland begins to secrete FSH and LH, so that their levels rise in the bloodstream. FSH and LH stimulate the maturation of the ovum and ovulation. After ovulation, LH in particular influences the maintenance of the corpus luteum and its production of estrogen and progesterone.

During pregnancy, the high levels of estrogen and progesterone affect the pituitary gland itself by shutting off its production of FSH and LH. This means that while a woman is pregnant, additional eggs do not mature and ovulation cannot occur. This hormonal interaction wherein a high level of hormones (estrogen and progesterone) acts to shut off the production of another set of hormones (FSH and LH) is called **negative feedback.** Negative feedback is the principle behind the action of birth control pills. The pills contain varying amounts of estrogen and progesterone. As they are taken, the level of hormones rises in the blood. Negative feedback occurs, and the pituitary does not release FSH or LH. Without FSH or LH, ovulation cannot occur and a woman does not become pregnant. Currently, subdermal implants containing estrogen and progesterone can be effective for up to 5 years. The most common device is called Norplant.

Other female contraceptive measures include the **IUD (intrauterine device)** and the **diaphragm.** The IUD is a small coil placed inside the uterus by a physician. It prevents implantation of the fertilized egg in the uterine lining. Use of the IUD carries risks including ectopic uterine pregnancy, infection, uterine perforation, and severely increased and painful menstrual flow. The diaphragm is a rubber, cup-shaped device inserted, before coitus, on the outside of the cervix to prevent the entrance of sperm into the uterus.

When the secretion of estrogen from the ovaries lessens and fewer egg cells are produced, **menopause** begins. Menopause is the gradual ending of the menstrual cycle and is a natural process resulting from the normal aging of the ovaries. Other names for menopause are change of life and **climacteric.** Premature menopause occurs before age 35, whereas delayed menopause occurs after age 58. Artificial menopause can occur if the ovaries are removed by surgery or made nonfunctional by radiation therapy or some types of chemotherapy.

During menopause, when estrogen levels fall, many women experience hot flashes (the temperature regulation mechanism in the brain is disturbed) and vaginal atrophy (the lining of the vagina dries and thins, predisposing it to irritation and discomfort during sexual intercourse). **Estrogen replacement therapy (ERT),** given orally or as a transdermal patch, is sometimes used to relieve uncomfortable symptoms of menopause, and when combined with progesterone in low doses, it is believed to protect a woman from uterine cancer, the development of porous bones (osteoporosis), and heart disease. ERT has been associated with an increased risk of breast cancer in younger women who take it for longer periods.

V. Vocabulary

This list will help you review many of the new terms introduced in the text. Short definitions will reinforce your understanding of the terms. See Section XII of this chapter for help in pronouncing the more difficult terms.

adnexa	Accessory parts of the uterus; the fallopian tubes and ovaries.
amnion	Innermost membrane around the developing embryo.
areola	Dark-pigmented area around the breast nipple.
Bartholin glands	Small exocrine glands at the vaginal orifice.
cervix	Lower, neck-like portion of the uterus.
chorion	Outermost layer of the two membranes surrounding the embryo; it is part of the placenta.
clitoris	Organ of sensitive erectile tissue anterior to the urinary meatus.

coitus	Sexual intercourse; copulation. Pronunciation is KŌ-ĭ-tus.
corpus luteum	Empty graafian follicle that secretes estrogen and progesterone after release of the egg cell; literally means yellow (luteum) body (corpus).
cul-de-sac	Region within the pelvis, midway between the rectum and the uterus.
embryo	Stage in development from fertilization of the ovum through the 2nd month of pregnancy.
endometrium	The inner mucous membrane lining the uterus.
estrogen	Hormone produced by the ovaries; responsible for female secondary sex characteristics and buildup of the uterine lining during the menstrual cycle.
fallopian tubes	Ducts through which the egg travels into the uterus.
fertilization	Union of the sperm and ovum (fusion of the two nuclei occurs).
fetus	The embryo from the 3rd month (after 8 weeks) to birth.
fimbriae (plural)	Finger-like ends of the fallopian tubes.
follicle-stimulating hormone (FSH)	Hormone produced by the pituitary gland; stimulates maturation of the ovum.
gamete	Sex cell; sperm or ovum.
genitalia	Reproductive organs; also called genitals.
gestation	Pregnancy.
gonads	Organs in the male and female that produce gametes; ovaries and testes.
graafian follicle	Developing sac enclosing each ovum within the ovary. Only about 400 of these sacs mature in a woman's lifetime.
human chorionic gonadotropin (HCG)	Hormone produced by the placenta to sustain pregnancy by stimulating (-tropin) the mother's ovaries to produce estrogen and progesterone.
hymen	Mucous membrane partially or completely covering the vaginal orifice.
labia	Lips of the vagina; labia majora are the larger, outermost lips, and labia minora are the smaller, innermost lips.
lactiferous ducts	Tubes that carry milk within the breast.
luteinizing hormone (LH)	Hormone produced by the pituitary gland; promotes ovulation.

menarche	The beginning of the first menstrual period during puberty.
menopause	The gradual ending of menstrual function; climacteric.
menstruation	The monthly shedding of the uterine lining; menses means month.
myometrium	The muscle layer lining the uterus.
orifice	An opening.
ovaries	Organs in the female lower abdomen that produce ova and hormones; female gonads. the ovaries are almond-shaped and about the size of large walnuts.
ovulation	Release of the ovum from the ovary.
ovum (plural: **ova)**	Egg cell; female gamete.
papilla	A small nipple-shaped projection or elevation. The mammary papilla is the nipple of the breast.
parturition	Act of giving birth.
perineum	In females, the area between the anus and the vagina.
placenta	Vascular organ that develops during pregnancy in the uterine wall and serves as a communication between the maternal and the fetal bloodstreams.
progesterone	Hormone produced by the corpus luteum in the ovary and the placenta of pregnant women. Progesterone means hormone (-one) for (pro-) pregnancy (gester).
puberty	Beginning of the fertile period when gametes are produced and secondary sex characteristics appear.
uterine serosa	Outermost layer surrounding the uterus.
uterus	Womb; muscular organ in which the embryo develops. The upper portion is the fundus; the middle portion is the corpus; and the lower, neck portion is the cervix. (See Fig. 8–3.)
vagina	A tube extending from the uterus to the exterior of the body.
vulva	External genitalia of the female; includes the labia, hymen, and clitoris.

VI. Terminology: Combining Forms, Suffixes, and Prefixes

Write the meanings of the medical terms in the spaces provided.

Combining Forms

Combining Form	Meaning	Terminology	Meaning
amni/o	amnion	amniocentesis	
		amniotic fluid	
cervic/o	cervix, neck	endocervicitis	
chori/o **chorion/o**	chorion	choriogenesis	
		chorionic	
colp/o	vagina	colporrhaphy	
		colposcopy	
culd/o	cul-de-sac	culdocentesis	

A needle is placed through the posterior wall of the vagina, and fluid is withdrawn from the cul-de-sac for diagnostic purposes.

episi/o	vulva	episiotomy	

An incision is made through the skin of the perineum to enlarge the vaginal orifice through which the baby will pass.

galact/o	milk	galactorrhea	

Abnormal, persistent discharge of milk, commonly seen with pituitary gland tumors.

gynec/o	woman, female	gynecomastia	

One or both breasts enlarge in a male. It often occurs with puberty or with aging or is drug related.

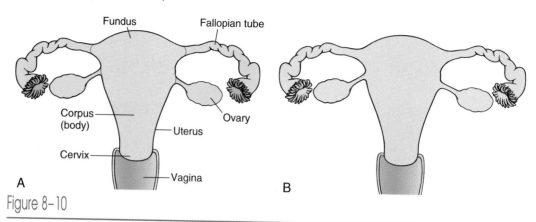

Fundus

Fallopian tube

Corpus (body)

Cervix

Uterus

Ovary

Vagina

A

B

Figure 8-10

(A) Total (complete) hysterectomy. The entire uterus (fundus, corpus, and cervix) is removed, but the ovaries and fallopian tubes remain. In a **laparoscopic assisted vaginal hysterectomy (LAVH),** the abdominal wall remains intact and the surgeon removes the uterus through an incision in the vagina with the aid of a laparoscope. **(B) Total hysterectomy with bilateral salpingo-oophorectomy** (fallopian tubes and ovaries are removed).

hyster/o	uterus, womb	hysterectomy _____
		Abdominal: removal through the abdominal wall; vaginal: removal through the vagina. A total abdominal hysterectomy (TAH) is removal of the entire uterus (including the cervix) through an abdominal incision (Fig. 8–10).
		hysteroscopy _____
		An endoscope (passed through the vagina) is used to view the uterine cavity.
lact/o	milk	lactogenesis _____
		lactation _____
		The normal secretion of milk.
mamm/o	breast	mammary _____
		mammoplasty _____
		Includes reduction and augmentation (enlargement) operations.
mast/o	breast	mastitis _____
		mastectomy _____
		Mastectomy procedures are discussed under carcinoma of the breast (see page 261, Section VII, Pathology).
men/o	menses, menstruation	amenorrhea _____
		Absence of menses for 6 months or for longer than 3 of the patient's normal menstrual cycles.
		dysmenorrhea _____

oligomenorrhea _____

Infrequent menstrual periods (interval varies from 36 days to 6 months).

menorrhagia _____

Profuse or prolonged menstrual bleeding occurring at regular intervals; fibroids (see page 260, Section VII, Pathology) are a leading cause of menorrhagia.

metr/o **metri/o**	uterus	metrorrhagia _____ *Uterine bleeding occurs between menses. Possible causes of metrorrhagia include ectopic pregnancy, cervical polyps, and ovarian and uterine tumors.* menometrorrhagia _____ *Excessive uterine bleeding at and between menstrual periods.* endometriosis _____ *See Section VII, Pathology.*
my/o	muscle	myometrium _____
myom/o	muscle tumor	myomectomy _____ *Fibroids are removed from the uterus.*
nat/i	birth	neonatal _____ *The neonatal period is the first 4 weeks of life after birth.*
obstetr/o	midwife	obstetric _____
o/o	egg	oogenesis _____
oophor/o	ovary	bilateral oophorectomy _____ *Oophor/o means to bear (phor/o) eggs (o/o).*
ov/o	egg	ovum _____
ovari/o	ovary	ovarian _____
ovul/o	egg	anovulatory _____
perine/o	perineum	perineorrhaphy _____
phor/o	to bear	oophoritis _____
salping/o	fallopian tubes	salpingectomy _____ *Figure 8–10B shows a total hysterectomy with bilateral salpingo-oophorectomy.*

| uter/o | uterus | uterine prolapse _____ |
| vagin/o | vagina | vaginal orifice _____ |

Orifice means opening. Colp/o also means vagina.

vaginitis _____

Bacteria and yeast (Candida) are common causes of infection. Use of antibiotics can change the internal environment (pH) of the vagina and destroy normally occurring bacteria, which allows yeast to grow.

| vulv/o | vulva | vulvovaginitis _____ |

Suffixes

Suffix	Meaning	Terminology	Meaning
-arche	beginning	menarche _____	
-cyesis	pregnancy	pseudocyesis _____	

Pseudo- means false. No pregnancy occurs, but symptoms such as weight gain and amenorrhea are present.

| **-gravida** | pregnancy | primigravida _____ | |

A woman during her first pregnancy (primi- means first). Gravida is also used as a noun to describe a pregnant woman, and it may be followed by numbers to indicate the number of pregnancies (gravida 1, 2, 3)

| **-parous** | to bear, bring forth | primiparous _____ | |

An adjective describing a woman who has borne (delivered) one child. Para is also used as a noun and may be followed by numbers to indicate the number of deliveries after the 20th week of gestation (para 1, 2, 3). When a woman arrives on the labor and delivery floor, her gravidity and parity are important facts to include in her medical and surgical history.

| **-rrhea** | discharge | leukorrhea _____ | |

This is a nonbloody vaginal discharge that may be mucoid or purulent (containing pus) and a sign of infection or cervicitis.

menorrhea _____

| **-salpinx** | uterine tube | pyosalpinx _____ | |
| **-tocia** | labor, birth | dystocia _____ | |

oxytocia _____

Oxy- means rapid. Oxytocin is a hormone released from the pituitary gland that stimulates the pregnant uterus to induce labor. It also causes milk to be secreted from the mammary glands.

-version	act of turning	cephalic version _____	

The fetal head turns or is turned toward the cervix. Presentation is the manner in which the fetus appears to the examiner during delivery. A breech presentation is buttocks first or feet first in a footling breech; a cephalic presentation is head first.

Prefixes			
Prefix	**Meaning**	**Terminology**	**Meaning**
ante-	before, forward	antenatal _____	
		anteversion _____	
		The normal position of the uterus—tilted anteriorly.	
dys-	painful	dyspareunia _____	
		Dĭs-pă-ROO-nē-ă. Pareunia means sexual intercourse.	
endo-	within	endometritis _____	
in-	in	involution of the uterus _____	
		Vol- means to roll. The uterus returns to its normal nonpregnant size.	
intra-	within	intrauterine device _____	
		Figure 8–11A shows an IUD in place in the uterus.	
multi-	many	multipara _____	
		multigravida _____	
		A woman who has been pregnant at least twice.	
nulli-	no, not, none	nulligravida _____	
		nullipara _____	
		Para 0. Figure 8–11B shows the cervix of a nulliparous woman and the cervix of a parous woman (who has had a vaginal delivery).	

Figure 8-11

(A) Intrauterine device (IUD) to prevent implantation of the fertilized egg. **(B) The cervix** of a **nulliparous woman** (the os, or opening, is small and perfectly round) and the cervix of a **parous woman** (the os is wide and irregular). These views would be visible under colposcopic examination.

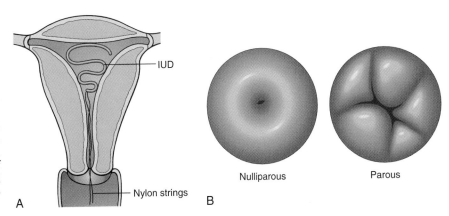

IUD

Nylon strings

A

Nulliparous   Parous

B

| **primi-** | first | primiparous _____ |
| **retro-** | backward | retroflexion _____ |

Flexion means to bend. The uterus is abnormally bent posteriorly.

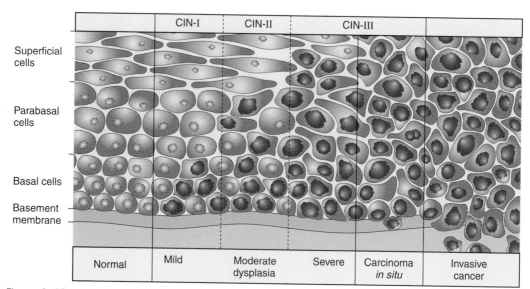

Figure 8-12

Carcinoma of the cervix. Notice the changes in cells from **normal** to preinvasive carcinoma, intraepithelial neoplasia, or **CIN** (dysplasia and carcinoma *in situ*), to **invasive cancer.** Normal epithelium contains mature, distinct layers of cells, whereas CIN epithelial layers are less distinct and have immature cells. Notice that the basement (foundation) membrane is intact in all forms of CIN, but cancerous cells have broken through in invasive cancer. (From Damjanov I: Pathology for the Health-Related Professions. Philadelphia, WB Saunders, 1996, p 381.)

VII. Pathology: Gynecological/Breast, Pregnancy, Neonatal

Gynecological and Breast

Uterus

carcinoma of the cervix

Malignant cells within the cervix (cervical cancer).

Cervical carcinoma is more common in women who have sexual intercourse at an early age, multiple sexual partners, a history of sexually transmitted diseases, and evidence of an **HPV (human papilloma virus)** infection. Early neoplastic changes in the cervix vary from **dysplasia** (abnormal cell growth) to **carcinoma *in situ* (CIS)** (localized cancer growth). Preinvasive neoplastic lesions (dysplasia and carcinoma *in situ*) are also called **CIN** (cervical intraepithelial neoplasia) and are graded from I to III as viewed on a **Pap smear** (microscopic examination of cells scraped off the cervical epithelium) (Fig. 8–12). Pap smears give important diagnostic information because CIN may be curable with resection. Further biopsy and resection **(conization)** may be necessary to diagnose and treat CIS. Surgery (hysterectomy) or radiation therapy (irradiation) or both are used to treat more extensive and metastatic disease.

cervicitis

Inflammation of the cervix.

This condition can become chronic because the lining of the cervix is not renewed each month as is the uterine lining during menstruation.

Common pathogens infecting the cervix are bacterial *(Chlamydia trachomatis* and *Neisseria gonorrhoeae)*, but many infections are nonspecific and the pathogenesis is not understood. Acute cervicitis is marked by **cervical erosions,** or ulcers, which appear as raw, red patches on the cervical mucosa. **Leukorrhea** (clear, white, or yellow pus-filled vaginal discharge) is also a symptom of cervical erosion.

After excluding the presence of malignancy (by Pap smear or biopsy), **cryocauterization** (destroying tissue by freezing) of the eroded area and treatment with antibiotics may be indicated.

carcinoma of the endometrium (endometrial cancer)

Malignant tumor of the uterus (inner lining).

The major symptom of adenocarcinoma of the uterus (endometrial cells lining the uterine cavity) is postmenopausal bleeding. Endometrial cancer is more common in women who are exposed to high levels of estrogen from exogenous estrogen (pills), estrogen-producing tumors, or obesity (estrogen is produced by fat tissue) and in nulliparous women. **Dilation** (opening the cervical canal) and **curettage** (scraping the inner lining of the uterus) is the best method of diagnosing the disease. If the tumor is confined to the uterus, it is curable by surgery (hysterectomy). Radiation therapy is prescribed for patients with more advanced disease.

endometriosis

Endometrial tissue is found in abnormal locations, including the ovaries, fallopian tubes, supporting ligaments, or small intestine.

Abnormal growth of endometrium can produce scar tissue, which causes dysmenorrhea, pelvic pain, infertility (inability to become pregnant), and dyspareunia. Most cases develop as a result of bits of menstrual endometrium that pass backward through the **lumen** (opening) of the fallopian tube and into the peritoneal cavity. Often, when the ovaries are involved, large blood-filled cysts, called chocolate cysts, may develop. Treatment ranges from symptomatic relief of pain and drugs that suppress the menstrual cycle to surgical removal of ectopic endometrial tissue and hysterectomy.

fibroids

Benign tumors in the uterus.

Fibroids, also called **leiomyomata** or **leiomyomas** (lei/o = smooth, my/o = muscle, and -oma = tumor), are composed of fibrous tissue and muscle. If fibroids grow too large and cause symptoms such as metrorrhagia, pelvic pain, or menorrhagia, hysterectomy or myomectomy is indicated. Figure 8–13 shows the location of uterine fibroids.

Ovaries

ovarian carcinoma

Malignant tumor of the ovary (adenocarcinoma).

Carcinomas of the ovary account for more deaths than those of cancers of the cervix or the uterus together. The tumor, which may be cystic or solid in consistency, is usually discovered in an advanced stage as an abdominal mass and may produce few symptoms in its early stages. In most patients, the disease metastasizes within or beyond the pelvic region before diagnosis. Surgery (oophorectomy and salpingectomy), radiotherapy, and more important, chemotherapy are used as therapeutic measures.

ovarian cysts

Collections of fluid within a sac (cyst) in the ovary.

Some cysts are lined by cells that are typical, normal lining cells of the ovary. These cysts originate in unruptured graafian follicles (follicle cysts) or in follicles that have ruptured and have immediately been sealed (luteal cysts). Other cysts may be lined with tumor cells (**cystadenomas** and **cystadenocarcinomas**). Occasionally it is necessary to remove these cysts to distinguish between benign and malignant tumors.

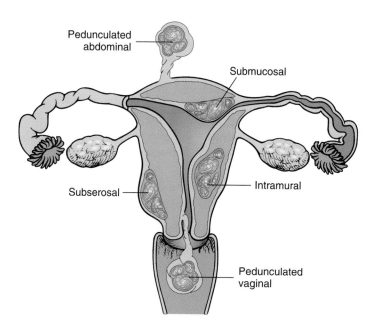

Figure 8-13

Location of uterine fibroids (leiomyomas). Pedunculated growths protrude on stalks. A **subserosal** mass lies under the serosal (outermost) layer of the uterus. A **submucosal** leiomyoma grows under the mucosal (innermost) layer. **Intramural** (mural means wall) masses arise within the muscular uterine wall. (From Damjanov I: Pathology for the Health-Related Professions. Philadelphia, WB Saunders, 1996, p 386.)

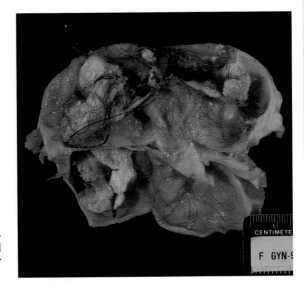

Figure 8-14

Dermoid cyst of the ovary with hair, skin, and teeth. (Courtesy of Dr. Elizabeth Chabner Thompson.)

Dermoid cysts are lined with a variety of cell types, including skin, hair, teeth, and cartilage, and arise from immature egg cells in the ovary. They are often called **benign cystic teratomas** (terat/o = monster) because of the strange assortment of tissue in the tumor (Fig. 8–14). Surgery to remove a dermoid cyst is curative.

Fallopian Tubes

pelvic inflammatory disease (PID)

Inflammation in the pelvic region; salpingitis.

The leading causes of PID are gonorrhea and chlamydial infection. They often occur at the same time, and repetitive episodes of these infections can lead to adhesions and scarring within the fallopian tubes. Women have an increased risk of ectopic pregnancies and difficulty getting pregnant after PID. Symptoms are vaginal discharge, pain in the abdomen (LLQ and RLQ), fever, and tenderness on **palpation** (examining by touch) of the cervix. An intrauterine device is the most common iatrogenic cause of PID. Antibiotics are used as treatment.

Breast

carcinoma of the breast

Malignant tumor of the breast (arising from milk glands and ducts).

This tumor first spreads to the lymph nodes located in the axilla (armpit) adjacent to the affected breast and then to the skin and chest wall. From the lymph nodes it may spread to any of the other body organs, including bone, liver, lung, or brain. The tumor is usually removed for purposes of diagnosis and as a primary means of treatment.

There are two objectives in the surgical treatment of breast cancer: first, to remove the tumor; and second, to sample the axillary lymph nodes to determine whether the tumor has spread beyond the breast. Various operations may be performed to accomplish these objectives. For small primary tumors the lump may be removed **(lumpectomy),** with the remainder of the breast left intact. This operation is usually followed by radiotherapy to the breast to kill remaining tumor cells. Alternatively, the surgeon may remove the entire breast **(simple** or **total mastectomy).** With either of these operations a separate incision is made to remove axillary lymph nodes to determine whether spread

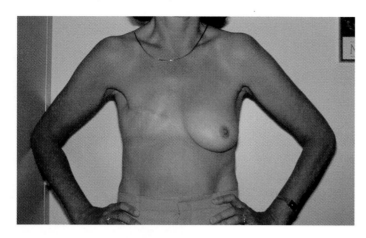

Figure 8-15

Surgical scar, modified radical mastectomy, right breast. (Courtesy of Dr. Elizabeth Chabner Thompson.)

beyond the breast has taken place. Another surgical procedure is removal of the breast, lymph nodes, and some adjacent chest wall muscles (pectorals) in a single procedure called a **modified radical mastectomy** (Fig. 8–15). If additional tumor is found in the axillary lymph nodes, the patient can then be treated with drugs (adjuvant chemotherapy) to prevent recurrence, and cure is possible.

After mastectomy, a plastic surgical procedure called a trans-rectus abdominis musculocutaneous flap **(TRAM flap)** may be performed to reconstruct the breast. A muscle from the lower abdomen is tunneled under the abdominal and thoracic wall to its new location at the mastectomy scar. Most surgeons perform the nipple reconstruction at a later time (Fig. 8–16).

It is also important to test the breast cancer tumor for the presence of **estrogen receptors.** These receptors are proteins that indicate that the tumor will respond to hormone therapy. If metastases should subsequently develop, this information will be valuable in selecting further treatment. **SERMs** are selective estrogen receptor modulators, a class of drugs that functions like estrogen in some tissues, but blocks estrogen's effect in others. The best known is **tamoxifen.** It blocks the potentially harmful action of estrogen in the breast (especially in women with estrogen receptor positive tumors), but preserves estrogen's benefits for bone maintenance and cardiovascular effects. Unfortunately, it retains estrogen's tendency to promote endometrial cancer. Another SERM, raloxifene, appears to have similar benefits but less risk of promoting uterine cancer.

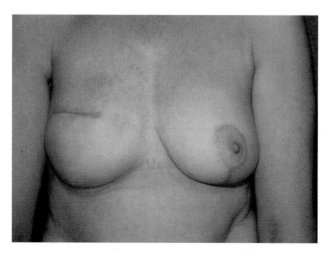

Figure 8-16

TRAM flap breast reconstruction. Right breast shows the results of TRAM flap reconstruction. Notice that the nipple reconstruction has not yet been performed. The left breast shows a lumpectomy scar. (Courtesy of Dr. Elizabeth Chabner Thompson.)

fibrocystic disease   **Small sacs of tissue and fluid in the breast.**

This is a common benign condition of the breast. The patient notices a nodular (lumpy) consistency of the breast, often associated with premenstrual tenderness and fullness. Mammography and then surgical biopsy may be indicated to differentiate fibrocystic changes from carcinoma of the breast.

Pregnancy

abruptio placentae   **Premature separation of the implanted placenta.**

Abruptio means a breaking or tearing away from, and placentae means of the placenta. This can occur secondary to trauma, such as a fall, seat belt injury, or assault or because of vascular insufficiency resulting from hypertension, cocaine use, or preeclampsia (see page 264). Symptoms of abruptio placentae include a sudden searing (burning) abdominal pain and bleeding. This is an obstetrical emergency.

choriocarcinoma   **Malignant tumor of the pregnant uterus.**

The tumor may appear following pregnancy or abortion. Cure is possible with surgery and chemotherapy.

ectopic pregnancy   **Implantation of the fertilized egg in any site other than the normal uterine location.**

The condition occurs in up to 1 per cent of pregnancies, and 90 per cent of these occur in the oviducts **(tubal pregnancy).** Rupture of the ectopic pregnancy within the fallopian tube can lead to massive hematosalpinx. Surgery is indicated to remove the implant and preserve the fallopian tube before rupture occurs. Other sites of ectopic pregnancies include the ovaries and abdominal cavity, and all are surgical emergencies.

placenta previa   **Placental implantation over the cervical os (opening) or in the lower region of the uterine wall (Fig. 8–17).**

This condition can result in less oxygen supply to the fetus and increased risk of hemorrhage and infection for the mother. Maternal symptoms include painless bleeding, hemorrhage, and premature labor. Cesarean delivery is usually recommended.

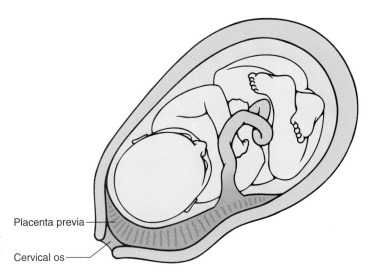

Figure 8–17

Placenta previa. Previa means before or in the front of.

Placenta previa

Cervical os

preeclampsia

A condition that occurs during pregnancy or shortly after and is marked by high blood pressure, proteinuria, and edema. If seizures occur, the condition is known as eclampsia or toxemia.

Mild preeclampsia can be managed by bed rest, but the more serious form of the illness is often more difficult to treat, and women are placed on medications such as magnesium sulfate and Dilantin to prevent seizures while in labor.

Neonatal

The following terms describe a few of the conditions or symptoms that may affect the newborn. The **Apgar score** is a system of scoring an infant's physical condition 1 and 5 minutes after birth. **Heart rate, respiration, color, muscle tone,** and **response to stimuli** are rated 0, 1, or 2. The maximum total score is 10. Infants with low Apgar scores require prompt medical attention (Fig. 8–18).

Down syndrome

Chromosomal abnormality (trisomy-21) results in mental retardation, retarded growth, a flat face with a short nose, low-set ears, and slanted eyes.

erythroblastosis fetalis

Hemolytic disease in the newborn caused by a blood group (Rh factor) incompatibility between the mother and the fetus.

hyaline membrane disease

Respiratory problem primarily in the premature neonate; lack of protein in the lining of the lung tissue causes collapse of the lungs.

This condition is also known as **respiratory distress syndrome.** Hyaline refers to the shiny (hyaline means glassy) membrane that forms in the lung sacs.

hydrocephalus

Accumulation of fluid in the spaces of the brain.

In an infant, the entire head can enlarge because the bones of the skull are never completely fused together at birth. The soft spot, normally present between the cranial bones of the fetus, is called a **fontanelle.** Hydrocephalus occurs because of a problem in the circulation of fluid within the brain and spinal cord.

APGAR SCORING CHART

SIGN	0	1	2
Heart rate	Absent	Below 100	Over 100
Respiratory effort	Absent	Slow, irregular	Good, crying
Muscle tone	Limp	Some flexion of extremities	Active motion
Response to catheter in nostril (tested after oropharynx is clear)	No response	Grimace	Cough or sneeze
Color	Blue, pale	Body pink, extremities blue	Completely pink

Figure 8–18

Apgar scoring chart. (Redrawn from O'Toole M [ed]: Miller-Keane Encyclopedia of Medicine, Nursing, and Allied Health, 6th ed. Philadelphia, WB Saunders, 1997, p 116.)

kernicterus   **High levels of bilirubin in the bloodstream of a neonate; leads to brain damage and mental retardation.**

Kern- means nucleus, referring to a collection of nerve cells in the brain. Icterus means yellow color or jaundice.

pyloric stenosis   **Narrowing of the opening of the stomach to the duodenum.**

Surgical repair of the pyloric opening may be necessary.

VIII. Clinical Tests, Procedures, and Abbreviations

Clinical Tests

Pap smear   The physician, after inserting a vaginal speculum (instrument to hold apart the vaginal walls), uses a wooden spatula and a cotton swab to take secretions from the cervix and vagina (Fig. 8–19). Microscopic analysis of the cell smear (spread on a glass slide) can detect the presence of cervical or vaginal carcinoma.

pregnancy test   Blood or urine test to detect the presence of HCG.

Procedures

X-Rays

hysterosalpingography   Contrast material is injected into the uterus and fallopian tubes, and x-rays are taken.

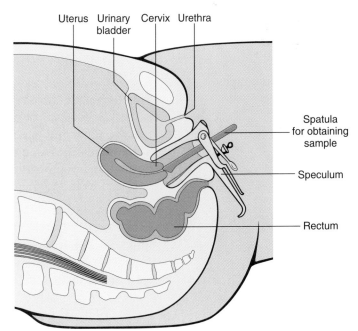

Uterus   Urinary bladder   Cervix   Urethra

Spatula for obtaining sample

Speculum

Rectum

Figure 8-19

Method of obtaining a sample for a **Pap smear.** The test is 95 per cent accurate in diagnosing early carcinoma of the cervix.

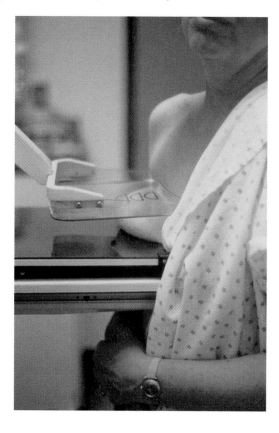

Figure 8-20

Mammography. The breast is compressed and x-rays (top to bottom and lateral) are taken. (Courtesy of Dr. Elizabeth Chabner Thompson.)

mammography	X-rays are taken of the breast. It is recommended that women have a baseline mammogram around the age of 50 for later comparisons if needed. Every 1 to 2 years a mammogram is recommended for women over the age of 50 to screen for breast cancer. Figure 8–20 illustrates mammography.

Ultrasound

pelvic ultrasonography	A record of sound waves as they bounce off organs in the pelvic region. This technique can evaluate fetal size, maturity, and organ development as well as fetal and placental position. Uterine tumors and other pelvic masses, including abscesses, can also be diagnosed by ultrasonography. **Transvaginal ultrasound** allows the radiologist a closer, sharper look at normal and pathological structures within the pelvis. The sound probe is placed in the vagina instead of across the pelvis or abdomen.

Gynecological Procedures

aspiration	Fluid is withdrawn by suction from a cavity or sac with a needle. Aspiration biopsy is a valuable technique for the evaluation of a patient with breast disease.
cauterization	Destruction of abnormal tissue with chemicals (silver nitrate) or an electrically heated instrument. It is used to treat cervical dysplasia or cervical erosion. **LEEP** is a loop electrocautery excision procedure to biopsy abnormal cervical tissue.

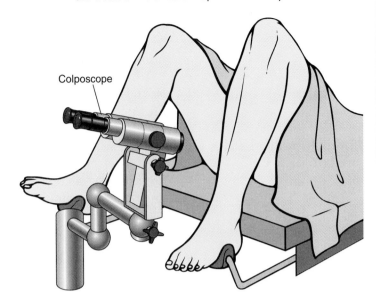

Figure 8-21

Colposcopy is used to evaluate a patient with an abnormal Pap smear. The female being examined is in the **dorsal lithotomy position.** This is so named because it is the same position used to remove a urinary tract stone (lithotomy means incision to remove a stone).

colposcopy

Visual examination of the vagina and cervix using a colposcope (a lighted, magnifying instrument resembling a small, mounted pair of binoculars). This procedure is more accurate than a Pap smear because it can identify the specific areas in which abnormal cells are located. A biopsy then can be taken from those areas for accurate diagnosis (Fig. 8–21).

conization

Removal of a cone-shaped section of the cervix for biopsy (diagnosis). The cone is cut out with a **cold knife** (blade) or **laser** (a device that produces a very thin beam of light in which high energies are concentrated) so as not to distort the tissue for histological examination (Fig. 8–22).

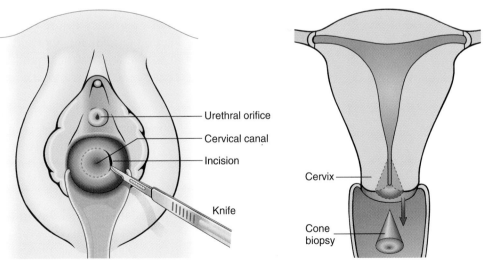

Urethral orifice

Cervical canal

Incision

Knife

Cervix

Cone biopsy

Figure 8-22

Two views of **conization of the cervix.**

cryosurgery Use of cold (cry/o means cold) temperatures to destroy tissue. The freezing temperature is produced by a probe containing liquid nitrogen. Also called **cryocauterization.**

culdocentesis Needle aspiration (through the vagina) of fluid from the cul-de-sac. Presence of blood may indicate a ruptured ectopic pregnancy.

dilation (dilatation) and curettage (D & C) Dilation (widening) of the cervical opening is accomplished by inserting a series of probes of increasing size. Curettage (scraping) is then performed using a curette (a metal loop at the end of a long, thin handle) to remove the lining of the uterus. This procedure is performed to diagnose uterine disease (obtaining tissue for microscopic examination) or to stop prolonged or heavy uterine bleeding. It is also used for the purpose of terminating a pregnancy or emptying the contents of the uterus (Fig. 8–23).

exenteration Removal of internal organs. Pelvic exenteration is the removal of the uterus, ovaries, fallopian tubes, vagina, bladder, rectum, and lymph nodes.

laparoscopy Visual examination of the abdominal cavity by making a small incision near a woman's navel and introducing a laparoscope (a thin tube containing a viewing instrument and light). The procedure is performed for diagnosis of disease or for tubal ligation.

tubal ligation Blocking of the fallopian tubes by burning or cutting them and tying them off. This **sterilization** (making an individual incapable of reproduction) technique involves making a small incision into the abdomen and inserting a laparoscope through which the instrument to block the tubes can be introduced.

Procedures During Pregnancy

abortion Premature termination of pregnancy before the embryo or fetus is able to exist on its own. Major methods for abortion are vaginal evacuation by D & C or vacuum aspiration (suction) and stimulation of uterine contractions by injecting saline (salt) into the amniotic cavity (second trimester).

amniocentesis Surgical puncture (transabdominal) of the amniotic sac to withdraw amniotic fluid for analysis. The cells of the fetus, found in the fluid, are cultured (grown), and cytological and biochemical studies are made (Fig. 8–24).

cesarean section Removal of the fetus by abdominal incision into the uterus (hysterotomy). Indications for cesarean section are cephalopelvic disproportion, hemorrhage from abruptio placentae or placenta previa, fetal distress (fetal hypoxia), and breech or shoulder presentation. The procedure takes its name from the Latin word *caedere,* to cut.

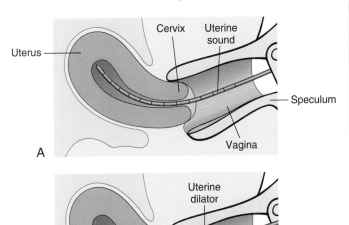

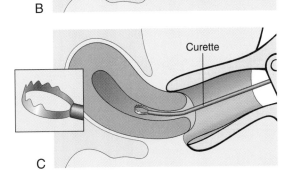

Figure 8-23

Dilation and curettage (D&C) of the uterus. **(A)** The uterine cavity is explored with a uterine sound (a slender instrument to measure the depth of the uterus to prevent perforation during dilation. **(B)** Uterine dilators (Hanks or Hagar) in graduated sizes are used to slowly dilate the cervix. **(C)** The uterus is gently curetted and specimens are collected.

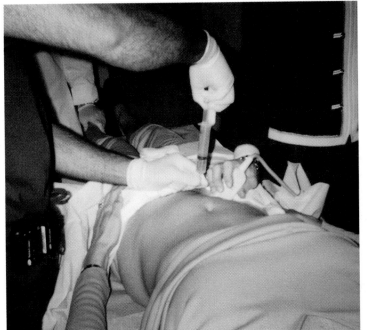

Figure 8-24

Amniocentesis. The obstetrician has placed a long needle through the patient's abdominal wall and into the amniotic cavity. His placement (avoiding the fetus and the placenta) is guided by concurrent ultrasound images produced by the transducer in the hand of the ultrasonographer. Amniotic fluid is the yellow liquid aspirated into the syringe attached to the needle. This patient was in her 16th week of pregnancy and the amniocentesis was performed because a low AFP (alpha-fetoprotein) level suggested that she was carrying a Down syndrome baby. Karyotype analysis (received 10 days later) showed normal chromosome configuration.

chorionic villus sampling   Transcervical sampling of chorionic villi (placental tissue) for prenatal diagnosis at 9–12 weeks of gestation. Fetal tissue is aspirated under ultrasound guidance.

fetal monitoring   Use of ultrasonography and electrocardiography to record the fetal heart rate (FHR) during labor.

pelvimetry   Measurement of the dimensions of the mother's pelvis to determine its capacity to allow passage of the fetus through the birth canal. Usually this is a part of the prenatal examination, but it is also of vital importance during protracted labor or with breech presentation.

ABBREVIATIONS

AB	abortion	**EDC**	estimated date of confinement
AFP	alpha-fetoprotein; high levels in amniotic fluid of fetus or maternal serum indicate increased risk of neurological birth defects in the infant.	**EMB**	endometrial biopsy
		ERT	estrogen replacement therapy
		FHR	fetal heart rate
BSE	breast self-examination	**FSH**	follicle-stimulating hormone
C-section	cesarean section	**G**	gravida (pregnant)
CIN	cervical intraepithelial neoplasia	**GYN**	gynecology
CIS	carcinoma *in situ*	**HCG; hCG**	human chorionic gonadotropin
CS	cesarean section	**HDN**	hemolytic disease of the newborn
CVS	chorionic villus sampling	**HPV**	human papilloma virus
Cx	cervix	**HSG**	hysterosalpingography
D & C	dilation (dilatation) and curettage	**IUD**	intrauterine device; contraceptive
DCIS	ductal carcinoma *in situ;* a precancerous breast lesion that indicates a higher risk for invasive ductal breast cancer	**LAVH**	laparoscopic assisted vaginal hysterectomy
DES	diethylstilbestrol; an estrogen compound used in the treatment of menopausal problems involving estrogen deficiency; if administered during pregnancy, it has been found to be related to subsequent tumors in the daughters (rarely in sons) of mothers so treated.	**LEEP**	loop electrocautery excision procedure
		LH	luteinizing hormone
		LMP	last menstrual period
		multip	multipara; multiparous
DUB	dysfunctional uterine bleeding	**OB**	obstetrics
ECC	endocervical curettage	**OCPs**	oral contraceptive pills

Para 2-0-1-2	woman's reproductive history: 2 full-term infants, 0 preterm, 1 abortion, and 2 living children	**SERMs**	selective estrogen receptor modulators
Pap smear	Papanicolaou smear (test for cervical or vaginal cancer)	**SLN biopsy**	sentinel node biopsy; blue dye or radioisotopes (or both) identifies the first lymph node draining the breast lymphatics
Path	pathology	**TAH-BSO**	total abdominal hysterectomy with bilateral salpingo-oophorectomy
PID	pelvic inflammatory disease	**TRAM flap**	trans-rectus abdominis musculocutaneous flap; breast reconstruction
PMS	premenstrual syndrome		
primip	primipara; primiparous		

IX. Practical Applications

This section contains medical terms that you have studied in this and previous chapters. Explanations of more difficult terms are added in brackets. Answers to the questions are on page 284 after Answers to Exercises.

Operative Report. Preoperative Diagnosis: Menorrhagia, Leiomyomata

Anesthetic: General
Material forwarded to laboratory for examination:

A. Endocervical curettings
B. Endometrial curettings

Operation performed: Dilation and curettage of the uterus

With the patient in the dorsal lithotomy position [legs are flexed on the thighs, thighs flexed on the abdomen and abducted] and sterilely prepped and draped, manual examination of the uterus revealed it to be 6- to 8-week size, retroflexed; no adnexal masses noted. The anterior lip of the cervix was then grasped with a tenaculum [a hook-like surgical instrument for grasping and holding parts]. The cervix was dilated up to a #20 Hank's dilator. The uterus was sounded [widened] up to 4 inches. A sharp curettage of the endocervix showed only a scant amount of tissue. With a sharp curettage, the uterus was curetted in a clockwise fashion with an irregularity noted in the posterior floor. A large amount of hyperplastic endometrial tissue was removed. The patient tolerated the procedure well.

Operative diagnosis: Leiomyomata uteri

Sentences Using Medical Terminology

1. Mammogram report: The breast parenchyma [essential tissue] is symmetrical bilaterally. There are no abnormal masses or calcifications in either breast. The axillae are normal.

2. This is a 43-year-old G3P2 with premature ovarian failure and now on ERT. She has history of endocervical atypia [cells are not normal or typical] secondary to chlamydial infection, which is now being treated.

3. The patient is a 40-year-old gravida II, para II, white female admitted for exploratory celiotomy [laparotomy] to remove and evaluate 10-cm left adnexal mass. Discharge diagnosis: (1) endometriosis, left ovary; (2) benign cystic teratoma [dermoid cyst], left ovary.

Operating Schedule: General Hospital

Match the surgery list in column I with a diagnosis or reason for the surgery in column II.

Column I—Surgery

1. Conization of the cervix _____

2. Vaginal hysterectomy with colporrhaphy _____

3. TAH-BSO, pelvic and periaortic lymphadenectomy _____

4. Exploratory laparotomy for uterine myomectomy _____

5. Excision of bilateral gynecomastia _____

6. Modified radical mastectomy _____

Column II—Diagnosis

A. Persistent, excessive breast tissue in a male
B. Fibroids
C. Endometrial carcinoma
D. Adenocarcinoma of the breast
E. Suspected cervical cancer
F. Uterine prolapse

X. Exercises

Remember to check your answers carefully with those given in Section XI, Answers to Exercises.

A. Match the following terms for structures or tissues with their meanings below.

fimbriae	cervix	vulva	mammary papilla
chorion	endometrium	perineum	ovaries
amnion	clitoris	fallopian tubes	placenta
areola	labia	uterine serosa	vagina

1. inner lining of the uterus _____

2. area between the anus and the vagina in females _____

3. dark-pigmented area around the breast nipple _____

4. finger-like ends of the fallopian tube _____

5. oviducts; ducts through which the egg travels into the uterus from the ovary

   _____

6. organ of sensitive erectile tissue in females; anterior to urethral orifice

   _____

7. nipple of the breast _____

8. blood-vessel–filled organ that develops during pregnancy in the uterine wall and serves as a communication between maternal and fetal bloodstreams _____

9. lower, neck-like portion of the uterus _____

10. innermost membrane around the developing embryo _____

11. outermost layer of the membranes around the developing embryo and forming part of the placenta _____

12. membrane surrounding the uterus _____

13. lips of the vagina _____

14. female gonads; producing ova and hormones _____

15. includes the perineum, labia, clitoris, and hymen; external genitalia _____

16. muscular tube extending from the uterus to the exterior of the body _____

B. Identify the following terms.

1. fetus _____

2. lactiferous ducts _____

3. gametes _____

4. gonads _____

5. adnexa _____

6. cul-de-sac _____

7. genitalia _____

8. Bartholin glands _____

9. graafian follicle _____

10. corpus luteum _____

C. Match the terms below with their descriptions.

menarche   coitus   human chorionic gonadotropin
luteinizing hormone   follicle-stimulating hormone   progesterone
myometrium   anteversion   fertilization
estrogen

1. a hormone produced by the ovaries; responsible for femaleness and buildup of the uterine lining

   during the menstrual cycle _____

2. a hormone produced by the pituitary gland to stimulate the maturation of the graafian follicle

   and ovum in the ovary _____

3. sexual intercourse _____

4. the normal bending forward of the uterus in the pelvic cavity _____

5. beginning of the first menstrual period during puberty _____

6. hormone produced by the placenta to sustain pregnancy by stimulating the ovaries to produce

   estrogen and progesterone _____

7. muscle layer lining the uterus _____

8. hormone produced by the corpus luteum in the ovary and also by the placenta of a pregnant

   woman _____

9. hormone produced by the pituitary gland to promote ovulation _____

10. fusion of the nuclei of the sperm and ovum _____

D. Give the meanings of the following.

1. galact/o and lact/o both mean _____

2. colp/o and vagin/o both mean _____

3. mamm/o and mast/o both mean _____

4. metr/o, uter/o, and hyster/o all mean _____

5. oophor/o and ovari/o both mean _____

6. o/o, ov/o, and ovul/o all mean _____

7. in- and endo- both mean _____

8. -cyesis and -gravida both mean _____

9. salping/o and -salpinx both mean _____

10. episi/o and vulv/o both mean _____

E. Complete the terms based on the meanings given.

1. inflammation of the cervix: _____ itis

2. suture of the vagina: colp _____

3. surgical puncture to remove fluid from the cul-de-sac: _____ centesis

4. surgical repair of the breast: mammo _____

5. removal of both fallopian tubes: bi _____ _____ ectomy

6. pertaining to newborn: neo _____

7. difficult labor: dys _____

8. first menstrual period: men _____

9. rapid labor: _____ tocia

10. production of milk: lacto _____

F. Give the meanings of the following symptoms.

1. amenorrhea _____

2. dysmenorrhea _____

3. leukorrhea _____

4. metrorrhagia _____

5. galactorrhea _____

6. menorrhagia _____

7. pyosalpinx _____

8. dyspareunia _____

9. menometrorrhagia _____

10. oligomenorrhea _____

G. State whether the following sentences are true or false and explain your answers.

1. After a total (complete) hysterectomy, a woman still has regular menstrual periods.

_____

2. After a total hysterectomy, a woman may still produce estrogen and progesterone.

_____

3. Birth control pills prevent pregnancy by reducing the levels of FSH and LH in the bloodstream.

_____

4. After a total hysterectomy with bilateral salpingo-oophorectomy, a doctor may advise estrogen

replacement therapy. _____

5. A total mastectomy involves removal of the entire breast, axillary nodes, and chest muscles.

_____

6. An episiotomy is an incision of the cervix and is part of a Pap smear. _____

7. Human chorionic gonadotropin is produced by the ovaries during pregnancy.

_____

8. Gynecomastia is a common condition in pregnant women. _____

9. Treatment for endometriosis is uterine myomectomy. _____

10. A gravida 3, para 2 is a woman who has given birth 3 times. _____

11. A nulligravida is a woman who has had several pregnancies. _____

12. Pseudocyesis is the same condition as a tubal pregnancy. _____

13. Fibrocystic changes in the breast are a malignant condition. _____

14. Cystadenomas occur in the ovaries. _____

15. FSH and LH are ovarian hormones. _____

H. Give the meanings of the following terms.

1. parturition _____

2. menopause _____

3. menarche _____

4. ovulation _____

5. gestation _____

6. anovulatory _____

7. sterilization _____

8. lactation _____

9. nulliparous _____

10. oophoritis _____

I. Match the following terms with their meanings as given below.

abruptio placentae	cervical carcinoma	cystadenocarcinoma
carcinoma *in situ*	cervicitis	choriocarcinoma
endometrial carcinoma	endometriosis	preeclampsia
placenta previa	leiomyomas	

1. a malignant tumor of the ovary _____

2. a chlamydial infection causing inflammation in the lower, neck-like portion of the uterus

    _____

3. cancerous tumor cells are localized in a small area _____

4. a condition during pregnancy or shortly thereafter, marked by hypertension, proteinuria, and

    edema _____

5. uterine tissue located outside the uterus (in the ovaries or cul-de-sac or attached to the perito-

    neum) _____

6. premature separation of a normally implanted placenta _____

7. placenta implantation over the cervical opening _____

8. a malignant tumor of the pregnant uterus _____

9. a malignant condition that can be diagnosed by a Pap smear, revealing dysplastic changes in cells

    _____

10. a malignant condition of the inner lining of the uterus _____

11. benign muscle tumors in the uterus _____

J. Give the name of the test or procedure described below. Parts of some terms are given.

1. destruction of abnormal tissue with chemicals or an electrically heated instrument:

    _____

2. contrast material is injected into the uterus and fallopian tubes, and x-rays are taken:

    _____ graphy

3. cold temperatures are used to destroy tissue:

    _____

4. visual examination of the vagina and cervix:

   _____ scopy

5. widening the cervical opening and scraping the lining of the uterus:

   _____

6. withdrawal of fluid by suction with a needle:

   _____

7. process of recording x-rays of the breast:

   mammo _____

8. a cone-shaped section of the cervix is removed for diagnosis or treatment of cervical dysplasia:

   _____

9. surgical puncture to remove fluid from the cul-de-sac:

   _____

10. echoes from sound waves are used to create an image of structures in the region of the hip:

    pelv _____ _____ ography

11. blocking the fallopian tubes by burning or cutting them and tying them off:

    _____

12. visual examination of the abdominal cavity:

    _____ scopy

13. HCG is measured in the urine or blood:

    _____ test

14. cells are taken from the cervix or vagina for microscopic analysis:

    _____ smear

15. complete removal of internal organs in the pelvic region:

    _____

K. Match the obstetrical and neonatal terms with the descriptions given below.

abortion	fontanelle	hydrocephalus
Apgar	cephalic version	cesarean section
pelvimetry	erythroblastosis fetalis	hyaline membrane disease
kernicterus	pyloric stenosis	fetal monitoring

1. Turning the fetus so that the head is toward the examiner is called _____ .

2. Measurement of the dimensions of the maternal pelvic bone is called

_____ .

3. The soft spot between the newborn's cranial bones is called a (an) _____ .

4. The evaluation of the newborn's physical condition is called a (an)

_____ score.

5. Premature termination of pregnancy is known as _____ .

6. Removal of the fetus by abdominal incision of the uterus is a (an) _____ .

7. A serious respiratory condition of the fetal lungs leading to collapse of the lungs is

_____ .

8. Use of a machine to electronically record fetal heart rate during labor is known as

_____ .

9. Narrowing of the opening of the stomach to the small intestine in the infant is called

_____ .

10. Hemolytic disease of the newborn is called _____ .

11. Accumulation of fluid in the spaces of a neonate's brain is called _____ .

12. The condition of high blood levels of bilirubin that can cause brain damage in the neonate is

called _____ .

L. Give medical terms for the following meanings. Pay careful attention to spelling.

1. benign muscle tumors in the uterus: _____

2. no menstrual discharge: _____

3. accessory organs: _____

4. suture of the vagina: _____

5. removal of an ovary: _____

6. condition of female breasts (in a male): _____

7. reproductive organs: _____

8. widening: _____

9. scraping: _____

10. ovarian hormone that sustains pregnancy: _____

11. nipple-shaped elevation: _____

12. inflammation of the vulva and vagina: _____

M. Give the meanings of the following abbreviations and then select the letter of the sentence that is the best association for each.

Column I

1. CIN _____ ____

2. FSH _____ ____

3. D & C _____ ____

4. multip _____ ____

5. CS _____ ____

6. AFP _____ ____

7. DCIS _____ ____

8. TAH-BSO _____ ____

9. primip _____ ____

10. SERMs _____ ____

Column II

A. This woman has given birth to three infants.

B. When levels of this protein are elevated, fetal spinal cord abnormalities are suspected.

C. This woman has given birth for the first time.

D. This is a secretion from the pituitary gland; it stimulates the ovaries.

E. This procedure is performed to stop abnormal uterine bleeding.

F. These are preinvasive changes in the lining of the neck of the uterus.

G. This surgical procedure is the removal of the uterus, fallopian tubes, and ovaries.

H. In this obstetrical procedure, the infant is delivered through an abdominal incision.

I. Tamoxifen is an example of these drugs that block estrogen's effect on breast tissue.

J. This is an example of a precancerous breast lesion.

N. Circle the term in parentheses that best completes the meaning of each sentence.

1. Dr. Hanson felt that it was important to do a **(culdocentesis, Pap smear, amniocentesis)** once yearly on each of her GYN patients to screen for abnormal cells.

2. When Doris missed her period, her doctor checked for the presence of **(LH, IUD, HCG)** in Doris' urine to see if she was pregnant.

3. Ellen was 34 weeks pregnant, experiencing bad headaches, a 10-pound weight gain in 2 days, and blurry vision. Dr. Murphy told her to go to the obstetrical emergency room because she suspected **(preeclampsia, pelvic inflammatory disease, fibroids)**.

4. Dr. Harris felt a breast mass when examining Mrs. Clark. She immediately ordered a **(dilation and curettage, hysterosalpingogram, mammogram)** for her 35-year-old patient.

5. Clara knew that she should not ignore her fevers and yellow vaginal discharge and the pain in her side. She had had a previous episode of **(PMS, PID, DES)** that was treated with IV antibiotics and was worried that she might have a recurrence.

XI. Answers to Exercises

A

1. endometrium
2. perineum
3. areola
4. fimbriae
5. fallopian tubes
6. clitoris
7. mammary papilla
8. placenta
9. cervix
10. amnion
11. chorion
12. uterine serosa
13. labia
14. ovaries
15. vulva
16. vagina

B

1. the embryo from the 3rd month (after 8 weeks) to birth
2. tubes that carry milk within the breast
3. sex cells; the egg and sperm cells
4. organs (ovaries and testes) in the female and male that produce gametes
5. accessory parts of an organ; the adnexa
   uteri are the ovaries, fallopian tubes, and supporting ligaments
6. the region of the abdomen between the rectum and the uterus
7. reproductive organs (genitals)
8. small exocrine glands at the vaginal orifice that secrete a lubricating fluid
9. the developing sac in the ovary that encloses the ovum
10. empty graafian follicle that secretes estrogen and progesterone after ovulation

C

1. estrogen
2. follicle-stimulating hormone
3. coitus
4. anteversion
5. menarche
6. human chorionic gonadotropin
7. myometrium
8. progesterone
9. luteinizing hormone
10. fertilization

D

1. milk
2. vagina
3. breast
4. uterus
5. ovary
6. egg
7. in, within
8. pregnancy
9. fallopian tube
10. vulva (external female genitalia)

E

1. cervicitis
2. colporrhaphy
3. culdocentesis
4. mammoplasty

5. bilateral salpingectomy
6. neonatal
7. dystocia
8. menarche

9. oxytocia
10. lactogenesis

F

1. no menstrual flow
2. painful menstrual flow
3. white discharge (from the vagina and associated with cervicitis)
4. bleeding from the uterus at irregular intervals

5. abnormal discharge of milk from the breasts
6. profuse or prolonged menstrual bleeding occurring at regular intervals
7. pus in the uterine tubes
8. painful sexual intercourse

9. heavy bleeding at and between menstrual periods
10. scanty menstrual flow

G

1. False. Total hysterectomy means removal of the entire uterus so that menstruation does not occur.
2. True. Total hysterectomy does not mean that the ovaries have been removed.
3. True. Birth control pills contain estrogen and progesterone, which cause negative feedback to the pituitary gland, lowering FSH and LH in the bloodstream and preventing ovulation.
4. True. This may be necessary to treat symptoms of estrogen loss (vaginal atrophy, hot flashes) and to prevent bone deterioration (osteoporosis).
5. False. A total (simple) mastectomy is removal of the breast and a sampling of axillary lymph nodes. A modified radical mastectomy involves removal of

the breast, axillary nodes, *and* some chest wall muscles.
6. False. An episiotomy is an incision of the perineum and is done during delivery to prevent the tearing of the perineum.
7. False. HCG is produced by the *placenta* during pregnancy.
8. False. Gynecomastia is a condition of increased breast development in *males*.
9. False. Myomectomy means removal of muscle tumors (fibroids). Endometriosis is abnormal location of uterine tissue outside the uterine lining.
10. False. A gravida 3, para 2 is a woman who has had 3 pregnancies but has given birth (delivered) twice.

11. False. A nulligravida is a woman who has had no pregnancies. A multigravida has had many pregnancies.
12. False. A pseudocyesis is a false pregnancy (no pregnancy occurs), and a tubal pregnancy is an ectopic pregnancy (pregnancy occurs in the fallopian tube, not in the uterus).
13. False. Fibrocystic changes in the breast are a benign condition.
14. True. Cystadenomas are glandular sacs lined with tumor cells; they occur in the ovaries.
15. False. FSH and LH are pituitary gland hormones. Estrogen and progesterone are secreted by the ovaries.

H

1. act of giving birth
2. gradual ending of menstrual function
3. beginning of the first menstrual period at puberty

4. release of the ovum from the ovary
5. pregnancy
6. pertaining to no ovulation (egg is not released from the ovary)

7. loss of ability to reproduce
8. production of milk
9. a woman who has never given birth
10. inflammation of the ovaries

I

1. cystadenocarcinoma
2. cervicitis
3. carcinoma *in situ*
4. preeclampsia

5. endometriosis
6. abruptio placentae
7. placenta previa
8. choriocarcinoma

9. cervical carcinoma
10. endometrial carcinoma
11. leiomyomas

J

1. cauterization
2. hysterosalpingography
3. cryosurgery
4. colposcopy
5. dilation (dilatation) and curettage

6. aspiration
7. mammography
8. conization
9. culdocentesis
10. pelvic ultrasonography

11. tubal ligation
12. laparoscopy
13. pregnancy test
14. Pap smear
15. pelvic exenteration

K

1. cephalic version
2. pelvimetry
3. fontanelle
4. Apgar

5. abortion
6. cesarean section
7. hyaline membrane disease
8. fetal monitoring

9. pyloric stenosis
10. erythroblastosis fetalis
11. hydrocephalus
12. kernicterus

Continued on following page

L

1. fibroids or leiomyomata
2. amenorrhea
3. adnexa
4. colporrhaphy

5. oophorectomy
6. gynecomastia
7. genitalia
8. dilation

9. curettage
10. progesterone
11. papilla
12. vulvovaginitis

M

1. cervical intraepithelial neoplasia. F
2. follicle-stimulating hormone. D
3. dilation (dilatation) and curettage. E
4. multipara. A
5. cesarean section. H

6. alpha-fetoprotein. B
7. ductal carcinoma *in situ*. J
8. total abdominal hysterectomy with bilateral salpingo-oophorectomy. G

9. primipara. C
10. selective estrogen receptor modulators. I

N

1. Pap smear
2. HCG
3. preeclampsia

4. mammogram
5. PID

Answers to Practical Applications

1. E
2. F
3. C

4. B
5. A
6. D

XII. Pronunciation of Terms

Pronunciation Guide

ā as in āpe
ē as in ēven
ī as in īce
ō as in ōpen
ū as in ūnit

ă as in ăpple
ĕ as in ĕvery
ĭ as in ĭnterest
ŏ as in pŏt
ŭ as in ŭnder

To test your understanding of the terminology in this chapter, write the meaning of each term in the space provided. In addition, you may wish to cover the terms and write them by looking at your definitions. Make sure your spelling is correct. The page number after each term indicates where it is defined or used in the text so you can easily check your responses.

Vocabulary and Terminology

Term	Pronunciation	Meaning
adnexa (250)	ăd-NĔK-să	
amenorrhea (254)	āmĕn-ō-RĒ-ă	
amniocentesis (268)	ăm-nē-ō-sĕn-TĒ-sĭs	
amniotic fluid (253)	ăm-nē-ŎT-ĭk FLOO-ĭd	
anovulatory (255)	ăn-ŎV-ū-lă-tōr-ē	

antenatal (257)	ăn-tē-NĀ-tăl	_____
anteversion (257)	ăn-tē-VĔR-shŭn	_____
areola (250)	ă-RĒ-ō-lă	_____
Bartholin glands (250)	BĂR-thō-lĭn glandz	_____
bilateral oophorectomy (255)	bī-LĂ-tĕr-ăl ō-ŏf-ō-RĔK-tō-mē or oo-fō-RĔK-tō-mē	_____
cephalic version (257)	sĕ-FĂL-lĭk VĔR-shŭn	_____
cervix (250)	SĔR-vĭkz	_____
choriogenesis (253)	kŏr-ē-ō-JĔN-ĕ-sĭs	_____
chorion (250)	KŌ-rē-ŏn	_____
chorionic (253)	kō-rē-ŎN-ĭk	_____
clitoris (250)	KLĬ-tō-rĭs	_____
coitus (251)	KŌ-ĭ-tŭs	_____
colporrhaphy (253)	kŏl-PŎR-ă-fē	_____
colposcopy (253)	kŏl-PŎS-kō-pē	_____
corpus luteum (251)	KŎR-pŭs LŪ-tē-ŭm	_____
cul-de-sac (251)	KŬL-dĕ-săk	_____
culdocentesis (253)	kŭl-dō-sĕn-TĒ-sĭs	_____
dysmenorrhea (254)	dĭs-mĕn-ō-RĒ-ă	_____
dyspareunia (257)	dĭs-pă-ROO-nē-ă	_____
dystocia (256)	dĭs-TŌ-sē-ă	_____
embryo (251)	ĔM-brē-ō	_____
endocervicitis (253)	ĕn-dō-sĕr-vĭs-SĪ-tĭs	_____
endometritis (251)	ēn-dō-mē-TRĪ-tis	_____
endometrium (251)	ĕn-dō-MĒ-trē-ŭm	_____
episiotomy (253)	ĕ-pĭs-ē-ŎT-ō-mē	_____
estrogen (251)	ĔS-trō-jĕn	_____

fallopian tubes (251)	fă-LŌ-pē-ăn tūbz	
fertilization (251)	fĕr-tĭl-ĭ-ZĀ-shŭn	
fetus (251)	FĒ-tŭs	
fimbriae (251)	FĬM-brē-ē	
follicle-stimulating hormone (251)	FŎL-lĭ-k'l STĬM-ū-lā-tĭng HŌR-mōn	
galactorrhea (253)	gă-lăk-tō-RĒ-ă	
gamete (251)	GĂM-ēt	
genitalia (251)	jĕn-ĭ-TĀ-lē-ă	
gestation (251)	jĕs-TĀ-shŭn	
gonads (251)	GŌ-nădz	
graafian follicle (251)	GRĂF-ē-ăn FŎL-lĭ-k'l	
gynecomastia (253)	gī-nĕ-kō-MĂS-tē-ă	
human chorionic gonadotropin (251)	HŪ-măn kō-rē-ŎN-ĭk gō-nă-dō-TRŌ-pĭn	
hymen (251)	HĪ-mĕn	
hysterectomy (254)	hĭs-tĕr-ĔK-tō-mē	
hysteroscopy (254)	hĭs-tĕr-ŎS-kō-pē	
intrauterine device (257)	ĭn-tră-Ū-tĕ-rĭn dĕ-VĪS	
involution (257)	ĭn-vō-LŪ-shŭn	
labia (251)	LĀ-bē-ă	
lactation (254)	lăk-TĀ-shŭn	
lactiferous ducts (251)	lăk-TĬ-fĕ-rŭs dŭkts	
lactogenesis (254)	lăk-tō-JĔN-ĕ-sĭs	
leukorrhea (256)	loo-kō-RĒ-ă	
luteinizing hormone (251)	LŪ-tĕ-nī-zĭng HŌR-mōn	
mammary (254)	MĂM-ŏr-ē	
mammoplasty (254)	MĂM-ō-plăs-tē	

mastectomy (254)	măs-TĒK-tō-mē	
mastitis (254)	măs-TĪ-tĭs	
menarche (252)	mĕ-NĂR-kē	
menometrorrhagia (255)	mĕn-ō-mĕt-rō-RĀ-jă	
menopause (252)	MĒN-ō-păwz	
menorrhea (256)	mĕn-ō-RĒ-ă	
menstruation (252)	mĕn-strū-Ā-shŭn	
metrorrhagia (255)	mĕ-trō-RĀ-jă	
multigravida (257)	mŭl-tē-GRĂV-ĭ-dă	
multipara (257)	mŭl-TĬP-ă-ră	
myomectomy (255)	mī-ō-MĔK-tō-mē	
myometrium (252)	mī-ō-MĒ-trē-ŭm	
neonatal (255)	nē-ō-NĀ-tăl	
nullipara (257)	nŭl-LĬP-ă-ră	
obstetric (255)	ŏb-STĔT-rĭk	
oligomenorrhea (255)	ŏl-ĭ-gō-mĕn-ō-RĒ-ă	
oogenesis (255)	ō-ō-JĔN-ĕ-sĭs	
oophoritis (255)	ō-ōf-ōr-Ī-tĭs	
orifice (252)	ŎR-ĭ-fĭs	
ovarian (255)	ō-VĂ-rē-an	
ovaries (252)	Ō-vă-rēz	
ovulation (252)	ōv-ū-LĀ-shŭn	
ovum; ova (252)	Ō-vŭm; Ō-vă	
oxytocia (256)	ŏks-ē-TŌ-sē-ă	
oxytocin (256)	ŏks-ē-TŌ-sĭn	
papilla (252)	pă-PĬL-ă	
parturition (252)	păr-tū-RĬSH-ŭn	

perineorrhaphy (255)   pĕ-rĭ-nē-ŎR-ră-fē   _____

perineum (252)   pĕ-rĭ-NĒ-ŭm   _____

placenta (252)   plă-SĔN-tă   _____

presentation (257)   prē-zĕn-TĀ-shŭn   _____

primigravida (256)   prī-mĭ-GRĂV-ĭ-dă   _____

primiparous (258)   prī-MĬP-ă-rŭs   _____

progesterone (252)   prō-JĔS-tĕ-rōn   _____

pseudocyesis (256)   sū-dō-sī-Ē-sĭs   _____

pyosalpinx (256)   pī-ō-SĂL-pĭnks   _____

retroflexion (258)   rĕ-trō-FLĔK-shŭn   _____

salpingectomy (255)   săl-pĭng-JĔK-tō-mē   _____

salpingitis (261)   săl-pĭng-JĪ-tĭs   _____

uterine serosa (252)   Ū-tĕr-ĭn sĕ-RŌ-să   _____

uterus (252)   Ū-tĕr-ŭs   _____

vagina (252)   vă-JĪ-nă   _____

vaginal orifice (256)   vā-jī-năl ŎR-ĭ-fĭs   _____

vaginitis (256)   vă-jĭ-NĪ-tĭs   _____

vulva (252)   VŬL-vă   _____

vulvovaginitis (256)   vŭl-vō-vă-jĭ-NĪ-tĭs   _____

Pathological Conditions, Clinical Tests, and Procedures

Term	Pronunciation	Meaning
abortion (268)	ă-BŎR-shŭn	
abruptio placentae (263)	ă-BRŬP-shē-ō plă-SĔN-tē	
Apgar score (264)	ĂP-găr skōr	
aspiration (266)	ăs-pĕ-RĀ-shŭn	
carcinoma *in situ* (259)	kăr-sĭ-NŌ-mă ĭn SĪ-tū	
carcinoma of the breast (261)	kăr-sĭ-NŌ-mă of the brĕst	

carcinoma of the cervix (259)	kăr-sĭ-NŌ-mă of the SĔR-vĭkz	_____
carcinoma of the endometrium (259)	kăr-sĭ-NŌ-mă of the ĕn-dō-MĒ-trē-ŭm	_____
cauterization (266)	kăw-tĕr-ĭ-ZĀ-shŭn	_____
cervical dysplasia (259)	SĔR-vĭ-kăl dĭs-PLĀ-zē-ă	_____
cervicitis (259)	sĕr-vĭ-SĪ-tĭs	_____
cesarean section (268)	sĕ-SĀ-rē-ăn SĔK-shŭn	_____
Chlamydia (259)	klă-MĬD-ē-ă	_____
choriocarcinoma (263)	kō-rē-ō-kăr-sĭ-NŌ-mă	_____
chorionic villus sampling (270)	kō-rē-ŎN-ik VĬL-us SĂMP-lĭng	_____
colposcopy (267)	kōl-PŎS-kō-pē	_____
conization (267)	kō-nĭ-ZĀ-shŭn	_____
cryocauterization (268)	krī-ō-kăw-tĕr-ĭ-ZĀ-shŭn	_____
culdocentesis (268)	kŭl-dō-sĕn-TĒ-sĭs	_____
cystadenocarcinoma (260)	sĭs-tăd-ĕ-nō-kăr-sĭ-NŌ-mă	_____
cystadenoma (260)	sĭs-tăd-ĕ-NŌ-mă	_____
dermoid cyst (261)	DĔR-moyd sĭst	_____
dilatation (268)	dĭ-lă-TĀ-shŭn	_____
dilation and curettage (268)	dī-LĀ-shŭn and kŭr-ĕ-TĂZH	_____
ectopic pregnancy (263)	ĕk-TŎP-ĭk PRĔG-năn-sē	_____
endometriosis (259)	ĕn-dō-mē-trē-Ō-sĭs	_____
erythroblastosis fetalis (264)	ĕ-rĭth-rō-blăs-TŌ-sĭs fĕ-TĂ-lĭs	_____
exenteration (268)	ĕks-ĕn-tĕ-RĀ-shŭn	_____
fetal monitoring (270)	FĒ-tăl MŎN-ĭ-tĕ-rĭng	_____
fibrocystic disease (263)	fī-brō-SĬS-tĭk dĭ-ZĒZ	_____
fibroids (260)	FĪ-broydz	_____

hyaline membrane disease (264)	HĪ-ă-lĭn MĔM-brān dĭ-ZĒZ	
hydrocephalus (264)	hī-drō-SĔF-ă-lŭs	
hysterosalpingography (265)	hĭs-tĕr-ō-săl-pĭng-ŎG-ră-fē	
kernicterus (265)	kĕr-NĬK-tĕr-ŭs	
laparoscopy (268)	lă-pă-RŎS-kō-pē	
leiomyoma (260)	lī-ō-mī-Ō-mă	
mammography (266)	măm-MŎG-ră-fē	
ovarian carcinoma (260)	ō-VĂR-ē-an kăr-sĭ-NŌ-mă	
ovarian cyst (260)	ō-VĂR-ē-an sĭst	
palpation (261)	păl-PĀ-shŭn	
Pap smear (265)	Păp smēr	
pelvic inflammatory disease (261)	PĔL-vĭk ĭn-FLĂM-mă-tō-rē dĭ-ZĒZ	
pelvic ultrasonography (266)	PĔL-vĭk ŭl-tră-sŏn-ŎG-ră-fē	
pelvimetry (270)	pĕl-VĬM-ĭ-trē	
placenta previa (263)	plă-SĔN-tă PRĒ-vē-ă	
preeclampsia (264)	prē-ĕ-KLĂMP-sē-ă	
pyloric stenosis (265)	pī-LŎR-ĭk stĕ-NŌ-sĭs	
respiratory distress syndrome (264)	RĔS-pĭr-ă-tō-rē dĭs-STRĔS SĬN-drōm	
tubal ligation (268)	TOO-băl lī-GĀ-shŭn	

XIII. Review Sheet

Write the meanings of the word parts in the spaces provided and test yourself. Check your answers with the information in the chapter or in the glossary (Medical Terms—English) at the end of the book.

COMBINING FORMS

Combining Form	Meaning	Combining Form	Meaning
amni/o	_____	myom/o	_____
cephal/o	_____	nat/i	_____
cervic/o	_____	obstetr/o	_____
chori/o	_____	olig/o	_____
colp/o	_____	oophor/o	_____
culd/o	_____	ov/o	_____
episi/o	_____	ovari/o	_____
galact/o	_____	ovul/o	_____
gynec/o	_____	perine/o	_____
hyster/o	_____	peritone/o	_____
lact/o	_____	phor/o	_____
mamm/o	_____	py/o	_____
mast/o	_____	salping/o	_____
men/o	_____	uter/o	_____
metr/o	_____	vagin/o	_____
metri/o	_____	vulv/o	_____
my/o	_____		

Continued on following page

SUFFIXES

Suffix	Meaning	Suffix	Meaning
-arche		-ptosis	
-cele		-rrhagia	
-cyesis		-rrhaphy	
-ectasis		-rrhea	
-ectomy		-salpinx	
-flexion		-scopy	
-genesis		-stenosis	
-gravida		-stomy	
-itis		-tocia	
-pareunia		-tomy	
-parous		-tresia	
-plasia		-version	
-plasty			

PREFIXES

Prefix	Meaning	Prefix	Meaning
ante-		nulli-	
bi-		oxy-	
dys-		peri-	
endo-		primi-	
in-		pseudo-	
intra-		retro-	
multi-		uni-	

CHAPTER 9

Male Reproductive System

This chapter is divided into the following sections

In this chapter you will

- Name, locate, and describe the functions of the organs of the male reproductive system;
- Define some abnormal and pathological conditions that affect the male system;
- Differentiate among several types of sexually transmitted diseases;
- Define many combining forms used to describe the structures of this system;
- Explain various laboratory tests, clinical procedures, and abbreviations that are pertinent to the system; and
- Apply your new knowledge to understanding medical terms in their proper contexts, such as medical reports and records.

I. Introduction

The male sex cell, the **spermatozoon** (sperm cell), is microscopic—in volume, only one third the size of a red blood cell, and less than 1/100,000th the size of the female ovum. It is a relatively uncomplicated cell, composed of a head region, which contains nuclear hereditary material (chromosomes), and a tail region, consisting of a **flagellum** (hair-like process) that makes the sperm motile, somewhat resembling a tadpole. The sperm cell contains relatively little food and cytoplasm, for it need live only long enough to travel from its point of release from the male to where the egg cell lies within the female (fallopian tube). Only one spermatozoon out of approximately 300 million sperm cells that may be released during a single **ejaculation** (ejection of sperm and fluid from the male urethra) can penetrate a single ovum and produce fertilization of the ovum.

If more than one egg is passing down the fallopian tube when sperm are present, multiple fertilizations are possible, and twins, triplets, quadruplets, and so forth may occur. Twins resulting from the fertilization of separate ova by separate sperm cells are called **fraternal twins.** Fraternal twins, developing *in utero* with separate placentas, can be of the same sex or different sexes and resemble each other no more than ordinary brothers and sisters. Fraternal twinning is hereditary; a gene is carried by the daughters of mothers of twins.

Identical twins are formed by the fertilization of a single egg cell by a single sperm. As the fertilized egg cell divides and forms many cells, it somehow splits and each part continues separately to undergo further division, each producing an embryo. Depending on when the embryo splits (day 1, 2, or 3), the fetuses will share the same gestational sac and/or placenta. Identical twins are always of the same sex and are very similar in form and feature.

The organs of the male reproductive system are designed to produce and release billions of spermatozoa throughout the lifetime of a male from puberty onward. In addition, the male reproductive system secretes a hormone called **testosterone** (-one= hormone). Testosterone is responsible for the production of the bodily characteristics of the male (such as beard, pubic hair, and deeper voice) and for the proper development of male gonads **(testes)** and accessory organs **(prostate gland** and **seminal vesicles)** that secrete fluids to ensure the lubrication and viability of sperm.

II. Anatomy

Label Figure 9–1 as you study the following description of the anatomy of the male reproductive system.

The male gonads consist of a pair (only one is pictured here) of **testes** (singular: **testis**), also called **testicles** [1], that develop in the abdomen at about the level of the kidneys before descending during embryonic development into the **scrotum** [2], a sac enclosing the testes on the outside of the body.

The scrotum, lying between the thighs, exposes the testes to a lower temperature than that of the rest of the body. This lower temperature is necessary for the adequate maturation and development of sperm **(spermatogenesis).** Lying between the anus and the scrotum, at the floor of the pelvic cavity in the male, is the **perineum** [3], which is analogous to the perineal region in the female.

The interior of a testis is composed of a large mass of narrow, coiled tubules called the **seminiferous tubules** [4]. These tubules contain cells that manufacture spermatozoa. The seminiferous tubules are the **parenchymal tissue** of the testis, which means that they perform the essential work of the organ (formation of sperm). Other cells in the testis, called **interstitial cells,** manufacture an important male hormone, **testosterone.**

All body organs contain **parenchyma** (parenchymal cells or tissue), which perform the essential functions of the organ. Organs also contain supportive, connective, and framework tissue, such as blood vessels, connective tissues, and sometimes muscle as well. This supportive tissue is called **stroma (stromal tissue).**

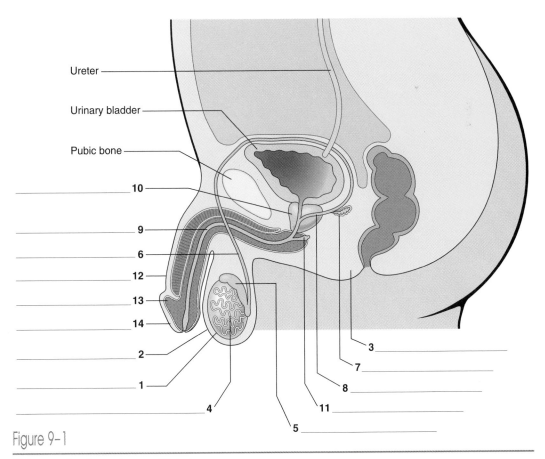

Ureter

Urinary bladder

Pubic bone

10

9

6

12

13

14

2

1

4

5

3

7

8

11

Figure 9–1

Male reproductive system, sagittal view.

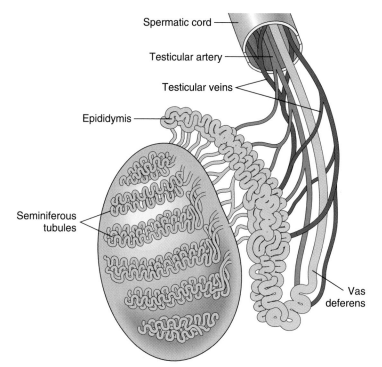

Spermatic cord

Testicular artery

Testicular veins

Epididymis

Seminiferous
tubules

Vas
deferens

Figure 9-2

**Internal structure of a testis
and the epididymis.**

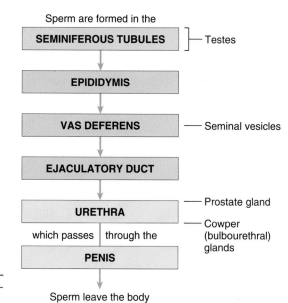

Sperm are formed in the

SEMINIFEROUS TUBULES ─── Testes

EPIDIDYMIS

VAS DEFERENS ─── Seminal vesicles

EJACULATORY DUCT

URETHRA ─── Prostate gland

─── Cowper
(bulbourethral)
glands

which passes | through the

PENIS

Sperm leave the body

Figure 9-3

The **passage of sperm** from the seminiferous tubules in the testes to the outside of the body.

As soon as the sperm cells are formed, they move through the seminiferous tubules and are collected in ducts that lead to a large tube at the upper part of each testis. This is the **epididymis** [5]. The spermatozoa mature and become motile in the epididymis and are temporarily stored there. An epididymis runs down the length of each testicle (the coiled tube is about 16 feet long) and then turns upward again and becomes a narrow, straight tube called the **vas deferens** [6] or **ductus deferens.** Figure 9–2 shows the internal structure of a testis and the epididymis. The vas deferens is about 2 feet long and carries the sperm up into the pelvic region, at the level of the urinary bladder, merging with ducts from the **seminal vesicles** [7] to form the **ejaculatory duct** [8] leading toward the urethra. Each vas deferens is cut and tied off when a **sterilization** procedure called a **vasectomy** is performed.

The seminal vesicles, two glands (only one is shown in Figure 9–1) located at the base of the bladder, open into the ejaculatory duct as it joins the **urethra** [9]. They secrete a thick, sugary, yellowish substance that nourishes the sperm cells and forms much of the volume of ejaculated semen. **Semen** is a combination of fluid and spermatozoa (sperm cells account for less than 1 per cent of the semen volume) that is ejected from the body through the urethra. In the male, as opposed to in the female, the genital orifice combines with the urinary (urethral) opening.

At the region where the vas deferens enters the urethra, and almost encircling the upper end of the urethra, is the **prostate gland** [10]. The prostate gland secretes a thick fluid that, as part of semen, aids the motility of the sperm. This gland is also supplied with muscular tissue that aids in the expulsion of sperm during ejaculation. **Cowper (bulbourethral) glands** [11] are just below the prostate gland and also secrete fluid into the urethra.

The urethra passes through the **penis** [12] to the outside of the body. The penis is composed of erectile tissue and at its tip expands to form a soft, sensitive region called the **glans penis** [13]. Ordinarily, a fold of skin called the **prepuce,** or **foreskin,** [14] covers the glans penis. Circumcision is the process whereby the foreskin is removed, leaving the glans penis visible at all times.

The flow diagram in Figure 9–3 traces the path of spermatozoa from their formation in the seminiferous tubules of the testes to the outside of the body.

III. Vocabulary

This list will help you review many of the new terms introduced in the text. Short definitions will reinforce your understanding of their terms. See Section X of this chapter for help in pronouncing the more difficult terms.

bulbourethral glands	Two exocrine glands near the male urethra.
Cowper glands	Bulbourethral glands.
ductus deferens	Vas deferens.
ejaculation	Ejection of sperm and fluid from the male urethra.
ejaculatory duct	Tube formed by the union of the vas deferens and the duct of the seminal vesicles, opening into the urethra at the prostate gland.

epididymis (plural: epididymides)	Tube located on top of each testis; it carries and stores the sperm cells before they enter the vas deferens. *Didymos* is a Greek word for testis.
flagellum	Hair-like process on a sperm cell that makes it motile (able to move).
fraternal twins	Twins resulting from two separate, concurrent fertilizations.
glans penis	Sensitive tip of the penis.
identical twins	Twins resulting from the separation of one fertilized egg into two distinct embryos.
interstitial cells of the testis	Cells that lie between the seminiferous tubules and produce the hormone testosterone. A pituitary gland hormone (luteinizing hormone [LH]) stimulates the interstitial cells to produce testosterone.
parenchymal tissue (parenchyma)	Tissue composed of the essential cells of any organ. In the testes, parenchymal tissue includes seminiferous tubules that produce sperm.
perineum	Area between the anus and scrotum in the male.
prepuce (foreskin)	Skin covering the tip of the penis.
prostate gland	Gland at the base of the urinary bladder that secretes a fluid into the urethra during ejaculation.
scrotum	External sac (double pouch) that contains the testes.
semen	Spermatozoa and fluid (prostatic and other glandular secretions).
seminal vesicles	Glands that secrete a fluid into the vas deferens.
seminiferous tubules	Narrow, coiled tubules in the testes that produce sperm.
spermatozoon (plural: spermatozoa)	Sperm cell.
sterilization	Any procedure rendering an individual incapable of reproduction; vasectomy and salpingectomy are examples.
stroma	Supportive, connective tissue of an organ.
testis (plural: testes)	Male gonad that produces spermatozoa and the hormone testosterone; testicle.
testosterone	Hormone secreted by the interstitial tissue of the testes; responsible for male sex characteristics.
vas deferens	Narrow tube (one on each side) that carries sperm from the epididymis into the body and toward the urethra.

IV. Combining Forms and Terminology

Write the meanings of the medical terms in the spaces provided.

Combining Form	Meaning	Terminology	Meaning
andr/o	male	androgen _____	
		Testosterone is an androgen. The testes in males and the adrenal glands in both men and women produce androgens.	
balan/o	glans penis	balanitis _____	
		Inflammation and infections of the male reproductive system are often caused by bacteria or viruses (Fig. 9–4A).	
cry/o	cold	cryogenic surgery _____	
		A method used to remove portions of the prostate gland during a transurethral resection of the prostate.	
crypt/o	hidden	cryptorchism _____	
		In this congenital condition, one or both testicles do not descend, by the time of birth, into the scrotal sac from the abdominal cavity (Fig. 9–4B).	

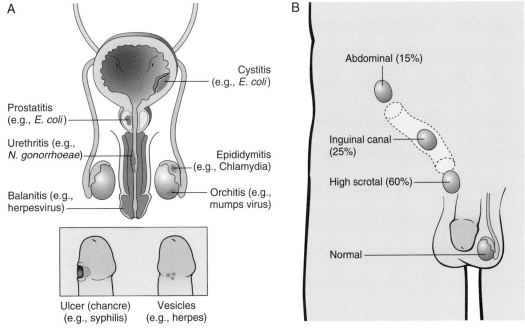

Figure 9-4

(A) Infections of the male reproductive system. E. coli (Escherichia coli) are bacteria commonly found in the large intestine; they are a common cause of urinary tract infections such as cystitis. **Chlamydia** are bacteria that invade the urethra and travel to the epididymis. **Gonococci (Neisseria gonorrhoeae)** are bacteria that affect the mucous membranes of genital and urinary organs. **Herpesvirus** affects the external genitalia, causing vesicles (blisters). **(B) Cryptorchism.** (From Damjanov I, Pathology for the Health-Related Professions. Philadelphia, WB Saunders, 1996, p 357.)

epididym/o	epididymis	epididymitis _____
gon/o	seed	gonorrhea _____
		See Sexually Transmitted Diseases, page 305.
hydr/o	water, fluid	hydrocele _____
		See Pathological Conditions, page 302.
orch/o, orchi/o, orchid/o	testis, testicle (the botanical name for orchid, the flower, is derived from the Greek word *orchis*, meaning testicle; it describes the fleshy tubers on the rootstocks of the plant)	orchiectomy _____ *Castration in males.* anorchism _____ orchitis _____ *Caused by injury or by the mumps virus, which also infects the salivary glands.*
prostat/o	prostate gland	prostatitis _____ *Bacterial* (E. coli) *prostatitis is often associated with urethritis and infection of the lower urinary tract.* prostatectomy _____
semin/i	semen, seed	seminiferous tubules _____ *-ferous means pertaining to bearing or carrying.* seminal vesicles _____
sperm/o **spermat/o**	spermatozoa, semen	spermolytic _____ *Noun suffixes ending in -sis, like -lysis, form adjectives by dropping the -sis and adding -tic.* oligospermia _____ aspermia _____ *Semen (sperm and fluid) is not formed or emitted.*

terat/o	monster	teratoma _____	

A tumor occurring in the testes composed of different types of tissue, such as bone, hair, cartilage, and skin cells. See page 302, Section V, under Pathological Conditions (carcinoma of the testes).

test/o	testis, testicle	testicular _____	

The term testis originates from a Latin term meaning witness. In ancient times men would take an oath with one hand on their testes, swearing by their manhood to tell the truth.

varic/o	varicose veins	varicocele _____	

A collection of varicose (swollen, twisted) veins above the testes.

vas/o	vessel, duct (referring to the vas deferens)	vasectomy _____	

See page 307, Section VI, under Clinical Procedures.

zo/o	animal life	azoospermia _____	

No sperm cells are found in the semen.

Suffixes			
Suffix	**Meaning**	**Terminology**	**Meaning**
-genesis	formation	spermatogenesis _____	
-one	hormone	testosterone _____	

ster/o means that this hormone is a type of chemical called a steroid.

-pexy	fixation, put in place	orchiopexy _____	

An operation to correct cryptorchism.

-stomy	new opening	vasovasostomy _____	

A reversal of vasectomy; the cut ends of the vas deferens are rejoined.

V. Pathological Conditions; Sexually Transmitted Diseases

Abnormal and Pathological Conditions

Testes

carcinoma of the testes

Malignant tumor of the testicles.

Testicular tumors are rare except in the 15- to 35-year-old age group. The most common tumor is a **seminoma,** which arises from embryonic (also called germ) cells in the testes. Nonseminomatous germ cell tumors are **embryonal carcinoma, teratoma,** and **teratocarcinoma** (combination of embryonal carcinoma and teratoma). Teratomas are composed of tissue such as bone, hair, cartilage, and skin cells (terat/o means monster).

Tumors of the testes are commonly treated and cured with surgery (orchiectomy), radiotherapy, and chemotherapy.

cryptorchism; cryptorchidism

Undescended testicles.

Orchiopexy is performed to bring the testes into the scrotum, if they do not descend on their own before the boy is 2 years old. Undescended testicles put the male at high risk of sterility and testicular cancer.

hydrocele

Sac of clear fluid (-cele means swelling or protrusion) **in the scrotum.**

Hydroceles may occur as a response to infection or tumors, or they may occur as a result of generalized edema. Often they are idiopathic. They can be differentiated from testicular masses by *transillumination* (shining a light source to the side of a scrotal enlargement). If the hydrocele does not resolve on its own, hydrocelectomy may be necessary. The sac is aspirated via needle and syringe or surgically removed through an incision in the scrotum (Fig. 9–5).

testicular torsion

Twisting of the spermatic cord (Fig. 9–5).

This condition can cut off the blood supply to a testis. It is a common testicular disorder in males around the age of puberty and arises suddenly,

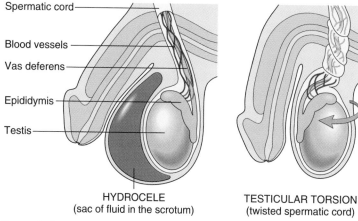
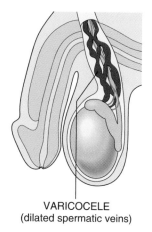

Spermatic cord
Blood vessels
Vas deferens
Epididymis
Testis

HYDROCELE
(sac of fluid in the scrotum)

TESTICULAR TORSION
(twisted spermatic cord)

VARICOCELE
(dilated spermatic veins)

Figure 9–5

Hydrocele, testicular torsion, and **varicocele.**

with acute scrotal swelling and severe pain. This is an emergency requiring surgical intervention within 6 to 12 hours. The spermatic cord is untwisted and the testicle is immobilized by suturing it to the scrotum (orchiopexy).

varicocele

Enlarged, dilated veins near the testicle.

This condition is often associated with oligospermia and azoospermia. Oligospermic men with varicoceles and scrotal pain should have a varicocelectomy. In this procedure, the internal spermatic vein is ligated (a segment is cut out and the ends are tied off), leading to a marked increase in fertility (Fig. 9–5).

Prostate Gland

carcinoma of the prostate

Malignant tumor of the prostate gland.

This cancer commonly occurs in men who are over 50 years of age. Careful rectal examination by a physician with digital (finger) palpation is a useful method of detection of early prostatic carcinoma (Fig. 9–6). Diagnosis requires identification by a pathologist of prostate cancer tissue in a prostate biopsy. Transrectal ultrasound (TRUS) is used to guide the precise placement of the biopsy needle. Computed tomography (CT) scans can detect lymph node metastases. Acid phosphatase (an enzyme) is normally released into the blood in small quantities by the prostate, and elevated levels are found in patients with metastatic disease.

Treatment consists of surgery (prostatectomy), radiation therapy, and hormonal chemotherapy. Because prostatic cells need androgens, antiandrogen hormones and estrogens are used to slow tumor growth by depriving the cells of testosterone.

Prostate-specific antigen (PSA) is a protein tumor marker that is elevated in carcinoma of the prostate. The normal PSA level is 4.0 ng/mL or less.

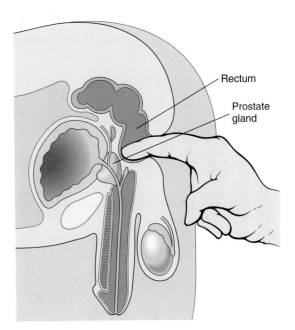

Rectum

Prostate gland

Figure 9–6

Digital rectal examination (DRE) of the prostate gland.

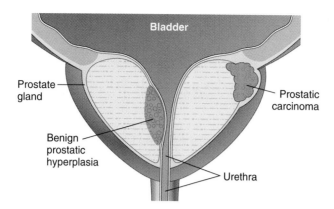

Figure 9-7

The prostate gland with carcinoma and benign prostatic hyperplasia (BPH). Carcinoma usually arises around the sides of the gland, whereas BPH occurs in the center of the gland. Because prostate cancers are located more peripherally, they can be palpated on digital rectal exam (DRE).

prostatic hyperplasia

Benign growth of cells (glandular and stromal tissue) **within the prostate gland; benign prostatic hyperplasia (BPH).**

BPH is a common occurrence in men over 60 years old. Urinary obstruction and inability to empty the bladder completely are symptoms. Figure 9–7 shows the prostate gland with BPH and with carcinoma. Surgical treatment by **transurethral resection (TURP)** is curative. An endoscope (resectoscope) is inserted into the penis and through the urethra. Prostatic tissue is removed by an electrical hot-loop attached to the resectoscope.

Several drugs to relieve BPH symptoms have been approved by the FDA. Finasteride (Proscar) inhibits production of a potent testosterone that is involved in the enlargement of the prostate. Other drugs, alpha-blockers such as tamsulosin (Flomax), act by relaxing the smooth muscle of the prostate and the neck of the bladder.

Penis

hypospadias; hypospadia

Congenital opening of the male urethra on the undersurface of the penis (Fig. 9–8A).

Hypospadias (-spadias means the condition of tearing or cutting) occurs in 1 of every 300 live male births and can be corrected surgically.

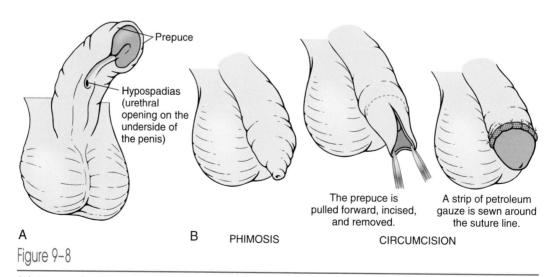

Figure 9-8

(A) Hypospadias. Surgical repair involves excising a portion of the prepuce, wrapping it (the graft) around a catheter, suturing it to the distal part of the urethra, and bringing it to exit at the tip of the penis. **(B) Phimosis** and **circumcision** to correct the condition.

phimosis	**Narrowing (stricture) of the opening of the prepuce over the glans penis; phim/o means to muzzle.**

This condition can interfere with urination and cause secretions to accumulate under the prepuce, leading to infection. Treatment is circumcision (cutting around the prepuce to remove it) (Fig. 9–8B).

Sexually Transmitted Diseases (STD, Venereal Diseases)

The following conditions, now also called **sexually transmitted infections,** occur in both men and women and are the most easily communicable diseases in the world. They are transmitted by sexual contact (the word venereal comes from Venus, the goddess of Love). AIDS (acquired immunodeficiency syndrome) is transmitted by sexual contact and is discussed in Chapter 14, under abnormal conditions of the lymphatic and immune systems.

chlamydial infection	**Bacteria (*Chlamydia trachomatis*) invade the urethra and reproductive tract of men and the vagina and cervix of women.**

Within 3 weeks after becoming infected, men may experience dysuria and a white or clear discharge from the penis. The term **nonspecific urethritis** is used to describe this condition in men.

Women may develop a yellowish endocervical discharge, but often the disease is asymptomatic. Treatment with tetracycline (an antibiotic) is curative.

gonorrhea	**Inflammation of the genital tract mucous membranes, caused by infection with gonococci (berry-shaped bacteria).**

Other areas of the body such as the eye, oral mucosa, rectum, and joints may be affected as well. Symptoms include dysuria and a yellow, muco**purulent** (purulent means pus-filled) discharge from the urethra. The ancient Greeks mistakenly thought that this discharge was a leakage of semen; hence they named the condition **gonorrhea,** meaning discharge of seed (gon/o).

Many women carry the disease asymptomatically, and others have pain, vaginal and urethral discharge, and salpingitis (pelvic inflammatory disease [PID]). As a result of sexual activity, men and women can acquire anorectal and pharyngeal gonococcal infections as well. Chlamydial infection and gonorrhea often occur together. When treating these infections, doctors give antibiotics for both and treat both partners.

herpes genitalis	**Infection of the skin and mucosa of the genitals, caused by the herpes simplex virus (HSV).**

Most cases of herpes genitalis are caused by HSV type II (although some are caused by HSV I, which is commonly associated with oral infections). Symptoms are reddening of skin with small, fluid-filled blisters and ulcers. Initial episodes can also involve inguinal lymphadenopathy, fever, headache, and malaise. Remissions and relapse periods occur; no drug is known to be effective as a cure. Neonatal herpes is a serious complication that affects infants born to women infected near the time of delivery, and studies suggest that women with herpes genitalis have a higher risk of developing vulvar and cervical cancer than do women not infected by HSV II.

syphilis	**Chronic STD infectious disease caused by a spirochete (spiral-shaped bacterium);** it can affect any organ of the body.

A **chancre** (hard ulcer) usually appears on the external genitalia a few weeks after bacterial infection. Lymphadenopathy follows as the infection spreads to internal organs. Later stages include damage to the brain, spinal cord, and heart. Syphilis (named after a shepherd in an Italian poem) can be congenital in the fetus if it is transmitted from the mother during pregnancy. Penicillin is the treatment.

VI. Laboratory Tests, Clinical Procedures, and Abbreviations

Laboratory Tests

PSA assay	This is a test to determine levels of prostate-specific antigen in the blood. PSA is found in normal seminal fluid and is produced by prostatic epithelial cells. Elevated levels of PSA are associated with prostatic enlargement and prostate cancer.
semen analysis	This test is done as a part of fertility studies and is also required to establish the effectiveness of vasectomy. The semen specimen is collected in a sterile container and is analyzed microscopically. Sperm cells are counted and examined for motility and shape. Men with fewer than 20 million sperm/mL of semen are usually sterile. Fever or infection of the testes may cause temporary sterility. In some cases of mumps in adult males, the testes become inflamed and sperm cells deteriorate, resulting in sterility.

Clinical Procedures

castration	Orchiectomy in males, and oophorectomy in females. When a male is castrated before puberty, he becomes a **eunuch. ■** His sex organs remain childlike and he does not develop secondary sex characteristics.
circumcision	A surgical procedure to remove the prepuce of the penis (see Fig. 9–8B).
digital rectal examination (DRE)	Examination of the prostate gland using finger palpation through the rectum (see Fig. 9–6).
transurethral resection of the prostate (TURP)	A resectoscope (an instrument similar to a cystoscope) is inserted into the urethra, and pieces of the prostate gland are removed using an electrical hot-loop attached to the resectoscope (Fig. 9–9). Another surgical procedure is **TUIP** (transurethral incision of the prostate) in which small cuts in the bladder neck widen the urethra. Laser surgery, which vaporizes prostate tissue, may be as effective as conventional surgery. Nonsurgical treatments that have recently been approved by the FDA are **TUMT** (transurethral microwave thermotherapy) and **TUNA** (transurethral needle ablation), using low-level radiofrequency energy through needles to burn away a defined region of an enlarged prostate.

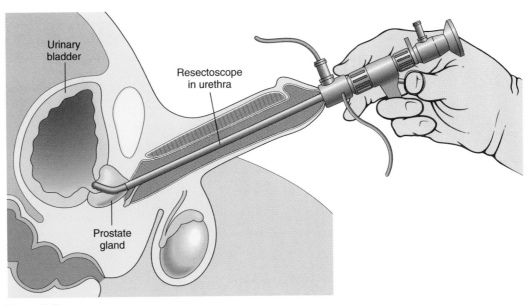

Figure 9-9

Transurethral resection of the prostate (TURP). The resectoscope contains a light, valves for controlling irrigating fluid, and an electrical loop that cuts tissue and seals blood vessels. The urologist uses a wire loop through the resectoscope to remove obstructing tissue one piece at a time. The pieces are carried by the fluid into the bladder and flushed out at the end of the operation.

vasectomy

The vas deferens on each side is cut, a piece is removed, and the free ends are folded and **ligated** (tied) with sutures. The procedure is performed under local anesthesia through an incision in the scrotal sac (Fig. 9–10). Vasectomy sterilizes the male, so that sperm are not released with the semen. It does not interfere with nerves or blood vessel supply to the testes or penis, so hormone secretion, sex drive, and **potency** (ability to have an erection) are not impaired. Unexpelled sperm degenerate and are reabsorbed within the epididymis and vas deferens. A small percentage of vasectomies are successfully reversed with vasovasostomy.

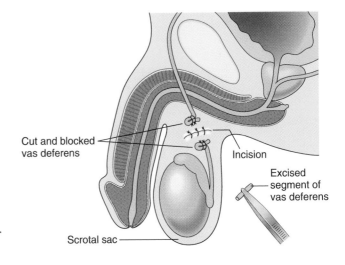

Figure 9-10

Vasectomy.

ABBREVIATIONS

BPH	benign prostatic hyperplasia	STI	sexually transmitted infections
DRE	digital rectal examination	TRUS	transrectal ultrasound (test to assess the prostate gland and to guide the precise placement of a biopsy needle)
GU	genitourinary		
HSV	herpes simplex virus	TUIP	transurethral incision of the prostate
PSA	prostate-specific antigen	TUMT	transurethral microwave thermotherapy
RPR	rapid plasma reagin (test for syphilis)	TUNA	transurethral needle ablation
STD	sexually transmitted diseases	TURP	transurethral resection of the prostate

VII. Practical Applications

Answers to the questions are on page 315 after Answers to Exercises.

Case Report: A Man with Post-TURP Complaints

The patient is a 70-year-old man who underwent a TURP for BPH 5 years ago and now has severe obstructive urinary symptoms with a large postvoid residual.

On DRE, his prostate was found to be large, bulky, and nodular, with palpable extension to the left seminal vesicle. His PSA level was 120 ng/mL [normal is 0–4 ng/mL] and a bone scan was negative. A pelvic sonogram revealed bilateral external iliac adenopathy with lymph nodes measuring 1.5 cm on average [normal lymph node size is less than 1 cm]. A prostatic biopsy revealed a poorly differentiated adenocarcinoma.

This patient most likely has at least stage D1 disease [distant metastases with pelvic lymph node involvement]. Recommendation is hormonal drug treatment to suppress secretion of testosterone, which stimulates prostatic tumor growth.

Questions on the Case Report

1. Five years previously, the patient had which type of surgery?
   (A) Removal of testicles
   (B) Perineal prostatectomy
   (C) Partial prostatectomy (transurethral)
2. What was the reason for the surgery then?
   (A) Cryptorchism
   (B) Benign overgrowth of the prostate gland
   (C) Testicular cancer

3. What symptom does he have now?
   (A) Burning pain on urination
   (B) Urinary retention
   (C) Premature ejaculation
4. What examination allowed the physician to feel the tumor?
   (A) Finger inserted into rectum
   (B) Pelvic sonogram
   (C) Prostate-specific antigen test
5. Where had the tumor spread?
   (A) Pelvic lymph nodes
   (B) Pelvic lymph nodes and left seminal vesicle
   (C) Pelvic bone
6. What is likely to stimulate prostatic adenocarcinoma growth?
   (A) Hormonal drug treatment
   (B) Prostatic biopsy
   (C) Testosterone secretion
7. Stage D1 means that the tumor
   (A) Is localized in the hip area
   (B) Is confined to the prostate gland
   (C) Has spread to lymph nodes and other organs
8. Why is staging of tumors important?
   (A) To classify the extent of spread of the tumor and to plan treatment
   (B) To make the initial diagnosis
   (C) To make an adequate biopsy of the tumor

FYI: Anabolic Steroids

Anabolic steroids are male hormones (androgens) that increase body weight and muscle size and may be used by doctors to increase growth in boys who do not mature physically as expected for their age. Steroids are also used by athletes in an effort to increase strength and enhance performance. However, there are significant detrimental side effects to their use:

1. High levels of anabolic steroids cause acne, hepatic tumors, and sterility (testicular atrophy and oligospermia).
2. In women, the androgenic effect of anabolic steroids leads to male hair distribution, deepening of voice, amenorrhea, and clitoral enlargement.
3. Anabolic steroid use also causes hypercholesterolemia, hypertension, jaundice (liver abnormalities), and salt and water retention (edema).

VIII. Exercises

Remember to check your answers carefully with those given in Section IX, Answers to Exercises.

A. *Build medical terms.*

1. inflammation of the testes _____

2. inflammation of the tube that carries the spermatozoa to the vas deferens

    _____

3. resection of the prostate gland _____

4. inflammation of the prostate gland _____

5. the process of producing (the formation of) sperm cells _____

6. fixation of undescended testicle _____

7. inflammation of the glans penis _____

8. condition of scanty sperm _____

9. no sperm or semen is produced _____

10. pertaining to a testicle _____

B. *Give the meanings of the following medical terms.*

1. hypospadias _____

2. parenchyma _____

3. stroma _____

4. cryogenic _____

5. interstitial cells of the testes _____

6. testosterone _____

7. phimosis _____

8. azoospermia _____

9. androgen_____

10. testicular seminoma _____

11. teratocarcinoma _____

C. Give medical terms for the descriptions below.

1. tube above each testis; carries and stores sperm _____

2. gland surrounding the urethra at the base of the urinary bladder _____

3. parenchymal tissue of the testes; produces spermatozoa _____

4. sperm cell _____

5. foreskin _____

6. male gonad; produces hormone and sperm cells _____

7. pair of sacs; secrete fluid into ejaculatory ducts _____

8. sac on outside of the body enclosing the testes _____

9. tube carrying sperm from the epididymis toward the urethra _____

10. pair of glands near the urethra; secrete fluid into the urethra _____

D. Match the term in column I with the letter of its meaning in column II.

Column I

1. castration   _____

2. semen analysis   _____

3. ejaculation   _____

4. purulent   _____

5. vasectomy   _____

6. circumcision   _____

7. ligation   _____

8. cryosurgery   _____

Column II

A. to tie off or bind
B. removal of a piece of the vas deferens
C. orchiectomy
D. removal of the prepuce
E. destruction of tissue by freezing
F. pus-filled
G. test of fertility (reproductive ability)
H. ejection of sperm and fluid from the urethra

E. Give medical terms for the following abnormal conditions.

1. prostatic enlargement, nonmalignant _____

2. opening of the urethra on the undersurface of the penis _____

3. sexually transmitted disease; infection with herpes virus _____

4. malignant tumor of the prostate gland _____

5. enlarged, swollen veins near the testes _____

6. sexually transmitted disease; primary stage marked by chancre _____

7. malignant tumor of the testes (three types) _____ ,

_____ , _____

8. venereal disease (etiologic agent is berry-shaped bacteria) marked by inflammation of genital

mucosa and mucopurulent discharge _____

9. undescended testicles _____

10. sac of clear fluid in the scrotum _____

F. Give the meanings of the following abbreviations and then select the letter from the sentence that is the best association for each.

Column I

1. PSA _____ ____

2. BPH _____ ____

3. TURP _____ ____

4. TRUS _____ ____

5. DRE _____ ____

6. HSV _____ ____

7. STD _____ ____

Column II

A. This is a manual diagnostic procedure to detect prostate cancer.
B. This procedure relieves symptoms of prostate gland enlargement.
C. This is an etiological agent of a venereal disease; characterized by blister formation.
D. This is a noncancerous enlargement of the prostate gland.
E. Chlamydia, gonorrhea, and syphilis are examples of this condition.
F. This procedure is helpful in guiding a prostatic biopsy needle.
G. High blood serum levels of this protein indicate prostatic carcinoma.

G. Review exercise. Give the meanings of the following.

1. -stasis _____

2. -sclerosis _____

3. -stenosis _____

4. -cele _____

5. -rrhagia _____

6. -ptosis _____

7. -plasia _____

8. -phagia _____

9. -rrhaphy _____

10. -pexy _____

11. -ectasis _____

12. -centesis _____

13. -genesis _____

14. balan/o _____

15. oophor/o _____

16. salping/o _____

17. hyster/o _____

18. metr/o _____

19. colp/o _____

20. mast/o _____

H. Match the following surgical procedures with the reasons they would be performed.

hydrocelectomy
orchiopexy
bilateral orchiectomy
TURP

vasectomy
vasovasostomy
radical (complete)
    prostatectomy

varicocelectomy
circumcision

1. carcinoma of the prostate gland _____

2. cryptorchism _____

3. sterilization (hormones remain and potency is not impaired) _____

4. benign prostatic hyperplasia _____

5. abnormal collection of fluid in a scrotal sac _____

6. reversal of sterilization procedure _____

7. teratocarcinoma of the testes _____

8. phimosis _____

9. swollen, twisted veins above the testes _____

I. Give the following medical terms based on their meanings and partial spellings. Check your answers carefully.

1. gland at the base of the urinary bladder in males: pro _____ gland

2. coiled tube on top of each testis: epi _____

3. the essential cells of an organ: par _____

4. the foreskin: pre _____

5. genus of bacteria that is the major cause of nonspecific urethritis in males and cervicitis in

    females: Ch _____

6. the ulcer that forms on genital organs after infection with syphilis: ch _____

7. androgen that is produced by the interstitial cells of the testis: test _____

8. fluid secreted by male reproductive gland and ejaculated with sperm: se _____

J. Circle the correct terminology to complete the following sentences.

1. Fred's doctors could feel only one testicle shortly after his birth and suggested close following of his condition of **(gonorrhea, cryptorchism, prostatic hyperplasia).**

2. Bob had many sexual partners, one of whom had been diagnosed with **(testosterone, phimosis, chlamydial infection),** a highly infectious STD.

3. At age 65, Mike had some difficulty with urgency and discomfort when urinating. His doctor did a digital rectal examination to examine his **(prostate gland, urinary bladder, vas deferens).**

4. Just after his birth, Nick's parents had a difficult time deciding whether to have the boy undergo **(TURP, castration, circumcision).**

5. Ted noticed a hard ulcer called a **(eunuch, chancre, seminoma)** on his penis and made an appointment with his doctor, who is a **(gastroenterologist, gynecologist, urologist).** The doctor viewed a specimen of the ulcer under the microscope and did a blood test, which revealed that Ted had contracted **(gonorrhea, herpes genitalis, syphilis).**

IX. Answers to Exercises

A

1. orchitis
2. epididymitis
3. prostatectomy
4. prostatitis
5. spermatogenesis
6. orchiopexy
7. balanitis
8. oligospermia
9. aspermia
10. testicular

B

1. Congenital anomaly in which the urethra opens on the underside of the penis.
2. The distinctive, essential tissue or cells of an organ, as for example, glomeruli and tubules of the kidney, seminiferous tubules of the testis.
3. The supportive and connective tissue of an organ.
4. Pertaining to producing cold or low temperatures.
5. The cells that produce the hormone testosterone. These cells are stimulated by luteinizing hormone from the pituitary gland.
6. A hormone made by the intestitial cells of the testes; responsible for secondary sex characteristics.
7. A narrowing, or stenosis, of the foreskin on the glans penis.
8. Lack of spermatozoa in the semen.
9. Hormone producing male characteristics.
10. Malignant tumor of the testes composed of germ or embryonic cells.
11. Malignant tumor of testes (composed of embryonic tissue forming bone, hair, skin, cartilage).

C

1. epididymis
2. prostate gland
3. seminiferous tubules (semin = semen, fer = to carry)
4. spermatozoon
5. prepuce
6. testis; testicle
7. seminal vesicles
8. scrotum; scrotal sac
9. vas deferens
10. bulbourethral or Cowper glands

D

1. C
2. G
3. H
4. F
5. B
6. D
7. A
8. E

E

1. benign prostatic hyperplasia
2. hypospadias
3. herpes genitalia
4. adenocarcinoma of the prostate
5. varicocele
6. syphilis
7. embryonal carcinoma; seminoma; teratoma or teratocarcinoma
8. gonorrhea
9. cryptorchism
10. hydrocele

F

1. prostatic-specific antigen. G
2. benign prostatic hyperplasia. D
3. transurethral resection of the prostate. B

4. transrectal ultrasound. F
5. digital rectal examination. A

6. herpes simplex virus. C
7. sexually transmitted disease. E

G

1. stopping, controlling
2. hardening
3. narrowing
4. hernia, swelling
5. hemorrhage
6. prolapse
7. formation

8. eating, swallowing
9. suture
10. fixation
11. widening
12. surgical puncture to remove fluid
13. producing
14. glans penis

15. ovary
16. fallopian tube
17. uterus
18. uterus
19. vagina
20. breast

H

1. radical (complete) prostatectomy
2. orchiopexy
3. vasectomy

4. TURP
5. hydrocelectomy
6. vasovasostomy

7. bilateral orchiectomy
8. circumcision
9. varicocelectomy

I

1. prostate
2. epididymis
3. parenchyma

4. prepuce
5. Chlamydia
6. chancre

7. testosterone
8. semen

J

1. cryptorchism
2. chlamydial infection
3. prostate gland

4. circumcision
5. chancre; urologist; syphilis

Answers to Practical Applications

1. C
2. B
3. B

4. A
5. B
6. C

7. C
8. A

X. Pronunciation of Terms

Pronunciation Guide

To test your understanding of the terminology in this chapter, write the meaning of each term in the space provided. In addition, you may wish to cover the terms and write them by looking at your definitions. Make sure your spelling is correct. The page number after each term indicates where it is defined or used in the text so you can easily check your responses.

ā as in āpe   ă as in ăpple
ē as in ēven   ě as in ěvery
ī as in īce   ĭ as in ĭnterest
ō as in ōpen   ŏ as in pŏt
ū as in ūnit   ŭ as in ŭnder

Term	Pronunciation	Meaning
androgen (299)	ĂN-drō-jĕn	_____
anorchism (300)	ăn-ŎR-kĭzm	_____

aspermia (300)   ā-SPĔR-mē-ă   _____

azoospermia (301)   ā-zō-ō-SPĔR-mē-ă   _____

balanitis (299)   băl-ă-NĪ-tĭs   _____

bulbourethral gland (297)   bŭl-bō-ū-RĒ-thrăl glănd   _____

castration (306)   kăs-TRĀ-shŭn   _____

chancre (306)   SHĂNG-kĕr   _____

chlamydial infection (305)   klă-MĬD-ē-al in-FĔK-shŭn   _____

circumcision (306)   sĕr-kŭm-SĬZH-ŭn   _____

cryogenic surgery (299)   krī-ō-GĔN-ik SŬR-jĕr-ē   _____

cryptorchism (299)   krĭp-TŎR-kĭzm   _____

ejaculation (297)   ē-jăk-ū-LĀ-shŭn   _____

embryonal carcinoma (302)   ĕm-brē-ŎN-ăl kăr-sĭ-NŌ-mă   _____

epididymis (298)   ĕp-ĭ-DĬD-ĭ-mĭs   _____

epididymitis (300)   ĕp-ĭ-dĭd-ĭ-MĪ-tĭs   _____

eunuch (306)   Ū-nŭk   _____

flagellum (298)   flă-JĔL-ŭm   _____

gonorrhea (305)   gŏn-ō-RĒ-ă   _____

herpes genitalis (305)   HĔR-pēz jĕn-ĭ-TĂL-ĭs   _____

hydrocele (302)   HĪ-drō-sēl   _____

hypospadias (304)   hī-pō-SPĀ-dē-ăs   _____

interstitial cells (298)   ĭn-tĕr-STĬSH-ăl sĕlz   _____

oligospermia (300)   ŏl-ĭ-gō-SPĔR-mē-ă   _____

orchiectomy (300)   ŏr-kē-ĔK-tō-mē   _____

orchiopexy (301)   ŏr-kē-ō-PĔK-sē   _____

orchitis (301)   ŏr-KĪ-tĭs   _____

parenchymal tissue (298)   pă-RĔNG-kĭ-măl TĬSH-ū   _____

perineum (298)   pĕr-ĭ-NĒ-ŭm   _____

phimosis (305)   fi-MŌ-sĭs   _____

prepuce (298)	PRĒ-pŭs	
prostatectomy (300)	prŏs-tă-TĔK-tō-mē	
prostate gland (298)	PRŎS-tāt glănd	
prostatic hyperplasia (304)	prŏs-TĂT-ĭk hĭ-pĕr-PLĀ-zē-ă	
prostatitis (300)	prŏs-tă-TĪ-tĭs	
purulent (305)	PŪR-ū-lent	
scrotum (298)	SKRŌ-tŭm	
semen (298)	SĒ-mĕn	
seminal vesicles (298)	SĔM-ĭn-ăl VĔS-ĭ-k'lz	
seminiferous tubules (298)	sĕ-mĭ-NĬF-ĕr-ŭs TŪB-ūlz	
seminoma (302)	sĕ-mĭ-NŌ-mă	
spermatogenesis (301)	spĕr-mă-tō-JĔN-ĕ-sĭs	
spermatozoa (298)	spĕr-mă-tō-ZŌ-ă	
spermatozoon (298)	spĕr-mă-tō-ZŌ-ōn	
spermolytic (300)	spĕr-mō-LĬT-ĭk	
sterilization (298)	stĕr-ĭ-lĭ-ZĀ-shŭn	
stroma (298)	STRŌ-mă	
syphilis (306)	SĬF-ĭ-lĭs	
teratoma (302)	tĕr-ă-TŌ-mă	
testicular (301)	tĕs-TĬK-ŭ-lăr	
testis (298)	TĔS-tĭs	
testosterone (298)	tĕs-TŎS-tĕ-rōn	
varicocele (303)	VĀR-ĭ-kō-sēl	
vas deferens (298)	văs DĔF-ĕr-ĕnz	
vasectomy (307)	vă-SĔK-tō-mē	
vasovasostomy (301)	vă-zō-vă-ZŎS-tō-mē	
venereal (305)	vĕ-NĒ-rē-ăl	

XI. Review Sheet

Write the meanings of the word parts in the spaces provided. Check your answers with the information in the chapter or in the glossary (Medical Terms—English) at the end of the book.

COMBINING FORMS

Combining Form	Meaning	Combining Form	Meaning
andr/o		prostat/o	
balan/o		semin/i	
cry/o		sperm/o	
crypt/o		spermat/o	
epididym/o		terat/o	
gon/o		test/o	
hydr/o		varic/o	
orch/o		vas/o	
orchi/o		vener/o	
orchid/o		zo/o	

SUFFIXES

Suffix	Meaning	Suffix	Meaning
-cele		-one	
-ectomy		-pexy	
-gen		-plasia	
-genesis		-rrhea	
-genic		-stomy	
-lysis		-tomy	
-lytic		-trophy	

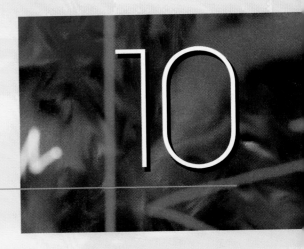

CHAPTER 10

Nervous System

This chapter is divided into the following sections

In this chapter you will

- Name, locate, and describe the functions of the major organs and parts of the nervous system;
- Recognize nervous system combining forms and make terms using them with new and familiar suffixes;
- Define several pathological conditions affecting the nervous system;
- Describe some laboratory tests, clinical procedures, and abbreviations that pertain to the system; and
- Apply your new knowledge to understanding medical terms in their proper contexts, such as medical reports and records.

I. Introduction

The nervous system is one of the most complex of all human body systems. More than 10 billion nerve cells are operating constantly all over the body to coordinate the activities we do consciously and voluntarily, as well as those that occur unconsciously or involuntarily. We speak, we move muscles, we hear, we taste, we see, we think, our glands secrete hormones, we respond to danger, pain, temperature, touch, we have memory, association, discrimination—all of these functions compose only a small number of the many activities controlled by our nervous systems.

Microscopic **nerve cells** collected into macroscopic bundles called **nerves** carry electrical messages all over the body. External stimuli, as well as internal chemicals such as **acetylcholine,** activate the cell membranes of nerve cells in order to release stored electrical energy within the cells. This energy, when released and passed through the length of the nerve cell, is called the **nervous impulse.** External **receptors** (sense organs) as well as internal receptors in muscles and blood vessels receive these impulses and transmit them to the complex network of nerve cells in the brain and spinal cord. Within this central part of the nervous system, impulses are recognized, interpreted, and finally relayed to other nerve cells that extend out to all parts of the body, such as muscles, glands, and internal organs.

II. General Structure of the Nervous System

The nervous system is classified into two major divisions: the **central nervous system (CNS)** and the **peripheral nervous system.** The central nervous system consists of the **brain** and **spinal cord.** The peripheral nervous system consists of 12 pairs of **cranial nerves** and 31 pairs of **spinal nerves.** The cranial nerves carry impulses between the brain and the head and neck. The one exception is the 10th cranial nerve, called the vagus nerve. It carries messages to and from the chest and abdomen, as well as the head and neck regions. Table 10–1 lists the cranial nerves and the parts of the body they affect. The spinal nerves carry messages between the spinal cord and the chest, abdomen, and extremities.

The spinal and cranial nerves are mainly composed of nerves that are **somatic** (som/o means body). These nerves help the body respond to changes in the outside world. They include sense receptors, such as the eye and the ear, and nerves (**sensory** or **afferent,** meaning carrying toward) that carry messages related to changes in the external environment to the CNS (groin and spinal cord). In addition, somatic nerves (**motor** or **efferent,** meaning to carry away from) travel from the CNS to voluntary muscles of the body, telling them how to respond.

Table 10-1. CRANIAL NERVES AND THEIR FUNCTIONS

A nerve is sensory when it carries messages toward the brain from sense organs and motor when it carries messages from the brain to muscles and internal organs. Mixed nerves carry both sensory and motor fibers.

Cranial Nerve	Function
I. Olfactory (sensory)	Smell
II. Optic (sensory)	Vision
III. Oculomotor (motor)	Eye movement
IV. Trochlear (motor)	Eye movement
V. Trigeminal	
Ophthalmic (sensory)	Face and scalp sensation
Maxillary (sensory)	Mouth and nose sensation
Mandibular (mixed)	Chewing
VI. Abducens (motor)	Eye movement
VII. Facial (mixed)	Face and scalp movement
	Tongue taste sensation
	Ear pain and temperature
VIII. Vestibulocochlear (sensory)	Hearing and equilibrium
IX. Glossopharyngeal (mixed)	Ear pain and temperature
	Tongue and throat sensations
	Throat movement
X. Vagus (mixed)	Throat, voice box, chest, abdominal sensations
	Voice box and throat movement
	Chest and abdominal viscera movement
XI. Accessory (motor)	Neck and back movement
XII. Hypoglossal (motor)	Tongue movement

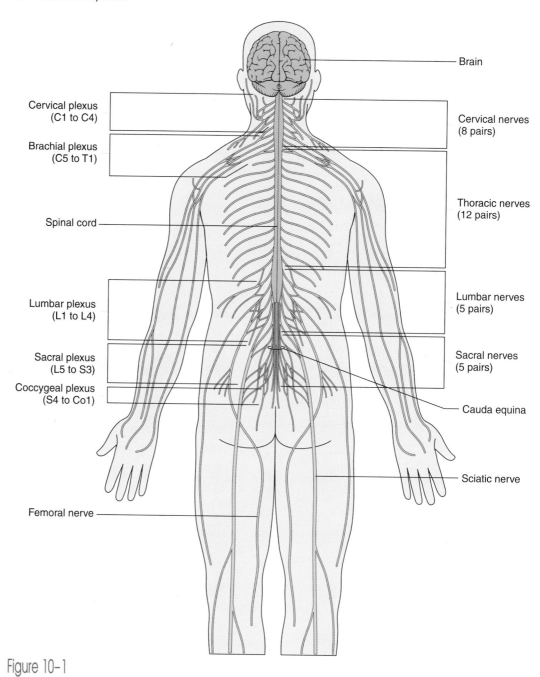

Figure 10-1

The brain and the spinal cord, spinal nerves, and spinal plexuses. The **femoral nerve** is a lumbar nerve leading to and from the thigh (femur). The **sciatic nerve** is a sacral nerve beginning in a region of the hip. The **cauda equina** ("horse's tail") is a bundle of spinal nerves below the end of the spinal cord.

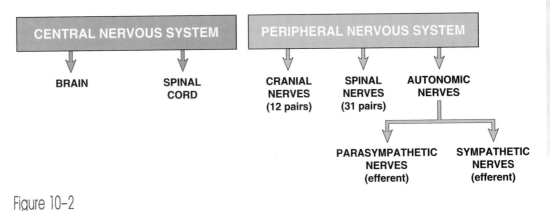

Figure 10-2

Divisions of the central nervous system (CNS) and peripheral nervous system (PNS). The autonomic nervous system is a part of the peripheral nervous system.

In addition to the spinal and cranial nerves (whose functions are mainly voluntary and involved with sensations of smell, taste, sight, hearing, and muscle movements), the peripheral nervous system consists of a large group of nerves that function involuntarily or automatically, without conscious control. These peripheral nerves are those of the **autonomic nervous system.** This system of nerve fibers carries impulses *from* the central nervous system to the glands, heart, blood vessels, and the involuntary muscles found in the walls of tubes like the intestines and hollow organs like the stomach and urinary bladder. These nerves are called **efferent,** since they carry (-ferent) impulses away from (ef-) the central nervous system.

Some of the autonomic nerves are called **sympathetic** nerves and others are called **parasympathetic** nerves. The sympathetic nerves stimulate the body in times of stress and crisis; that is, they increase heart rate and forcefulness, dilate (relax) airways so more oxygen can enter, increase blood pressure, stimulate the adrenal glands to secrete epinephrine (adrenaline), and inhibit intestinal contractions so that digestion is slower. The parasympathetic nerves normally act as a balance for the sympathetic nerves. Parasympathetic nerves slow down heart rate, contract the pupils of the eye, lower blood pressure, stimulate peristalsis to clear the rectum, and increase the quantity of secretions like saliva.

A **plexus** is a large network of nerves in the peripheral nervous system. The cervical, brachial (brachi/o means arm), lumbar, sacral, and coccygeal plexuses are examples. Figure 10–1 illustrates the relationship of the brain and spinal cord to the spinal nerves and plexuses.

Figure 10–2 summarizes the divisions of the central and peripheral nervous systems.

III. Neurons, Nerves, and Neuroglia

A **neuron** is an individual nerve cell, a microscopic structure. Impulses are passed along the parts of a nerve cell in a definite manner and direction. The parts of a neuron are pictured in Figure 10–3; label it as you study the following.

A **stimulus** begins a wave of excitability in the receptive branching fibers of the neuron, which are called **dendrites** [1]. A change in the electrical charge of the dendrite membranes is thus begun, and the nervous impulse wave moves along the dendrites like the movement of falling dominoes. The impulse, traveling in only one direction, next reaches the **cell body** [2], which contains the **cell nucleus** [3]. Small collections of nerve cell bodies outside the brain and spinal cord are called **ganglia** (singular: **ganglion**). Extending from the cell body is the **axon** [4], which carries the impulse away from the cell body. Axons are covered with a fatty tissue called a **myelin sheath** [5]. The myelin sheath gives a white appearance to the nerve fiber—hence the term white matter, as in parts of the spinal cord and the white matter of the brain and most peripheral nerves. The gray matter of the brain and spinal cord is composed of the cell bodies of neurons that appear gray because they are not covered by a myelin sheath.

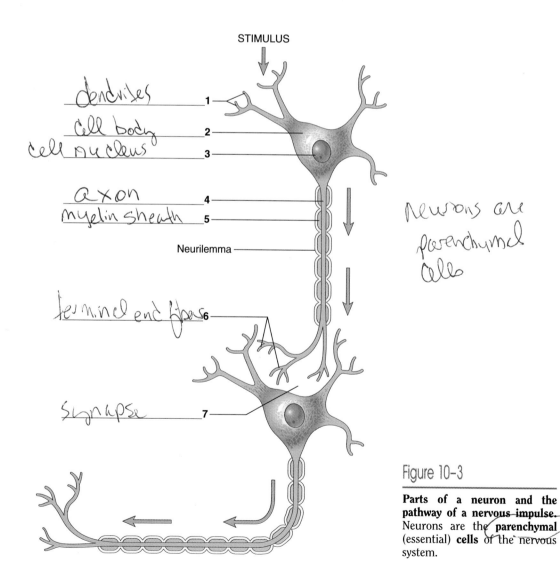

STIMULUS

1 — *dendrites*
2 — *cell body*
3 — *cell nucleus*
4 — *axon*
5 — *myelin sheath*

Neurilemma

6 — *terminal end fibers*

7 — *synapse*

Neurons are parenchymal cells

Figure 10–3

Parts of a neuron and the pathway of a nervous impulse. Neurons are the **parenchymal** (essential) **cells** of the nervous system.

Another axon covering, called the **neurilemma,** is a membranous sheath outside the myelin sheath on the nerve cells of peripheral nerves. The nervous impulse passes through the axon to leave the cell via the **terminal end fibers** [6] of the neuron. The space where the nervous impulse jumps from one neuron to another is called the **synapse** [7]. The transfer of the impulse across the synapse depends upon the release of a chemical substance, called a **neurotransmitter,** by the neuron that brings the impulse to the synapse. Tiny sacs containing the neurotransmitter are located at the ends of neurons, and they release the neurotransmitter into the synapse. Acetylcholine, epinephrine (adrenaline), dopamine, and serotonin are examples of **neurotransmitters.**

Whereas a neuron is a microscopic structure within the nervous system, a **nerve** is macroscopic, able to be seen with the naked eye. A nerve consists of a bundle of dendrites and axons that travel together like strands of rope. Peripheral nerves that carry impulses to the brain and spinal cord from stimulus receptors like the skin, eye, ear, and nose are called **afferent (sensory) nerves;** those that carry impulses *from* the CNS to organs that produce responses, for example, muscles and glands, are called **efferent (motor) nerves.**

Neurons and nerves are the **parenchymal** tissue of the nervous system; that is, they do the essential work of the system by conducting impulses throughout the body. The **stromal** tissue of the nervous system consists of other cells called **neuroglia.** Neuroglial cells are supportive and connective in function, as well as phagocytic, and are able to help the nervous system ward off infection and injury. Neuroglial cells do not transmit impulses but are far more numerous than neurons and are capable of reproduction.

There are three types of neuroglial cells. **Astrocytes (astroglial cells)** are star-like (astr/o means star) and transport water and salts between capillaries and neurons. **Microglia (microglial cells)** are small cells with many branching processes. As phagocytes, they protect neurons in response to inflammation. **Oligodendroglia (oligodendroglial cells)** have few (olig/o means few or scanty) dendrites. These cells form the myelin sheath that protects axons in the CNS. Another cell, called an **ependymal cell** (*ependyma* in Greek means upper garment) lines membranes within the brain and around the spinal cord and helps form the fluid that circulates within the brain and spinal cord.

Neuroglial cells, particularly the astrocytes, are associated with blood vessels and regulate the passage of potentially harmful substances from the blood into the nerve cells of the brain. This protective barrier between the blood and brain cells is called the **blood-brain barrier.** Figure 10–4 illustrates neuroglial cells and an ependymal cell.

Figure 10-4

Neuroglial cells and an ependymal cell. These are the supportive, protective, and connective cells of the CNS. Neuroglial cells and ependymal cells are **stromal** (framework) **tissue,** whereas neurons are parenchymal tissue of the nervous system.

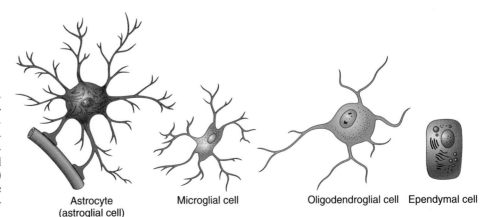

Astrocyte
(astroglial cell)   Microglial cell   Oligodendroglial cell   Ependymal cell

IV. The Brain

The brain is the primary center for regulating and coordinating body activities. In the human adult, it weighs about 3 pounds and has many different parts, all of which control different aspects of body functions.

The largest part of the brain is the **cerebrum.** The outer nervous tissue of the cerebrum, known as the **cerebral cortex,** is arranged in folds to form elevated portions known as **convolutions** (also called **gyri**) and depressions or grooves known as **fissures** (also called **sulci**). The **cerebral hemispheres** are the paired halves of the cerebrum. Each hemisphere is subdivided into four major lobes named for the cranial (skull) bones that overlie them. Figure 10–5 shows these areas as well as the gyri and sulci.

The cerebrum has many functions. All thought, judgment, memory, association, and discrimination take place within it. In addition, sensory impulses are received through afferent cranial nerves, and when registered in the cortex, they are the basis for perception. Efferent cranial nerves carry motor impulses from the cerebrum to muscles and glands, and these produce movement and activity. Figure 10–5 shows the location of some of the centers in the cerebral cortex that control speech, vision, smell, movement, hearing, and thought processes.

Within the middle region of the cerebrum are spaces, or canals, called **ventricles** (pictured in Fig. 10–6). They contain a watery fluid that flows throughout the brain and around the spinal cord. This fluid is called **cerebrospinal fluid (CSF)** and it protects the brain and spinal cord from shock as might a cushion. CSF is usually clear and colorless and contains lymphocytes, sugar, chlorides, and protein. Spinal fluid can be withdrawn for diagnosis or relief of pressure on the brain; this is called a **lumbar puncture (LP).** A hollow needle is inserted in the lumbar region of the spinal column

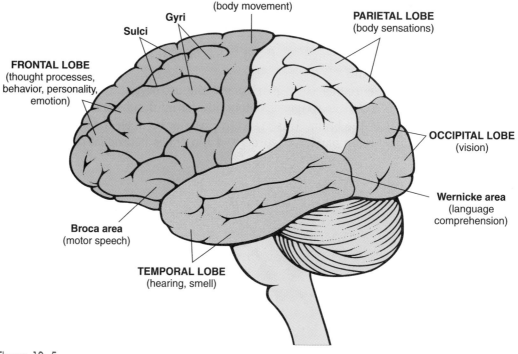

Figure 10–5

Left cerebral hemisphere (lateral view). Gyri (convolutions) and sulci (fissures) are indicated. Notice the lobes of the cerebrum and the functional centers that control speech, vision, movement, hearing, thinking, and other processes.

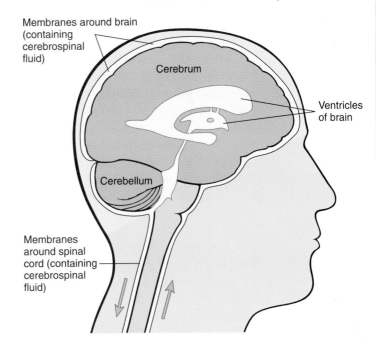

Figure 10-6

Circulation of cerebrospinal fluid (CSF) in the brain (ventricles) and around the spinal cord. CSF is formed within the ventricles and circulates between the membranes around the brain and spinal cord. CSF empties into the bloodstream through the membranes surrounding the brain and spinal cord.

Membranes around brain (containing cerebrospinal fluid)

Cerebrum

Ventricles of brain

Cerebellum

Membranes around spinal cord (containing cerebrospinal fluid)

below the region where the nervous tissue of the spinal cord ends, and fluid is withdrawn.

Two other important parts of the brain, the **thalamus** and **hypothalamus,** are below the cerebrum (Fig. 10–7). The thalamus is a large mass of gray matter that acts as a relay center for impulses that travel from receptors such as the eye, ear, and skin

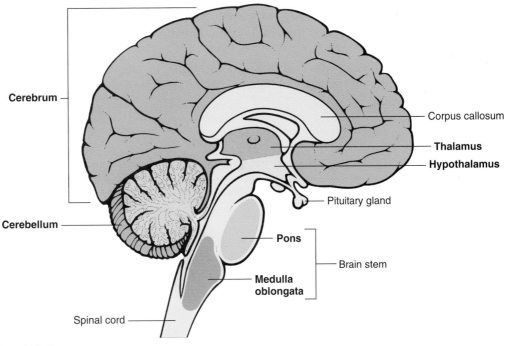

Cerebrum

Cerebellum

Corpus callosum

Thalamus

Hypothalamus

Pituitary gland

Pons

Brain stem

Medulla oblongata

Spinal cord

Figure 10-7

Parts of the brain: cerebrum, thalamus, hypothalamus, cerebellum, pons, and medulla oblongata. Note the location of the pituitary gland below the hypothalamus. The corpus callosum is a mass of tissue that lies in the center of the brain and connects the two hemispheres.

to the cerebrum. The thalamus integrates and monitors these sensory impulses, suppressing some and magnifying others. Perception of pain is controlled by this area of the brain. The hypothalamus (below the thalamus) contains neurons that control body temperature, sleep, appetite, sexual desire, and emotions such as fear and pleasure. The hypothalamus also regulates the release of hormones from the pituitary gland at the base of the brain and integrates the activities of the sympathetic and parasympathetic nervous systems.

The following structures within the brain lie below the posterior portion of the cerebrum and connect the cerebrum with the spinal cord; the cerebellum, pons, and medulla oblongata. The pons and medulla are part of the **brain stem.**

The **cerebellum** is located beneath the posterior part of the cerebrum. Its function is to aid in the coordination of voluntary movements and to maintain balance, posture, and muscular tone.

The **pons** is a part of the brain that literally means bridge. It contains nerve fiber tracts that connect the cerebellum and cerebrum with the rest of the brain.

The **medulla oblongata,** located at the base of the brain, connects the spinal cord with the rest of the brain. Nerve tracts cross over in the medulla oblongata. For example, nerve cells that control the movement of the left side of the body are found in the right half of the cerebrum. These cells send out axons that cross over (decussate) to the opposite side of the brain in the medulla oblongata and then travel down the spinal cord.

In addition, the medulla oblongata contains important vital centers that regulate internal activities of the body. These are:

1. Respiratory center, which controls muscles of respiration in response to chemicals or other stimuli;
2. Cardiac center, which slows the heart rate when the heart is beating too rapidly; and
3. Vasomotor center, which affects (constricts or dilates) the muscles in the walls of blood vessels, thus influencing blood pressure.

Figure 10–7 shows the locations of the thalamus, hypothalamus, cerebellum, pons, and medulla oblongata. Table 10–2 reviews the functions of these parts of the brain.

Table 10-2. FUNCTIONS OF THE PARTS OF THE BRAIN

Part of the Brain	Functions
Cerebrum	Thinking, reasoning, sensations, movements, memory
Thalamus	Relay station for body sensations; pain
Hypothalamus	Body temperature, sleep, appetite, emotions, control of the pituitary gland
Cerebellum	Coordination of voluntary movements
Pons	Connection of nerve fiber tracts
Medulla oblongata	Nerve fibers cross over, left to right and right to left; contains centers to regulate heart, blood vessels, and respiratory system

V. The Spinal Cord and Meninges

Spinal Cord

The **spinal cord** is a column of nervous tissue extending from the medulla oblongata to the second lumbar vertebra within the vertebral column. It ends as the **cauda equina** (horse's tail), a fan of nerve fibers found below the second lumbar vertebra of the spinal column (see Fig. 10–1). It carries all the nerves that affect the limbs and lower part of the body, and it is the pathway for impulses going to and from the brain. A cross section of the spinal cord (Fig. 10–8) reveals an inner section of **gray matter** (containing cell bodies and dendrites of peripheral nerves) and an outer region of **white matter** (containing the nerve fiber tracts with myelin sheaths) conducting impulses to and from the brain.

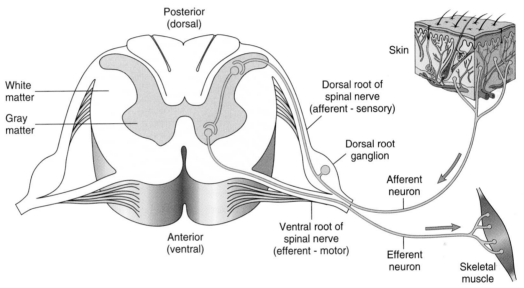

Figure 10-8

The spinal cord, showing gray and white matter (transverse view). Afferent neurons bring impulses from a sensory receptor (such as the skin) into the spinal cord. Efferent neurons carry impulses from the spinal cord to effector organs (such as a skeletal muscle).

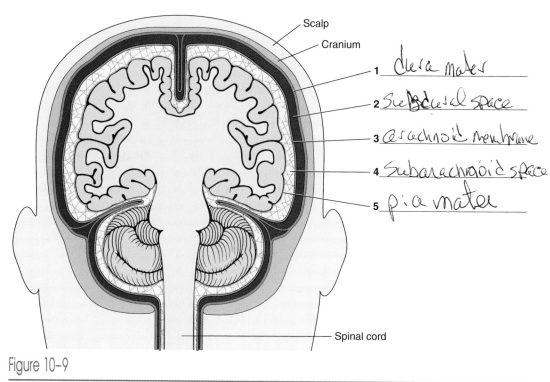

Scalp
Cranium
1 *dura mater*
2 *subdural space*
3 *arachnoid membrane*
4 *subarachnoid space*
5 *pia mater*
Spinal cord

Figure 10-9

The meninges, frontal view.

Meninges

The **meninges** are three layers of connective tissue membranes that surround the brain and spinal cord. Label Figure 10–9 as you study the following description of the meninges.

The outermost membrane of the meninges is called the **dura mater** [1]. It is a thick and tough membrane and contains channels through which blood can enter the brain tissue. The **subdural space** [2] is a space below the dura membrane that contains many blood vessels. The second layer around the brain and spinal cord is called the **arachnoid membrane** [3]. The arachnoid (spider-like) membrane is loosely attached to the other meninges by web-like fibers so there is a space for fluid between the fibers and the third membrane. This space is called the **subarachnoid space** [4], and it contains the CSF. The third layer of the meninges, closest to the brain and spinal cord, is called the **pia mater** [5]. It is made of delicate (pia) connective tissue with a rich supply of blood vessels.

VI. Vocabulary

This list will help you review many of the new terms introduced in the text. Short definitions will reinforce your understanding of the terms. See Section XIII of this chapter for help in pronouncing the most difficult terms.

acetylcholine	Neurotransmitter chemical released at the ends of some nerve cells.
afferent nerves	Nerves that carry impulses *toward* (af- means toward) the brain and spinal cord; sensory nerves.
arachnoid membrane	Middle layer of the three membranes (meninges) that surround the brain and spinal cord. The Greek *arachne* means spider.
astrocyte	A type of neuroglial cell; connective, supporting cell of the nervous system. Astrocytes transport water and salts between capillaries and nerve cells.
autonomic nervous system	Nerves that control involuntary body functions; automatically carry impulses from the brain and spinal cord to muscles, glands, and internal organs.
axon	Microscopic fiber that carries the nervous impulse along a nerve cell.
blood-brain barrier	Blood vessels (capillaries) that selectively let certain substances enter the brain tissue and keep other substances out.
brain stem	Lower portion of the brain that connects the cerebrum with the spinal cord. The pons and medulla oblongata are part of the brain stem.
cauda equina	Horse's tail; collection of spinal nerves below the end of the spinal cord at the level of the 2nd lumbar vertebra.
cell body	Part of a nerve cell that contains the nucleus.
central nervous system (CNS)	The brain and the spinal cord.
cerebellum	The posterior part of the brain; it is responsible for coordinating voluntary muscle movements and maintaining balance.
cerebral cortex	Outer region of the cerebrum; also called the gray matter of the brain.
cerebrospinal fluid (CSF)	Liquid that circulates throughout the brain and spinal cord.
cerebrum	Largest part of the brain; responsible for voluntary muscular activity, vision, speech, taste, hearing, thought, memory, and many other functions.

convolution   Elevated portion of the cerebral cortex; gyrus.

dendrite   Microscopic branching fiber of a nerve cell that is the first part to receive the nervous impulse.

dura mater   Outermost layer of the meninges surrounding the brain and spinal cord; from the Latin, meaning hard mother.

efferent nerves   Nerves that carry impulses away from the brain and spinal cord to the muscles, glands, and organs; motor nerves.

ependymal cell   A cell that lines parts of the brain and spinal cord and produces cerebrospinal fluid.

fissure   Depression, or groove, in the surface of the cerebral cortex; sulcus.

ganglion (plural: **ganglia**)   A collection of nerve cell bodies in the peripheral nervous system.

gyrus (plural: **gyri**)   Elevation in the surface of the cerebral cortex; convolution.

hypothalamus   Portion of the brain beneath the thalamus; controls sleep, appetite, body temperature, and the secretions from the pituitary gland.

medulla oblongata   The part of the brain just above the spinal cord; controls breathing, heartbeat, and the size of blood vessels; nerve fibers cross over here.

meninges   Three protective membranes that surround the brain and spinal cord.

microglial cell   One type of neuroglial cell. A microglial cell is a phagocyte.

motor nerves   Nerves (controlling motion) that carry messages away from the brain and spinal cord to muscles and organs.

myelin sheath   Fatty tissue that surrounds and protects the axon of a nerve cell.

nerve   Macroscopic structure consisting of axons and dendrites in bundles like strands of rope.

neuroglial cells   Cells in the nervous system that do not carry impulses but are supportive and connective in function. Examples are astrocytes, microglial cells, and oligodendroglia. There are about 100 billion neuroglial cells.

neuron   A nerve cell; carries impulses throughout the body. There are about 10 billion neurons.

neurotransmitter   Chemical messenger, released at the end of a nerve cell, that stimulates or inhibits another cell. The second cell affected may be another nerve cell, a muscle cell, or a gland cell. Examples of neurotransmitters are acetylcholine, epinephrine, dopamine, and serotonin.

oligodendroglial cell A neuroglial cell that forms the myelin sheath covering axons.

parasympathetic nerves Involuntary, autonomic nerves that help regulate body functions like heart rate and respiration.

parenchyma The essential, distinguishing cells of an organ. Neurons are the parenchymal tissue of the brain.

peripheral nervous system Nerves outside the brain and spinal cord; cranial, spinal, and autonomic nerves.

pia mater Thin, delicate inner membrane of the meninges.

plexus (plural: plexuses) A large, interlacing network of nerves. Examples are cervical, lumbar, and brachial (brachi/o means arm) plexuses. The term originated from the Indo-European *plek* meaning to weave together.

pons Bridge; the part of the brain anterior to the cerebellum and between the medulla and the rest of the brain.

receptor An organ that receives a nervous stimulation and passes it on to nerves within the body. The skin, ears, eyes, and taste buds are receptors.

sensory nerves Nerves that carry messages to the brain and spinal cord from a receptor.

stimulus (plural: stimuli) A change in the internal or external environment that evokes a response.

stroma The connective and framework tissue of an organ. Neuroglial cells are the stromal tissue of the brain.

sulcus (plural: sulci) Depression in the surface of the cerebral cortex; fissure.

sympathetic nerves Autonomic nerves that influence body functions involuntarily in times of stress.

synapse The space (juncture) through which a nervous impulse is transmitted from one neuron to another or from a neuron to another cell, such as a muscle or gland cell. From the Greek *synapsis,* a point of contact.

thalamus Main relay center of the brain. It conducts impulses between the spinal cord and the cerebrum; incoming sensory messages are relayed through the thalamus to appropriate centers in the cerebrum. The name thalamus, meaning room, comes from the Romans who thought this part of the brain was hollow—therefore resembling a room.

ventricles of the brain Reservoirs (canals) in the interior of the brain that are filled with cerebrospinal fluid.

VII. Combining Forms and Terminology

This section is divided into terms that describe organs and structures of the nervous system and those that relate to neurological symptoms. Write the meanings of the medical terms in the spaces provided.

Organs and Structures

Combining Form	Meaning	Terminology	Meaning
cerebell/o	cerebellum	cerebellar _____	
cerebr/o	cerebrum	cerebrospinal fluid _____	
		cerebral cortex _____	

Cortical means pertaining to the cortex, or outer area of an organ.

dur/o	dura mater	subdural hematoma _____	
		epidural hematoma _____	

Figure 10–10 shows subdural, epidural, and intracerebral hematomas.

encephal/o	brain	encephalitis _____	
		encephalopathy _____	
		anencephaly _____	

This is the most common congenital brain malformation; it is incompatible with extrauterine survival.

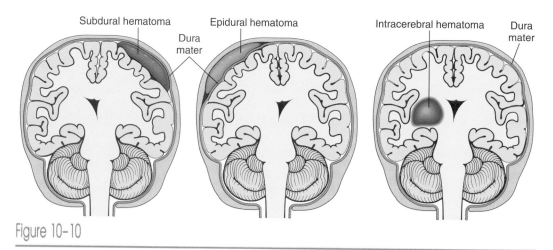

Figure 10-10

Hematomas. A **subdural hematoma** results from the tearing of veins between the dura and arachnoid membranes. It is often the result of blunt trauma, such as in boxing lesions and in elderly patients who have fallen out of bed. An **epidural hematoma** occurs between the skull and the dura as the result of a ruptured meningeal artery. An **intracerebral hematoma** is caused by bleeding directly into brain tissue, such as can occur in the case of uncontrolled hypertension (high blood pressure).

encephalomalacia _____

This is often caused by ischemia or infarction.

gli/o	glue, parts of the nervous system that support and connect	neuroglial cells _____ *Stromal or connective tissue of the nervous system.* glioma _____
lept/o	thin, slender	leptomeningitis _____ *The pia and arachnoid membranes are known as the leptomeninges because of their thin, delicate structure.*
mening/o, meningi/o	membranes, meninges	meningeal _____ meningioma _____ meningomyelocele _____ *This abnormality occurs in infants born with spina bifida. See Section VIII, Pathological Conditions.*
my/o	muscle	myoneural _____
myel/o	spinal cord	myelogram _____
	(means bone marrow in other contexts)	poliomyelitis _____ *Polio means gray matter. This is a viral disease in which the gray matter of the spinal cord is affected, leading to paralysis of the muscles that rely on the damaged neurons. "Polio" is relatively uncommon nowadays because of the effectiveness of vaccines developed in the 20th century.*
neur/o	nerve	neuropathy _____ polyneuritis _____
pont/o	pons	cerebellopontine _____ *-ine means pertaining to.*
radicul/o	nerve root (of spinal nerves)	radiculopathy _____
thalam/o	thalamus	thalamic _____
thec/o	sheath (refers to the meninges)	intrathecal injection _____ *Chemicals, such as chemotherapeutic drugs, are delivered into the subarachnoid space.*

| vag/o | vagus nerve (10th cranial nerve) | vagal _____ |

This cranial nerve has branches to the head and neck as well as to the chest (larynx, trachea, bronchial tubes, lungs, and heart) and abdomen (esophagus, stomach, and intestines).

| Symptoms | | | |
Combining Form or Suffix	Meaning	Terminology	Meaning
alges/o -algesia	excessive sensitivity to pain	analgesia _____	
-algia	pain	neuralgia _____	
caus/o	burning	causalgia _____	

This is intense burning pain following an injury to a sensory (afferent) nerve.

cephalalgia _____

*Also written **cephalgia**. Most headaches result from vasodilation (widening) of blood vessels in tissues surrounding the brain or from tension in neck and scalp muscles. A **migraine** is a severe headache often accompanied by nausea and vomiting. Prodromal symptoms sometimes include sensitivity to light and sound and an aura phase of flashes before the eyes and partial blindness.*

| comat/o | deep sleep (coma) | comatose _____ | |

A coma is a state of unconsciousness from which the patient cannot be aroused. An irreversible coma is one in which there is complete unresponsivity to stimuli, no spontaneous breathing or movement, and a flat EEG. Also called brain death.

| esthesi/o
-esthesia | feeling, nervous sensation | anesthesia _____ | |

Lack of nervous sensation—for example, absence of sense of touch or pain. Two common types of regional anesthesia are spinal and epidural (caudal) blocks (Fig. 10–11).

hyperesthesia _____

A light touch with a pin may provoke increased sensation.

paresthesia _____

Par- (from para-) means abnormal here. Examples are sensations such as burning, prickling, tingling, or numbness for no apparent reason.

| kines/o
-kinesia | movement | bradykinesia _____ | |

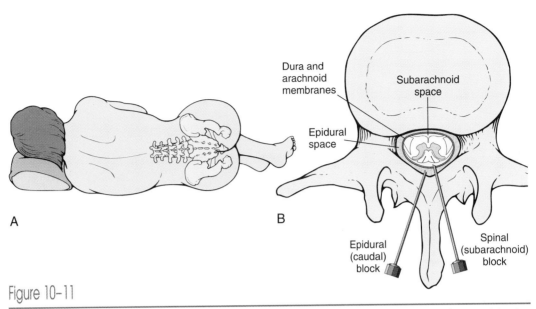

Figure 10-11

(A) Positioning of a patient for spinal anesthesia. (B) Cross-section of the spinal cord showing injection sites for **epidural** and **spinal blocks (anesthesia).** Epidural (caudal) anesthesia is achieved by injecting an agent into the epidural space in the sacral region and is commonly used in obstetrics. Spinal anesthesia is achieved by injecting local anesthetics into the subarachnoid space. Patients experience loss of sensation and paralysis of feet, legs, and abdomen.

| **kinesi/o** | movement | hyperkinesis |
| **-kinesis** | | |

Amphetamines (CNA stimulants) are used to treat hyperkinesis in children, but the mechanism of their action is not understood.

kinesiology

| **-lepsy** | seizure | epilepsy |

See page (340), Section VIII, Pathological Conditions.

narcolepsy

Sudden, uncontrollable compulsion to sleep (narc/o = stupor, sleep).

| **lex/o** | word, phrase | dyslexia |

Reading, writing, and learning disorders.

| **-paresis** | slight paralysis | hemiparesis |

Affects either right or left side (half) of the body. Paresis is also used by itself to mean partial paralysis or weakness of muscles.

| **-phasia** | speech | aphasia |

***Motor** (also called Broca or expressive) **aphasia** is present when a patient knows what she or he wants to say but cannot move muscles properly to speak. **Sensory aphasia** is present when the patient articulates (pronounces) words easily but uses them inappropriately. The patient has difficulty in understanding written and verbal commands and cannot repeat them.*

-plegia	paralysis (loss or impairment of the ability to move parts of the body)	hemiplegia _____
		Affects right or left half of the body and results from a stroke or other brain injury. The hemiplegia is contralateral to the brain lesion because motor nerve fibers from the right half of the brain cross to the left side of the body (in the medulla oblongata).
		paraplegia _____
		Originally, the term paraplegia meant a stroke (paralysis) on one side (para-). Now, however, the term means paralysis of both legs and the lower part of the body due to injury or disease of the spinal cord at the lumbar level.
		quadriplegia _____
		Quadri- means four. All four extremities are affected. Injury is at the cervical level of the spinal cord.
-praxia	action	apraxia _____
		Movements and behavior are not purposeful.
-sthenia	strength	neurasthenia _____
		Nervous exhaustion; weakness and irritability. Asthenia is used as a noun to describe loss or lack of bodily strength.
syncop/o	to cut off, cut short	syncopal _____
		Syncope (SĬN-kō-pē) is fainting; sudden and temporary loss of consciousness caused by inadequate flow of blood to the brain. The term syncope comes from a Greek word meaning a cutting into pieces. The implication is that a fainting spell meant one was cut off from strength.
tax/o	order, coordination	ataxia _____
		Persistent unsteadiness on the feet can be caused by a disorder involving the cerebellum.

VIII. Pathological Conditions

The CNS is protected from external injury by the bones of the skull and the vertebral column and by the meninges containing CSF, which provides a cushion around the brain and spinal cord. In addition, neuroglial cells, which surround neurons, help to form a blood-brain barrier that prevents many potentially harmful substances in the bloodstream from gaining access to nerve cells. However, these protective factors are counterbalanced by the sensitivity of nerve cells to oxygen deficiency (brain cells die in a few minutes when deprived of oxygen) and by the inability of neurons to regenerate (adult nerve cells do not undergo cell division and cannot replace themselves).

Neurological diseases may be classified in the following categories of disorders:

1. Congenital
2. Degenerative, Movement, and Seizure
3. Infectious

4. Neoplastic
5. Traumatic
6. Vascular

Congenital Disorders

hydrocephalus

Abnormal accumulation of fluid (CSF) in the brain.

If circulation of CSF in the brain or spinal cord is impaired, it accumulates under pressure in the ventricles of the brain. Characteristic features in infants are enlarged head and small face. To relieve pressure on the brain, a catheter (shunt) is placed from the ventricle of the brain into the peritoneal space (ventriculoperitoneal shunt) so that the CSF is continuously drained from the brain.

Hydrocephalus can also occur in an adult as a result of tumors and infections.

spina bifida

Congenital defect in the spinal column due to imperfect union of vertebral parts.

Spina bifida (bi- = two, fid = split) usually occurs in the lumbar region and there are several forms:

Spina bifida occulta — The vertebral lesion is covered over with skin and evident only on x-ray examination. In its most minor form, there is no defect in the skin, and the only evidence of its presence may be a small dimple with a tuft of hair.

Spina bifida cystica — The more severe type of spina bifida, involving protrusion of the meninges **(meningocele)** or protrusion of the meninges and spinal cord **(meningomyelocele)** (Fig. 10–12A and B.)

Spina bifida cystica can involve hydrocephalus, paraplegia, and lack of control of bladder and rectum. Surgery may be indicated to remove the herniated tissue.

Figure 10-12

(A) Spina bifida with meningocele and with meningomyelocele. (B) Meningomyelocele. Both the meninges and spinal cord are included in a cystlike structure visible just above the buttocks. This condition is commonly associated with hydrocephalus. Because meningomyelocele exposes the CNS to the outside environment, infection is a common complication. (**A,** Modified from Damjanov I: Pathology for the Health-Related Professions. Philadelphia, WB Saunders, 1996, p 502; **B,** from Kumar V, Cotran R, Robbins SL: Basic Pathology, 6th ed. Philadelphia, WB Saunders, 1997, p 724.)

A   MENINGOCELE

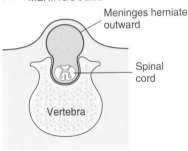

MYELOMENINGOCELE

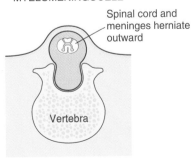

B

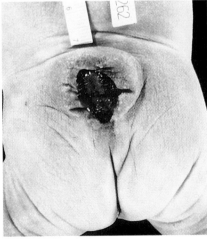

Degenerative, Movement, and Seizure Disorders

Alzheimer disease (AD)

Brain disorder marked by deterioration of mental capacity (dementia) beginning in middle age.

The disorder develops gradually; and an early sign is loss of memory for recent events, persons, and places, followed by impairment of judgment, comprehension, and intellect. Anxiety, depression, and emotional disturbances can occur as well. On autopsy of the brain there is atrophy of the cerebral cortex and widening of the cerebral sulci, especially in the frontal and temporal regions (Fig. 10–13A). Microscopic examination shows **senile plaques** resulting from degeneration of neurons and **neurofibrillary tangles** (bundles of fibrils in the cytoplasm of a neuron) in the cerebral cortex. Deposits of **amyloid** (a protein) occur and are a component of both the neurofibrillary tangles and the senile plaques. The cause of AD remains unknown, although genetic factors may play a role. A mutation on chromosome 14 has been linked to familial cases. There is as yet no effective treatment.

amyotrophic lateral sclerosis (ALS)

A progressive disorder characterized by degeneration of motor neurons in the spinal cord and brain stem; also called **Lou Gehrig disease.**

Named for a famous baseball player, Lou Gehrig, who became a victim of the disease, ALS presents in adulthood and affects men more often than women. Symptoms are weakness in skeletal muscles, difficulty in swallowing and talking, and dyspnea as the respiratory muscles become affected. Eventually muscles atrophy, and the patient becomes a quadriplegic. Etiology (cause) and cure for ALS are both unknown.

epilepsy

A chronic brain disorder characterized by recurrent seizure activity.

A seizure is an abnormal, sudden excessive discharge of electrical activity within the brain. Seizures are often symptoms of underlying brain pathological conditions, such as brain tumors, meningitis, vascular disease, or scar tissue from a head injury. **Tonic-clonic seizures (grand mal seizures)** are characterized by a sudden loss of consciousness, falling down, and then tonic contractions (stiffening of muscles) followed by clonic contractions (twitching and jerking movements of the limbs). Often, these convulsions are preceded by an **aura,** which is a peculiar sensation appearing before more definite symptoms. Dizziness, numbness, or visual disturbances are examples of an aura. **Absence seizures (petit mal seizures)** are a minor form of seizure consisting of momentary clouding of consciousness and loss of contact with the environment. Drug therapy (anticonvulsants) is used for control of epileptic seizures.

The term comes from the Greek *epilepsis,* meaning a laying hold of. The Greeks thought a victim of a seizure was laid hold of by some mysterious force.

Huntington disease

A hereditary nervous disorder due to degenerative changes in the cerebrum and involving bizarre, abrupt, involuntary, dance-like movements.

This condition begins in adulthood (between the ages of 30 and 45) and results in mental decline with choreic (meaning dance) movements (uncontrollable, irregular, jerking movements of the arms, legs, and face).

The recent discovery that the genetic defect in patients with Huntington disease is located on chromosome 4 has made it possible to test and identify

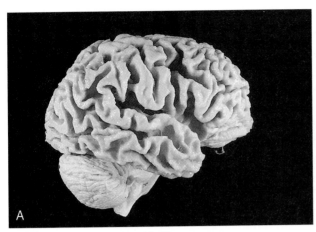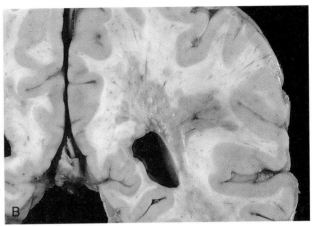

Figure 10-13

(A) Alzheimer disease. Generalized loss of brain parenchyma (neuronal tissue) results in the narrowing of the cerebral cortical gyri and the widening of the sulci. **(B) Multiple sclerosis** (MS). The typical MS plaque is a well-defined, gray-pink lesion that can occur anywhere in the brain or spinal cord. Common sites are the white matter around the ventricles of the brain, the optic nerves, and the white matter of the spinal cord. (From Kumar V, Cotran RS, Robbins SL: Basic Pathology, 6th ed. Philadelphia, WB Saunders, pp 740 and 736.)

those who will eventually develop the disease. There is no cure; management is symptomatic.

multiple sclerosis (MS)

Destruction of the myelin sheath on neurons in the CNS and its replacement by plaques of sclerotic (hard) tissue (Fig. 10–13B).

One of the leading causes of neurological disability in persons 20–40 years of age, MS is a chronic disease often marked by long periods of remission and then relapse. **Demyelination** prevents the conduction of nerve impulses through the axon and causes paresthesias, muscle weakness, unsteady **gait** (manner of walking), and paralysis. There may be visual (blurred and double vision) and speech disturbances as well. Etiology is unknown, but it is likely to be an autoimmune disease in which lymphocytes react against myelin. Immunosuppressive agents are often given with some benefit.

myasthenia gravis

A neuromuscular disorder characterized by relapsing weakness (-asthenia) of skeletal muscles (attached to bones).

Myasthenia gravis means grave muscle weakness and is a chronic autoimmune disorder. Antibodies block the ability of acetylcholine (a neurotransmitter) to transmit the nervous impulse from nerve to muscle cell, and normal muscle contraction fails to occur. Muscles on the outside of the eye (extraocular) are affected (causing ptosis of the eyelid) as well as those of the face, tongue, and extremities. Therapy to reverse symptoms includes anticholinesterase drugs, which inhibit the enzyme that breaks down acetylcholine. Corticosteroids (prednisone) and immunosuppressive drugs (azathioprine, methotrexate, and cyclophosphamide) are also used in treatment. **Thymectomy** (removal of the thymus gland, the source of antibody-producing white blood cells) is an alternative method of treatment and is beneficial to many patients.

palsy

Paralysis (partial or complete loss of motor function).

Cerebral palsy is partial paralysis and lack of muscular coordination caused by damage to the cerebrum during gestation or in the perinatal period. **Bell palsy** involves unilateral facial paralysis, which is due to a disorder of the facial nerve. Etiology is unknown, but complete recovery is possible.

Parkinson disease

Degeneration of nerves in the brain, occurring in later life and leading to tremors, weakness of muscles, and slowness of movement.

This slowly progressive condition is caused by a deficiency of **dopamine** (a neurotransmitter) that is made by cells in the midbrain (below the cerebrum and above the pons and medulla oblongata). Motor disturbances include stooped posture, shuffling gait, muscle stiffness (rigidity), and often a tremor of the hands. In patients with mild symptoms, anticholinergic agents (they block the effects of acetylcholine) and antidepressants (they block the reuptake of dopamine from nerve synapses) are effective.

Drugs such as levodopa plus carbidopa (Sinemet) that increase dopamine levels in the brain are useful **palliative** (relieving but not curative) measures to control the most severe symptoms. Implantation of fetal brain tissue containing dopamine-producing cells has been used as an experimental treatment but has produced uncertain results.

Tourette syndrome

Neurological disorder marked by involuntary, spasmodic, twitching movements; uncontrollable vocal sounds; and inappropriate words.

These involuntary movements, usually beginning with twitching of the eyelid and muscles of the face, are called **tics.** Although the cause of Tourette syndrome is not known, it is associated with either an excess of dopamine or a hypersensitivity to dopamine. Psychological problems do not cause Tourette syndrome, but physicians have had some success in treating it with the antipsychotic drug haloperidol (Haldol), antidepressants, and mood stabilizers.

Infectious Disorders

meningitis

Inflammation of the meninges; leptomeningitis.

This condition can be caused by meningococcal or streptococcal bacteria **(pyogenic meningitis)** or viruses **(viral meningitis).** Symptoms are fever and signs of meningeal irritation, such as headache, photophobia (sensitivity to light), and a stiff neck. Antibiotics are used to treat the more serious pyogenic form, and the viral form is treated symptomatically until it runs its course.

shingles

Viral disease affecting peripheral nerves.

Blisters and pain spread in a band-like pattern over the skin, following the peripheral nerves that are affected. Shingles is caused by a herpes virus **(herpes zoster),** the same virus that causes chickenpox. Reactivation of the chickenpox virus (herpes varicella-zoster), which remained in the body after the person had chickenpox, occurs.

Neoplastic Disorders

brain tumors

Abnormal growths of brain tissue and meninges.

Most of the primary intracranial tumors arise from neuroglial cells (**gliomas**) or the meninges (**meningiomas**). Examples of gliomas are **astrocytoma** (Fig. 10–14A) and **oligodendroglioma.** The most malignant form of the astrocytoma is **glioblastoma multiforme** (-blast means immature) (Fig. 10–14B). Tumors can cause swelling (**cerebral edema**) and hydrocephalus. If there is increased CSF pressure, swelling can also occur near the optic nerve (at the back of the eye). Gliomas are removed surgically, and radiotherapy is used for those that are not completely resected. Steroids are given to reduce swelling after surgery.

Meningiomas are usually benign and surrounded by a capsule, but they may cause compression and distortion of the brain.

About 25–30 per cent of tumors in the brain are metastatic growths. Most arise in the lung, breast, skin (melanoma), kidney, and gastrointestinal tract.

Traumatic Disorders

cerebral concussion

Temporary brain dysfunction (brief loss of consciousness) after injury, usually clearing within 24 hours.

There is no evidence of structural damage to the brain tissue. Severe concussions may lead to coma.

cerebral contusion

Bruising of brain tissue as a result of direct trauma to the head; neurological deficits persist longer than 24 hours.

A contusion is usually associated with a fracture of the skull. Subdural and epidural hematomas occur and can lead to permanent brain injury or epilepsy.

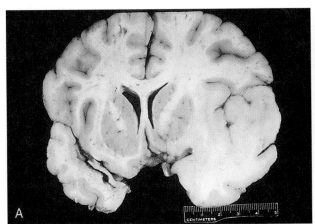 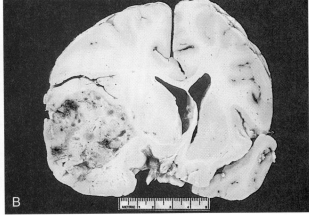

Figure 10–14

(A) This is a well-differentiated infiltrating **astrocytoma** located in the right temporal lobe of the brain (above the ruler). It has obscured the normal boundaries between white and gray matter. Because of the ill-defined borders, surgical resection seldom removes all of the tumor. **(B)** A **glioblastoma multiforme** containing discoloration and cystic changes reflecting the presence of necrosis and hemorrhage. These lesions are infiltrative and are associated with considerable mass effect. Note the shift of the midline structures to the right. (From Kumar V, Cotran RS, Robbins SL: Basic Pathology, 6th ed. Philadelphia, WB Saunders, 1997, pp 731 and 732.)

Vascular Disorders

cerebrovascular accident (CVA)

Disruption in the normal blood supply to the brain.

This condition, also known as **stroke** or **cerebral infarction,** is the result of a localized area of ischemia (and ultimately infarction or necrosis) in the brain. There are three types of strokes (Fig. 10–15):

1. **Thrombotic**—blood clot **(thrombus)** in the arteries leading to the brain, resulting in **occlusion** (blocking) of the vessel. Atherosclerosis leads to this common type of stroke as blood vessels become blocked over time. Before total occlusion occurs, a patient may experience symptoms that point to the gradual occlusion of blood vessels. These short episodes of neurological dysfunction are known as **TIAs (transient ischemic attacks).**
2. **Embolic**—an **embolus** (a clot that breaks off from an area of the body) travels to the cerebral arteries and occludes a small vessel. This type of stroke occurs very suddenly.
3. **Hemorrhagic**—bursting forth of blood from a cerebral artery. This type of stroke is often fatal and results from advancing age, atherosclerosis, or high blood pressure—all of which result in degeneration of cerebral blood vessels. If the hemorrhage is small, the blood is reabsorbed and the patient can make a good recovery with only slight disability. In a younger patient, cerebral hemorrhage is usually due to mechanical injury associated with skull fracture or bursting of an arterial **aneurysm** (weakness in the vessel wall that balloons and eventually bursts).

Three major risk factors for stroke are hypertension, diabetes, and heart disease. Other risk factors include smoking, obesity, substance abuse (cocaine), and elevated cholesterol levels.

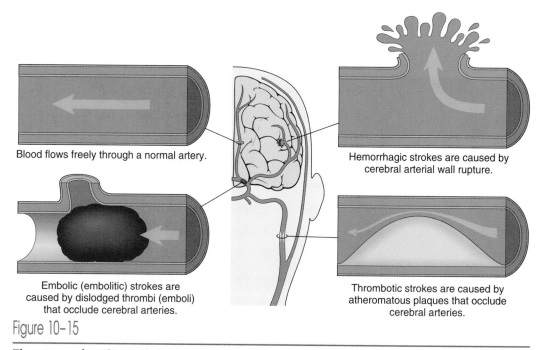

Blood flows freely through a normal artery.

Hemorrhagic strokes are caused by cerebral arterial wall rupture.

Embolic (embolitic) strokes are caused by dislodged thrombi (emboli) that occlude cerebral arteries.

Thrombotic strokes are caused by atheromatous plaques that occlude cerebral arteries.

Figure 10–15

Three types of strokes: embolic, hemorrhagic, and thrombotic. (Modified from Ignatavicius DD, Workman ML, Mishler MA: Medical-Surgical Nursing Across the Health Care Continuum, 3rd ed. Philadelphia, WB Saunders, 1999, p 1109.)

Thrombotic strokes are treated medically with anticoagulant (clot-dissolving) drug therapy (tissue plasminogen activator, or tPA, is started within 3 hours after the onset of a stroke) and surgically with carotid endarterectomy (removal of the atherosclerotic plaque from the inner lining of an artery in the neck).

▪ STUDY SECTION

The following is a review of new terms used in Section VIII, Pathological Conditions. Practice spelling each term and know its meaning.

absence seizure	Minor (petit mal) form of seizure, consisting of momentary clouding of consciousness and loss of contact with the environment.
aneurysm	Abnormal widening of a blood vessel; can lead to hemorrhage and CVA (stroke).
astrocytoma	Malignant tumor of neuroglial brain cells (astrocytes).
aura	Peculiar sensation appearing before more definite symptoms.
-blast	Immature cells (as in glio*blast*oma).
dementia	Mental decline and deterioration.
demyelination	Destruction of myelin on axons of nerves (as in multiple sclerosis).
dopamine	A neurotransmitter that is deficient in Parkinson disease.
embolus	A mass (clot) of material travels through the bloodstream and suddenly blocks a vessel.
gait	Manner of walking.
herpes zoster	Type of herpes virus that causes shingles—eruption of blisters in a pattern that follows the path of peripheral nerves around the trunk of the body; zoster means girdle.
occlusion	Blockage.
palliative	Relieving symptoms but not curing.
thymectomy	Removal of the thymus gland (a lymphocyte-producing gland in the chest); used as treatment for myasthenia gravis.
TIA	Transient ischemic attack; mini-stroke.
tonic-clonic seizure	Major convulsive seizure marked by sudden loss of consciousness, stiffening of muscles, and twitching and jerking movements.

IX. Laboratory Tests, Clinical Procedures, and Abbreviations

Laboratory Tests

cerebrospinal fluid analysis

Cell counts, bacterial smears, and cultures of samples of CSF are done when disease of the meninges or brain is suspected. Normal constituents of CSF are water, glucose, sodium, chloride, and protein, and changes in their concentrations are helpful in the diagnosis of brain disease. CSF normally has more chloride and less glucose than blood.

Clinical Procedures

X-Rays

cerebral angiography

Contrast medium is injected into an artery (usually the femoral) and x-rays are taken of the blood vessel system of the brain. The purpose of the test is to diagnose vascular disease (aneurysm, occlusion, hemorrhage) in the brain.

computed tomography (CT)

X-rays are used to compose a computerized cross-sectional picture of the brain and spinal cord. Contrast medium may also be injected intravenously to see abnormalities. The contrast material leaks through the **blood-brain barrier** from blood vessels into the brain tissue and shows areas of tumor, hemorrhage, and blood clots (Fig. 10–16).

myelography

Contrast medium is injected into the subarachnoid space, and x-rays are taken of the spinal cord. Myelography is becoming less commonly performed as CT and magnetic resonance imaging (MRI) replace this more invasive technique.

Magnetic Imaging

MRI of the brain

The use of magnetic and radio waves to create an image of the brain (frontal, cross-sectional, and sagittal planes can be viewed). MRI and CT are used to complement each other in diagnosing brain and spinal cord lesions. MRI is excellent for viewing soft tissues.

Radiologic Study

positron emission tomography (PET)

An isotope (radioactive chemical) that gives off particles called positrons is injected intravenously, combined with a form of glucose. The uptake

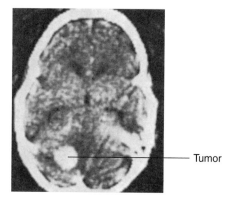

Tumor

Figure 10-16

CT scan of a 40-year-old woman with carcinoma of the lung, who developed occipital headache and gait unsteadiness. The scan (performed after contrast agent infusion) shows a round, high-density (white) area in the left cerebellar hemisphere. This is probably a metastatic lung carcinoma in the brain. (From Weisberg LA, Nice C, Katz M: Cerebral Computed Tomography: A Text-Atlas. Philadelphia, WB Saunders, 1978, p 153.)

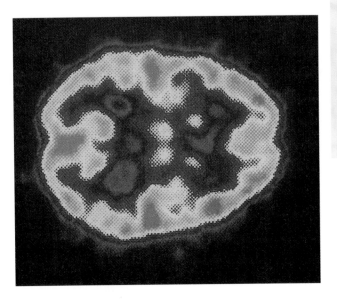

Figure 10-17

A **PET scan of the brain** showing decreased metabolic activity after a seizure (noted as green areas on the scan). (From Black JM, Matassarin-Jacobs E: Medical-Surgical Nursing: Clinical Management for Continuity of Care, 5th ed. Philadelphia, WB Saunders, 1997, p 253.)

of the radioactive material is then recorded on a television screen. The cross-sectional images show how the brain uses glucose and give information about brain function. PET scans provide valuable information about patients with Alzheimer disease, stroke, schizophrenia, and epilepsy (Fig. 10–17).

Other Procedures

electroencephalography (EEG)   Recording of the electrical activity of the brain. EEG is used to demonstrate seizure activity in the brain, brain tumors, and other diseases and injury to the brain.

lumbar (spinal) puncture   CSF is withdrawn from between two lumbar vertebrae (Fig. 10–18). A device to measure the pressure of the CSF can be attached to the end of the needle after it has been inserted. Contrast medium for x-ray studies (myelography) or intrathecal medicines may be administered through the lumbar puncture as well. Leakage of CSF around the puncture site can sometimes lead to lower pressure in the subarachnoid space and cause headache.

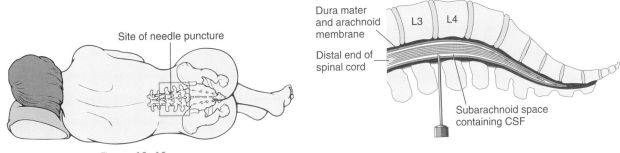

Figure 10-18

Lumbar (spinal) puncture. The patient lies laterally, with the knees drawn up to the abdomen and the chin brought down to the chest. This position increases the spaces between the vertebrae. The lumbar puncture needle is inserted between the 3rd and 4th (or 4th and 5th) lumbar vertebrae, and it enters the subarachnoid space.

stereotactic radiosurgery

Use of a stereotactic instrument that, when fixed onto the skull, can locate a target by three-dimensional measurement. **Stereotactic radiosurgery** with a **gamma knife** (high-energy radiation beams) has been used to treat deep and often inaccessible intracranial brain tumors and abnormal blood vessel masses (arteriovenous malformations) without surgical incision (Fig. 10–19).

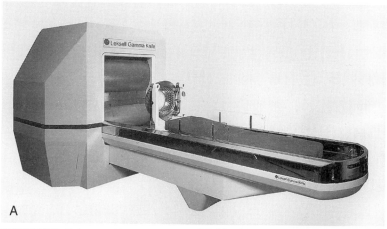

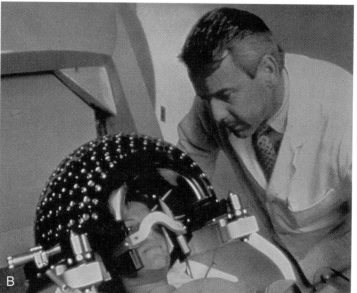

Figure 10–19

(A) The Leksell Gamma Knife Radiosurgery System. (B) Stereotactic frame in place to allow accurate focus of the radiotherapy beams. (Courtesy of Elekta Instruments, Norcross, GA.)

ABBREVIATIONS

AD	Alzheimer disease
AFP	alpha-fetoprotein (elevated levels in amniotic fluid and maternal blood are associated with congenital malformations of the nervous system, such as anencephaly and spina bifida)
ALS	amyotrophic lateral sclerosis
AVM	arteriovenous malformation (congenital tangle of arteries and veins in the cerebrum)
CNS	central nervous system
CSF	cerebrospinal fluid
CT	computed tomography
CVA	cerebrovascular accident
EEG	electroencephalogram
ICP	intracranial pressure; normal pressure is 5 to 15 mmHg
LP	lumbar puncture
MRI	magnetic resonance imaging
MS	multiple sclerosis
PET	positron emission tomography
RIND	reversible, ischemic neurological deficit
TENS	transcutaneous electrical nerve stimulation (a battery-powered device used to relieve acute and chronic pain)
TIA	transient ischemic attack (temporary interference with the blood supply to the brain)
tPA	tissue plasminogen activator (a clot-dissolving drug used as therapy for strokes)

X. Practical Applications

Answers to the questions are on page (360) after Answers to Exercises.

Case Report

This patient was admitted on January 14 with a history of progressive right hemiparesis for the previous 1–2 months; fluctuating numbness of the right arm, thorax, and buttocks; jerking of the right leg; periods of speech arrest; diminished comprehension in reading; and recent development of a spastic hemiplegic gait [partial hemiplegia with spasmodic contractions of muscles when walking]. He is suspected of having a left parietal tumor [the parietal lobes of the cerebrum are on either side under the roof of the skull].

Examinations done prior to hospitalization included skull films, EEG, brain scan, and CSF analysis, which were all normal. After admission, the brain scan was abnormal in the left parietal region, as was the EEG.

Left percutaneous common carotid angiography [the carotid arteries are in the neck and supply the brain with blood] was attempted, but the patient became progressively more restless and agitated after receiving the sedation, so that it was impossible to do the procedure. During the recovery phase from the sedation, the patient was alternately somnolent [sleepy] and violent, but it was later apparent that he had developed almost a complete aphasia and right hemiplegia.

In the next few days, he became more alert although he remained dysarthric [from arthroun—to utter distinctly] and hemiplegic.

Continued on following page

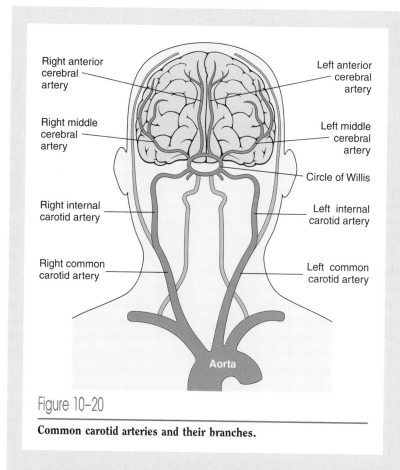

Figure 10-20

Common carotid arteries and their branches.

Bilateral carotid angiograms under general anesthesia on January 19 showed complete occlusion of the left internal carotid artery with cross-filling of the left anterior and middle cerebral arteries from the right internal carotid circulation.

Final diagnosis: Left cerebral infarction due to left internal carotid artery occlusion.

[Fig. 10–20 shows the common carotid arteries and their branches within the head and brain.]

Questions on the Case Report

1. **The patient was admitted with a history of**
   (A) right-sided paralysis due to a previous stroke
   (B) paralysis on the left side of his body
   (C) increasing slight paralysis on the right side of his body

2. **The patient has also experienced periods of**
   (A) aphasia and dyslexia
   (B) dysplastic gait
   (C) apraxia and aphasia

3. **After his admission, where did the brain scan show an abnormality?**
   (A) right posterior region of the brain
   (B) left and right sides of the brain
   (C) left side of the brain

> 4. **What test determined the final diagnosis?**
>   (A) EEG for both sides of the brain
>   (B) CSF analysis
>   (C) x-ray of arteries in the neck and brain after injecting contrast
> 5. **What was the final diagnosis?**
>   (A) a stroke; necrotic tissue in the left cerebrum due to blockage of an artery
>   (B) cross-filling of blood vessels from the left to the right side of the brain
>   (C) cerebral palsy on the left side of the brain with cross-filling of two cerebral arteries

XI. Exercises

Remember to check your answers carefully with those given in Section XII, Answers to Exercises.

A. *Match the following neurological structures with their meanings as given below.*

dendrite   meninges   astrocyte
cauda equina   axon   plexus
myelin sheath   cerebral cortex   neuron
oligodendroglial cell

1. microscopic fiber leading from the cell body that carries the nervous impulse along a nerve cell

   axon

2. a large, interlacing network of nerves *plexus*

3. three protective membranes surrounding the brain and spinal cord *meninges*

4. microscopic branching fiber of a nerve cell that is the first part to receive the nervous impulse

   dendrite

5. outer region of the largest part of the brain; composed of gray matter *cerebral cortex*

6. neuroglial cell that transports water and salts between capillaries and nerve cells *astrocyte*

7. neuroglial cell that produces myelin *oligodendroglial cell*

8. a nerve cell that transmits a nervous impulse *neuron*

9. collection of spinal nerves below the end of the spinal cord at the level of the second lumbar

   vertebra *cauda equina*

10. protective fatty tissue that surrounds the axon of a nerve cell *myelin sheath*

B. Give the meanings of the following terms.

1. dura mater _____

2. central nervous system _____

3. peripheral nervous system _____

4. arachnoid membrane _____

5. hypothalamus _____

6. synapse _____

7. sympathetic nerves _____

8. medulla oblongata _____

9. pons _____

10. cerebellum _____

11. thalamus _____

12. ventricles of the brain _____

13. brain stem _____

14. cerebrum _____

15. ganglion _____

C. Match the following terms with the meanings or associated terms below.

convolutions	neuroglial cell	afferent nerves
neurotransmitter	pia mater	efferent nerves
fissures	parenchymal cell	subarachnoid space

1. innermost meningeal membrane _pia mater_____

2. motor nerves; carry messages away from the brain and spinal cord to muscles and glands

    (effectors) _efferent nerves_____

3. sensory nerves; carry messages toward the brain and spinal cord from receptors _afferent nerve_

4. sulci; grooves in the cerebral cortex _fissures_____

5. contains cerebrospinal fluid _subarachnoid space_____

6. gyri; elevations in the cerebral cortex _Convolutions_

7. acetylcholine is an example of this chemical that is released at the end of a nerve cell and stimulates or inhibits another cell _Neurotransmitter_

8. essential cell of the nervous system; a neuron _Parenchymal cell_

9. connective and supportive (stromal) cell _Neuroglial cell_

D. Choose the correct term to fit the definition given.

1. softening of the brain (encephalopathy, encephalomalacia)

2. part of the brain that controls muscular coordination and balance (cerebrum, cerebellum)

3. collection of blood above the dura mater (subdural hematoma, epidural hematoma)

4. inflammation of the pia and arachnoid membranes (leptomeningitis, causalgia)

5. condition of absence of a brain (encephalopathy, anencephaly)

6. inflammation of the gray matter of the spinal cord (poliomyelitis, polyneuritis)

7. pertaining to the membranes around the brain and spinal cord (cerebellopontine, meningeal)

8. disease of nerve roots (of spinal nerves) (neuropathy, radiculopathy)

9. hernia of the meninges and the spinal cord (meningomyelocele, meningioma)

10. pertaining to a cranial nerve (thalamic, vagal)

E. Give the meanings of the following terms.

1. cerebral cortex _____

2. intrathecal _____

3. polyneuritis _____

4. thalamic _____

5. myelogram _____

6. meningioma _____

7. glioma _Brain tumor; tumor of neuroglial cells_

8. subdural hematoma _Below dura mater_

F. Match the following neurological symptoms with the meanings below.

causalgia   bradykinesia   ataxia
hyperesthesia   neurasthenia   apraxia
paraplegia   narcolepsy   hemiparesis
aphasia   dyslexia   syncope

1. reading, writing, or learning disorder _dyslexia_

2. condition of no coordination _ataxia_

3. condition of slow movement _bradykinesia_

4. condition of increased nervous sensation _hyperesthesia_

5. seizure of sleep; uncontrollable compulsion to sleep _narcolepsy_

6. inability to speak _aphasia_

7. movements and behavior that are not purposeful _apraxia_

8. slight paralysis in the right or left half of the body _hemiparesis_

9. burning pain _causalgia_

10. paralysis in the lower part of the body (damage to lower part of the spinal cord) _paraplegia_

11. fainting _syncope_

12. nervous exhaustion (lack of strength) and irritability _neurasthenia_

G. Give the meanings of the following terms.

1. analgesia _____

2. motor aphasia _____

3. paresis _____

4. quadriplegia _____

5. asthenia _no strength (weakness)_

6. comatose _____

7. paresthesia _____

8. hyperkinesis _excessive movement_

9. anesthesia _____

10. causalgia _intense burning pain_

H. Match the following terms with their descriptions below. The terms in boldface should give you a clue to the pathological condition described.

spina bifida cystica   Alzheimer disease   myasthenia gravis
amyotrophic lateral sclerosis epilepsy   Parkinson disease
hydrocephalus   Huntington disease   multiple sclerosis
Bell palsy

1. Destruction of myelin sheaths (demyelination) and their replacement by plaques of **hard** tissue lead to this condition. _Multiple scleross_

2. Sudden, transient disturbances of brain function cause **seizures** in this abnormal condition.
   epilepsy

3. The **spinal** column is imperfectly joined (a **split** in a vertebra occurs), and part of the meninges and spinal cord can herniate out of the spinal cavity in this congenital condition.
   spina bifida

4. This condition involves **atrophy** of muscles and paralysis due to damage to motor neurons in the spinal cord and brain stem. _amyotrophic_

5. In this hereditary condition, the patient displays bizarre, abrupt, involuntary, **dance**-like movements, as well as decline in mental functions. _Huntington's_

6. Cerebrospinal **fluid** accumulates in the **head** (in the ventricles of the brain) in this condition.
   hydrocephalus

7. This neuromuscular disorder is marked by **loss of muscle strength** because of the inability of a neurotransmitter (acetylcholine) to transmit impulses from nerve cells to muscle cells.
   Myasthenia gravis

8. Degeneration of nerves in the brain occur in later life, leading to tremors, shuffling gait, and muscle stiffness; **dopamine** (neurotransmitter) is deficient in the brain. _Parkinson_

9. This condition begins in middle age and is marked by deterioration of mental capacity (**dementia**); autopsy shows cerebral cortex atrophy, widening of cerebral sulci, and microscopic neurofibrillary tangles. _Alzheimer_

10. Unilateral facial **paralysis** characterizes this condition. _Bell palsy_

I. Give the meanings of the following abnormal conditions.

1. astrocytoma _____

2. pyogenic meningitis _____

3. Tourette syndrome _____

4. cerebral contusion _____

5. cerebrovascular accident _____

6. cerebral concussion _____

7. shingles _____

8. cerebral embolus _____

9. cerebral thrombosis _____

10. cerebral hemorrhage _____

11. cerebral aneurysm _____

J. Match the term in column I with the letter of its associated term or meaning in column II.

Column I

1. ataxia _____

2. aura _____

3. transient ischemic attack _____

4. tonic-clonic seizure _____

5. herpes zoster _____

6. palliative _____

7. dopamine _____

8. occlusion _____

9. absence seizure _____

10. glioblastoma multiforme _____

Column II

A. relieving, but not curing
B. virus that causes chickenpox and shingles
C. uncoordinated gait
D. neurotransmitter
E. peculiar symptoms appearing before more definite symptoms
F. malignant brain tumor of immature neuroglial cells
G. major convulsive epileptic seizure; grand mal
H. interruption of blood supply to the cerebrum; mini-stroke
I. minor form of epileptic seizure; petit mal
J. blockage

K. Describe what happens in the following two procedures.

1. MRI of the brain _____

2. stereotactic radiosurgery with gamma knife _____

_____

L. Give the meanings of the following abbreviations and then select the letter from the sentence that is the best association for each.

Column I

1. EEG *electroencephalography*   E

2. PET *positron emission tomography*   I

3. AFP *alpha-feto protein*   G

4. MS *multiple sclerosis*   J

5. MRI *magnetic resonance imaging*   H

6. LP *lumbar puncture*   C

7. CVA *cerebrovascular accident*   B

8. AD *Alzheimer disease*   A

9. TIA *transient ischemic accident*   F

10. CSF *cerebrospinal fluid*   D

Column II

A. In this condition, dementia begins in middle age.

B. This is a stroke; embolus, hemorrhage, or thrombosis are etiological factors.

C. Intrathecal medications can be administered through this procedure.

D. This fluid is analyzed by means of cell counts, bacterial smears, and cultures.

E. This procedure is used to diagnose abnormal electrical activity in the brain.

F. Mini-stroke; caused by temporary interference with the blood supply to the brain.

G. High levels in amniotic fluid and maternal blood are associated with spina bifida.

H. This diagnostic procedure allows excellent visualization of soft tissue in the brain.

I. An intravenous isotope is taken up by organs, and images are recorded.

J. Destruction of the myelin sheath in the CNS occurs with plaques of hard scar tissue.

M. Select the terms that complete the meanings of the sentences.

1. Suzy had such severe headaches that she could find relief only with strong analgesics. Her condition of **(spina bifida, migraine, epilepsy)** was debilitating.

2. Paul was in a coma after his high-speed car accident. His physicians were concerned that he had suffered a **(palsy, meningomyelocele, concussion and subdural hematoma)** as a result of the accident.

3. Dick went to the ER complaining of dizziness, nausea, and headache. The physician, suspecting ICP, prescribed corticosteroids, and Dick's symptoms disappeared. Symptoms returned when the steroids were discontinued. **(MRI of the brain, electroencephalography, CSF analysis)** revealed a lesion that was removed surgically and proved to be a(an) **(hydrocele, astrocytoma, herpes zoster)**.

4. Dorothy felt tingling sensations in her hands, and noticed blurred vision and numbness in her arm, all signs of **(shingles, meningitis, TIA)**. Her physician requested **(myelography, cerebral angiography, lumbar puncture)** to assess any damage to cerebral blood vessels and possible stroke.

5. When Bill noticed ptosis and muscle weakness in his face, he reported these symptoms to his doctor. The doctor diagnosed his condition as **(Tourette syndrome, Huntington disease, myasthenia gravis)** and prescribed **(dopamine, anticonvulsants, immunosuppressants),** which relieved his condition.

N. Complete the spelling of the following terms based on their meanings.

1. the part of the brain that controls sleep, appetite, temperature, and secretions of the pituitary gland: hypo _____

2. pertaining to fainting: syn _____

3. abnormal sensations: par _____

4. slight paralysis: par _____

5. inflammation of a spinal nerve root: _radiculitis_____ itis

6. inability to speak: a _physia_____

7. movements and behavior that are not purposeful: a _taxia_____

8. lack of muscular coordination: a _____

9. reading, writing, and learning disorders: dys _____

10. excessive movement: hyper _____

11. paralysis in one half (right or left) of the body: _____ plegia

12. paralysis in the lower half of the body: _____ plegia

13. paralysis in all four limbs: _____ plegia

14. nervous exhaustion and weakness: neur _____

XII. Answers to Exercises

A

1. axon
2. plexus
3. meninges
4. dendrite
5. cerebral cortex
6. astrocyte
7. oligodendroglial cell
8. neuron
9. cauda equina
10. myelin sheath

B

1. outermost meningeal layer surrounding the brain and spinal cord
2. the brain and the spinal cord
3. nerves outside the brain and spinal cord; cranial, spinal, and autonomic nerves
4. middle meningeal membrane surrounding the brain and spinal cord
5. the part of the brain below the thalamus; controls sleep, appetite, body temperature, and secretions from the pituitary gland
6. space through which a nervous impulse is transmitted from a nerve cell to another nerve cell or to a muscle or gland cell
7. autonomic nerves that influence body functions involuntarily in times of stress
8. part of the brain just above the spinal cord that controls breathing, heartbeat, and the size of blood vessels
9. part of the brain anterior to the cerebellum and between the medulla and the upper parts of the brain; connects these parts of the brain
10. posterior part of the brain that coordinates voluntary muscle movements
11. part of the brain below the cerebrum; relay center that conducts impulses
between the spinal cord and the cerebrum
12. canals in the interior of the brain that are filled with CSF
13. lower portion of the brain that connects the cerebrum with the spinal cord (includes the pons and the medulla)
14. largest part of the brain; controls voluntary muscle movement, vision, speech, hearing, thought, memory
15. a collection of nerve cell bodies outside the brain and spinal cord

C

1. pia mater
2. efferent nerves
3. afferent nerves
4. fissures
5. subarachnoid space
6. convolutions
7. neurotransmitter
8. parenchymal cell
9. neuroglial cell

D

1. encephalomalacia
2. cerebellum
3. epidural hematoma
4. leptomeningitis
5. anencephaly
6. poliomyelitis
7. meningeal
8. radiculopathy
9. meningomyelocele
10. vagal

E

1. the outer region of the cerebrum (contains gray matter)
2. pertaining to within a sheath—through the meninges and into the subarachnoid space
3. inflammation of many nerves
4. pertaining to the thalamus
5. record (x-ray) of the spinal cord (after contrast is injected via lumbar puncture)
6. tumor of the meninges
7. tumor of neuroglial cells (a brain tumor)
8. mass of blood below the dura mater (outermost meningeal membrane)

F

1. dyslexia
2. ataxia
3. bradykinesia
4. hyperesthesia
5. narcolepsy
6. aphasia
7. apraxia
8. hemiparesis
9. causalgia
10. paraplegia
11. syncope
12. neurasthenia

G

1. lack of sensitivity to pain
2. inability to speak (cannot articulate words, but can understand speech and knows what she or he wants to say)
3. slight paralysis
4. paralysis in all four extremities (damage is to the cervical part of the spinal cord)
5. no strength (weakness)
6. pertaining to coma (loss of consciousness from which the patient cannot be aroused)
7. condition of abnormal sensations (prickling, tingling, numbness, burning) for no apparent reason
8. excessive movement
9. condition of no sensation or nervous feeling
10. intense burning pain

H

1. multiple sclerosis
2. epilepsy
3. spina bifida cystica
4. amyotrophic lateral sclerosis
5. Huntington disease
6. hydrocephalus
7. myasthenia gravis
8. Parkinson disease
9. Alzheimer disease
10. Bell palsy

I

1. tumor of neuroglial brain cells (astrocytes)
2. inflammation of the meninges (bacterial infection with pus formation)
3. involuntary spasmodic, twitching movements (tics), uncontrollable vocal sounds, and inappropriate words
4. bruising of brain tissue as a result of direct trauma to the head
5. disruption of the normal blood supply to the brain; stroke or cerebral infarction
6. temporary brain dysfunction; loss of consciousness that usually clears within 24 hours
7. neurological condition caused by infection with herpes zoster virus; blisters form along the course of peripheral nerves
8. blockage of a blood vessel in the cerebrum caused by material from another part of the body that suddenly occludes the vessel
9. blockage of a blood vessel in the cerebrum caused by the formation of a clot within the vessel
10. bursting forth of blood from a cerebral artery (can cause a stroke)
11. a widening of a blood vessel (artery) in the cerebrum; the aneurysm can burst and lead to a CVA

J

1. C
2. E
3. H
4. G
5. B
6. A
7. D
8. J
9. I
10. F

K

1. Use of magnetic and radio waves to create an image (in frontal, transverse, or sagittal plane) of the brain.
2. an instrument (stereotactic) is fixed onto the skull and locates a target by three-dimensional measurement; gamma radiation beams are used to treat deep brain lesions

L

1. electroencephalography. E
2. positron emission tomography. I
3. alpha-fetoprotein. G
4. multiple sclerosis. J
5. magnetic resonance imaging. H
6. lumbar puncture. C
7. cerebrovascular accident. B
8. Alzheimer disease. A
9. transient ischemic attack. F
10. cerebrospinal fluid. D

M

1. migraine
2. concussion and subdural hematoma
3. MRI of the brain; astrocytoma
4. TIA; cerebral angiography
5. myasthenia gravis; immunosuppressants

N

1. hypothalamus
2. syncopal
3. paresthesias
4. paresis
5. radiculitis
6. aphasia
7. apraxia
8. ataxia
9. dyslexia
10. hyperkinesis
11. hemiplegia
12. paraplegia
13. quadriplegia
14. neurasthenia

Answers to Practical Applications

1. C
2. A
3. C
4. C
5. A

XIII. Pronunciation of Terms

Pronunciation Guide

ā as in āpe   ă as in ăpple
ē as in ēven   ĕ as in ĕvery
ī as in īce   ĭ as in ĭnterest
ō as in ōpen   ŏ as in pŏt
ū as in ūnit   ŭ as in ŭnder

To test your understanding of the terminology in this chapter, write the meaning of each term in the space provided. In addition, you may wish to cover the terms and write them by looking at your definitions. Make sure your spelling is correct. The page number after each term indicates where it is defined or used in the text so you can easily check your responses.

Vocabulary and Combining Forms and Terminology

Term	Pronunciation	Meaning
acetylcholine (331)	ăs-ĕ-tĭl-KŌ-lēn	_____
afferent nerves (331)	ĂF-ĕr-ĕnt nĕrvz	_____
analgesia (336)	ăn-ăl-JĒ-zē-ă	_____
anencephaly (334)	ăn-ĕn-SĔF-ă-lē	_____
anesthesia (336)	ăn-ĕs-THĒ-zē-ă	_____
aphasia (337)	ă-FĀ-zē-ă	_____
apraxia (338)	ā-PRĂK-sē-ă	_____
arachnoid membrane (331)	ă-RĂK-noyd MĔM-brān	_____
astrocyte (331)	ĂS-trō-sīt	_____
ataxia (338)	ă-TĂK-sē-ă	_____
autonomic nervous system (331)	ăw-tō-NŌM-ĭk NĔR-vŭs SĬS-tĕm	_____
axon (331)	ĂK-sŏn	_____
blood-brain barrier (331)	blŭd-brān BĂ-rē-ĕr	_____
bradykinesia (336)	brā-dē-kĭ-NĒ-zē-ă	_____
brain stem (331)	brān stĕm	_____
cauda equina (331)	KĂW-dă ĕ-QUĪ-nă	_____
causalgia (336)	kăw-ZĂL-jē-ă	_____
cephalalgia (cephalgia) (336)	sēf-ăl-ĂL-jă (sĕ-FĂL-jă)	_____

cerebellar (334)   sĕr-ĕ-BĔL-ăr   _____

cerebellopontine (335)   sĕr-ĕ-bĕl-ō-PŎN-tēn   _____

cerebellum (331)   sĕr-ĕ-BĔL-ŭm   _____

cerebral   sĕ-RĒ-brăl (or SĔR-ĕ-brăl)   _____
  cortex (331)   KŎR-tĕks

cerebrospinal fluid (331) sĕ-rē-brō-SPĪ-năl FLŪ-ĭd   _____

cerebrum (331)   sĕ-RĒ-brŭm   _____

coma (336)   KŌ-mă   _____

comatose (336)   KŌ-mă-tōs   _____

convolution (332)   kŏn-vō-LŪ-shŭn   _____

dendrite (332)   DĔN-drīt   _____

dura mater (332)   DŪ-ră MĀ-tĕr   _____

dyslexia (337)   dĭs-LĔK-sē-ă   _____

efferent nerves (332)   ĔF-ĕr-ĕnt nĕrvz   _____

encephalitis (334)   ĕn-sĕf-ă-LĪ-tĭs   _____

encephalomalacia (335)   ĕn-sĕf-ă-lō-mă-LĀ-shē-ă   _____

encephalopathy (334)   ĕn-sĕf-ă-LŎP-ă-thē   _____

ependymal cell (332)   ĕp-ĔN-dĭ-măl sĕl   _____

epidural hematoma (334) ĕp-ĕ-DŪ-răl hē-mă-TŌ-mă   _____

epilepsy (340)   ĔP-ĭ-lĕp-sē   _____

fissure (333)   FĬSH-ŭr   _____

glioma (335)   glē-Ō-mă   _____

gyrus; gyri (332)   JĪ-rŭs; JĪ-rē   _____

hemiparesis (337)   hĕm-ē-pă-RĒ-sĭs   _____

hemiplegia (338)   hĕm-ē-PLĒ-jă   _____

hyperesthesia (336)   hī-pĕr-ĕs-THĒ-zē-ă   _____

hyperkinesis (337)   hī-pĕr-kĭ-NĒ-sĭs   _____

hypothalamus (332)   hī-pō-THĂL-ă-mŭs   _____

intrathecal (335)	ĭn-tră-THĒ-kăl	
leptomeningitis (335)	lĕp-tō-mĕn-ĭn-JĪ-tĭs	
medulla oblongata (332)	mĕ-DŪL-ă (or mĕ-DŬL-ă) ŏb-lŏn-GĂ-tă	
meningeal (335)	mĕ-NĬN-jē-ăl or mĕ-nĭn-JĒ-ăl	
meninges (332)	mĕ-NĬN-jēz	
meningioma (335)	mĕ-nĭn-jē-Ō-mă	
meningomyelocele (335)	mĕ-nĭng-gō-MĪ-ĕ-lō-sēl	
microglial cell (332)	mĭ-krō-GLĒ-ăl sĕl	
motor nerves (332)	MŌ-tĕr nĕrvz	
myelin sheath (332)	MĪ-ĕ-lĭn shēth	
myelogram (335)	MĪ-ĕ-lō-grăm	
myoneural (335)	mī-ō-NŪ-răl	
narcolepsy (337)	NĂR-kō-lĕp-sē	
neuralgia (336)	nū-RĂL-jă	
neurasthenia (338)	nū-răs-THĒ-nē-ă	
neuroglial cells (332)	nū-rō-GLĒ-ăl sĕlz	
neuron (332)	NŪ-rŏn	
neuropathy (335)	nū-RŎP-ă-thē	
neurotransmitter (332)	nū-rō-trăns-MĬ-tĕr	
oligodendroglial cell (333)	ŏl-ĭ-gō-dĕn-drō-GLĒ-ăl sĕl	
paraplegia (338)	păr-ă-PLĒ-jă	
parasympathetic nerves (333)	păr-ă-sĭm-pă-THĔT-ĭk nervz	
parenchyma (333)	păr-ĔN-kĭ-mă	
paresis (337)	pă-RĒ-sĭs	
paresthesia (336)	păr-ĕs-THĒ-zē-ă	
peripheral nervous system (333)	pĕ-RĬF-ĕr-ăl NĔR-vŭs SĬS-tĕm	

pia mater (333)	PĒ-ă MĂ-tĕr	_____
plexus (333)	PLĔK-sŭs	_____
poliomyelitis (335)	pō-lē-ō-mī-ĕ-LĪ-tĭs	_____
polyneuritis (335)	pōl-ē-nū-RĪ-tĭs	_____
pons (333)	pŏnz	_____
quadriplegia (338)	kwŏd-rĭ-PLĒ-jă	_____
radiculopathy (335)	ră-dĭk-ū-LŎP-ă-thē	_____
sensory nerves (333)	SĔN-sō-rē nĕrvz	_____
stimulus (333)	STĬM-ū-lŭs	_____
stroma (333)	STRŌ-mă	_____
subdural hematoma (334)	sŭb-DŪ-răl hē-mă-TŌ-mă	_____
sulcus; sulci (333)	SŬL-kŭs; SŬL-sī	_____
sympathetic nerves (333)	sĭm-pă-THĔT-ĭk nĕrvz	_____
synapse (333)	SĬN-ăps	_____
syncopal (338)	SĬN-kō-păl	_____
syncope (338)	SĬN-kō-pē	_____
thalamic (335)	THĂL-ă-mĭk or thă-LĂM-ĭk	_____
thalamus (333)	THĂL-ă-mŭs	_____
vagal (336)	VĀ-găl	_____
ventricles of the brain (333)	VĔN-trĭ-k'lz of the brān	_____

Pathological Conditions, Laboratory Tests, and Clinical Procedures

Term	Pronunciation	Meaning
absence seizures (345)	ĂB-sĕns SĒ-zhŭrz	_____
Alzheimer disease (340)	ĂLZ-hī-mĕr dĭ-ZĒZ	_____
amyotrophic lateral sclerosis (340)	ā-mī-ō-TRŌ-fĭk LĂ-tĕr-ăl sklĕ-RŌ-sis	_____
aneurysm (345)	ĂN-ūr-ĭ-zĭm	_____
astrocytoma (345)	ăs-trō-sī-TŌ-mă	_____

aura (345)	ĂW-ră	
Bell palsy (342)	běl PĂL-zē	
cerebral angiography (346)	sě-RĒ-brăl ăn-jē-ŌG-ră-fē	
cerebral concussion (343)	sě-RĒ-brăl kŏn-KŬS-shŭn	
cerebral contusion (343)	sě-RĒ-brăl kŏn-TŪ-shŭn	
cerebral hemorrhage (344)	sě-RĔ-brăl HĔM-ŏr-ĭj	
cerebral palsy (342)	sě-RĒ-brăl (or SĔR-ě-brăl) PĂL-zē	
cerebrospinal fluid analysis (346)	sě-rē-brō-SPĪ-năl FLOO-ĭd ă-NĂL-ĭ-sĭs	
cerebrovascular accident (344)	sě-rē-brō-VĂS-kū-lăr ĂK-sĭ-děnt	
dementia (345)	dě-MĔN-shē-ă	
demyelination (345)	dē-mī-ě-lĭ-NĀ-shun	
dopamine (345)	DŌ-pă-mēn	
electroencephalography (347)	ě-lěk-trō-ěn-sěf-ă-LŎG-ră-fē	
embolus (345)	ĔM-bō-lŭs	
gait (345)	GĀT	
glioblastoma multiforme (343)	glē-ō-blăs-TŌ-mă mŭl-tē-FŎR-mă	
grand mal seizure (340)	grăn măl SĒ-zhŭr	
herpes zoster (345)	HĔR-pēz ZŎS-těr	
Huntington disease (340)	HŬN-ting-tŏn dĭ-ZĒZ	
hydrocephalus (339)	hī-drō-SĔF-ă-lŭs	
lumbar puncture (347)	LŬM-băr PŬNK-shŭr	
magnetic resonance imaging (346)	măg-NĔT-ĭk rě-zō-NĂNCE ĬM-ă-jĭng	
meningitis (342)	měn-ĭn-JĪ-tĭs	
migraine (336)	MĪ-grān	
multiple sclerosis (341)	mŭl-tĭ-p'l sklě-RŌ-sĭs	

myasthenia gravis (341)	mī-ăs-THĒ-nē-ă GRĂ-vĭs	_____
palliative (345)	PĂ-lē-ă-tĭv	_____
palsy (342)	PĂWL-zē	_____
Parkinson disease (342)	PĂR-kĭn-sŭn dĭ-ZĒZ	_____
petit mal seizures (340)	pĕ-TĒ măl SĒ-zhŭrz	_____
positron emission tomography (346)	PŎS-ĭ-trŏn ē-MĬ-shŭn tō-MŎG-ră-fē	_____
shingles (342)	SHĬNG-ălz	_____
spina bifida (339)	SPĬ-nă BĬF-ĭ-dă	_____
stereotactic radiosurgery (348)	stĕ-rē-ō-TĂK-tĭk rā-dē-ō SŬR-gĕr-ē	_____
thrombosis (344)	thrŏm-BŌ-sĭs	_____
tonic-clonic seizures (345)	TŎN-ĭk-KLŌ-nĭk SĒ-zhŭrz	_____
Tourette syndrome (342)	Tŭ-RĔT SĬN-drōm	_____
transient ischemic attack (344)	TRĂN-zē-ĕnt ĭs-KĒ-mĭk ă-TĂK	_____

XIV. Review Sheet

Write the meanings of the word parts in the spaces provided. Check your answers with the information in the chapter or in the glossary (Medical Terms—English) at the end of the book.

COMBINING FORMS

Combining Form	Meaning	Combining Form	Meaning
alges/o		lept/o	
angi/o		lex/o	
caus/o		mening/o, meningi/o	
cephal/o		my/o	
cerebell/o		myel/o	
cerebr/o		narc/o	
comat/o		neur/o	
crani/o		pont/o	
cry/o		radicul/o	
dur/o		spin/o	
encephal/o		syncop/o	
esthesi/o		tax/o	
gli/o		thalam/o	
hydr/o		thec/o	
kines/o		troph/o	
kinesi/o		vag/o	

Continued on following page

PREFIXES

Prefix	Meaning	Prefix	Meaning
a-, an-	_____	micro-	_____
dys-	_____	para-	_____
epi-	_____	polio-	_____
hemi-	_____	poly-	_____
hyper-	_____	quadri-	_____
hypo-	_____	sub-	_____
intra-	_____		

SUFFIXES

Suffix	Meaning	Suffix	Meaning
-algesia	_____	-ose	_____
-algia	_____	-paresis	_____
-blast	_____	-pathy	_____
-cele	_____	-phagia	_____
-esthesia	_____	-phasia	_____
-gram	_____	-plegia	_____
-graphy	_____	-praxia	_____
-ine	_____	-ptosis	_____
-itis	_____	-sclerosis	_____
-kinesia, -kinesis	_____	-sthenia	_____
-lepsy	_____	-tomy	_____
-oma	_____	-trophy	_____

CHAPTER 11

Cardiovascular System

This chapter is divided into the following sections

In this chapter you will

- Name the parts of the heart and associated blood vessels and their functions in the circulation of blood;
- Trace the pathway of blood through the heart;
- List the meanings of major pathological conditions affecting the heart and blood vessels;
- Define combining forms that relate to the cardiovascular system;
- Recognize the meaning of many laboratory tests, clinical procedures, and abbreviations pertaining to the cardiovascular system; and
- Apply your new knowledge to understand medical terms in their proper context, such as in medical reports and records.

I. Introduction

In previous chapters we have discussed the diverse and important functions of many organs of the body. These functions include conduction of nerve impulses, production of hormones and reproductive cells, excretion of waste materials, and digestion and absorption of food substances into the bloodstream. In order to perform these functions reliably and efficiently, the body organs are powered by a unique energy source. The cells of each organ receive energy from the food substances that reach them after being taken into the body. Food contains stored energy that can be converted into the energy of movement and work. This conversion of stored energy into the active energy of work occurs when food and oxygen combine in cells during the chemical process of catabolism. It is obvious, then, that each cell of each organ is dependent on a constant supply of food and oxygen in order to receive sufficient energy to work well.

How does the body assure that oxygen and food will be delivered to all its cells? The cardiovascular system, consisting of a fluid called blood, vessels to carry the blood, and a hollow, muscular pump called the heart, transports food and oxygen to all organs and cells of the body. Blood vessels in the lungs absorb the oxygen that has been inhaled from the air, and blood vessels in the small intestine absorb food substances from the digestive tract. In addition, blood vessels carry cellular waste materials such as carbon dioxide and urea and transport these substances to the lungs and kidneys, respectively, where they can be eliminated from the body.

The heart and blood vessels and the terminology related to their anatomy, physiology, and disease conditions will be explored in this chapter. The nature of blood and another body fluid called lymph will be discussed in a later chapter.

II. Blood Vessels and the Circulation of Blood

Blood Vessels

There are three types of blood vessels in the body. These are arteries, veins, and capillaries.

Arteries are the large blood vessels that lead away from the heart. Their walls are made of connective tissue, muscle tissue, elastic fibers, and an innermost layer of epithelial cells called **endothelium.** Endothelial cells, which line all blood vessels, secrete factors that affect the size of blood vessels, reduce blood clotting, and promote the growth of blood vessels. Because arteries carry blood away from the heart, they must be strong enough to withstand the high pressure of the pumping action of the heart. Their elastic walls allow them to expand as the heartbeat forces blood into the arterial system throughout the body. Smaller branches of arteries are called **arterioles.** Arterioles are thinner than arteries and carry the blood to the tiniest of blood vessels, the capillaries.

Capillaries have walls that are only one endothelial cell thick. These delicate, microscopic vessels carry nutrient-rich, oxygenated blood from the arteries and arterioles to the body cells. Their walls are thin enough to allow passage of oxygen and nutrients out of the bloodstream and into the tissue fluid surrounding the cells. Once inside the cells, the nutrients are burned in the presence of oxygen (catabolism) to release needed energy within the cell. At the same time, waste products such as carbon dioxide and water pass out of the cells and into the thin-walled capillaries. The waste-filled blood then flows back to the heart in small veins called **venules,** which branch to form larger vessels called veins.

Veins are thinner walled than arteries. They conduct blood (that has given up most of its oxygen) toward the heart from the tissues. Veins have little elastic tissue and less connective tissue than arteries, and blood pressure in veins is extremely low compared with pressure in arteries. In order to keep blood moving back toward the heart, veins have valves that prevent the backflow of blood and keep the blood moving in one direction. Muscular action also helps the movement of blood in veins. Figure 11–1 illustrates the differences in blood vessels.

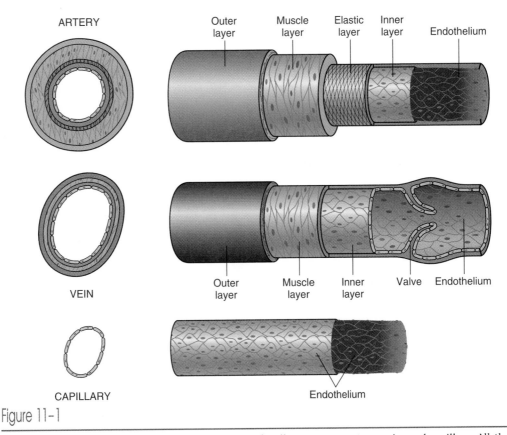

Figure 11-1

Blood vessels. Observe the differences in thickness of walls among an artery, vein, and capillary. All three vessels are lined with endothelium. Endothelial cells actively secrete substances that prevent clotting and regulate the tone of blood vessels. Examples of endothelial secretions are endothelium-derived relaxing factor (EDRF) and endothelin (a vasoconstrictor). (Some parts modified from Damjanov I: Pathology for the Health-Related Professions. Philadelphia, WB Saunders, 1996, p. 155.)

Circulation of Blood

Arteries, arterioles, veins, venules, and capillaries, together with the heart, form a circulatory system for the flow of blood. Figure 11–2 is a schematic representation of this circulatory system. Refer to it as you read the following paragraphs. (Note that the numbers in the following paragraphs correspond with those in Fig. 11–2.)

Blood deficient in oxygen flows through two large veins, the **venae cavae** [1], on its way from the tissue capillaries to the heart. The blood became oxygen-poor at the tissue capillaries when oxygen left the blood and entered the body cells.

Oxygen-poor blood enters the **right side of the heart** [2] and travels through that side and into the **pulmonary artery** [3], a vessel that divides in two, one branch leading to the left lung, the other to the right lung. The arteries continue dividing and subdividing within the lungs, forming smaller and smaller vessels (arterioles) and finally reaching the **lung capillaries** [4]. The pulmonary artery is unusual in that it is the only artery in the body that carries blood deficient in oxygen.

While passing through the lung (pulmonary) capillaries, blood absorbs the oxygen that entered the body during inhalation. The newly oxygenated blood next returns immediately to the heart through **pulmonary veins** [5]. The pulmonary veins are unusual in that they are the only veins in the body that carry oxygen-rich **(oxygenated)** blood. The circulation of blood through the vessels from the heart to the lungs and then back to the heart again is known as the **pulmonary circulation.**

Oxygen-rich blood enters the **left side of the heart** [6] from the pulmonary veins. The muscles in the left side of the heart pump the blood out of the heart through the largest single artery in the body, the **aorta** [7]. The aorta moves up at first (ascending

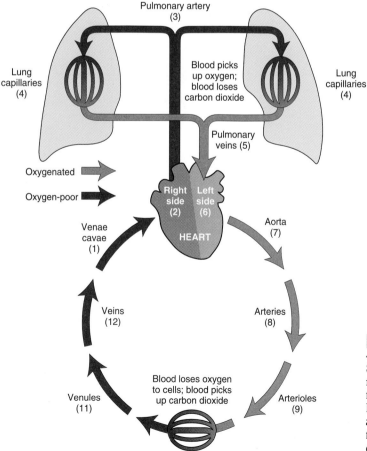

Figure 11–2

Schematic diagram of the pulmonary circulation (blood flow from the heart to lung capillaries and back to the heart) and **systemic circulation** (blood flow from the heart to tissue capillaries and back to the heart).

aorta) but then arches over dorsally and runs downward (descending aorta) just in front of the vertebral column. The aorta divides into numerous branches called **arteries** [8] that carry the oxygenated blood to all parts of the body. The names of some of these arterial branches will be familiar to you: brachial (brachi/o means arm), axillary, splenic, gastric, and renal arteries. The **carotid** arteries supply blood to the head and neck.

The relatively large arterial vessels branch further to form smaller **arterioles** [9]. The arterioles, still containing oxygenated blood, branch into smaller **tissue capillaries** [10], which are near the body cells. Oxygen leaves the blood and passes through the thin capillary walls to enter the body cells. There, food is broken down, in the presence of oxygen, and energy is released.

One metabolic product of this chemical process is **carbon dioxide** (CO_2). CO_2 is produced in the cell but is harmful to the cell if it remains. It must thus pass out of the cells and into the capillary bloodstream at the same time that oxygen is entering the cell. As the blood makes its way back from the tissue capillaries toward the heart in **venules** [11] and **veins** [12] it is full of CO_2 and is oxygen-poor.

The circuit is thus completed when oxygen-poor blood enters the heart from the venae cavae. This circulation of blood from the body organs (except the lungs) to the heart and back again is called the **systemic circulation.** Figure 11–3 shows the aorta, selected arteries, and pulse points (the beat of the heart as it is felt through the walls of arteries).

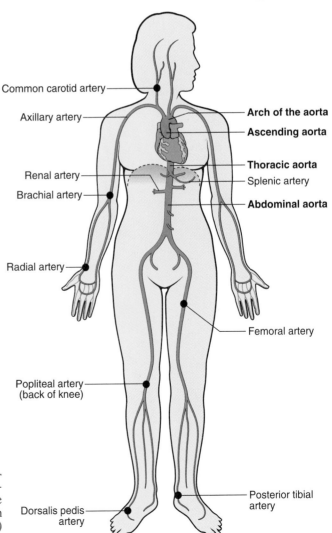

Figure 11-3

The aorta and arteries. Bold dots indicate **pulse points** in arteries. These are areas in which the pulse (expansion and contraction of a superficial artery) can be felt.

III. Anatomy of the Heart

The human heart weighs less than a pound, is roughly the size of an adult fist, and lies in the thoracic cavity, just behind the breastbone in the mediastinum (between the lungs).

The heart is a pump, consisting of four chambers: two upper chambers called **atria** (singular: **atrium**) and two lower chambers called **ventricles.** It is actually a double pump, bound into one organ and synchronized very carefully. Blood passes through each pump in a definite pattern. Pump station number one, on the right side of the heart, sends oxygen-deficient blood to the lungs, where the blood picks up oxygen and releases its carbon dioxide. The newly oxygenated blood returns to the left side of the heart to pump station number two and does not mix with the oxygen-poor blood in pump station number one. Pump station number two then forces the oxygenated blood out to all parts of the body. At the body tissues, the blood loses its oxygen, and on returning to the heart, to pump station number one, blood poor in oxygen (rich in carbon dioxide) is sent out to the lungs to begin the cycle anew.

Label Figure 11–4 as you learn the names of the parts of the heart and the vessels that carry blood to and from it.

Oxygen-poor blood enters the heart through the two largest veins in the body, the **venae cavae.** The **superior vena cava** [1] drains blood from the upper portion of the body, and the **inferior vena cava** [2] carries blood from the lower part of the body.

The venae cavae bring oxygen-poor blood that has passed through all of the body to the **right atrium** [3], the thin-walled upper right chamber of the heart. The right atrium contracts to force blood through the **tricuspid valve** [4] (cusps are the flaps of the valves) into the **right ventricle** [5], which is the lower right chamber of the heart. The cusps of the tricuspid valve form a one-way passage designed to keep the blood flowing in only one direction. As the right ventricle contracts to pump oxygen-poor blood through the **pulmonary valve** [6] into the **pulmonary artery** [7], the tricuspid valve stays shut, thus preventing blood from pushing back into the right atrium. The pulmonary artery then branches to carry oxygen-deficient blood to each lung.

The blood that enters the lung capillaries from the pulmonary artery soon loses its large quantity of carbon dioxide into the lung tissue, and the carbon dioxide is expelled. At the same time, oxygen enters the capillaries of the lungs and is brought back to the heart via the **pulmonary veins** [8]. The newly oxygenated blood enters the **left atrium** [9] of the heart from the pulmonary veins. The walls of the left atrium contract to force blood through the **mitral valve** [10] into the **left ventricle** [11].

The left ventricle has the thickest walls of all four heart chambers (three times the thickness of the right ventricle). It must pump blood with great force so that the blood travels through arteries to all parts of the body. The blood is pumped out of the left ventricle through the **aortic valve** [12] and into the **aorta** [13], which branches to carry blood all over the body. The aortic valve prevents the return of aortic blood to the left ventricle once it has been pumped out.

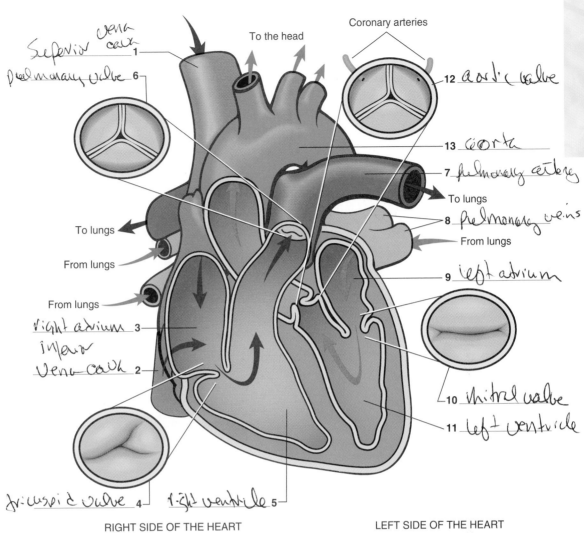

Superior vena cava 1
pulmonary valve 6
right atrium 3
inferior
vena cava 2
tricuspid valve 4

12 aortic valve
13 aorta
7 pulmonary artery
8 pulmonary veins
9 left atrium
10 mitral valve
11 left ventricle

right ventricle 5

Coronary arteries

To the head

To lungs

From lungs

From lungs

To lungs

From lungs

RIGHT SIDE OF THE HEART   LEFT SIDE OF THE HEART

Figure 11-4

Structure of the heart. Blue arrows indicate oxygen-poor blood flow. Red arrows show oxygenated blood flow. (Modified from Damjanov I: Pathology for the Health-Related Professions. Philadelphia, WB Saunders, 1996, p. 154.)

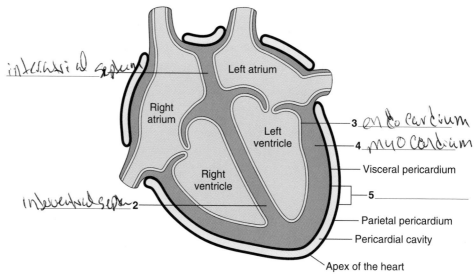

interatrial septum

Left atrium

Right atrium

Left ventricle

3 endocardium

4 myocardium

Visceral pericardium

Right ventricle

interventricular septum 2

5 _____

Parietal pericardium

Pericardial cavity

Apex of the heart

Figure 11-5

The walls of the heart and pericardium. Note that the apex of the heart is the conical (shaped like a cone) lower tip of the heart.

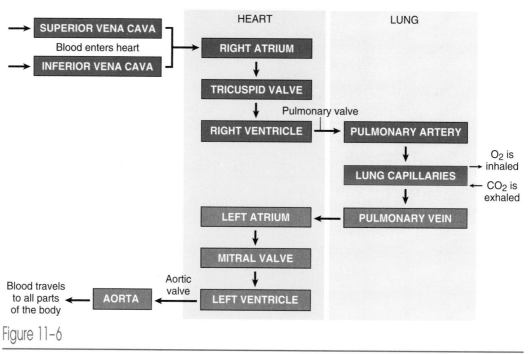

Figure 11-6

Pathway of blood through the heart.

In Figure 11–5 it can be seen that the four chambers of the heart are separated by partitions called **septa** (singular: **septum**). (Label Fig. 11–5 as you read these paragraphs.) The **interatrial septum** [1] separates the two upper chambers (atria), and the **interventricular septum** [2] is a muscular wall that comes between the two lower chambers (ventricles).

The heart wall is composed of three layers, as shown in Figure 11–5. The **endocardium** [3] is a smooth layer of endothelial cells that lines the interior of the heart and the heart valves. The **myocardium** [4] is the middle, muscular layer of the heart wall and is its thickest layer. The **pericardium** [5] is a fibrous and membranous sac surrounding the heart. It is composed of two layers, the **visceral pericardium,** which adheres to the heart, and the **parietal** (parietal means wall) **pericardium,** which lines the outer fibrous coat. The **pericardial cavity** (between the visceral and the parietal pericardia) normally contains 10–15 ml of fluid, which lubricates the membranes as the heart beats.

Figure 11–6 schematically traces the flow of blood through the heart.

IV. Physiology of the Heart

Heartbeat and Heart Sounds

There are two phases of the heartbeat. These phases are called **diastole** (relaxation) and **systole** (contraction). Diastole occurs when the ventricle walls relax and blood flows into the heart from the venae cavae and the pulmonary veins. The tricuspid and mitral valves are open in diastole, as blood passes from the right and left atria into the ventricles. The pulmonary and aortic valves are closed during diastole (Fig. 11–7).

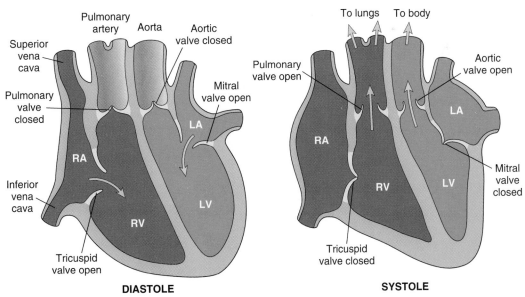

Figure 11-7

Phases of the heartbeat: diastole and systole. During diastole, the tricuspid and mitral valves are open as blood enters the ventricles. During systole, the pulmonary and aortic valves are open as blood is pumped to the pulmonary artery and aorta. RA = right atrium; RV = right ventricle; LA = left atrium; LV = left ventricle.

Systole occurs next, as the walls of the right and left ventricles contract to pump blood into the pulmonary artery and the aorta. Both the tricuspid and the mitral valves are closed during systole, thus preventing the flow of blood back into the atria (see Fig. 11–7).

This diastole-systole cardiac cycle occurs between 70 and 80 times per minute (100,000 times a day). The heart pumps about 3 ounces of blood with each contraction. This means that about 5 quarts of blood are pumped by the heart in 1 minute (75 gallons an hour and about 2000 gallons a day).

Closure of the heart valves is associated with audible sounds, such as "lub, dub, lub, dub," that can be heard when listening to a normal heart with a stethoscope. The "lub" is associated with closure of the tricuspid and mitral valves at the beginning of systole and the "dub" with the closure of the aortic and pulmonary valves at the end of systole. The "lub" sound is called the first heart sound and the "dub" is the second heart sound because the normal cycle of the heartbeat starts with the beginning of the systole. An abnormal heart sound is known as a **murmur.**

Conduction System of the Heart

What keeps the heart at its perfect rhythm? Although the heart does have nerves that can affect its rate, they are not primarily responsible for its beat. It is known that the heart starts beating in the embryo before the heart is supplied with nerves, and it will continue to beat in experimental animals even when the nerve supply is cut.

Primary responsibility for initiating the heartbeat rests with a small region of specialized muscle tissue in the posterior portion of the right atrium, where an electrical impulse originates. This region of the right atrium is called the **sinoatrial node (SA node).** The SA node is also called the **pacemaker** of the heart. The current of electricity generated by the pacemaker causes the walls of the atria to contract and force blood into the ventricles (ending diastole).

Almost like ripples in a pond of water when a stone is thrown, the wave of electricity passes from the pacemaker to another region of the myocardium. This

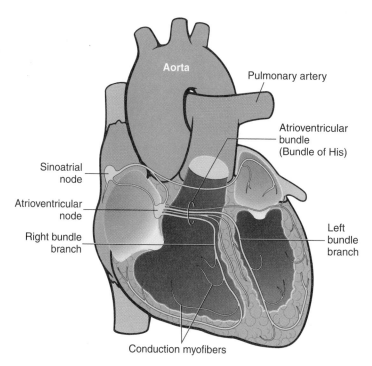

Figure 11-8

Conduction system of the heart.

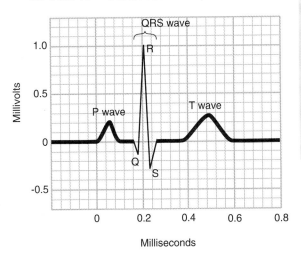

Figure 11-9

Electrocardiogram. P wave = spread of excitation wave over the atria just before contraction; **QRS wave** = spread of excitation wave over the ventricles as the ventricles contract; **T wave** = electrical recovery and relaxation of ventricles. (From Applegate MS: The Anatomy and Physiology Learning System: Textbook. Philadelphia, WB Saunders, 1997, p. 253.)

region is at the posterior portion of the interatrial septum and is called the **atrioventricular node (AV node).** The AV node immediately sends the excitation wave to a bundle of specialized muscle fibers called the **atrioventricular bundle** or **bundle of His** (pronounced hiss). Within the interventricular septum, the bundle of His divides into **right and left bundle branches,** which form the conduction myofibers that extend through the ventricle walls and stimulate them to contract. Thus, systole occurs and blood is pumped away from the heart. A short rest period follows, and then the pacemaker begins the wave of excitation across the heart again. Figure 11-8 shows the conduction system of the heart.

The record used to detect these electrical changes in heart muscle as the heart beats is called an **electrocardiogram** (ECG or EKG, from the Greek root *kardia*). The normal ECG shows five waves, or **deflections,** that represent the electrical changes as a wave of excitation spreads through the heart. The deflections are called P, QRS, and T waves. The P wave represents electrical activity of the SA node impulse formation and the change in the electrical activity in the wall of the atria (atrial depolarization). The QRS wave represents ventricular depolarization as electricity passes through the atrioventricular bundle and the ventricular wall. This is the largest wave because the ventricle contains the most muscle. The T wave represents ventricular repolarization, which is when the ventricular wall relaxes and recovers from contraction. Figure 11-9 illustrates P, QRS, and T waves in a normal ECG. The ECG is used to diagnose a heart attack (myocardial infarction), which causes abnormal deflections.

Normal heart rhythm (originating in the SA node and traveling through the heart) is called **sinus rhythm.** Sympathetic nerves speed up the heart rate during conditions of emotional stress or vigorous exercise. Parasympathetic nerves slow the heart rate when the need for extra pumping is past.

V. Blood Pressure

Blood pressure is the force that the blood exerts on the arterial walls. This pressure is measured by a device called a **sphygmomanometer.**

The sphygmomanometer consists of a rubber bag inside a cloth cuff that is wrapped around the upper arm, just above the elbow. The rubber bag is inflated with air by means of a rubber bulb. As the bag is pumped up, the pressure within it increases and is measured on a recording device attached to the cuff.

The vessels in the upper arm are compressed by the air pressure in the bag. When there is sufficient air pressure in the bag to stop the flow of blood in the main artery of the arm (brachial artery), the pulse in the lower arm (where the observer is listening with a stethoscope) obviously drops.

Air is then allowed to escape from the bag and the pressure is lowered slowly, allowing the blood to begin to make its way through the gradually opening artery. At the point when the person listening with the stethoscope first hears the sounds of the pulse beats, the reading on the device attached to the cuff shows the higher, systolic, blood pressure (pressure in the artery when the left ventricle is contracting to force the blood into the aorta and other arteries).

As air continues to escape, the sounds become progressively louder. Finally, when a change in sound from loud to soft occurs, the observer makes note of the pressure on the recording device. This is called the diastolic blood pressure (pressure in the artery when the ventricles are relaxing and the heart is filling, receiving blood from the venae cavae and pulmonary veins).

Blood pressure is usually expressed as a fraction: for example, 120/80, in which 120 represents the systolic pressure and 80 the diastolic pressure.

VI. Vocabulary

This list will help you review many of the new terms introduced in the text. Short definitions will reinforce your understanding of the terms. See Section XIII of this chapter for help in pronouncing the more difficult terms.

aorta	Largest artery in the body.
arteriole	Small artery.
artery	Largest type of blood vessel; carries blood away from the heart to all parts of the body.
atrioventricular bundle (bundle of His)	Specialized muscle fibers in the wall between the ventricles that carry the electric impulses to the ventricles.
atrioventricular node (AV node)	Specialized tissue at the base of the wall between the two upper heart chambers. Electrical impulses pass from the pacemaker (SA node) through the AV node to the bundle of His.
atrium (plural: **atria**)	Upper chamber of the heart.
capillary	Smallest blood vessel. Materials pass to and from the bloodstream through the thin capillary walls.
carbon dioxide (CO_2)	A gas (waste) released by body cells and transported via veins to the heart and then to the lungs to be expelled.
coronary arteries	The blood vessels that branch from the aorta and carry oxygen-rich blood to the heart muscle.

deoxygenated blood	Blood that is oxygen-poor.
diastole	Relaxation phase of the heartbeat. From the Greek *diastole,* meaning dilation.
endocardium	Inner lining of the heart.
endothelium	Innermost lining of blood vessels.
mitral valve	Valve found between the left atrium and the left ventricle of the heart (Fig. 11–10). This valve is also known as the bicuspid valve.
murmur	An abnormal heart sound caused by improper closure of the heart valves.
myocardium	Muscle layer of the heart.
oxygen	Gas that enters the blood through the lungs and travels to the heart to be pumped via arteries to all body cells.
pacemaker	Sensitive tissue in the right atrium that begins the heartbeat; also called the **sinoatrial node.**
pericardium	Sac-like membrane surrounding the heart.
pulmonary artery	An artery carrying oxygen-poor blood from the heart to the lungs.
pulmonary circulation	The flow of blood from the heart to the lungs and back to the heart.

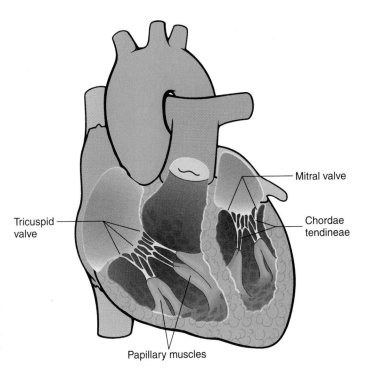

Figure 11-10

Tricuspid and mitral valves. These valves work like parachutes. The chordae tendineae are the connective tissue strings that attach to the papillary muscles projecting from the lining of the ventricles and anchor the valve in place. As blood rushes into the ventricles, it strikes the valves (parachute), which swing up, meet in the midline, and fit together so that the valve is shut tight.

pulmonary valve   Valve between the right ventricle and the pulmonary artery.

pulmonary vein   A vein carrying oxygenated blood from the lungs to the heart.

pulse   The beat of the heart as felt through the walls of the arteries.

septum (plural: **septa**)   A partition; in the cardiovascular system, a partition between the right and the left sides of the heart.

sinoatrial node (SA node)   The pacemaker of the heart.

sphygmomanometer   Instrument to measure blood pressure.

systemic circulation   The flow of blood from the body cells to the heart and then back out from the heart to the cells.

systole   The contraction phase of the heartbeat. From the Greek *systole*, meaning a contracting.

tricuspid valve   Valve located between the right atrium and the right ventricle; it has three (tri-) leaflets, or cusps (see Fig. 11–10).

valve   A structure in veins or in the heart that temporarily closes an opening so that blood flows in only one direction.

vein   Thin-walled blood vessel that carries blood from the body tissues and lungs to the heart.

vena cava (plural: **venae cavae**)   Largest vein in the body. The superior and inferior venae cavae bring blood into the right atrium of the heart.

ventricle   Lower and larger chamber of the heart.

venule   Small vein.

VII. Combining Forms and Terminology

Write the meaning of the medical term in the space provided.

Combining Form	Meaning	Terminology	Meaning
angi/o	vessel	angiogram _____	
		angioplasty _____	
aort/o	aorta	aortic stenosis _____	

arter/o   artery   arteriosclerosis _____
arteri/o
                                     arterial anastomosis _____

                                     arteriography _____

                                     endarterectomy _____

                                     See Section IX, page (400), under Clinical Procedures.

ather/o   yellowish   atheroma _____
                     plaque, fatty
                     substance (the *The suffix -oma means mass or collection. Atheromas are*
                     Greek *athere*, *collections of plaque that protrude into the lumen (opening) of an*
                     means   *artery, weakening the muscle lining.*
                     porridge)
                                     atherosclerosis _____

                                     The major form of arteriosclerosis in which deposits of yellow
                                     plaque containing cholesterol and lipids are found within the lining
                                     of the artery (Fig. 11–11).

                                     atherectomy _____

Figure 11-11

Atherosclerosis leading to **(A)** plaque formation from lipid collection; **(B)** rupture or erosion of the plaque, causing platelet aggregation on the plaque; **(C)** formation of a thrombus that is occlusive, totally blocks the artery, and produces an acute myocardial infarction (heart attack) or sudden cardiac death; or **(D)** formation of a partially occlusive mural thrombus (mural means pertaining to a wall), which causes unstable angina (chest pain that is variable, usually increasing in frequency and intensity and with irregular timing). (Modified from Kumar V, Cotran RS, Robbins SL: Basic Pathology, 6th ed. Philadelphia, WB Saunders, 1997, p. 319.)

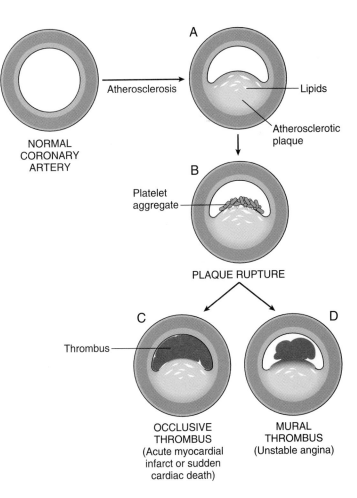

atri/o	atrium, upper heart chamber	atrial _____
		atrioventricular _____
brachi/o	arm	brachial artery _____
cardi/o	heart	cardiomegaly _____
		cardiomyopathy _____

*Toxic or infectious agents may be the cause, but often the etiology is unknown (idiopathic). **Hypertrophic cardiomyopathy** is an increase in heart muscle weight, especially along the septum, which causes narrowing (stenosis) of the aortic valve.*

bradycardia _____

Slower than 60 beats per minute. Normal pulse is about 60–80 beats per minute.

tachycardia _____

Faster than 100 beats per minute.

| **cholesterol/o** | cholesterol (a lipid substance) | hypercholesterolemia _____ |
| **coron/o** | heart | coronary arteries _____ |

These arteries come down over the top of the heart like a crown (corona) (Fig. 11–12).

| **cyan/o** | blue | cyanosis _____ |

This bluish discoloration of the skin indicates diminished oxygen content of the blood.

| **myx/o** | mucus | myxoma _____ |

A benign tumor derived from connective tissue, with cells embedded in soft mucoid stromal tissue. These tumors occur most frequently in the left atrium.

ox/o	oxygen	hypoxia _____
pericardi/o	pericardium	pericardiocentesis _____
phleb/o	vein	phlebotomy _____
		phlebitis _____
sphygm/o	pulse	sphygmomanometer _____

A manometer measures pressure.

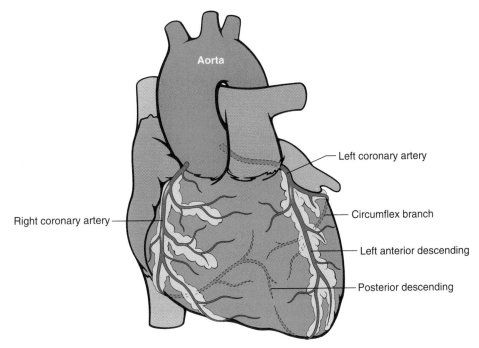

Figure 11-12

Coronary arteries supplying blood to the myocardium.

steth/o	chest	stethoscope _____
		A misnomer because the examination is by ear, not by eye. Auscultation means listening to sounds within the body using a stethoscope.
thromb/o	clot	thrombolysis _____
valvul/o	valve	valvuloplasty _____
valv/o		mitral valvulitis _____
		valvotomy _____
vas/o	vessel	vasoconstriction _____
		Constriction means to tighten or narrow.
		vasodilation _____
vascul/o	vessel	vascular _____
ven/o	vein	venous _____
ventricul/o	ventricle, lower heart chamber	ventriculotomy _____
		interventricular septum _____

VIII. Pathological Conditions: The Heart and Blood Vessels

Heart

arrhythmias

Abnormal heart rhythms (dysrhythmias).

Examples of cardiac arrhythmias are:

**1. heart block
   (atrioventricular block)**

Failure of proper conduction of impulses through the AV node to the atrioventricular bundle (bundle of His).

Damage to the SA node may cause its impulses to be too weak to activate the AV node and impulses fail to reach the ventricles. If the failure occurs only occasionally, the heart will miss a beat in a rhythm at regular intervals (partial heart block). If no impulses reach the AV node from the SA node, the ventricles contract slower than the atria and are not coordinated. This is complete heart block.

Implantation of a **cardiac pacemaker** can overcome heart block and establish a normal rhythm. Most pacemakers are powered with batteries that will function at a normal heart rate for 5–10 years (Fig. 11–13).

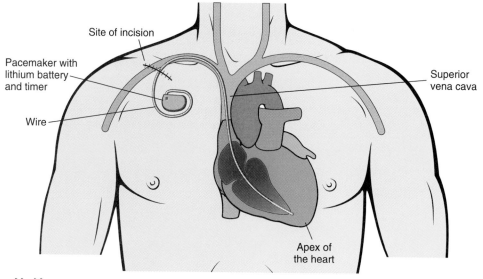

Site of incision

Pacemaker with lithium battery and timer

Superior vena cava

Wire

Apex of the heart

Figure 11-13

Permanent **pacemaker** is placed within the chest.

2. flutter

Rapid but regular contractions of atria or ventricles.

This condition can occur in patients with heart disease. The heart rhythm may reach up to 300 beats per minute.

3. fibrillation

Rapid, random, ineffectual, and irregular contractions of the heart (350 beats or more per minute).

In atrial fibrillation, the wave of excitation passes through the atrial myocardium even more quickly than in atrial flutter. In order to restore normal heart rhythm, an electrical device called a **defibrillator** is applied to the chest wall. The electric shock stops the heart and reverses its abnormal rhythm. This is also called **cardioversion.** Drugs, such as **digoxin** may also be used to convert fibrillation into regular rhythm.

A device, called an **automatic implantable cardioverter/defibrillator (AICD),** can now be implanted in the chest to sense arrhythmias and correct them. These are pacemaker-sized devices that give shocks to change abnormal rhythms, such as ventricular fibrillation. **Radiofrequency catheter ablation (RFA)** is a nonsurgical treatment used to treat arrhythmias, such as paroxysmal (sharp, sudden spasms) tachycardia. A catheter, placed in blood vessels leading up against heart muscle, delivers a high-frequency current to burn a small portion of the muscle. This injury (ablation) to the muscle destroys the arrhythmia.

Cardiac arrest is the sudden and often unexpected stoppage of heart movement, caused by heart block or ventricular fibrillation (resulting from underlying heart disease).

Palpitations are uncomfortable sensations in the chest associated with different types of arrhythmias. Palpitations do not necessarily indicate serious heart disease (smoking, caffeine, and drugs such as antidepressants can produce palpitations). Two cardiac causes of palpitations are **premature ventricular contractions (PVCs)** and **premature atrial contractions (PACs).**

congenital heart disease

Abnormalities in the heart at birth.

The following conditions are congenital anomalies resulting from some failure in the development of the fetal heart.

1. coarctation of the aorta (CoA)

Narrowing (coarctation) of the aorta.

Figure 11–14A shows one form of coarctation of the aorta. Surgical treatment consists of removal of the constricted region and end-to-end anastomosis of the aortic segments.

2. patent ductus arteriosus (PDA)

A small duct (ductus arteriosus) between the aorta and the pulmonary artery, which normally closes soon after birth, remains open (patent).

This condition, illustrated in Figure 11–14B, means that oxygenated blood flows from the aorta to the pulmonary artery. The anomaly occurs most often in females and is commonly associated with intrauterine rubella (German measles) infection, prematurity, and infantile respiratory distress syndrome. Treatment is surgery to close the ductus arteriosus. Alternative measures include minimally invasive surgery (a metal clip is used to close the PDA) and use of indomethacin, a drug that blocks the effects of prostaglandin, which naturally keeps the ductus arteriosus open.

3. septal defects

Small holes in the septa between the atria (atrial septal defects [ASDs]) or the ventricles (ventricular septal defects [VSDs]). Figure 11–15A shows a ventricular septal defect.

Although many septal defects will close spontaneously, others will require surgery. Septal defects can be closed while maintaining a general circulation by means of a **heart-lung machine.** This machine is connected to the patient's circulatory system and relieves the heart and lungs of pumping and oxygenation functions during heart surgery.

Two recent procedures as alternatives to traditional surgery are **trans-catheter closure** (a "clamshell" device is threaded through the blood via a catheter into the heart and into the septal defect, where it is fixed in place to block the hole) and **minimally invasive heart surgery** (through 3 or 4 small "puncture" holes in the chest; special instruments are used to repair the defect).

4. tetralogy of Fallot (fã-LŌ)

A congenital malformation of the heart involving four (tetra-) distinct defects.

The condition, named for Etienne Fallot, the French physician who described it in 1888, is illustrated in Figure 11–15B. The four defects are:

1. **Pulmonary artery stenosis.** This means that blood is not adequately passed to the lungs for oxygenation.
2. **Ventricular septal defect.** The gap in the septum allows deoxygenated blood to pass into the left ventricle, and from there to the aorta.
3. **Shift of the aorta to the right,** so that the aorta overrides the interventricular septum. Oxygen-poor blood passes even more easily from the right ventricle to the aorta.
4. **Hypertrophy of the right ventricle.** The myocardium has to work harder to pump blood through a narrowed pulmonary artery.

An infant with this condition is described as a "blue baby" because of the extreme degree of **cyanosis** present at birth (other congenital conditions that

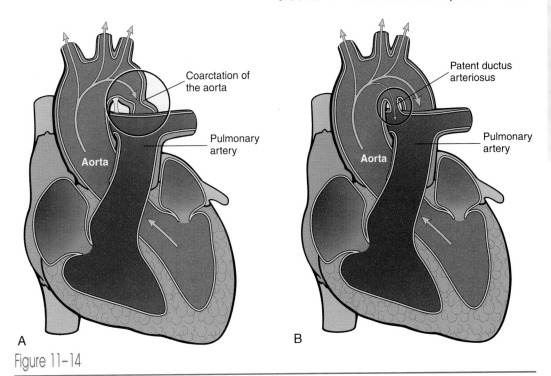

Figure 11-14

(A) **Coarctation of the aorta.** Localized narrowing of the aorta reduces the supply of blood to the lower part of the body. (B) **Patent ductus arteriosus.** The ductus arteriosus fails to close after birth, and blood from the aorta flows through it into the pulmonary artery.

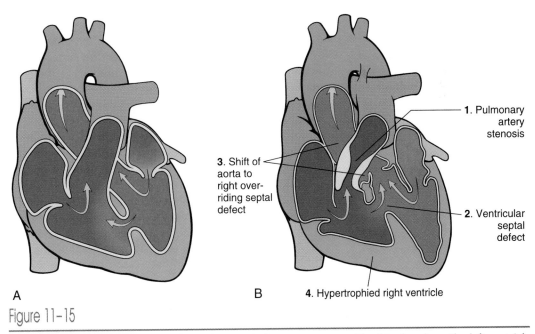

Figure 11-15

(A) **Ventricular septal defect.** A hole in the ventricular septum causes blood to flow from the left ventricle to the right and into the lungs via the pulmonary artery. (B) **Tetralogy of Fallot** showing the four defects. The flow of blood is indicated by the arrows. (Part B modified from Kumar V, Cotran RS, Robbins SL: Basic Pathology, 6th ed. Philadelphia, WB Saunders, 1997, p. 335.)

involve a shunt of blood from the right to the left without passing through the lungs and receiving proper oxygenation can lead to cyanosis as well). Surgery is required to repair the various heart defects.

congestive heart failure

The heart is unable to pump its required amount of blood (more blood enters the heart from the veins than leaves through the arteries).

Blood accumulates in the lungs (left-sided heart failure) causing **pulmonary edema** (fluid seeps out of capillaries into the tiny air sacs of the lungs). Damming back of blood resulting from right-sided heart failure results in accumulation of fluid in the abdominal organs (liver and spleen) and subcutaneous tissue of the legs. Congestive heart failure often develops gradually over several years, although it can be acute. Therapy includes lowering dietary intake of sodium and diuretics to promote loss of fluids.

Recent studies have shown that drugs known as **angiotensin-converting enzyme (ACE) inhibitors** can improve the performance of the heart and its pumping activity. These drugs also decrease pressure inside blood vessels and are used to treat hypertension (high blood pressure). If drug therapy and life-style changes fail to control congestive heart failure, heart transplantation may be the only treatment option. While waiting for a transplant, patients may need a device to assist the heart's pumping. A **left ventricular assist device (LVAD)** is a booster pump implanted in the abdomen, with a cannula (tube) inserted into the left ventricle. It pumps blood out of the heart to all parts of the body. The LVAD is sometimes called a "bridge to transplant."

coronary artery disease (CAD)

Disease of the arteries surrounding the heart.

The coronary arteries are three large vessels that arise from the aorta and supply oxygenated blood to the heart. It is interesting that the blood that constantly flows through the four hollow chambers of the heart does not itself nourish the myocardial tissue. Instead, after blood leaves the heart via the aorta, a portion is at once led back over the surface of the heart through the coronary arteries, so that the heart muscle receives blood before any other organ. This seems logical because the energy requirements of the heart are greater than those of any other organ. Figure 11–12 shows the right and left coronary arteries as they branch from the aorta.

Coronary artery disease is usually the result of **atherosclerosis.** This is the deposition of fatty compounds on the inner lining of the coronary arteries (any other artery can be similarly affected). The ordinarily smooth lining of the artery becomes roughened as the atherosclerotic plaque collects in the artery.

Atherosclerosis is dangerous for two important reasons. First, narrowing of the vessel due to atherosclerosis can cause inflexibility and plugging up of the vessel. Second, the roughened lining of the artery may rupture or cause abnormal clotting of blood, leading to a **thrombotic occlusion** (blocking of the coronary artery by a clot). In both cases, blood flow is decreased **(ischemia)** or stopped entirely, leading to death **(necrosis)** of a part of the myocardium. The area of dead myocardial tissue is known as an **infarction.** The infarcted area is eventually replaced by scar tissue. Figure 11–16 illustrates coronary artery occlusion leading to ischemia and infarction of heart muscle. Figure 11–17 is a photograph of myocardium after an acute myocardial infarction.

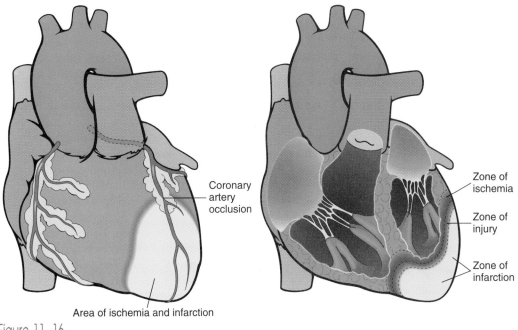

Coronary
artery
occlusion

Zone of
ischemia

Zone of
injury

Zone of
infarction

Area of ischemia and infarction

Figure 11-16

(A) **Ischemia** and **infarction** produced by coronary artery occlusion. **(B)** Internal view of the ventricles of the heart showing an area damaged by myocardial infarction.

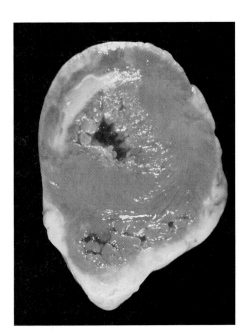

Figure 11-17

Acute myocardial infarction (MI), 5 to 7 days old. The infarct is visible as a well-demarcated, pale yellow lesion in the posterolateral region of the left ventricle. The border of the infarct is surrounded by a dark red zone of acute inflammation. (From Kumar V, Cotran RS, Robbins SL: Basic Pathology, 6th ed. Philadelphia, WB Saunders, 1997, p. 315.)

The severity of a **myocardial infarction** (also known as **heart attack**) depends on the size of the artery that is blocked and the extent of the blockage. If the blocked artery is small, the result may be death of only a small portion of the heart immediately fed by the artery. After scar tissue forms, the patient may be able to resume completely normal activity.

Angina pectoris is an episode of chest pain, often called precordial pain (precordial means in front of the chest), resulting from a temporary difference between the supply and the demand of oxygen to the heart muscle. Angina can be the result of low oxygen levels in the blood (from smoking or respiratory disease), restricted blood flow to the heart (coronary artery disease), or an increase in the work of the heart beyond normal levels. For acute attacks of angina, **nitroglycerin** is given sublingually. This drug, one of several called **nitrates,** is a powerful vasodilator and muscle relaxant.

Treatment guidelines for CAD begin with controlling risk factors, such as smoking, obesity, and lack of exercise. Daily aspirin therapy (to prevent formation of clots) and drug therapy to lower cholesterol (HMGs or "statins" reduce the production of cholesterol in the liver) are also important to prevent heart disease. After the occurrence of an MI, patients may require maintenance and anti-ischemic therapy with drugs called **beta-blockers,** which reduce the force and speed of the heartbeat and lower blood pressure. Other drugs, such as **nitrates** and **calcium channel blockers,** cause dilation of blood vessels, making it easier for the heart to pump blood through vessels.

Surgical treatment of CAD is an open heart operation called **coronary artery bypass grafting,** or **CABG.** See page (400). Cardiologists perform **percutaneous transluminal coronary angioplasty (PTCA),** in which catheterization with balloons and stents opens clogged coronary arteries. See page (402).

An innovative method of treatment is **transmyocardial laser revascularization (TMLR).** A laser makes holes in the heart muscle to induce **angiogenesis** (growth of new blood vessels). Gene therapy (giving DNA or viruses containing DNA to promote expression of factors that lead to angiogenesis) is another new technique to restore damaged heart muscle.

endocarditis

Inflammation of the inner lining of the heart caused by bacteria (bacterial endocarditis).

This condition may be a complication of another infectious disease, an operation, or an injury. Damage to the heart valves produces lesions called **vegetations** (they resemble cauliflower) that break off into the bloodstream as **emboli** (material that travels through the blood). When the emboli lodge in the small vessels of the skin, multiple pinpoint hemorrhages known as **petechiae** (from the Italian *petechio,* meaning a fleabite) form. Antibiotics are effective in curing bacterial endocarditis.

hypertensive heart disease

High blood pressure affecting the heart.

This condition is caused by the contraction of arterioles leading to increased pressure in arteries. The heart itself is affected because it has to pump more vigorously to overcome the increased resistance in the arteries. Vessels lose their elasticity, become like solid pipes, and place increased burden on the heart to pump blood through the body.

mitral valve prolapse (MVP)

Improper closure of the mitral valve when the heart is pumping blood (Fig. 11–18).

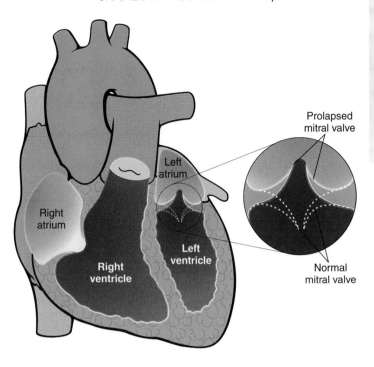

Figure 11-18

Position of a normal mitral valve and prolapsed mitral valve.

This condition, found most frequently in otherwise healthy young women, occurs because the mitral valve enlarges and prolapses into the left atrium during systole. The physician hears a midsystolic click on auscultation (listening with a stethoscope). Most people with MVP live normal lives, but because prolapsed valves can on rare occasions become infected, persons with MVP are advised to have preventive antibiotics at the time of dental procedures if the murmur is present.

murmur

An extra heart sound, heard between normal beats.

Murmurs are heard with the aid of a stethoscope and are usually caused by a valvular defect or disease that disrupts the smooth flow of blood in the heart. They are also heard in cases of interseptal defects when blood flows abnormally between chambers through holes in the septa. A functional murmur is one that is not caused by a valve or septal defect and is not a serious danger to the patient's health.

A **bruit** (brū-Ē) is an abnormal sound or murmur heard on auscultation. A **thrill,** which is a vibration felt on palpation of the chest, often accompanies a murmur.

pericarditis

Inflammation of the membrane (pericardium) surrounding the heart.

In most instances, pericarditis is secondary to disease elsewhere in the body (such as pulmonary infection). Bacteria and viruses cause the condition, or the etiology may be idiopathic. Malaise, fever, and chest pain occur, as well as accumulation of fluid within the pericardial cavity. Compression of the heart due to collection of fluid is called **cardiac tamponade** (tăm-pŏ-NĀD). If a considerable amount of fluid is present, pressure on the pulmonary veins may slow the return of blood from the lungs. Excess fluid is drained by pericardiocentesis.

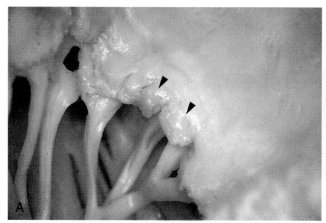 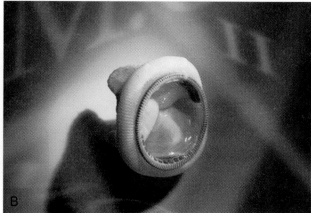

Figure 11-19

(A) Acute rheumatic mitral valvulitis with chronic rheumatic heart disease. Small vegetations are visible along the line of closure of the mitral valve leaflet *(arrows)*. Previous episodes of rheumatic valvulitis have caused fibrous thickening and fusion of the chordae tendineae of the valves. **(B) Porcine xenograft valve.** A xenograft (*xen/o* means stranger) is tissue that is transferred from an animal of one species (pig) to one of another species (human). (Part A from Kumar V, Cotran RS, Robbins SL: Basic Pathology, 6th ed. Philadelphia, WB Saunders, 1997, p. 323; Part B from Lewis SM, Collier IC, Heitkemper MM: Medical-Surgical Nursing: Assessment and Management of Clinical Problems, 4th ed. St. Louis, Mosby, 1996, p. 1029.)

rheumatic heart disease

Heart disease caused by rheumatic fever.

Rheumatic fever is a disease, usually occurring in childhood, that can follow a few weeks after a streptococcal infection. Damage is done to the heart, particularly the heart valves, by one or more attacks of rheumatic fever. The valves, especially the mitral valve, become inflamed and scarred (with **vegetations**), so that they do not open and close normally. Figure 11-19A is a photograph of a damaged heart valve with chronic rheumatic heart disease. **Mitral stenosis,** atrial fibrillation, and congestive heart failure, due to weakening of the myocardium, are other aspects of rheumatic heart disease. Treatment consists of reduced activity, drugs to control arrhythmia, surgery to repair a damaged valve, and anticoagulant therapy to prevent emboli from forming. Mechanical or porcine (pig) valve implants are also used to replace deteriorated heart valves. Figure 11-19B shows a porcine (pig) valve implant.

Blood Vessels

aneurysm

Local widening (ballooning out of a small area) of an artery caused by weakness in the arterial wall or breakdown of the wall owing to atherosclerosis.

Aneurysm literally means to widen (-eurysm) up (ana-). It may occur anywhere in the body but most commonly in the aorta. The danger of an aneurysm is that as the wall of the artery pushes outward it becomes progressively thinner and may eventually rupture. Treatment of an aneurysm depends on the particular vessel involved, the site, and the health of the patient. In aneurysms of small vessels in the brain (berry aneurysms), treatment is occlusion of the vessel with small clips. For larger arteries, such as the aorta, the aneurysm is resected and a synthetic graft is sewn within the aneurysm. Figure 11-20A shows an abdominal aortic aneurysm, and Figure 11-20B illustrates a synthetic graft in place.

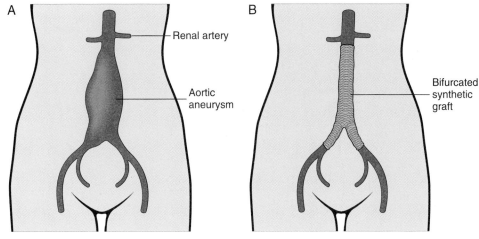

Figure 11-20

(A) Abdominal aortic aneurysm. A dissecting aortic aneurysm is splitting or dissection of the wall of the aorta by blood entering a tear or hemorrhage within the walls of the vessel. (B) Bifurcated synthetic graft in place.

hypertension	**High blood pressure.**

Most high blood pressure is **essential hypertension,** in which the cause of the increased pressure is idiopathic. In adults, a blood pressure equal to or greater than 140/90 mmHg is considered high. Diuretics, beta-blockers, ACE inhibitors, and calcium channel blockers are used as treatment for essential hypertension. Losing weight, limiting sodium (salt) intake, stopping smoking, and reducing fat in the diet are also important in therapy.

In **secondary hypertension,** there is always some associated lesion, such as glomerulonephritis, pyelonephritis, or disease of the adrenal glands, that is responsible for the elevated blood pressure.

peripheral vascular disease   **Blockage of blood vessels (arteries) in the lower extremities due to atherosclerosis.**

When arteries in the groin or upper leg narrow or become blocked, blood flow to the lower leg and foot is reduced. Often, the **femoral** (thigh) **artery** or the **popliteal** (back of the knee) **artery** is involved. An early sign of the problem is **intermittent claudication** (absence of pain or discomfort in a leg at rest, but pain, tension, and weakness after walking has begun). Treatment is exercise, avoidance of nicotine, which causes vessel constriction, and control of risk factors such as hypertension, hyperlipidemia, and diabetes. Surgical treatment includes endarterectomy and bypass grafting (from the normal proximal vessel around the diseased area to a normal vessel distally).

Raynaud phenomenon   **Short episodes of pallor and numbness in the fingers and toes due to temporary constriction of arterioles in the skin.**

This condition is usually idiopathic, but it may also be secondary to some other, more serious disorder. The episodes can be triggered by cold temperatures, emotional stress, or cigarette smoking. Protecting the body from cold and use of vasodilators are effective treatment.

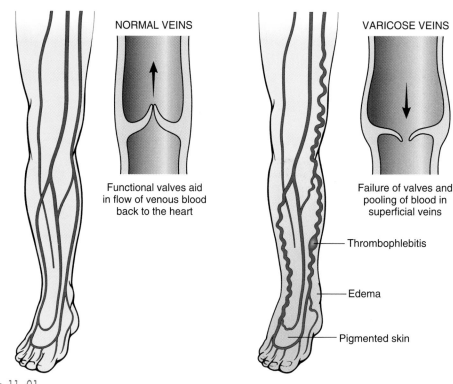

NORMAL VEINS

Functional valves aid
in flow of venous blood
back to the heart

VARICOSE VEINS

Failure of valves and
pooling of blood in
superficial veins

—— Thrombophlebitis

—— Edema

—— Pigmented skin

Figure 11-21

Normal and varicose veins. The slow flow in veins makes an individual susceptible to clot formation. Thrombotic occlusion of varicose veins is known as thrombophlebitis. If a thrombus becomes loosened from its place in the vein, it can travel to the lungs **(pulmonary embolism)** and block a blood vessel there. When blood pools in the lower parts of the leg, fluid leaks from distended small capillaries, causing **edema.**

varicose veins

Abnormally swollen and twisted veins, usually occurring in the legs.

This condition is due to damaged valves that fail to prevent the backflow of blood (Fig. 11–21). The blood then collects in the veins, which distend to many times their normal size. Because of the slow flow of blood in the varicose veins and frequent injury to the vein, thrombosis may occur as well. **Hemorrhoids** (piles) are varicose veins near the anus. Surgical treatment of hemorrhoids includes injection of sclerosing solutions, ligation with rubber bands, and cryosurgery.

Treatment of varicose veins includes wearing elastic stockings, elevation of the legs if edema occurs, and surgery to ligate (tie off) and strip (remove) the twisted, swollen veins. The surgical procedure is called vein stripping.

STUDY SECTION

Practice spelling each term and know its meaning.

angina pectoris

Chest pain resulting from a temporary difference between the supply and the demand of oxygen to the heart muscle.

angiotensin-converting enzyme (ACE) inhibitors

These drugs block the conversion of angiotensin I to angiotensin II and thus reduce blood vessel constriction. They are antihypertensive drugs.

auscultation

Listening with a stethoscope.

beta-blockers

Drugs used to treat angina, hypertension, and arrhythmias. They block the action of epinephrine (Adrenalin) at receptor sites on cells so that the heart beats more slowly and with less force and requires less oxygen.

bruit

An abnormal sound (murmur) heard on auscultation.

calcium channel blockers

Drugs used to treat angina and hypertension. They dilate blood vessels by blocking the influx of calcium into muscles that line the vessels.

claudication

Pain, tension, and weakness in a leg after walking has begun, but absence of pain at rest.

digoxin

A drug used to correct arrhythmias and improve the strength of the heartbeat.

emboli (singular: embolus)

Collections of material (clots or other substances) that travel to and suddenly block a blood vessel.

infarction

Area of dead tissue.

nitrates

Drugs used in the treatment of angina pectoris. They dilate blood vessels, so that a patient is less likely to develop myocardial oxygen deficit.

nitroglycerin

A nitrate drug used in the treatment of angina pectoris.

occlusion

Closure of a blood vessel.

palpitations

Uncomfortable sensations in the chest related to cardiac arrhythmias.

patent

Open.

petechiae

Small, pinpoint hemorrhages.

thrill

A vibration felt on palpation of the chest.

vegetations

Collections of platelets, clotting proteins, microorganisms, and red blood cells that attach to the endocardium in conditions such as bacterial endocarditis and rheumatic heart disease.

IX. Laboratory Tests, Clinical Procedures, and Abbreviations

Laboratory Tests

lipid tests

Lipids are fatty substances found in foods and in the body. Examples of lipids are **cholesterol** and **triglycerides.** Lipid tests measure the amounts of these substances in a blood sample. High levels of triglycerides and cholesterol in the blood are associated with a greater risk of atherosclerosis. A cholesterol level below 200 mg/dL in a middle-aged adult is associated with a relatively low risk for coronary artery disease (CAD). A diet high in **saturated fat** (solid fats of animal origin, such as milk, butter, and meats) tends to increase the amount of cholesterol in the blood. **Polyunsaturated fats** (such as corn oil and safflower oil) do not raise blood cholesterol.

The mainstay of treatment for people with hyperlipidemia is proper diet (low fat and high fiber intake with fresh fruits and vegetables) and exercise. Niacin (a vitamin) is also helpful in reducing lipids. Drug therapy includes HMG reductase inhibitors (HMGs), which lower cholesterol by reducing its production in the liver. These are known as "statins," and examples are simvastatin, lovastatin, and pravastatin.

lipoprotein electrophoresis

Lipoproteins are proteins that carry lipids (fats) in the bloodstream. Protein electrophoresis is the process of physically separating lipoproteins from a blood sample. High levels of **low-density lipoproteins (LDL)** and **very-low-density lipoproteins (VLDL)** are associated with atherosclerosis. High levels of **high-density lipoproteins (HDL),** which remove cholesterol and transport it to the liver, protect adults from the development of atherosclerosis. Factors that increase HDL are estrogen, exercise, and alcohol in moderation.

serum enzyme tests

During a myocardial infarction, enzymes are released into the bloodstream from the dying heart muscle. These enzymes can be measured and are useful as evidence of an infarction. The enzymes tested for are **creatine phosphokinase (CPK)** and **lactate dehydrogenase (LDH).** Other blood tests measure levels of muscle proteins, myoglobin, and troponin-T.

Clinical Procedures

X-Ray

angiography

Dye is injected into the bloodstream or heart chamber, and x-ray films are taken of the heart and large blood vessels in the chest. If dye is injected into the aorta or an artery in the groin, the procedure is called **arteriography.**

digital subtraction angiography (DSA)

Video equipment and a computer are used to produce x-ray pictures of blood vessels. First, an x-ray is produced of the area to be studied, and the results are stored in a computer. Next, contrast material is injected into a vein, and a second image is produced that is also recorded in the computer. The computer then compares the two images and subtracts the first image from the second (removing parts not being studied such as bone, muscle, and fat), leaving nothing but an image of the contrast medium and vessels.

Ultrasound Tests

Doppler ultrasound

An instrument is used to focus sound waves on a blood vessel; blood flow is measured as echoes bounce off red blood cells. Velocity of blood flow increases in areas of stenosis. Arteries or veins in the arms, neck, or legs are examined to detect vascular occlusion (blockage due to clots or atherosclerosis).

echocardiography (ECHO)

Pulses of high-frequency sound waves (ultrasound) are transmitted into the chest, and echoes returning from the valves, chambers, and surfaces of the heart are electronically plotted and recorded. This procedure can show the structure and movement of the heart. In **transesophageal echocardiography (TEE),** a transducer attached to a fiberoptic endoscope is placed in the esophagus to provide images or Doppler information. It is especially useful to detect cardiac masses, prosthetic valve function, aneurysm, and posterior pericardial effusions.

Nuclear Cardiology

positron emission tomography (PET) scan

An IV radiopharmaceutical is administered, followed by an injection of glucose. These localize in the myocardium. Uptake is proportional to the glucose metabolic activity of myocardial cells. Images showing blood flow and functional activity of the myocardium are obtained. Indications for PET scanner use include detection of CAD, assessment of myocardial viability, and differentiation of ischemia and cardiomyopathy.

thallium 201 scintigraphy

Thallium 201 is a radioactive isotope that is taken up by myocardial tissue. After intravenous injection, the concentration of thallium 201 is measured (by perfusion scanning). Infarcted or scarred myocardium does not extract any isotope, showing up as "cold spots." Thallium 201 imaging can be performed before or after an exercise ECG study or as a resting study only.

technetium 99m ventriculography (multiple-gated acquisition scan, or MUGA scan)

This radioactive test studies the motion of the left ventricular wall and measures the ventricle's ability to eject blood. It is a test of the functioning of the heart and cardiac output.

Magnetic Resonance Imaging (MRI)

cardiac MRI

Magnetic waves are beamed at the heart, and an image is produced. The procedure is used to obtain detailed information about congenital heart disease, cardiac masses, and lesions of large blood vessels prior to surgery.

Other Procedures

cardiac catheterization

A thin, flexible tube (catheter) is introduced into a vein or artery and is guided into the heart for purposes of detecting pressures and patterns of blood flow. Contrast can also be injected and x-ray films made (angiography). Figure 11–22 shows catheterization of the heart.

cardioversion (defibrillation)

Very brief discharges of electricity are applied across the chest to stop a cardiac arrhythmia and to allow a more normal rhythm to begin.

coronary bypass surgery (CABG)

Vessel grafts, consisting of veins taken from other parts of the body, are anastomosed (connected) to existing coronary arteries to detour around blockages in the coronary arteries and keep the myocardium supplied with oxygenated blood (Fig. 11–23). Minimally invasive CABG surgery is performed with smaller incisions instead of the traditional sternotomy to open the chest.

electrocardiography (ECG, EKG)

Process of recording the electricity flowing through the heart and thus the rhythm of the heartbeat. A normal sinus rhythm begins in the SA node and is between 60 and 100 beats per minute, with normal intervals and no ectopic beats. Figure 11–24 shows normal sinus rhythm and ventricular tachycardia on ECG strips.

endarterectomy

This procedure involves surgical removal of the innermost (end-) lining of an artery when it is thickened by fatty deposits (atheromas) and thromboses.

extracorporeal circulation (ECC)

A heart-lung machine (pump oxygenator) is used as a bypass to divert blood from the heart and lungs while the heart is being repaired. Blood leaves the body, enters the heart-lung machine, where it is oxygenated,

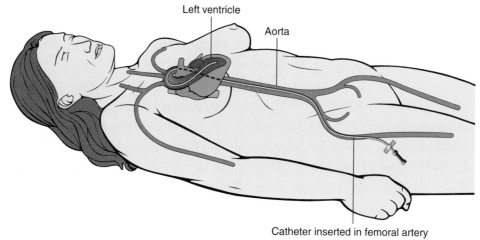

Left ventricle

Aorta

Catheter inserted in femoral artery

Figure 11-22

Left-sided cardiac catheterization. The catheter is passed retrograde (backward) from the femoral artery into the aorta and then into the left ventricle. For right-sided cardiac catheterization, the cardiologist inserts a catheter through the femoral vein and advances it to the right atrium and right ventricle and into the pulmonary artery.

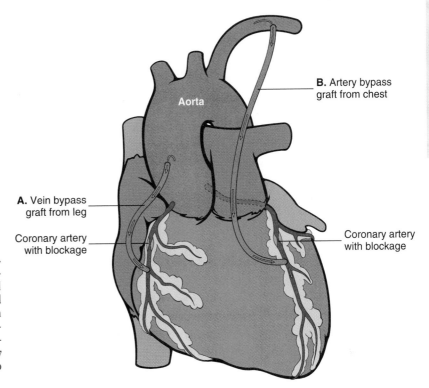

A. Vein bypass graft from leg

Coronary artery with blockage

B. Artery bypass graft from chest

Aorta

Coronary artery with blockage

Figure 11-23

Coronary artery bypass graft (CABG) surgery with anastomosis of vein and arterial grafts. **(A)** Section of a vein is removed from the leg and anastomosed (upside down because of its directional valves) to a coronary artery to bypass an area of arteriosclerotic blockage. **(B)** An internal mammary artery is grafted to a coronary artery to bypass a blockage.

and then returns to a blood vessel (artery) to circulate through the bloodstream. Extracorporeal means outside (extra-) the body (corpor/o).

heart transplantation

A donor heart is transferred to a recipient. The surgery consists of removal of the diseased heart (from cardiomyopathy or heart failure), leaving the posterior walls of the recipient's atria, and anastomosis of the atria, aorta, and pulmonary arteries. While waiting for a transplant, a patient may need a **left ventricular assist device (LVAD),** which is a booster pump implanted in the abdomen with a cannula to the left ventricle.

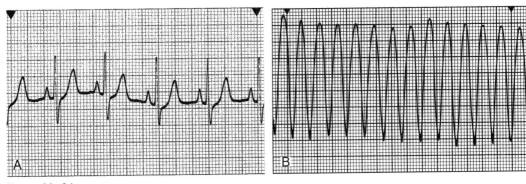

Figure 11-24

(A) Normal sinus rhythm as seen on ECG (EKG) strip. **(B) Ventricular tachycardia** as seen on an ECG strip. Ventricular tachycardia is a cardiac dysrhythmia with a rate range of 100 to 220 beats per minute. (Modified from Wiederhold R: Electrocardiography: The Monitoring and Diagnostic Leads, 2nd ed. Philadelphia, WB Saunders, 1999, pp. 37 and 70.)

Holter monitoring

A compact version (about the size of a portable tape player) of an electrocardiograph (instrument to measure the electricity flowing through the heart) is worn during a 24-hour period to detect cardiac arrhythmias.

percutaneous transluminal coronary angioplasty (PTCA)

In this procedure, also called **balloon angioplasty,** a balloon-tipped catheter is inserted via the femoral (thigh) artery and threaded up the aorta into a coronary artery. The balloon is inflated, compressing fatty deposits or plaque against the side of the artery and opening the artery to allow for the passage of blood. **Balloon valvuloplasty** is used to open narrowed cardiac valves and is seen as a possible alternative to surgery for valvular stenosis.

Stents (expandable slotted tubes) are now used instead of PTCA to create wider lumens and make restenosis less likely. Figure 11–25 shows placement of an intracoronary stent.

stress test

Also known as **exercise tolerance test (ETT),** this procedure determines the heart's response to physical exertion (stress). An ECG and other measurements (blood pressure and heart rate) are taken while the patient is exercising on a treadmill. Changes in the ECG during increasing workload or stress indicate the presence and severity of ischemia.

thrombolytic therapy

Drugs such as **tPA** (tissue-type plasminogen activator) and **streptokinase,** which dissolve clots, are injected into the bloodstream in patients

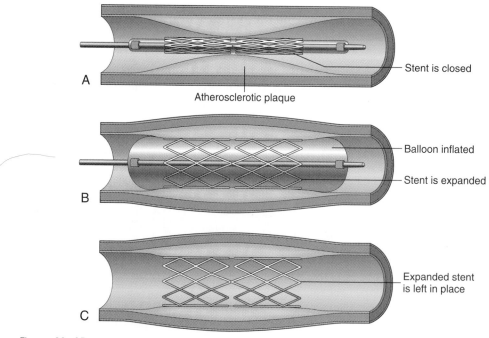

Figure 11-25

Placement of an intracoronary artery stent. (A) The stent is positioned at the site of the lesion. **(B)** The balloon is inflated, expanding the stent. **(C)** The balloon is then deflated and removed, and the implanted stent is left in place. Coronary stents are stainless-steel scaffolding devices that help hold open arteries, such as the coronary, renal, and carotid arteries.

diagnosed as having a coronary thrombosis. This technique, which restores blood flow to the heart and limits irreversible damage to heart muscle, must be undertaken within 12 hours after the onset of a heart attack. Thrombolytic agents reduce mortality in patients with myocardial infarction by 25 per cent.

ABBREVIATIONS

ACE inhibitors	Angiotensin-converting enzyme inhibitors	**HMG**	Hydroxymethyl glutaryl CoA reductase, an enzyme that blocks the synthesis of cholesterol
AF	Atrial fibrillation	**LDH**	Lactate dehydrogenase (enzyme released from dying heart muscle)
AICD	Automatic implantable cardioverter/defibrillator	**LDL**	Low-density lipoproteins
AS	Aortic stenosis	**LV**	Left ventricle
ASD	Atrial septal defect	**LVAD**	Left ventricular assist device
AV, A-V	Atrioventricular	**LVH**	Left ventricular hypertrophy
BBB	Bundle branch block	**MI**	Myocardial infarction
BP	Blood pressure	**MR**	Mitral regurgitation
CABG	Coronary artery bypass graft	**MUGA**	Multiple-gated acquisition scan; a radioactive test of heart function
CAD	Coronary artery disease	**MVP**	Mitral valve prolapse
CCU	Coronary care unit	**PAC**	Premature atrial contraction
Cath	Catheterization	**PDA**	Patent ductus arteriosus
CHF	Congestive heart failure	**PTCA**	Percutaneous transluminal coronary angioplasty
CoA	Coarctation of the aorta		
CPK	Creatine phosphokinase; released into the bloodstream following injury to heart or skeletal muscles	**PVC**	Premature ventricular contraction
		RFA	Radiofrequency catheter ablation
CVP	Central venous pressure (measured with a catheter in the superior vena cava)	**SA, S-A**	Sinoatrial
DSA	Digital subtraction angiography	**TEE**	Transesophageal echocardiography
DVT	Deep venous thrombosis	**TMLR**	Transmyocardial laser revascularization
ECC	Extracorporeal circulation	**tPA**	Tissue-type plasminogen activator; a drug used to prevent thrombosis
ECG, EKG	Electrocardiogram	**VFib**	Ventricular fibrillation
ECHO	Echocardiography	**VSD**	Ventricular septal defect
ETT	Exercise tolerance test	**VT**	Ventricular tachycardia
HDL	High-density lipoproteins; high blood levels are associated with lower incidence of coronary artery disease	**WPW**	Wolff-Parkinson-White syndrome; an abnormal ECG pattern often associated with paroxysmal tachycardia

X. Practical Applications

Operating Schedule: General Hospital

Match the operation in column I with a diagnosis in column II. Answers are found at the end of Answers to Exercises, page (417).

Column I—Operation

1. Coronary artery bypass _____ 6
2. Left carotid endarterectomy _____ C
3. Varicose vein bilateral ligation and stripping _____ H
4. LV aneurysmectomy _____ I
5. Atrial septal defect repair _____ D
6. Pulmonary balloon valvuloplasty _____ A
7. Pericardiocentesis _____ B
8. Aortic valve replacement _____ J
9. Pacemaker implantation _____ G
10. Femoral-popliteal bypass graft _____ F

Column II—Diagnosis

A. stenosis of the pulmonary valve
B. cardiac tamponade (fluid in the space surrounding the heart)
C. atherosclerotic occlusion of a main artery leading to the head
D. congenital hole in the wall of the upper chamber of the heart
E. disabling angina pectoris and extensive coronary atherosclerosis despite medical therapy
F. peripheral vascular disease
G. heart block
H. swollen, twisted blood vessels in the leg
I. protrusion of the wall of a lower heart chamber
J. aortic stenosis

Medical Language As Written

1. The main determinants of death after acute myocardial infarction are the extent of left ventricular damage and occurrence of arrhythmias.

2. Evaluation of risk factors for sudden cardiac death is important in patients with coronary artery disease. Risk factors include a family history of sudden cardiac death and early myocardial infarction (before age 50 years), hypertension and left ventricular hypertrophy, smoking, diabetes mellitus, and markedly elevated serum cholesterol levels.

3. A 24-year-old woman with a history of palpitations [heartbeat is unusually strong, rapid, or irregular, so that patient is aware of it] and vague chest pains enters the hospital. With the patient supine, you hear a midsystolic click that

is followed by a grade 3/6 [moderately loud—6/6 is loud and 1/6 is quiet] honking murmur. Your diagnosis: mitral valve prolapse (click-murmur syndrome).

4. A 47-year-old man had a myocardial infarction in November 1984. On March 3, 1985, he was readmitted to the hospital with an acute inferior myocardial infarction, documented by electrocardiograms and blood enzyme elevations. On April 8, the patient developed a loud systolic murmur and his blood pressure fell sharply. A diagnosis of rupture of the ventricular septum was made, and he was transferred to the surgical service. Right cardiac catheterization confirmed the presence of a left-to-right shunt [of blood] at the ventricular level. Emergency surgery was attempted, but the patient died suddenly. Autopsy diagnosis: ruptured ventricular septum secondary to myocardial infarction.

XI. Exercises

Remember to check your answers carefully with those given in Section XII, Answers to Exercises.

A. Match the following terms with their meanings below.

arteriole	venule	tricuspid valve
aorta	atrium	pulmonary artery
mitral valve	superior vena cava	pulmonary vein
capillary	inferior vena cava	ventricle

1. valve that lies between the right atrium and the right ventricle _tricusp. valve_

2. smallest blood vessel _Capillary_

3. carries oxygenated blood from the lungs to the heart _Pulmonary Vein_

4. largest artery in the body _aorta_

5. brings oxygen-poor blood into the heart from the upper parts of the body _Sup vena Cava_

6. upper chamber of the heart _atrium_

7. carries oxygen-poor blood to the lungs from the heart _Pulmonary artery_

8. small artery _arteriole_

9. valve that lies between the left atrium and the left ventricle _Mitral valve_

10. brings blood from the lower half of the body to the heart _inferior vena cava_

11. a small vein _venule_

12. lower chamber of the heart _ventricle_

B. Trace the path of blood through the heart. Begin as the blood enters the right atrium from the venae cavae (and include the valves within the heart).

1. _____   7. _____

2. _____   8. _____

3. _____   9. _____

4. _____   10. _____

5. _____   11. _____

6. capillaries of the lung   12. aorta

C. Complete the following sentences.

1. The pacemaker of the heart is the _sino atrial node_ .

2. The sac-like membrane surrounding the heart is the _pericardium_ .

3. The wall of the heart between the right and the left atria is the _interatrial septa_ .

4. The relaxation phase of the heartbeat is called _diastole_ .

5. Specialized conductive tissue in the wall between the ventricles is the _atrioventricular bundle_ _bundle of His_ .

6. The inner lining of the heart is the _endocardium_ .

7. The contractive phase of the heartbeat is called _systole_ .

8. A gas released as a metabolic product of catabolism is _CO₂_ .

9. Specialized conductive tissue at the base of the wall between the two upper heart chambers is the _atrioventricular node_ .

10. The inner lining of the pericardium, adhering to the outside of the heart, is the _visceral pericardium_ .

11. An abnormal heart sound caused by improper closure of heart valves is a _murmur_ .

12. The beat of the heart as felt through the walls of arteries is called the _auscultation pulse_ .

D. *Complete the following terms from their definitions.*

1. hardening of arteries: arterio _____

2. disease condition of heart muscle: cardio _____

3. enlargement of the heart: cardio *megly* _____

4. inflammation of a vein: phleb _____

5. condition of rapid heartbeat: _____ *tachy* _____ cardia

6. condition of slow heartbeat: _____ *brady* _____ cardia

7. high levels of cholesterol in the blood: hyper *cholesterol* _____

8. surgical repair of a valve: valvulo _____

9. condition of deficient oxygen: hyp *oxia* _____

10. pertaining to an upper heart chamber: _____ *atri* _ al

11. narrowing of the mitral valve: mitral *stenosis* _____

12. breakdown of a clot: thrombo *lysis* _____

E. *Give the meanings for the following terms.*

1. cyanosis _____

2. phlebotomy _____

3. arterial anastomosis _____

4. aneurysmorrhaphy _____

5. atheroma _____

6. arrhythmia _____

7. sphygmomanometer _____

8. stethoscope _____

9. mitral valvulitis _____

10. atherosclerosis _____

11. vasoconstriction _____

12. vasodilation _____

F. Match the following pathological conditions of the heart with their meanings below.

fibrillation   tetralogy of Fallot   endocarditis
hypertensive heart disease   atrial septal defect   pericarditis
coarctation of the aorta   congestive heart failure   mitral valve prolapse
patent ductus arteriosus   coronary artery disease   flutter

1. inflammation of the inner lining of the heart _____

2. rapid but regular atrial or ventricular contractions _____

3. small hole between the upper heart chambers; congenital anomaly _____

4. improper closure of the valve between the left atrium and ventricle during systole

_____

5. blockage of the arteries surrounding the heart leading to ischemia _____

6. high blood pressure affecting the heart _____

7. rapid, random, ineffectual, and irregular contractions of the heart _____

8. inflammation of the sac surrounding the heart _____

9. inability of the heart to pump its required amount of blood _____

10. congenital malformation involving four separate heart defects _____

11. congenital narrowing of the large artery leading from the heart _____

12. a small duct between the aorta and the pulmonary artery, which normally closes soon after birth,

remains open _____

G. Give the meanings for the following terms.

1. heart block _____

2. cardiac arrest _____

3. palpitations _____

4. artificial cardiac pacemaker _____

5. thrombotic occlusion _____

6. angina pectoris _____

7. myocardial infarction _____

8. necrosis _____

9. infarction _____

10. ischemia _____

11. nitroglycerin _____

12. digoxin _____

13. bruit _____

14. thrill _____

H. Match the following terms with their descriptions.

rheumatic heart disease	vegetations	emboli
Raynaud phenomenon	essential hypertension	secondary hypertension
petechiae	auscultation	peripheral vascular disease
aneurysm	claudication	murmur

1. lesions that form on heart valves after damage by infection _____

2. clots that travel to and suddenly block a blood vessel _____

3. small, pinpoint hemorrhages _____

4. an extra heart sound, heard between normal beats and caused by a valvular defect or condition

   that disrupts the smooth flow of blood through the heart _____

5. listening with a stethoscope _____

6. heart disease caused by rheumatic fever _____

7. high blood pressure in arteries when the etiology is idiopathic _____

8. high blood pressure related to kidney disease _____

9. short episodes of pallor and numbness in fingers and toes due to a temporary constriction of

   arterioles in the skin _____

10. local widening of an artery _____

11. pain, tension, and weakness in a limb after walking has begun _____

12. blockage of arteries in the lower extremities; etiology is atherosclerosis

_____

I. Give short answers for the following.

1. Name three types of drugs used to treat angina _____

_____ .

2. When damaged valves in veins fail to prevent the backflow of blood, the condition that results is

called _____ .

3. If veins are swollen and twisted in the rectal region, the condition is known as _____ .

4. Name the four defects in tetralogy of Fallot from their descriptions:

A. Narrowing of the artery leading to the lungs from the heart _____ .

B. Gap in the wall between the ventricles _____ .

C. The large vessel leading from the left ventricle moves over the interventricular septum

_____ .

D. Excessive development of the wall of the right lower heart chamber

_____ .

J. Select from the following terms to complete the definitions below.

lipid test	angiography	cardiac MRI
lipoprotein electrophoresis	echocardiography	cardioversion
serum enzyme test	cardiac scan	coronary bypass surgery
electrocardiography	endarterectomy	stress test

1. surgical removal of the innermost lining of an artery when it is thickened with fatty deposits

_____

2. very brief discharges of electricity are applied across the chest to stop a cardiac arrhythmia;

defibrillation _____

3. measurement of levels of fatty substances (cholesterol and triglycerides) in the bloodstream

_____

4. measurement of the heart's response to physical exertion (patient is monitored while jogging on a

treadmill) _____

5. blood measurement of creatine phosphokinase (CPK) and lactate dehydrogenase (LDH) after myocardial infarction _____

6. contrast material is injected into vessels and x-ray films are produced _____

7. process of recording the electricity in the heart _____

8. a radioactive substance is injected intravenously, and its accumulation in heart muscle is measured with a special detection device _____

9. pulses of high-frequency sound waves are transmitted into the chest, and echoes are electronically recorded to show the structure and movement of the heart _____

10. process of physically separating HLD, VLDL, and LDL from a blood sample

    _____

11. vessel grafts are anastomosed to existing coronary arteries to keep the myocardium supplied with oxygenated blood _____

12. magnetic waves are beamed at the heart, and an image is produced to show the structure of the heart _____

K. Give the meanings for the following terms.

1. digital subtraction angiography _____

2. heart transplantation _____

3. balloon angioplasty _____

4. Doppler ultrasound _____

5. Holter monitoring _____

6. thrombolytic therapy _____

7. extracorporeal circulation _____

8. cardiac catheterization _____

L. Identify the following cardiac dysrhythmias from their abbreviations.

1. AF _____

2. VT _____

3. VFib _____

4. PVC _____

5. PAC _____

M. Identify the following abnormal cardiac conditions from their abbreviations.

1. CHF _____

2. VSD _____

3. MI _____

4. PDA _____

5. MVP _____

6. AS _____

7. CAD _____

8. ASD _____

N. Match the following abbreviations for cardiac procedures with their explanations below.

ECHO	TEE	LVAD
MUGA	RFA	TMLR
AICD	ETT	

1. A laser makes a hole in heart muscle to induce growth of new blood vessels (angiogenesis).

_____

2. A booster pump implanted in the abdomen with a cannula leading to the heart is a "bridge to transplant." _____

3. Ultrasound images of the heart are taken through the esophagus. _____

4. A new device to sense arrhythmias and give shocks that correct them can be implanted in the

chest. _____

5. A catheter, placed in blood vessels leading up against the heart muscle, delivers a high-frequency
current to burn a small portion of the heart muscle, which reverses an abnormal heart rhythm.

_____

6. This procedure determines the heart's response to physical exertion (stress).

_____

7. High-frequency sound waves are pulsed through the chest wall and bounce off heart structures,

creating an image of heart structure. _____

8. This is a radioactive test of heart function. _____

O. Spell the term correctly from its definition.

1. pertaining to the heart: _____ ary

2. not a normal heart rhythm: arr _____

3. abnormal condition of blueness: _____ osis

4. relaxation phase of the heartbeat: _____ tole

5. chest pain: _____ pectoris

6. inflammation of a vein: _____ itis

7. widening of a vessel: vaso _____

8. enlargement of the heart: cardio _____

9. hardening of arteries with fatty plaque: _____ sclerosis

10. swollen veins in the rectal region: _____ oids

P. Match the following surgical terms with their meanings below.

CABG
embolectomy
endarterectomy

atherectomy
valvotomy
pericardiocentesis

PTCA
aneurysmorrhaphy

1. incision of a heart valve _____

2. removal of a clot that has traveled into a blood vessel and suddenly caused occlusion

_____

3. coronary bypass surgery (to relieve ischemia) _____

4. surgical puncture to remove fluid from the pericardial space _____

5. percutaneous transluminal coronary angioplasty _____

6. removal of the inner lining of an artery to make it wider _____

7. suture (repair) of a ballooned-out portion of an artery _____

8. removal of plaque from an artery _____

Q. Select the term that best completes each sentence.

1. Simon was having pain in his chest that radiated up his neck and down his arm. He called Dr. Dan, who thought Simon should report to the emergency department immediately. The first test they performed was a(an) **(stress test, ECG, balloon angioplasty).**

2. Dr. Kelly explained to the family that their observation about the bluish color of baby Charles' skin helped him make the diagnosis of a(an) **(thrombotic, aneurysmal, septal)** defect in the baby's heart, which needed immediate attention.

3. Mr. Duggan had a fever of unknown origin. When the doctors completed an echocardiogram and saw vegetations on his mitral valve, they suspected **(bacterial endocarditis, hypertensive heart disease, angina pectoris).**

4. Claudia's hands turned red, almost purple, whenever she went out into the cold or became stressed. Her physician thought it might be wise to evaluate her for **(varicose veins, Raynaud phenomenon, intermittent claudication).**

5. Daisy's heart felt like it was skipping beats every time she drank coffee. Her physician suggested that she wear a **(Holter monitor, PTCA, CABG)** for 24 hours to assess the nature of the arrhythmia.

XII. Answers to Exercises

A

1. tricuspid valve
2. capillary
3. pulmonary vein
4. aorta
5. superior vena cava
6. atrium
7. pulmonary artery
8. arteriole
9. mitral valve
10. inferior vena cava
11. venule
12. ventricle

B

1. right atrium
2. tricuspid valve
3. right ventricle
4. pulmonary valve
5. pulmonary artery
6. capillaries of the lung
7. pulmonary veins
8. left atrium
9. mitral valve
10. left ventricle
11. aortic valve
12. aorta

C

1. sinoatrial (SA) node
2. pericardium
3. interatrial septum
4. diastole
5. atrioventricular bundle or bundle of His
6. endocardium
7. systole
8. carbon dioxide (CO_2)
9. atrioventricular (AV) node
10. visceral pericardium (the outer lining is the parietal pericardium)
11. murmur
12. pulse

D

1. arteriosclerosis
2. cardiomyopathy
3. cardiomegaly
4. phlebitis
5. tachycardia
6. bradycardia
7. hypercholesterolemia
8. valvuloplasty
9. hypoxia
10. atrial
11. mitral stenosis
12. thrombolysis

E

1. bluish discoloration of the skin owing to deficient oxygen in the blood
2. incision of a vein
3. new connection between arteries
4. suturing (repair) of an aneurysm
5. mass of yellowish plaque (fatty substance)
6. abnormal heart rhythm
7. instrument to measure blood pressure
8. instrument to listen to sounds within the chest
9. inflammation of the mitral valve
10. hardening of arteries with a yellowish, fatty substance (plaque)
11. narrowing of a vessel
12. widening of a vessel

F

1. endocarditis
2. flutter
3. atrial septal defect
4. mitral valve prolapse
5. coronary artery disease
6. hypertensive heart disease
7. fibrillation
8. pericarditis
9. congestive heart failure
10. tetralogy of Fallot
11. coarctation of the aorta
12. patent ductus arteriosus

G

1. failure of proper conduction of impulses through the AV node to the atrioventricular bundle (bundle of His)
2. sudden stoppage of heart movement
3. uncomfortable sensations in the chest associated with arrhythmias
4. battery-operated device that is placed in the chest and wired to send electrical current to the heart to establish a normal rhythm
5. blockage of a vessel by a clot
6. chest pain resulting from insufficient oxygen being supplied to the heart muscle
7. area of necrosis (dead tissue) in the heart muscle; heart attack
8. abnormal condition of death (dead tissue)
9. tissue that dies because of deprivation of oxygen
10. blood is held back from an area of the body
11. a nitrate drug used in the treatment of angina pectoris
12. a drug that increases the strength and regularity of the heartbeat
13. abnormal sound (murmur) heard on auscultation
14. vibration felt on palpation of the chest

H

1. vegetations
2. emboli
3. petechiae
4. murmur
5. auscultation
6. rheumatic heart disease
7. essential hypertension
8. secondary hypertension
9. Raynaud phenomenon
10. aneurysm
11. claudication
12. peripheral vascular disease

Continued on following page

I

1. nitrates, beta-blockers, calcium channel blockers
2. varicose veins
3. hemorrhoids

4. A pulmonary artery stenosis
   B ventricular septal defect
   C shift of the aorta to the right
   D hypertrophy of the right ventricle

J

1. endarterectomy
2. cardioversion
3. lipid test
4. stress test

5. serum enzyme test (-ase means enzyme)
6. angiography (arteriography)
7. electrocardiogram
8. cardiac scan

9. echocardiography
10. lipoprotein electrophoresis
11. coronary bypass surgery
12. cardiac MRI

K

1. Video equipment and a computer produce x-ray pictures of blood vessels by taking two pictures (without and with contrast) and subtracting the first image (without contrast) from the second.
2. A donor heart is transferred to a recipient.
3. A catheter is threaded into a coronary artery, and a balloon is inflated that compresses the fatty deposits and opens the artery so that more blood can pass

through (also called percutaneous transluminal coronary angioplasty).
4. An instrument that focuses sound waves on a blood vessel to measure blood flow.
5. A compact version of an electrocardiograph is worn during a 24-hour period to detect cardiac arrhythmias.
6. Treatment with drugs (streptokinase and tPA) to dissolve clots after a heart attack.

7. A heart-lung machine is used to divert blood from the heart and lungs during surgery. The machine oxygenates the blood and sends it back into the bloodstream.
8. A catheter (tube) is inserted into an artery or vein and threaded into the heart chambers. Dye can be injected to take x-ray pictures, patterns of blood flow can be detected, and blood pressures can be measured.

L

1. atrial fibrillation
2. ventricular tachycardia
3. ventricular fibrillation

4. premature ventricular contraction
5. premature atrial contraction

M

1. congestive heart failure
2. ventricular septal defect
3. myocardial infarction

4. patent ductus arteriosus
5. mitral valve prolapse
6. aortic stenosis

7. coronary artery disease
8. atrial septal defect

N

1. TMLR; transmyocardial laser revascularization
2. LVAD; left ventricular assist device
3. TEE; transesophageal echocardiography

4. AICD; automatic implantable cardioverter/defibrillator
5. RFA; radiofrequency catheter ablation
6. ETT; exercise tolerance test

7. ECHO; echocardiography
8. MUGA; multiple-gated acquisition scan

O

1. coronary
2. arrhythmia
3. cyanosis
4. diastole

5. angina pectoris
6. phlebitis
7. vasodilation
8. cardiomegaly

9. atherosclerosis
10. hemorrhoids

P

1. valvotomy
2. embolectomy
3. CABG

4. pericardiocentesis
5. PTCA
6. endarterectomy

7. aneurysmorrhaphy
8. atherectomy

Q

1. ECG
2. septal
3. bacterial endocarditis

4. Raynaud phenomenon
5. Holter monitor

Answers to Practical Applications

1. E	5. D	8. J
2. C	6. A	9. G
3. H	7. B	10. F
4. I		

XIII. Pronunciation of Terms

Pronunciation Guide

ā as in āpe   ă as in ăpple
ē as in ēven   ĕ as in ĕvery
ī as in īce   ĭ as in ĭnterest
ō as in ōpen   ŏ as in pŏt
ū as in ūnit   ŭ as in ŭnder

To test your understanding of the terminology in this chapter, write the meaning of each term in the space provided. In addition, you may wish to cover the terms and write them by looking at your definitions. Make sure your spelling is correct. The page number after each term indicates where it is defined or used in the text so you can easily check your responses.

Vocabulary and Terminology

Term	Pronunciation	Meaning
angiogram (382)	ĂN-jē-ō-grăm	
angioplasty (382)	ĂN-jē-ō-plăs-tē	
aorta (380)	ā-ŎR-tă	
aortic stenosis (382)	ā-ŎR-tĭk stĕ-NŌ-sĭs	
arrhythmia (386)	ā-RĬTH-mē-ă	
arterial anastomosis (383)	ăr-TĒ-rē-ăl ă-năs-tō-MŌ-sĭs	
arteriography (383)	ăr-tē-rē-ŎG-ră-fē	
arteriole (380)	ăr-TĒ-rē-ōl	
arteriosclerosis (383)	ăr-tē-rē-ō-sklĕ-RŌ-sĭs	
artery (380)	ĂR-tĕ-rē	
atherectomy (383)	ă-thĕ-RĔK-tō-mē	
atheroma (383)	ăth-ĕr-Ō-mă	
atherosclerosis (383)	ăth-ĕr-ō-sklĕ-RŌ-sĭs	
atrial (384)	Ā-trē-ăl	

atrioventricular bundle (380)	ā-trē-ō-věn-TRĬK-ū-lăr BŬN-dl	_____
atrioventricular node (380)	ā-trē-ō-věn-TRĬK-ū-lăr nōd	_____
atrium (plural: atrial) (380)	Ā-trē-ŭm (Ā-trē-ă)	_____
brachial artery (384)	BRĀ-kē-ăl ĀR-tě-rē	_____
bradycardia (384)	brād-ē-KĂR-dē-ă	_____
bundle of His (380)	BŬN-dl of Hĭs	_____
capillary (380)	KĂP-ĭ-lăr-ē	_____
carbon dioxide (380)	kăr-bŏn dī-ŎK-sīd	_____
cardiomegaly (384)	kăr-dē-ō-MĔG-ă-lē	_____
cardiomyopathy (384)	kăr-dē-ō-mī-ŎP-ă-thē	_____
coronary arteries (380)	KŎR-ō-năr-ē ĂR-tě-rēz	_____
cyanosis (384)	sī-ă-NŌ-sĭs	_____
deoxygenated blood (381)	dē-ŎK-sĭ-jě-NĀ-těd blŭd	_____
diastole (381)	dī-ĂS-tō-lē	_____
endocardium (381)	ěn-dō-KĂR-dē-ŭm	_____
endothelium (381)	ěn-dō-THĒ-lē-um	_____
hypercholesterolemia (384)	hī-pěr-kō-lěs-těr-ŏl-Ē-mē-ă	_____
hypoxia (384)	hī-PŎK-sē-ă	_____
interventricular septum (385)	ĭn-těr-věn-TRĬK-ū-lăr SĔP-tŭm	_____
mitral valve (381)	MĪ-trăl vălv	_____
mitral valvulitis (385)	MĪ-trăl văl-vū-LĪ-tĭs	_____
myocardium (381)	mī-ō-KĂR-dē-ŭm	_____
myxoma (384)	mĭk-SŌ-mă	_____
oxygen (381)	ŎK-sĭ-jěn	_____
pacemaker (381)	PĀS-mā-kěr	_____
pericardiocentesis (384)	pěr-ĭ-kăr-dē-ō-sěn-TĒ-sĭs	_____
pericardium (381)	pěr-ĭ-KĂR-dē-ŭm	_____

phlebitis (384)   flē-BĪ-tĭs   _____

phlebotomy (384)   flĕ-BŎT-ō-mē   _____

pulmonary artery (381)   PŬL-mō-nĕr-ē ĂR-tĕr-ē   _____

pulmonary circulation (381)   PŬL-mō-nĕr-ē sĕr-kŭ-LĀ-shŭn   _____

pulmonary valve (382)   PŬL-mō-nĕr-ē vălv   _____

pulmonary vein (382)   PŬL-mō-nĕr-ē vān   _____

septum (plural: septa) (382)   SĔP-tŭm (SĔP-tă)   _____

sinoatrial node (382)   sī-nō-Ā-trē-ăl nōd   _____

sphygmomanometer (382)   sfĭg-mō-mă-NŌM-ĕ-tĕr   _____

stethoscope (385)   STĔTH-ō-skōp   _____

systemic circulation (382)   sĭs-TĔM-ĭk sĕr-kū-LĀ-shŭn   _____

systole (382)   SĬS-tō-lē   _____

tachycardia (384)   tăk-ē-KĂR-dē-ă   _____

thrombolysis (385)   thrŏm-BŎL-ĭ-sĭs   _____

tricuspid valve (382)   trī-KŬS-pĭd vălv   _____

valvotomy (385)   văl-VŎT-ō-mē   _____

valvuloplasty (385)   văl-vū-lō-PLĂS-tē   _____

vascular (385)   VĂS-kū-lăr   _____

vasoconstriction (385)   văz-ō-kŏn-STRĬK-shŭn   _____

vasodilation (385)   văz-ō-dī-LĀ-shŭn   _____

vein (382)   vān   _____

vena cava (plural: venae cavae) (382)   VĒ-nă KĀ-vă (VĒ-nē KĀ-vē)   _____

venous (385)   VĒ-nŭs   _____

ventricle (382)   VĔN-trĭ-k'l   _____

ventriculotomy (385)   vĕn-trĭk-ū-LŎT-ō-mē   _____

venule (382)   VĔN-ū'l   _____

Pathology, Laboratory Tests, and Clinical Procedures

Term	Pronunciation	Meaning
ACE inhibitors (397)	ĀCE ĭn-HĬB-ĭ-tŏrz	
aneurysm (394)	ĂN-ū-rĭzm	
angina pectoris (397)	ăn-JĪ-nă PĔK-tŏr-ĭs or ĂN-jĭ-nă PĔK-tŏr-ĭs	
angiography (398)	ăn-jē-ŎG-ră-fē	
atrioventricular block (386)	ā-trē-ō-vĕn-TRĬK-ū-lăr blŏk	
auscultation (397)	ăw-skŭl-TĀ-shŭn	
beta-blocker (397)	BĀ-tă-BLŎK-ĕr	
bruit (397)	BRŪ-ē	
calcium channel blocker (397)	KĂL-sē-ŭm CHĂ-nĕl BLŎK-ĕr	
cardiac arrest (387)	KĂR-dē-ăk ā-RĔST	
cardiac catheterization (400)	KĂR-dē-ăk kăth-ĕ-tĕr-ĭ-ZĀ-shŭn	
cardioversion (400)	kăr-dē-ō-VĔR-zhŭn	
claudication (397)	klăw-dĕ-KĀ-shŭn	
coarctation of the aorta (388)	kō-ărk-TĀ-shŭn of the ā-ŎR-tă	
congenital heart disease (388)	kŏn-GĔN-ĭ-tăl hărt dĭ-ZĒZ	
congestive heart failure (390)	kŏn-GĔS-tĭv hărt FĀL-ŭr	
coronary artery disease (390)	kŏr-ō-NĂR-ē ĂR-tĕ-rē dĭ-ZĒZ	
coronary bypass surgery (400)	kŏr-ō-NĂR-ē BĪ-păs SŬR-jĕr-ē	
digoxin (397)	dĭg-ŎK-sĭn	
digital subtraction angiography (398)	DĬJ-ĭ-tăl sŭb-TRĂK-shŭn ăn-jē-ŎG-ră-fē	
Doppler ultrasound (399)	DŎP-lĕr ŬL-tră-sŏnd	

echocardiography (399)	ĕk-ō-kăr-dē-ŌG-ră-fē	_____
electrocardiography (400)	ē-lĕk-trō-kăr-dē-ŌG-ră-fē	_____
embolus (plural: emboli) (397)	ĔM-bō-lŭs (ĔM-bō-lī)	_____
endarterectomy (400)	ĕnd-ăr-tĕr-ĔK-tō-mē	_____
endocarditis (392)	ĕn-dō-kăr-DĪ-tĭs	_____
extracorporeal circulation (400)	ĕks-tră-kŏr-PŎR-ē-ăl sĕr-kū-LĀ-shŭn	_____
fibrillation (387)	fĭb-rĭ-LĀ-shŭn	_____
flutter (387)	FLŬ-tĕr	_____
hemorrhoids (396)	HĔM-ō-roydz	_____
Holter monitoring (402)	HŎL-tĕr MŎN-ĭ-tĕ-rĭng	_____
hypertension (395)	hī-pĕr-TĔN-shŭn	_____
infarction (397)	ĭn-FĂRK-shŭn	_____
ischemia (390)	ĭs-KĒ-mē-ă	_____
lipid tests (398)	LĬ-pĭd tĕsts	_____
lipoprotein electrophoresis (398)	lī-pō-PRŌ-tēn ē-lĕk-trō-fŏr-Ē-sĭs	_____
mitral stenosis (394)	MĪ-trăl stĕ-NŌ-sĭs	_____
mitral valve prolapse (392)	MĪ-trăl vălv PRŌ-laps	_____
murmur (393)	MŬR-mĕr	_____
myocardial infarction (390)	mī-ō-KĂR-dē-ăl ĭn-FĂRK-shŭn	_____
nitroglycerin (397)	nī-trō-GLĬS-ĕr-ĭn	_____
peripheral vascular disease (395)	pĕ-RĬ-fĕr-ăl VĂS-kū-lăr dĭ-ZĒZ	_____
palpitations (397)	păl-pĭ-TĀ-shŭnz	_____
patent ductus arteriosus (388)	PĀ-tĕnt DŬK-tŭs ăr-tĕr-ē-Ō-sŭs	_____

percutaneous transluminal coronary angioplasty (402)	pĕr-kū-TĀ-nē-ŭs trăns-LŪ-mĭ-năl KŎR-ō-năr-ē ĂN-jē-ō-plăs-tē	_____
pericarditis (393)	pĕr-ĭ-kăr-DĪ-tĭs	_____
petechiae (397)	pĕ-TĒ-kē-ē	_____
positron emission tomography (399)	pŏs-ĭ-tron ē-MĬSH-un tō-MŎG-ră-fē	_____
Raynaud phenomenon (395)	rā-NŌ fĕ-NŎM-ĕ-nŏn	_____
rheumatic heart disease (394)	roo-MĂT-ik hărt dĭ-ZĒZ	_____
septal defects (388)	SĔP-tăl DĒ-fĕkts	_____
serum enzyme tests (398)	SĔ-rum ĔN-zīm tĕsts	_____
stress test (402)	STRĔS tĕst	_____
tetralogy of Fallot (388)	tĕ-TRĂL-ō-jē of fă-LŌ	_____
technetium 99m ventriculography (399)	tĕk-NĒ-shē-ŭm 99m vĕn-trĭk-ū-LŎG-ră-fē	_____
thallium 201 scintigraphy (399)	THĂL-ē-um 201 sĭn-TĬG-ră-fē	_____
thrill (397)	thrĭl	_____
thrombolytic therapy (402)	thrŏm-bō-LĬ-tĭk THĔ-ră-pē	_____
thrombotic occlusion (390)	thrŏm-BŎT-ĭk ō-KLŪ-zhŭn	_____
varicose veins (396)	VĂR-ĭ-kōs vānz	_____
vegetations (397)	vĕj-ĕ-TĀ-shŭnz	_____

XIV. Review Sheet

Write the meanings of each word part in the space provided. Check your answers with the information in the chapter or in the Glossary (Medical Terms—English) at the end of the book.

COMBINING FORMS

Combining Form	Meaning	Combining Form	Meaning
aneurysm/o	_____	myx/o	_____
angi/o	_____	ox/o	_____
aort/o	_____	pericardi/o	_____
arter/o, arteri/o	_____	phleb/o	_____
ather/o	_____	pulmon/o	_____
atri/o	_____	sphygm/o	_____
axill/o	_____	steth/o	_____
brachi/o	_____	thromb/o	_____
cardi/o	_____	valv/o	_____
cholesterol/o	_____	valvul/o	_____
coron/o	_____	vas/o	_____
cyan/o	_____	vascul/o	_____
isch/o	_____	ven/o	_____
my/o	_____	ventricul/o	_____

Continued on following page

SUFFIXES

Suffix	Meaning	Suffix	Meaning
-constriction	_____	-oma	_____
-dilation	_____	-osis	_____
-emia	_____	-plasty	_____
-graphy	_____	-sclerosis	_____
-lysis	_____	-stenosis	_____
-megaly	_____	-tomy	_____
-meter	_____		

PREFIXES

Prefix	Meaning	Prefix	Meaning
a-, an-	_____	hypo-	_____
brady-	_____	inter-	_____
de-	_____	peri-	_____
dys-	_____	tachy-	_____
endo-	_____	tetra-	_____
hyper-	_____	tri-	_____

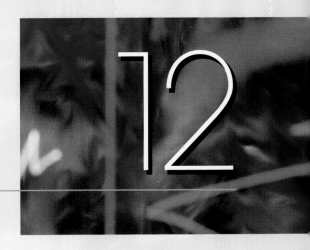

CHAPTER 12

Respiratory System

This chapter is divided into the following sections

In this chapter you will

- Name the organs of the respiratory system and describe their location and function;
- Identify various pathological conditions that affect the system;
- Recognize medical terms that pertain to respiration;
- Identify clinical procedures and abbreviations related to the system; and
- Apply your new knowledge to understanding medical terms in their proper contexts, such as medical reports and records.

I. Introduction

We usually think of **respiration** as the mechanical process of breathing, that is, the repetitive and, for the most part, unconscious exchange of air between the lungs and the external environment. This exchange of air at the lungs is also called **external respiration.** In external respiration, oxygen is inhaled (inhaled air contains about 21 per cent oxygen) into the air spaces (sacs) of the lungs and immediately passes into tiny capillary blood vessels surrounding the air spaces. Simultaneously, carbon dioxide, a gas produced when oxygen and food combine in cells, passes from the capillary blood vessels into the air spaces of the lungs to be exhaled (exhaled air contains about 16 per cent oxygen).

While external respiration occurs between the outside environment and the capillary bloodstream of the lungs, another form of respiration is occurring simultaneously between the individual body cells and the tiny capillary blood vessels that surround them. This process is called **internal (cellular) respiration.** Internal respiration is the exchange of gases not at the lungs but at the cells within all the organs of the body. In this process, oxygen passes out of the bloodstream and into the tissue cells. At the same time, carbon dioxide passes from the tissue cells into the bloodstream and is carried by the blood back to the lungs to be exhaled.

II. Anatomy and Physiology of Respiration

Label Figure 12–1 as you read the following paragraphs.

Air enters the body through the **nose** [1] and passes through the **nasal cavity** [2], which is lined with a mucous membrane and fine hairs **(cilia)** to help filter out foreign bodies, as well as to warm and moisten the air. **Paranasal sinuses** [3] are hollow, air-containing spaces within the skull that communicate with the nasal cavity. They, too, have a mucous membrane lining and function to provide the lubricating fluid mucus, as well as to lighten the bones of the skull and help produce sound.

After passing through the nasal cavity, the air next reaches the **pharynx (throat).** There are three divisions of the pharynx. The **nasopharynx** [4] is the first division, and it is nearest to the nasal cavities. It contains the **pharyngeal tonsils,** or **adenoids** [5], which are collections of lymphatic tissue. They are more prominent in children, and if enlarged, can obstruct air passageways. Below the nasopharynx and closer to the mouth is the second division of the pharynx, the **oropharynx** [6]. The **palatine tonsils** [7], two rounded masses of lymphatic tissue, are located in the oropharynx. The third division of the pharynx is the **laryngopharynx** [8]. It is in this region that the pharynx, serving as a common passageway for food from the mouth and air from the nose, divides into two branches, the **larynx (voice box)** [9] and the **esophagus** [10].

The esophagus leads into the stomach and carries food to be digested. The larynx contains the vocal cords and is surrounded by pieces of cartilage for support. The thyroid cartilage is the largest and is commonly referred to as the Adam's apple. Sounds are produced as air is expelled past the vocal cords, and the cords vibrate. The tension of the vocal cords determines the high or low pitch of the voice.

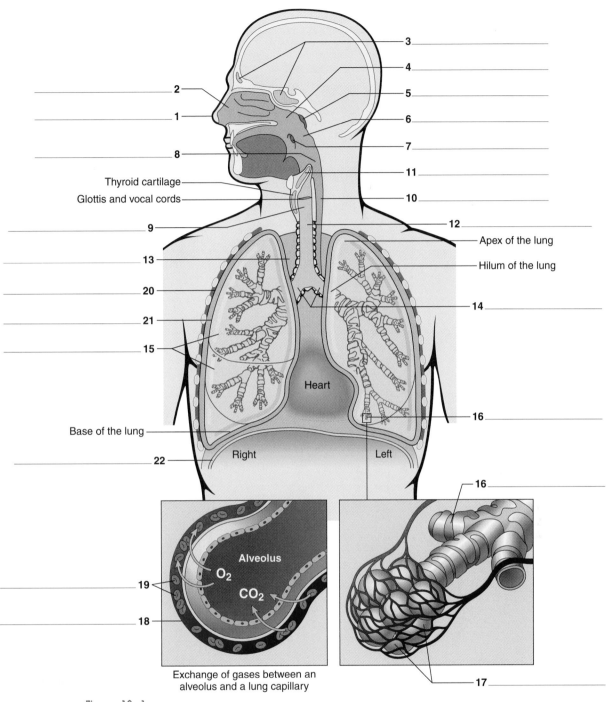

Thyroid cartilage

Glottis and vocal cords

Apex of the lung

Hilum of the lung

Heart

Base of the lung

Right

Left

Alveolus

O$_2$

CO$_2$

Exchange of gases between an
alveolus and a lung capillary

Figure 12-1

Organs of the respiratory system.

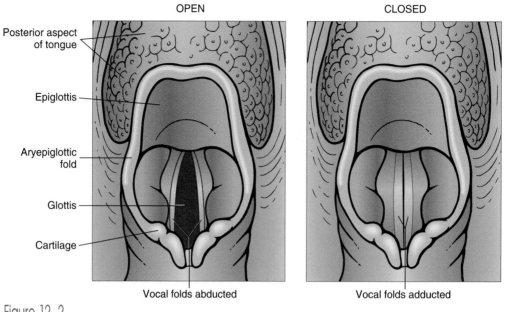

OPEN   CLOSED

Posterior aspect of tongue

Epiglottis

Aryepiglottic fold

Glottis

Cartilage

Vocal folds abducted   Vocal folds adducted

Figure 12-2

The larynx from a superior view.

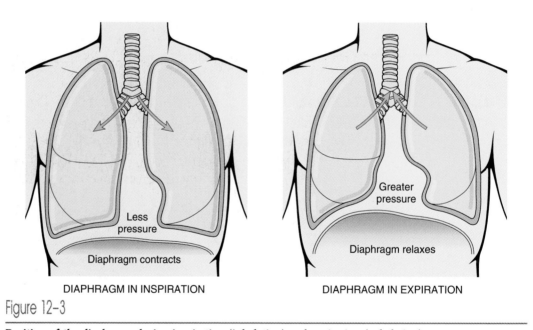

Less pressure

Diaphragm contracts

DIAPHRAGM IN INSPIRATION

Greater pressure

Diaphragm relaxes

DIAPHRAGM IN EXPIRATION

Figure 12-3

Position of the diaphragm during inspiration (inhalation) and expiration (exhalation).

Since food entering from the mouth and air entering from the nose mix in the pharynx, what prevents the passing of food or drink into the larynx and respiratory system after it has been swallowed? Even if a small quantity of solid or liquid matter finds its way into the air passages, breathing can be seriously blocked and the aspirated food can cause irritation in the lungs. A special deterrent to this event is provided by a flap of cartilage attached to the root of the tongue that acts as a lid over the larynx. This flap of cartilage is called the **epiglottis** [11]. It covers the **glottis,** which is the opening to the larynx. In the act of swallowing, when food and liquid move through the throat, the epiglottis closes off the larynx so that these cannot enter. Figure 12–2 shows the larynx from a superior view.

On its way to the lungs, air passes from the larynx to the **trachea (windpipe)** [12], a vertical tube about 4½ inches long and 1 inch in diameter. The trachea is kept open by 16–20 C-shaped rings of cartilage separated by fibrous connective tissue that stiffen the front and sides of the tube.

In the region of the **mediastinum** [13], the trachea divides into two branches called **bronchial tubes,** or **bronchi** [14] (singular: **bronchus**). Each bronchus leads to a separate **lung** [15] and divides and subdivides into smaller and finer tubes, somewhat like the branches of a tree.

The smallest of the bronchial branches are called **bronchioles** [16]. At the end of the bronchioles are clusters of air sacs called **alveoli** [17] (singular: **alveolus**). Each alveolus is made of a one-cell layer of epithelium. The very thin wall allows for the exchange of gases between the alveolus and the **capillary** [18] that surrounds and comes in close contact with it. The blood that flows through the capillaries accepts the oxygen from the alveolus and deposits carbon dioxide into the alveolus to be exhaled. Oxygen is bound to a protein (hemoglobin) in red blood cells called **erythrocytes** [19] and carried to all parts of the body.

Each lung is enveloped in a double-folded membrane called the **pleura.** The outer layer of the pleura, nearest the ribs, is the **parietal pleura** [20], and the inner layer, closest to the lung, is the **visceral pleura** [21]. The pleura is moistened with a serous (thin, watery fluid) secretion that facilitates the movements of the lungs within the chest (thorax).

The two lungs are not quite mirror images of each other. The right lung, which is the slightly larger of the two, is divided into three **lobes** and the left lung is divided into two lobes. It is possible for one lobe of the lung to be removed without damage to the rest, which can continue to function normally. The uppermost part of the lung is called the **apex,** and the lower area is the **base.** The **hilum** or **hilus** of the lung is the midline region where blood vessels, nerves, lymphatic tissue, and bronchial tubes enter and exit the organ.

The lungs extend from the collarbone to the **diaphragm** [22] in the thoracic cavity. The diaphragm is a muscular partition that separates the thoracic from the abdominal cavity and aids in the process of breathing. The diaphragm contracts and descends with each **inhalation (inspiration).** The downward movement of the diaphragm enlarges the area in the thoracic cavity and reduces the internal air pressure, so that air flows into the lungs to equalize the pressure. When the lungs are full, the diaphragm relaxes and elevates, making the area in the thoracic cavity smaller, and thus increasing the air pressure in the thorax. Air then is expelled out of the lungs to equalize the pressure; this is called **exhalation (expiration).** Figure 12–3 shows the position of the diaphragm in inspiration and expiration.

Figure 12–4 is a flow diagram reviewing the pathway of air from the nose, where air enters the body, to the capillaries of the lungs, where oxygen enters the bloodstream.

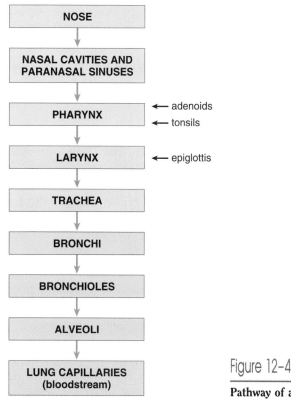

Figure 12-4

Pathway of air from the nose to the capillaries of the lungs.

III. Vocabulary

This list will help you review many of the new terms introduced in the text. Short definitions will reinforce your understanding of the terms. See Section X of this chapter for help in pronouncing the more difficult terms.

adenoids	Collections of lymph tissue in the nasopharynx; also called pharyngeal tonsils.
alveolus (plural: **alveoli**)	Air sac in the lung.
apex of the lung	Uppermost portion of the lung. **Apical** means pertaining to the apex.
base of the lung	Lower portion of the lung.
bronchioles	Smallest branches of the bronchi.
bronchus (plural: **bronchi**)	Branch of the trachea (windpipe) that acts as a passageway into the air spaces of the lung; bronchial tube.
carbon dioxide (CO$_2$)	A gas produced by body cells when oxygen and food combine; exhaled through the lungs.
cilia	Thin hairs attached to the mucous membrane epithelium lining the respiratory tract.

diaphragm	Muscle separating the chest and abdomen. It is the most important muscle for breathing.
epiglottis	Lid-like piece of cartilage that covers the larynx.
exhalation	Breathing out (expiration).
external respiration	Exchange of gases in the lungs.
glottis	The opening to the larynx.
hilum (of lung)	Midline region where the bronchi, blood vessels, and nerves enter and exit the lungs. **Hilar** means pertaining to the hilum.
inhalation	Breathing in (inspiration).
internal respiration	Exchange of gases at the tissue cells.
larynx	Voice box.
lobes	Divisions of the lungs.
mediastinum	Region between the lungs in the chest cavity. It contains the trachea, heart, aorta, esophagus, and bronchial tubes.
oxygen (O$_2$)	Gas that passes into the bloodstream at the lungs and travels to all body cells.
palatine tonsils	Rounded masses of lymph tissue in the oropharynx (palatine means roof of the mouth).
paranasal sinuses	Air-containing cavities in the bones near the nose.
parietal pleura	The outer fold of pleura lying closest to the ribs and wall of the thoracic cavity.
pharynx	Throat; composed of the nasopharynx, oropharynx, and laryngopharynx.
pleura	Double-folded membrane surrounding each lung.
pleural cavity	Space between the folds of the pleura.
pulmonary parenchyma	The essential cells of the lung, those performing its main function; the air sacs (alveoli) and small bronchioles.
trachea	Windpipe.
visceral pleura	The inner fold of pleura lying closest to the lung tissue.

IV. Combining Forms, Suffixes, and Terminology

Write the meanings of the medical terms in the spaces provided.

Combining Forms

Combining Form	Meaning	Terminology	Meaning
adenoid/o	adenoids	adenoidectomy _____	
		adenoid hypertrophy _____	
alveol/o	alveolus, air sac	alveolar _____	
bronch/o **bronchi/o**	bronchial tube, bronchus	bronchospasm _____	
		bronchiectasis _____	
		Caused by weakening of the bronchial wall by infection.	
		bronchodilator _____	
		This is a drug that causes dilation, or enlargement, of the opening of a bronchus (for example, epinephrine).	
bronchiol/o	bronchiole, small bronchus	bronchiolitis _____	
		Figure 12–5 shows the relationship among bronchioles, alveoli, and the blood vessels surrounding them.	
capn/o	carbon dioxide	hypercapnia _____	
coni/o	dust	pneumoconiosis _____	
		See page 440, Section V, under Pathological Terms.	
cyan/o	blue	cyanosis _____	
		Caused by deficient oxygen in the blood; hemoglobin in red blood cells is deoxygenated.	
epiglott/o	epiglottis	epiglottitis _____	
laryng/o	larynx, voice box	laryngeal _____	
		laryngospasm _____	
		laryngitis _____	
lob/o	lobe of the lung	lobectomy _____	
		Figure 12–6 shows four different types of lung resections.	
mediastin/o	mediastinum	mediastinoscopy _____	

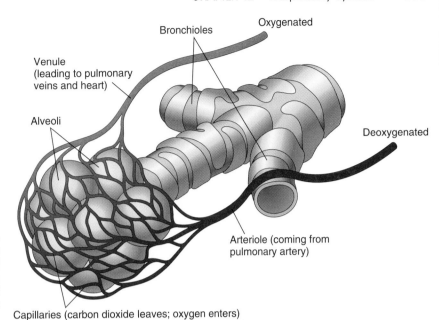

Figure 12-5

Bronchioles, alveoli, and blood vessels that surround the alveoli. Exchange of gases takes place as carbon dioxide leaves the capillaries to enter the alveoli and oxygen enters the capillaries from the alveoli.

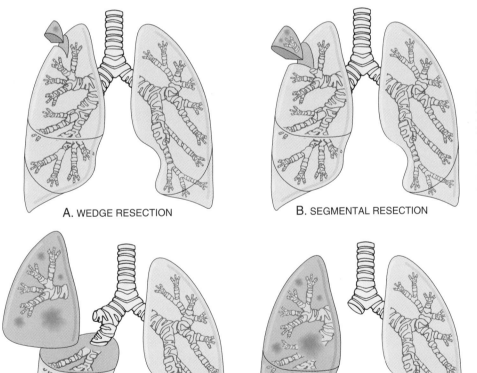

A. WEDGE RESECTION

B. SEGMENTAL RESECTION

C. LOBECTOMY

D. PNEUMONECTOMY

Figure 12-6

Pulmonary resections. (A) Wedge resection is the removal of a small, localized area of diseased tissue near the surface of the lung. Pulmonary function and structure are relatively unchanged after healing. **(B)** Segmental resection is the removal of a bronchiole and its alveoli (one or more lung segments). The remaining lung tissue expands to fill the previously occupied space. **(C)** Lobectomy is the removal of an entire lobe of the lung. Following lobectomy, the remaining lung increases in size to fill the space in the thoracic cavity. **(D)** Pneumonectomy is the removal of an entire lung. Techniques (removal of ribs and elevation of the diaphragm) are used to reduce the size of the empty thoracic space.

nas/o	nose	paranasal sinuses _____
		Para- means near in this term.
		nasogastric tube _____
orth/o	straight, upright	orthopnea _____
		Breathing (-pnea) is easier in the upright position. A major cause of orthopnea is congestive heart failure (the lungs fill with fluid when the patient is lying flat). Physicians assess the degree of orthopnea by the number of pillows a patient requires to sleep comfortably (e.g., two-pillow orthopnea).
ox/o	oxygen	hypoxia _____
		Tissues have a decreased amount of oxygen, and cyanosis can result.
pector/o	chest	expectoration _____
		Expectorated sputum can contain mucus, blood, cellular debris, pus, and microorganisms.
pharyng/o	pharynx, throat	pharyngeal _____
		nasopharyngitis _____
phon/o	voice	dysphonia _____
		Hoarseness or other voice impairment.
phren/o	diaphragm	phrenic nerve _____
pleur/o	pleura	pleuritic _____
		pleurodynia _____
		-dynia means pain.
		pleural effusion _____
		An effusion is the escape of fluid from blood vessels or lymphatics into a cavity or into tissue spaces.
pneum/o **pneumon/o**	air, lung	pneumothorax _____
		-thorax means chest. Air accumulates in the pleural cavity, between the pleura (Fig. 12–7).
		pneumonitis _____
		pneumonectomy _____
pulmon/o	lung	pulmonary _____
rhin/o	nose	rhinorrhea _____
		rhinoplasty _____

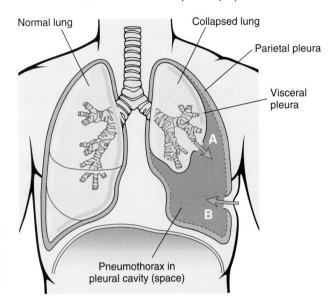

Figure 12-7

Pneumothorax. Air gathers in the pleural cavity. This condition **(A)** can occur with lung disease or **(B)** can follow trauma to and perforation of (a hole through) the chest wall.

sinus/o	sinus, cavity	sinusitis _____
spir/o	breathing	spirometer _____
		expiration _____

Note that the s is omitted.

respiration _____

Cheyne-Stokes respiration is marked by rhythmic changes in the depth of breathing. The pattern occurs every 45 seconds to 3 minutes. The cause is heart failure or brain damage, both of which affect the respiratory center in the brain.

tel/o	complete	atelectasis _____

Incomplete expansion (-ectasis) of a lung; collapsed lung. Atelectasis may occur after surgery when a patient experiences pain and does not take deep breaths (Fig. 12–8).

Figure 12-8

Two forms of atelectasis. (A) An obstruction prevents air from reaching distal airways, and alveoli collapse. The most frequent cause is blockage of a bronchus by a mucous or mucopurulent (pus-filled) plug, as might occur postoperatively. **(B)** Accumulations of fluid, blood, or air within the pleural cavity collapse the lung. This can occur with congestive heart failure (poor circulation leads to fluid build up in the pleural cavity) or because of leakage of air caused by a pneumothorax.

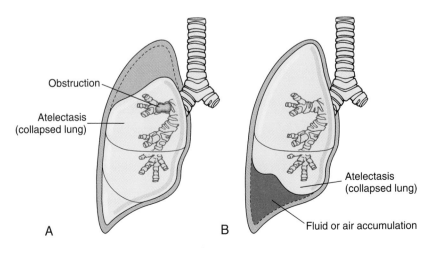

thorac/o	chest	thoracotomy _____	
		thoracic _____	
tonsill/o	tonsils	tonsillectomy _____	
		The oropharyngeal (palatine) tonsils are removed.	
trache/o	trachea, windpipe	tracheotomy _____	
		tracheal stenosis _____	
		Having an endotracheal tube in place for a prolonged period may lead to tracheal trauma or the formation of scar tissue.	

Suffixes			
Suffix	**Meaning**	**Terminology**	**Meaning**
-ema	condition	empyema _____	
		Em- means in. Empyema is a collection of pus, and it most commonly occurs in the pleural cavity as pyothorax.	
-osmia	smell	anosmia _____	
-pnea	breathing	apnea _____	
		dyspnea _____	
		Paroxysmal (sudden) nocturnal (at night) dyspnea may occur in patients with congestive heart failure when they recline in bed. Patients often describe the sensation as "air hunger."	
		hyperpnea _____	
		An increase in the depth of breathing.	
		tachypnea _____	
		Excessively rapid and shallow breathing; hyperventilation.	
-ptysis	spitting	hemoptysis _____	
-sphyxia	pulse	asphyxia _____	
		Interference with respiration can ultimately lead to the absence of pulse.	

-thorax	pleural cavity, chest	hemothorax _____
		pyothorax _____

Empyema of the chest.

V. Diagnostic and Pathological Terms

Diagnostic Terms

auscultation

Listening to sounds within the body.

This procedure, performed with a stethoscope, is used chiefly for diagnosing conditions of the lungs, pleura, heart, and abdomen, as well as to determine the condition of the fetus during pregnancy.

percussion

Tapping on a surface to determine the difference in the density of the underlying structure.

Tapping over a solid organ produces a dull sound without resonance. Percussion over an air-filled structure, such as the lung, produces a resonant, hollow note. As the lungs are filled with fluid and become more dense, as in pneumonia, resonance is replaced by dullness.

pleural rub

Grating sound produced by the motion of pleural surfaces rubbing against each other; also called a friction rub.

Pleural rub occurs when the pleura are thickened by inflammation, scarring or neoplastic cells. It is heard by auscultation and can be felt by placing the fingers on the chest wall.

rales (crackles)

Abnormal crackling sounds heard during inspiration when there is fluid, blood, or pus in the alveoli.

Rhonchi are coarse, loud rales usually caused by secretions in the bronchial tubes.

sputum

Material expelled from the chest by coughing or clearing the throat.

Purulent (containing pus) sputum results from infection and is often green or brown in color. Blood-tinged sputum makes physicians suspicious of tuberculosis.

stridor

A strained, high-pitched, noisy sound made on inspiration; it is associated with obstruction of the larynx, trachea, or a bronchus.

wheezes **Musical sounds usually heard during expiration.**

Wheezes occur in patients with bronchial constriction and inflammation (as in asthma or bronchitis).

Pathological Terms

Upper Respiratory Disorders

croup **Acute respiratory syndrome in children and infants; characterized by obstruction of the larynx, barking cough, and stridor.**

Croup may result from infection, allergy, or the presence of a foreign body in the larynx.

diphtheria **Acute infection of the throat and upper respiratory tract caused by diphtheria bacteria (*Corynebacterium*).**

Inflammation occurs, and a leathery, opaque membrane forms in the pharynx and respiratory tract.

Immunity to diphtheria (by production of antibodies) is induced by the administration of weakened toxins (antigens) beginning between the 6th and the 8th weeks of life. These injections are usually given in combination with pertussis and tetanus toxins and are called **DPT** injections.

epistaxis **Nosebleed.**

Epistaxis (from the Greek meaning to let fall, drop by drop) results from traumatic or spontaneous rupture of blood vessels in the mucous membrane of the nose.

pertussis **Bacterial infection of the pharynx, larynx, and trachea caused by *Bordetella pertussis*, a highly contagious bacterium. Also known as whooping cough.**

Bronchial Tube Disorders

asthma **Spasm and narrowing of bronchi, which leads to bronchial airway obstruction.**

Associated symptoms are **paroxysmal** (sudden) dyspnea, wheezing, and cough. Etiology may involve allergy or infection, and asthma may be aggravated by anxiety, cold, and exercise. Asthma (the term comes from a Greek word meaning panting) is treated with drugs, including inhaled agents that dilate the bronchi.

bronchiectasis **Chronic dilation of a bronchus or bronchi; secondary to infection that usually involves the lower portion of the lung.**

This disease is often caused by recurrent infections, especially pneumonia. It may also be congenital. Bronchiectasis commonly leads to chronic obstruction of a bronchus. Treatment is palliative (noncurative) and includes antibiotics, bronchodilators, and respiratory therapy.

Figure 12-9

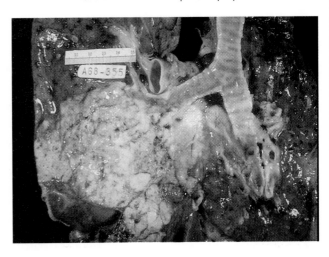

Bronchogenic carcinoma. The gray-white tumor tissue is infiltrating the substance of the lung. This tumor was identified as a squamous cell carcinoma. Squamous cell carcinomas arise in major bronchi and spread to local hilar lymph nodes. (From Kumar V, Cotran RS, Robbins SL: Basic Pathology, 6th ed. Philadelphia, WB Saunders, 1997, p 433.)

bronchogenic carcinoma	**Cancerous tumors arising from a bronchus; lung cancer (Fig. 12–9).**

This group of malignant tumors, associated with cigarette smoking, is responsible for 31 per cent of cancer deaths in males and 25 per cent of cancer deaths in females (United States, 1999). Lung cancers are divided into two main categories: small cell (10 per cent) and non-small cell (90 per cent). **Small cell lung cancer (SCLC)** derives from small, round to oval secretory cells in pulmonary epithelium. It tends to grow rapidly and spread distantly. Surgical resection is not curative. Treatment is radiation therapy (irradiation) and chemotherapy.

There are two main types of **non-small cell lung cancer (NSCLC): adenocarcinoma** (derived from mucus-secreting cells) and **squamous cell carcinoma** (derived from the lining of a bronchus). For localized tumors, surgery may be curative. When disease is locally advanced (lymph nodes or mediastinum), chemotherapy and radiation therapy are options. Metastatic disease (to the liver, brain, and bones) is also treated with chemotherapy and irradiation.

chronic bronchitis	**Inflammation of the bronchi that persists for a long time.**

This disease is often caused by infection or cigarette smoking and is characterized by increased secretion from the bronchial mucosa and obstruction of the respiratory passages. Chronic bronchitis, asthma, and emphysema (see Lung Disorders) are known as **chronic obstructive pulmonary diseases (COPDs).**

cystic fibrosis	**Inherited disease of exocrine glands (pancreas, sweat glands, and mucous membranes of the respiratory tract) that leads to airway obstruction.**

Chronic respiratory infections are common, as is pancreatic insufficiency (fats are improperly digested). Therapy involves replacement of pancreatic enzymes and treatment of pulmonary obstruction and infection. The gene responsible for the condition has been found, and persons carrying the gene can be identified.

Lung Disorders

atelectasis

Incomplete (atel/o) expansion (-ectasis) of alveoli; collapsed, functionless, airless lung or portion of a lung.

In atelectasis, the bronchioles and alveoli (pulmonary parenchyma) resemble a collapsed balloon. Common causes of atelectasis include poor inspiration effort in the postoperative period, blockage of a bronchus or smaller bronchial tube by secretions, and a tumor or a chest wound that permits air, fluid, or blood to accumulate in the pleural cavity. Acute atelectasis requires removal of the underlying cause (tumor, foreign body, excessive mucous secretions) and therapy to open airways.

emphysema

Hyperinflation of air sacs with destruction of alveolar walls.

Loss of elasticity and the breakdown of the alveoli walls result in loss of air movement in the air sacs. There is a strong association between cigarette smoking and emphysema. Chronic bronchitis is often associated with emphysema. As a result of the destruction of lung parenchyma, including blood vessels, pulmonary artery pressure rises and the right side of the heart must work harder to pump blood. This leads to right ventricular hypertrophy and heart failure **(cor pulmonale).**

pneumoconiosis

Abnormal condition caused by dust in the lungs, with chronic inflammation, infection, and bronchitis.

Various forms are named according to the type of dust particle inhaled: **anthracosis**—coal (anthrac/o) dust (black lung disease); **asbestosis**—asbestos (asbest/o) particles (in shipbuilding and construction trades); **silicosis**—silica (silic/o = rocks) or glass (grinder's disease).

pneumonia

Acute inflammation and infection of alveoli, which fill with pus or products of the inflammatory reaction.

Etiological agents are most often pneumococci and less frequently staphylococci, fungi, or viruses. Infection damages alveolar membranes, so that fluid, blood cells, and debris consolidate in the alveoli. **Lobar pneumonia** involves one or more lobes of a lung. When both lungs are affected, the disease is called bilateral, or "double," pneumonia. **Bronchopneumonia** begins in the terminal bronchioles and affects a smaller area. Symptoms appear gradually and are milder. Pneumonia is treated with appropriate antibiotics and, if necessary, supplemental oxygen and respiratory therapy.

pulmonary abscess

A large collection of pus (bacterial infection) in the lungs.

pulmonary edema

Swelling and fluid in the air sacs and bronchioles.

This condition is often caused by the inability of the heart to pump blood (congestive heart failure). Blood then backs up in the pulmonary blood vessels, and fluid seeps out into the alveoli and bronchioles. This is a condition that requires immediate medical attention, including drugs (diuretics, vasodilators, digitalis), oxygen in high concentrations, and keeping the patient in a sitting position (to decrease venous return to the heart).

pulmonary embolism

Clot (thrombus) or other material lodges in vessels of the lung.

The clot travels from distant veins, usually in the legs. Occlusion can produce an area of dead (necrotic) lung tissue called a **pulmonary infarction.**

sarcoidosis	**Inflammatory disease in which small nodules or tubercles develop in lungs, lymph nodes, and other organs.**

Lesions develop on the skin and in the lungs, lymph nodes, spleen, and liver. The condition resembles the tubercles of tuberculosis, but the cause is unknown. Many patients are asymptomatic and retain adequate pulmonary function. Others have more active disease and impaired pulmonary function. Corticosteroid drugs are used to prevent progression in these patients.

tuberculosis	**An infectious disease caused by *Mycobacterium tuberculosis*; lungs are usually involved, but any organ in the body may be affected.**

Rod-shaped bacteria called **bacilli** invade the lungs, producing small tubercles (from the Latin word *tuber* meaning a swelling) of infection. Early tuberculosis (TB) is usually asymptomatic and is detected on routine chest x-ray. Symptoms of advanced disease are cough, weight loss, night sweats, hemoptysis, and pleuritic pain. Antituberculous chemotherapy (isoniazid, rifampin) is effective in most cases. Immunocompromised patients are particularly susceptible to antibiotic-resistant tuberculosis. It is important and often necessary to treat TB with many drugs at the same time to prevent drug resistance.

The PPD skin test (see page 447, Section VI, under Clinical Procedures) is given to most hospital and medical employees because TB can be transmitted very easily.

Pleural Disorders

mesothelioma	**A malignant tumor arising in the pleura;** composed of mesothelium, which is epithelium that covers the surfaces of membranes such as the pleura, peritoneum, and pericardium.

This is a rare tumor and is associated with exposure to asbestos.

pleural effusion	**Escape of fluid into the pleural cavity.**

Pleural effusions are typically categorized on the basis of whether they are transudates (fluid that has passed through a membrane or tissue) or exudates (fluid, high in protein, that oozes from blood vessels and wounds).

pleurisy (pleuritis)	**Inflammation of the pleura.**

This condition causes pleurodynia and dyspnea and, in chronic cases, escape of fluid into the pleural cavity.

pneumothorax	**Accumulation of air or gas in the pleural cavity.**

Pneumothorax may occur in the course of a pulmonary disease (emphysema, carcinoma, tuberculosis, or lung abscess) when rupture of any pulmonary lesions near the pleural surface allows communication between an alveolus or bronchus and the pleural cavity. It may also follow trauma and perforation of the chest wall or prolonged high-flow oxygen delivered by a respirator in an intensive care unit (ICU).

■ STUDY SECTION

Practice spelling each term and know its meaning.

anthracosis Coal dust accumulation in the lungs; a pneumoconiosis.

asbestosis Asbestos particles accumulate in the lungs.

bacilli (singular: **bacillus**) Rod-shaped bacteria.

chronic obstructive pulmonary disease (COPD) A chronic condition of persistent obstruction of air flow through the bronchial tubes and lungs. Chronic bronchitis and emphysema are the two conditions mainly associated with COPD. Patients with COPD are referred to as *blue bloaters* (bronchitic, cyanotic, stocky build) or *pink puffers* (emphysemic, no change in skin color, short of breath).

cor pulmonale Failure of the right side of the heart to pump a sufficient amount of blood to the lungs; occurs as a complication of lung disease.

hydrothorax Collection of fluid in the pleural cavity.

paroxysmal Pertaining to a sudden occurrence, such as a spasm or seizure; oxysm/o means sudden.

pulmonary infarction An area of dead (necrotic) tissue in the lung.

purulent Pertaining to containing pus.

silicosis Silica or glass dust in the lungs; occurs in mining occupations.

VI. Clinical Procedures and Abbreviations

Clinical Procedures

X-Rays

chest x-ray An x-ray picture of the chest (Fig. 12–10) can be taken in the frontal (coronal) plane (AP or PA view) or in the sagittal plane (lateral view). **Chest tomograms** are a series of x-rays that show pictures of the chest region at various depths; tomograms are able to detect small masses not seen on a regular film.

CT scan of the chest A computerized reconstruction of a series of x-ray pictures of the chest taken as slices in a transverse (axial or cross-sectional) plane.

pulmonary angiography Dye is injected into a blood vessel, and x-rays are taken of the arteries or veins in the lung.

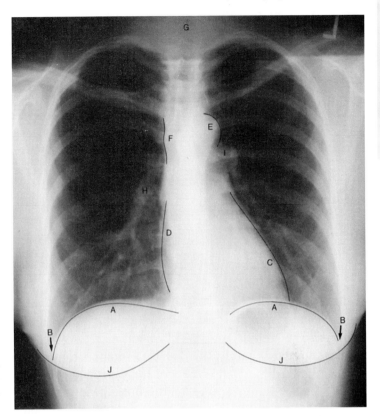

Figure 12-10

A **normal chest x-ray** taken from the posteroanterior (PA) view. The backwards L in the upper corner is placed on the film to indicate the left side of the patient's chest. **(A)** diaphragm; **(B)** costophrenic angle; **(C)** left ventricle; **(D)** right atrium; **(E)** aortic arch; **(F)** superior vena cava; **(G)** trachea; **(H)** right bronchus; **(I)** left bronchus; **(J)** breast shadows. (From Black JM, Matassarin-Jacobs E: Medical Surgical Nursing, 6th ed. Philadelphia, WB Saunders, 1997, p 1059.)

Magnetic Imaging

MRI scan of the chest

Magnetic resonance imaging of the chest. Magnetic waves are used to create detailed images of the chest in the frontal, sagittal, and transverse planes (Fig. 12–11).

Radioactive Test

lung scan or V/Q scan

Radioactive material is injected intravenously or inhaled, and images are recorded of its distribution in lung tissue, to show air flow (ventilation) and blood supply (perfusion) to the lungs.

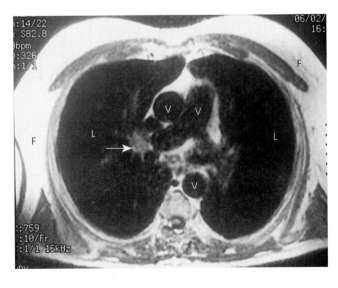

Figure 12-11

MRI of the upper chest, transverse (axial) view. Notice the lungs (L), fat (F), and vessels (V). A hilar tumor (arrow) is easily identified. (From Ballinger PW, Frank ED: Merrill's Atlas of Radiographic Positions and Radiologic Procedures, 9th ed. Vol. 3. St. Louis, Mosby, 1999, p 338.)

Other Procedures

bronchoscopy

Examination of the bronchial tubes by passing a lighted, flexible fiber-optic tube through the nose, throat, larynx, and trachea and into the bronchi. Specimens can be obtained through the tube for cytological and bacterial studies by aspirating bronchial secretions or by injecting fluid and retrieving fluid **(bronchial alveolar lavage, or bronchial washing).** Biopsies can be performed on suspicious areas by means of a forceps (an instrument that can grasp tissue) or brush **(bronchial brushing)** that is inserted through the bronchoscope (Fig. 12–12).

endotracheal intubation

A tube is placed through the nose or mouth, through the pharynx and larynx, and into the trachea to establish an airway and allow a person to be placed on a **ventilator** (an apparatus that moves air in and out of the lungs) (Fig. 12–13). This typically occurs during surgery or in the ICU.

laryngoscopy

Visual examination of the larynx. A lighted, flexible tube is passed through the mouth or nose into the larynx.

mediastinoscopy

Visual examination of the mediastinum. This procedure is done in the operating room with local or general anesthesia. A suprasternal (above the breastbone) incision is made and the procedure is used to remove biopsy samples of lymph nodes, tumors, and tuberculosis.

pulmonary function tests

This group of tests measures ventilation (breathing) mechanics of the lungs, that is, the quantity of air moved into and out of the lungs under normal conditions. A **spirometer** measures the air taken in and

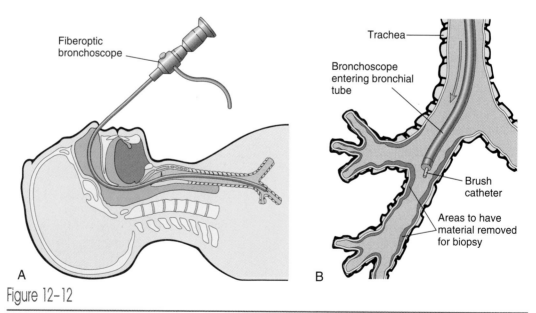

Figure 12-12

(A) Fiberoptic bronchoscopy. A bronchoscope is passed through the nose, throat, larynx, and trachea into a bronchus. **(B)** A **bronchoscope,** with brush catheter, in place in a bronchial tube.

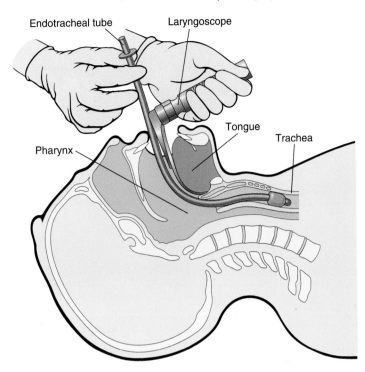

Endotracheal tube

Laryngoscope

Tongue

Trachea

Pharynx

Figure 12-13

Endotracheal intubation. The patient is in a supine position; the head is hyperextended, the lower portion of the neck is flexed, and the mouth is opened. A **laryngoscope** is used to hold the airway open, to expose the vocal cords, and as a guide for placing the ET tube into the trachea.

out of the lungs. The **forced vital capacity (FVC)** of the lungs is measured by asking the patient to inspire to the maximum and then exhale into the spirometer as forcefully and rapidly as possible. **Incentive spirometry** (Fig. 12–14) is used to promote alveolar inflation and restore and maintain lung capacity.

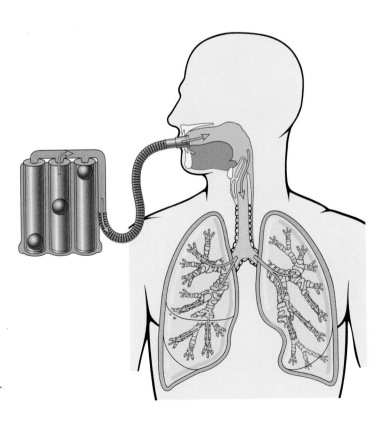

Figure 12-14

Incentive spirometer.

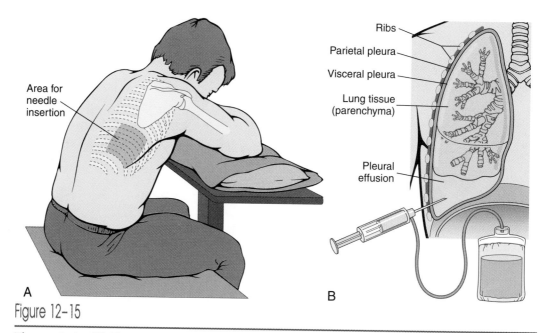

Figure 12–15

Thoracentesis. (A) The patient is sitting in the correct position for the procedure; it allows the chest wall to be pulled outward in an expanded position. **(B)** The needle is inserted close to the base of the effusion so the gravity can help with drainage, but it is kept as far away from the diaphragm as possible.

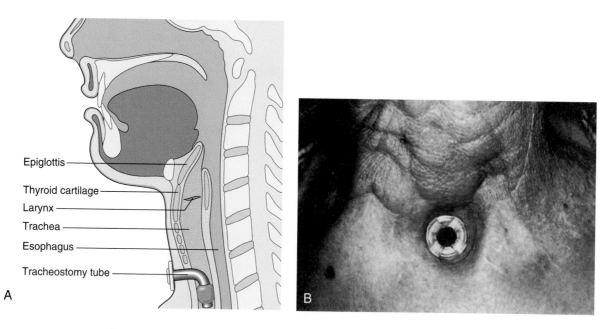

Figure 12–16

(A) Tracheostomy with tube in place. **(B) Healed tracheostomy incision** after laryngectomy. (**B** from Black JM, Matassarin-Jacobs E: Medical-Surgical Nursing, 6th ed. Philadelphia, WB Saunders, 1997, p 1099.)

thoracentesis Insertion of a needle or catheter through the skin and between the ribs into the pleural space in order to obtain fluid from the pleural cavity for analysis, to drain pleural effusions, or to re-expand a collapsed lung (Fig. 12–15).

thoracoscopy Examination of the pleural space, pleura, and lungs with a scope that is inserted through a small incision between the ribs. Thoracoscopy can be used for taking biopsies of the lungs, repairing leaks in the lungs, and diagnosing a variety of diseases of the pleura.

thoracotomy A major surgical procedure in which the chest is opened, by making an incision, for diagnostic or therapeutic procedures. Thoracotomy is necessary for **lung biopsy** and lung resections (lobectomy, pneumonectomy).

tracheostomy The creation of an opening into the trachea through the neck and the insertion of a tube to create an airway. A tracheostomy tube may be a permanent as well as an emergency device (Fig. 12–16).

tuberculin tests Agents such as **PPD** (purified protein derivative) are applied to the surface of the skin with multiple punctures **(Heaf and tine tests)** or by intradermal injection **(Mantoux test).** A local cutaneous inflammatory reaction (redness, swelling) is observed in persons who are sensitive to the test substance; a positive test indicates prior or present infection with tuberculosis.

tube thoracostomy A **chest tube** is passed through a small incision in the skin to continuously drain pleural spaces after thoracotomy.

ABBREVIATIONS

AFB	acid-fast bacillus (organism causing tuberculosis)	**CTA**	clear to auscultation
ARDS	adult (or acute) respiratory distress syndrome (a group of symptoms—tachypnea, dyspnea, tachycardia, hypoxemia, cyanosis—resulting in acute respiratory failure)	**CXR**	chest x-ray
		DOE	dyspnea on exertion
		DPT	diphtheria, pertussis, tetanus (injection in an infant to provide immunity to these diseases)
Bronch	bronchoscopy		
COPD	chronic obstructive pulmonary disease (airway obstruction associated with emphysema and chronic bronchitis)	**FVC**	forced vital capacity
		ICU	intensive care unit
CPR	cardiopulmonary resuscitation (three basic steps: airway opened by tilting the head, breathing restored by mouth-to-mouth breathing, circulation restored by external cardiac compression)	**IMV**	intermittent mandatory ventilation
		LLL	left lower lobe (of lung)
		LUL	left upper lobe (of lung)

MDI	metered-dose inhaler; used to deliver aerosolized medications to patients with respiratory disease
NSCLC	non-small cell lung cancer
pCO₂	carbon dioxide partial pressure; amount of carbon dioxide in arterial blood
pO₂	oxygen partial pressure; amount of oxygen in arterial blood
PCP	*Pneumocystis carinii* pneumonia (a type of pneumonia seen in patients with AIDS)
PEEP	positive end expiratory pressure (a common mechanical ventilator setting in which airway pressure is maintained above atmospheric pressure)
PFT	pulmonary function tests
PND	paroxysmal nocturnal dyspnea

PPD	purified protein derivative (substance used in a tuberculosis test)
RDS	respiratory distress syndrome (condition of the newborn marked by dyspnea and cyanosis and related to absence of surfactant, a substance that permits normal expansion of lungs); also called hyaline membrane disease
RLL	right lower lobe (of lung)
RUL	right upper lobe (of lung)
SCLC	small cell lung cancer
SOB	shortness of breath
TB	tuberculosis
URI	upper respiratory infection
V/Q scan	ventilation-perfusion scan. Radioactive test of lung ventilation space and blood perfusion throughout the lung capillaries (lung scan).

VII. Practical Applications

This section contains actual medical reports using terms that you have studied in this and previous chapters. Explanations of more difficult terms are added in brackets. Answers to the questions are on page 457 after Answers to Exercises.

Case Report

A 22-year-old known heroin abuser was admitted to an emergency room comatose with shallow respirations. Routine laboratory studies and chest x-rays were done after the patient was aroused. He was then transferred to the ICU. He complained of left-sided chest pain. Examination of the chest x-ray showed three fractured ribs on the right and a large right pleural effusion. Further questioning of a friend revealed that he had fallen and struck the corner of a table after injecting heroin.

The diagnosis was traumatic hemothorax secondary to fractured ribs, and a thoracotomy tube was inserted into the right pleural space. No blood could be obtained despite maneuvering of the tube. Another chest x-ray showed that the tube was correctly placed in the right pleural space but the fractured ribs and pleural effusion were on the left. The radiologist then realized that he had reversed the first film. A second tube was inserted into the left pleural space, and 1500 mL (6–7 cups) of blood were evacuated.

Necropsy Report and Questions

Adenocarcinoma, bronchogenic, left lung, with extensive mediastinal, pleural, and pericardial involvement. Metastasis to tracheobronchial lymph nodes, liver, lumbar vertebrae. Pulmonary emboli, multiple, recent, with recent infarct of left lower lobe. The tumor apparently originated at the left main bronchus and extends peripherally. Parenchyma (alveoli) is particularly atelectatic with a centrally located area of hemorrhage in the lower lobe.

Questions on the Case Report

1. What was the patient's primary disease?
   (A) blood clots in the lung
   (B) mediastinal, pleural, and pericardial inflammation
   (C) lung cancer
2. Which was *not* an area of metastasis?
   (A) backbones
   (B) bone marrow
   (C) hepatocytes
3. What event was probably the cause of death?
   (A) infarction of lung tissue due to pulmonary emboli
   (B) COPD
   (C) myocardial infarction
4. What best describes the pulmonary parenchyma in the lower left lobe?
   (A) alveoli are filled with tumor
   (B) alveoli are collapsed, with central area of bleeding
   (C) alveoli are filled with pus and blood

X-Ray Reports and Bronchoscopy

1. CXR: Complete opacification of left hemithorax with deviation of mediastinal structures of right side. Massive pleural effusion.
2. Chest tomograms: Mass most compatible with LUL bronchogenic carcinoma. Possible left paratracheal adenopathy or direct involvement of mediastinum.
3. Bronchoscopy: Larynx, trachea, carina [area of bifurcation or forking of the trachea], and left lung all within normal limits. On the right side there was irregularity and roughening of the bronchial mucosa on the lateral aspect of the bronchial wall. This irregularity extended into the RUL, and the apical and posterior segments [divisions of lobes of the lung] each contained inflamed irregular mucosa. Conclusion: suspicious for infiltrating tumor, but may be nonspecific inflammation. Bronchial washings, brushings, and bxs [biopsies] taken. Bronchial biopsy diagnosis: squamous cell carcinoma. Washings and brushings showed no malignant cells.

VIII. Exercises

Remember to check your answers carefully with those given in Section IX, Answers to Exercises.

A. Select from the following anatomical structures to complete the sentences below.

mediastinum	cilia	paranasal sinuses
alveoli	bronchioles	palatine tonsils
larynx	parietal pleura	visceral pleura
pharynx	hilum	adenoids
trachea	epiglottis	bronchi

1. The outer fold of pleura lying closest to the ribs is called _____ .

2. Collections of lymph tissue in the nasopharynx are the _____ .

3. The windpipe is known as the _____ .

4. The lid-like piece of cartilage that covers the voice box is the _____ .

5. Branches of the windpipe that lead into the lungs are the _____ .

6. The region between the lungs in the chest cavity is the _____ .

7. Air-containing cavities in the bones around the nose are the _____ .

8. Thin hairs attached to the mucous membrane lining the respiratory tract are called _____ .

9. The inner fold of pleura closest to lung tissue is called _____ .

10. The throat is known as the _____ .

11. Air sacs of the lung are called _____ .

12. The voice box is called the _____ .

13. Smallest branches of bronchi are the _____ .

14. Collections of lymph tissue in the oropharynx are the _____ .

15. The midline region of the lungs where the bronchi, blood vessels, and nerves enter and exit the

lungs is called the _____ .

B. Complete the following sentences.

1. The apical part of the lung is the _____ .

2. The gas that passes into the bloodstream at the lungs is _____ .

3. Breathing in air is called _____ .

4. Divisions of the lungs are known as _____ .

5. The gas produced by cells and exhaled through the lungs is called _____ .

6. The space between the visceral and the parietal pleura is called the _____ .

7. Breathing out air is called _____ .

8. The essential cells of the lung that perform its main function are known as the pulmonary

_____ .

9. The exchange of gases in the lung is called _____ respiration.

10. The exchange of gases at the tissue cells is called _____ respiration.

C. Give the meanings of the following medical terms.

1. bronchiectasis _____

2. pleuritis _____

3. pneumothorax _____

4. anosmia _____

5. laryngectomy _____

6. nasopharyngitis _____

7. phrenic _____

8. alveolar _____

9. glottis _____

10. tracheal stenosis _____

D. Complete the medical terms for the following respiratory symptoms.

1. excessive carbon dioxide in the blood: hyper _____

2. breathing is possible only in an upright position: _____ pnea

3. difficult breathing: _____ pnea

4. condition of blueness of skin: _____ osis

5. spitting up blood: hemo _____

6. deficiency of oxygen: hyp _____

7. condition of pus in the pleural cavity: pyo _____ or em _____

8. hoarseness; voice impairment: dys _____

9. blood in the pleural cavity: hemo _____

10. nosebleed: epi _____

E. Give the meanings of the following medical terms.

1. rales (crackles) _____

2. auscultation _____

3. sputum _____

4. percussion _____

5. rhonchi _____

6. pleural rub _____

7. purulent _____

8. paroxysmal nocturnal dyspnea _____

9. hydrothorax _____

10. pulmonary infarction _____

11. stridor _____

F. Match the following terms with their descriptions below.

chronic bronchitis   atelectasis   diphtheria
pertussis   emphysema   asthma
asbestosis   croup   bronchogenic carcinoma
cystic fibrosis   sarcoidosis

  1. acute infectious disease of the throat caused by *Corynebacterium* _____

  2. acute respiratory syndrome in children and infants that is marked by obstruction of the larynx

     and stridor _____

  3. hyperinflation of air sacs with destruction of alveolar walls _____

  4. inflammation of tubes that lead from the trachea; lasts for a long period of time _____

  5. spasm and narrowing of bronchi, leading to obstruction _____

  6. lungs or a portion of a lung is collapsed _____

  7. malignant neoplasm originating in a bronchus _____

  8. whooping cough _____

  9. inherited disease of exocrine glands that leads to airway obstruction _____

10. type of pneumoconiosis; dust particles are inhaled _____

11. inflammatory disease in which small nodules form in lungs and lymph nodes _____

G. Give the meanings of the following medical terms.

  1. pulmonary abscess _____

  2. pulmonary edema _____

  3. pneumoconiosis _____

  4. pneumonia _____

  5. pulmonary embolism _____

  6. tuberculosis _____

  7. pleural effusion _____

  8. pleurisy _____

9. anthracosis _____

10. mesothelioma _____

11. adenoid hypertrophy _____

12. pleurodynia _____

13. expectoration _____

14. tachypnea _____

H. Match the clinical procedure or abbreviation with its description.

pulmonary function tests	mediastinoscopy	tube thoracostomy
tuberculin tests	bronchial alveolar lavage	thoracentesis
endotracheal intubation	bronchoscopy	lung scan (V/Q scan)
tracheostomy	laryngoscopy	pulmonary angiography

1. tube is placed through the mouth into the trachea to establish an airway _____

2. radioactive material is injected or inhaled, and images are recorded of its distribution in the

   lungs _____

3. PPD, tine, and Mantoux tests _____

4. chest wall is punctured with a needle to obtain fluid from the pleural cavity _____

5. tests that measure the ventilation mechanics of the lung _____

6. an opening is made into the trachea through the neck to establish an airway _____

7. visual examination of the bronchi _____

8. fluid is injected into the bronchi and then removed for examination _____

9. tube is inserted through the nose into the larynx to view the voice box _____

10. contrast material is injected into a blood vessel; x-rays are taken of arteries or veins in the lung

   _____

11. visual examination of the area between the lungs _____

12. a chest tube is passed through a small skin incision to continuously drain the pleural spaces

   _____

I. Give the meanings of the following abbreviations and then select the letter of the sentences that follow that is the best association for each.

Column I

1. DOE _____ ____

2. PND _____ ____

3. MDI _____ ____

4. CPR _____ ____

5. NSCLC _____ ____

6. ARDS _____ ____

7. COPD _____ ____

8. PFT _____ ____

9. PPD _____ ____

10. DPT _____ ____

Column II

A. Patients with congestive heart failure and pulmonary edema experience this symptom when they recline in bed.
B. Examples of this condition are chronic bronchitis and emphysema.
C. This is a substance used in the test for tuberculosis.
D. Examples of this condition are adenocarcinoma and squamous cell carcinoma.
E. This instrument delivers aerosolized medication to patients with respiratory disease.
F. This is an injection in an infant to provide immunity.
G. A spirometer is used for these respiratory tests.
H. This symptom means that a patient has difficulty breathing and is short of breath when exercising.
I. The three basic steps are airway opened by tilting the head; breathing restored by mouth-to-mouth breathing; circulation restored by external cardiac compression.
J. A group of symptoms resulting in acute respiratory failure.

J. Match the respiratory system procedures with their meanings.

pneumonectomy   thoracotomy   thoracentesis
rhinoplasty   tonsillectomy   thoracoscopy
laryngectomy   lobectomy

1. removal of lymph tissue in the oropharynx _____

2. surgical puncture of the chest to remove fluid from the pleural space _____

3. surgical repair of the nose _____

4. incision of the chest for lung biopsy _____

5. removal of the voice box _____

6. removal of a region of a lung _____

7. endoscopic examination of the pleural space, pleura, and lungs _____

8. pulmonary resection _____

K. Circle the terms that best complete the meanings of the sentences.

1. Ruth was having difficulty taking a deep breath and her chest x-ray showed accumulation of fluid in her pleural spaces. Dr. Smith ordered **(PPD, tracheotomy, thoracentesis)** to relieve the pressure on her lungs.

2. Dr. Wong used her stethoscope to perform **(percussion, auscultation, thoracentesis)** on the patient's chest.

3. Before surgery on Mrs. Hope, an 80-year-old-woman with lung cancer, her physicians ordered **(COPD, bronchoscopy, PFTs)** to determine the functioning of her lungs.

4. Sylvia was bringing up yellow-colored sputum and had a high fever. Her physician told her that she had **(pneumonia, pulmonary embolism, pneumothorax)** and needed antibiotics.

5. The night before her thoracotomy for lung biopsy, Mrs. White was told by her anesthesiologist that he would place a (an) **(thoracostomy tube, mediastinoscope, endotracheal tube)** down her throat to keep her airways open during surgery.

IX. Answers to Exercises

A

1. parietal pleura	6. mediastinum	11. alveoli
2. adenoids	7. paranasal sinuses	12. larynx
3. trachea	8. cilia	13. bronchioles
4. epiglottis	9. visceral pleura	14. palatine tonsils
5. bronchi	10. pharynx	15. hilum

B

1. uppermost part	5. carbon dioxide	9. external
2. oxygen	6. pleural cavity	10. internal
3. inspiration; inhalation	7. expiration; exhalation	
4. lobes	8. parenchyma	

C

1. chronic dilation of a bronchus	5. removal of the voice box	9. opening to the larynx
2. inflammation of pleura	6. inflammation of the nose and throat	10. narrowing of the windpipe
3. air in the chest (pleural cavity)	7. pertaining to the diaphragm	
4. lack of sense of smell	8. pertaining to an air sac	

D

1. hypercapnia	5. hemoptysis	9. hemothorax
2. orthopnea	6. hypoxia	10. epistaxis
3. dyspnea	7. pyothorax; empyema	
4. cyanosis	8. dysphonia	

E

1. abnormal crackling sounds heard on inspiration when there is fluid, blood, or pus in the alveoli
2. listening to sounds within the body
3. material expelled from the chest by coughing or clearing the throat
4. tapping on the surface to determine the underlying structure
5. coarse, loud rales caused by bronchial secretions
6. abnormal grating sound produced by the motion of pleural surfaces rubbing against each other (caused by inflammation or tumor cells)
7. pus-filled
8. sudden attack of difficult breathing
associated with lying down at night (caused by congestive heart failure and pulmonary edema as the lungs fill with fluid)
9. fluid in the pleural cavity
10. area of dead tissue in the lung
11. strained, high-pitched inspirational sound

F

1. diphtheria
2. croup
3. emphysema
4. chronic bronchitis
5. asthma
6. atelectasis
7. bronchogenic carcinoma
8. pertussis
9. cystic fibrosis
10. asbestosis
11. sarcoidosis

G

1. collection of pus in the lungs
2. swelling, fluid collection in the air sacs and bronchioles
3. abnormal condition of dust in the lungs
4. acute inflammation and infection of alveoli; they become filled with fluid and blood cells
5. floating clot or other material blocking the blood vessels of the lung
6. an infectious disease caused by
rod-shaped bacilli and producing tubercules (nodes) of infection
7. collection of fluid in the pleural cavity
8. inflammation of pleura
9. abnormal condition of coal dust in the lungs (black-lung disease)
10. malignant tumor arising in the pleura; composed of mesothelium (epithelium that covers the surfaces of membranes such as pleura and peritoneum)
11. excessive growth of cells in the adenoids (lymph tissue in the nasopharynx)
12. pain of the pleura (irritation of pleural surfaces leads to intercostal pain)
13. coughing up of material from the chest
14. rapid breathing; hyperventilation

H

1. endotracheal intubation
2. lung scan
3. tuberculin tests
4. thoracentesis
5. pulmonary function tests
6. tracheostomy
7. bronchoscopy
8. bronchial alveolar lavage
9. laryngoscopy
10. pulmonary angiography
11. mediastinoscopy
12. tube thoracostomy

I

1. dyspnea on exertion. H
2. paroxysmal nocturnal dyspnea. A
3. metered-dose inhaler. E
4. cardiopulmonary resuscitation. I
5. non-small cell lung cancer. D
6. acute (adult) respiratory distress syndrome. J
7. chronic obstructive pulmonary disease. B
8. pulmonary function tests. G
9. purified protein derivative. C
10. diphtheria, pertussis, and tetanus. F

J

1. tonsillectomy
2. thoracentesis
3. rhinoplasty
4. thoracotomy
5. laryngectomy
6. lobectomy
7. thoracoscopy
8. pneumonectomy

K

1. thoracentesis
2. auscultation
3. PFTs
4. pneumonia
5. endotracheal tube

Answers to Practical Applications

1. C
2. B
3. A
4. B

X. Pronunciation of Terms

Pronunciation Guide

To test your understanding of the terminology in this chapter, write the meaning of each term in the space provided. In addition, you may wish to cover the terms and write them by looking at your definitions. Make sure your spelling is correct. The page number after each term indicates where it is defined or used in the text so you can easily check your responses.

ā as in āpe   ă as in ăpple
ē as in ēven   ĕ as in ĕvery
ī as in īce   ĭ as in ĭnterest
ō as in ōpen   ŏ as in pŏt
ū as in ūnit   ŭ as in ŭnder

Vocabulary and Terminology

Term	Pronunciation	Meaning
adenoidectomy (432)	ăd-ĕ-noyd-ĔK-tō-mē	_____
adenoid hypertrophy (432)	ĂD-ĕ-noyd hī-PĔR-trō-fē	_____
adenoids (430)	ĂD-ĕ-noydz	_____
alveolar (432)	ăl-VĒ-ō-lăr	_____
alveolus (alveoli) (430)	ăl-VĒ-ō-lŭs (ăl-VĒ-ō-lī)	_____
anosmia (436)	ăn-ŎS-mē-ă	_____
apex of the lung (430)	Ā-pĕkz of the lŭng	_____
apical (430)	Ā-pĭ-kăl	_____
apnea (436)	ăp-NĒ-ă	_____
asphyxia (436)	ăs-FĬK-sē-ă	_____
atelectasis (435)	ă-tĕ-LĔK-tă-sĭs	_____
bronchiectasis (432)	brŏng-kē-ĔK-tă-sĭs	_____
bronchiole (430)	BRŎNG-kē-ŏl	_____
bronchiolitis (432)	brŏng-kē-ō-LĪ-tĭs	_____
bronchodilator (432)	brŏng-kō-DĪ-lā-tĕr	_____
bronchospasm (432)	BRŎNG-kō-spăzm	_____
carbon dioxide (430)	KĂR-bŏn dī-ŎK-sīd	_____
cilia (430)	SĬL-ē-ă	_____

cyanosis (432)	sī-ă-NŌ-sĭs	_____
diaphragm (431)	DĪ-ă-frăm	_____
dysphonia (434)	dĭs-FŌ-nē-ă	_____
dyspnea (436)	DĬSP-nē-ă	_____
empyema (436)	ĕm-pī-Ē-mă	_____
epiglottis (431)	ĕp-ĭ-GLŎT-ĭs	_____
epiglottitis (432)	ĕp-ĭ-glŏ-TĪ-tĭs	_____
expectoration (434)	ĕk-spĕk-tō-RĀ-shŭn	_____
glottis (431)	GLŎ-tĭs	_____
hemoptysis (436)	hē-MŎP-tĭ-sĭs	_____
hemothorax (437)	hē-mŏ-THŌ-răks	_____
hilum of the lung (431)	HĪ-lŭm of the lŭng	_____
hypercapnia (432)	hī-pĕr-KĂP-nē-ă	_____
hyperpnea (436)	hī-PĔRP-nē-ă	_____
hypoxia (434)	hī-PŎK-sē-ă	_____
laryngeal (432)	lă-RĬN-jē-ăl or lăr-ĭn-JĒ-ăl	_____
laryngospasm (432)	lă-RĬNG-gō-spăzm	_____
laryngitis (432)	lă-rĭn-JĪ-tĭs	_____
larynx (431)	LĂR-ĭnks	_____
lobectomy (432)	lō-BĔK-tō-mē	_____
mediastinum (431)	mē-dē-ă-STĪ-nŭm	_____
nasogastric tube (434)	nā-zō-GĂS-trĭk toob	_____
nasopharyngitis (434)	nā-zō-făr-ĭn-JĪ-tĭs	_____
orthopnea (434)	ŏr-thŏp-NĒ-ă	_____
oxygen (431)	ŎKS-ĭ-jĕn	_____
palatine tonsils (431)	PĂL-ĭ-tīn TŎN-sĭlz	_____
paranasal sinuses (431)	pă-ră-NĀ-zăl SĪ-nĭ-sĕz	_____

parietal pleura (431)	pă-RĪ-ĕ-tăl PLOO-răh	_____
pharyngeal (434)	fă-RĬN-jē-ăl or făr-ĭn-JĒ-ăl	_____
pharynx (431)	FĂR-ĭnkz	_____
phrenic nerve (434)	FRĔN-ĭk nĕrv	_____
pleura (431)	PLOOR-ă	_____
pleural cavity (431)	PLOOR-ăl KĂ-vĭ-tē	_____
pleuritic (434)	ploo-RĬT-ĭk	_____
pneumoconiosis (432)	nū-mō-kō-nē-Ō-sĭs	_____
pneumonectomy (434)	nū-mō-NĔK-tō-mē	_____
pneumonitis (434)	nū-mō-NĪ-tĭs	_____
pneumothorax (434)	nū-mō-THŌ-răks	_____
pulmonary (434)	PŬL-mō-năr-ē	_____
pulmonary parenchyma (431)	pŭl-mō-NĂR-ē pă-RĔN-kă-mă	_____
pyothorax (437)	pī-ō-THŌ-răks	_____
rhinoplasty (434)	RĪ-nō-plăs-tē	_____
rhinorrhea (434)	rī-nō-RĒ-ăh	_____
sinusitis (435)	sī-nū-SĪ-tĭs	_____
spirometer (435)	spī-RŎM-ĕ-tĕr	_____
tachypnea (436)	tăk-ĭp-NĒ-ă	_____
thoracic (436)	thŏr-RĂ-sĭk	_____
thoracoscopy (447)	thŏr-ră-KŎS-kō-pē	_____
thoracotomy (436)	thŏr-ră-KŎT-ō-mē	_____
tonsillectomy (436)	tŏn-sĭ-LĔK-tō-mē	_____
trachea (431)	TRĀ-kē-ă	_____
tracheal stenosis (436)	TRĀ-kē-ăl stĕ-NŌ-sĭs	_____
tracheotomy (436)	trā-kē-ŎT-ō-mē	_____
visceral pleura (431)	VĬ-šer-ăl PLOO-ră	_____

Pathological Conditions, Laboratory Tests, and Clinical Procedures

Term	Pronunciation	Meaning
anthracosis (442)	ăn-thră-KŌ-sĭs	
asbestosis (442)	ăs-bĕs-TŌ-sĭs	
asthma (438)	ĂZ-mă	
atelectasis (440)	ă-tĕ-LĔK-tă-sĭs	
auscultation (437)	ăw-skŭl-TĀ-shŭn	
bacilli (442)	bă-SĬL-ī	
bronchial alveolar lavage (444)	BRŎNG-kē-ăl ăl-vē-Ō-lar lă-VĂJ	
bronchogenic carcinoma (439)	brŏng-kō-JĔN-ĭk kăr-sĭ-NŌ-mă	
bronchoscopy (444)	brŏng-KŎS-kō-pē	
chest tomograms (442)	chĕst TŌ-mō-grămz	
chronic bronchitis (439)	KRŎ-nĭk brŏng-KĪ-tĭs	
chronic obstructive pulmonary disease (442)	KRŎ-nĭk ŏb-STRŬK-tĭv PŬL-mō-nă-rē dĭ-ZĒZ	
cor pulmonale (442)	kŏr pŭl-mō-NĂ-lē	
croup (438)	kroop	
cystic fibrosis (439)	SĬS-tĭk fī-BRŌ-sĭs	
diphtheria (438)	dĭf-THĔR-ē-ă	
emphysema (440)	ĕm-fĭ-ZĒ-mă	
endotracheal intubation (444)	ĕn-dō-TRĀ-kē-ăl ĭn-tū-BĀ-shŭn	
epistaxis (438)	ĕp-ĭ-STĂK-sĭs	
hydrothorax (442)	hī-drō-THŎR-ăks	
laryngoscopy (444)	lăr-ĭng-GŎS-kō-pē	
lung scan (443)	lŭng skăn	
mediastinoscopy (444)	mē-dē-ă-stī-NŎS-kō-pē	
mesothelioma (441)	mĕz-ō-thē-lē-Ō-mă	

paroxysmal (442)	păr-ŏk-SĬZ-măl	
percussion (437)	pĕr-KŬSH-ŭn	
pertussis (438)	pĕr-TŬS-ĭs	
pleural effusion (441)	PLOOR-ăl ĕ-FŪ-zhŭn	
pleurisy (441)	PLOOR-ă-sē	
pneumonia (440)	nū-MŌ-nē-ă	
pulmonary abscess (440)	PŬL-mō-nă-rē ĂB-sĕs	
pulmonary angiography (442)	PŬL-mō-nă-rē ăn-jē-ŎG-ră-fē	
pulmonary edema (440)	PŬL-mō-nă-rē ĕ-DĒ-mă	
pulmonary embolism (440)	PŬL-mō-nă-rē ĔM-bō-lĭzm	
pulmonary function tests (444)	PŬL-mō-nă-rē FŬNK-shŭn tĕstz	
pulmonary infarction (442)	PŬL-mō-nă-rē ĭn-FĂRK-shŭn	
purulent (442)	PŪ-roo-lĕnt	
rales (437)	răhlz	
rhonchi (437)	RŎNG-kī	
sarcoidosis (441)	săr-koy-DŌ-sĭs	
silicosis (442)	sĭ-lĭ-KŌ-sĭs	
sputum (437)	SPŬ-tŭm	
stridor (437)	STRĪ-dŏr	
thoracentesis (447)	thō-ră-sĕn-TĒ-sĭs	
thoracoscopy (447)	thō-ră-KŎS-kō-pē	
tracheostomy (447)	trā-kē-ŎS-tō-mē	
tuberculin tests (447)	too-BĔR-kū-lĭn tĕstz	
tuberculosis (441)	too-bĕr-kū-LŌ-sĭs	
tube thoracostomy (447)	tūb thŏr-ă-KŎS-tō-mē	
wheezes (438)	wēz-ĕz	

XI. Review Sheet

Write the meanings of the word parts in the spaces provided. Check your answers with the information in the chapter or in the glossary (Medical Terms—English) at the end of the book.

COMBINING FORMS

Combining Form	Meaning	Combining Form	Meaning
adenoid/o	_____	pector/o	_____
alveol/o	_____	pharyng/o	_____
bronch/o	_____	phon/o	_____
bronchi/o	_____	phren/o	_____
bronchiol/o	_____	pleur/o	_____
capn/o	_____	pneum/o	_____
coni/o	_____	pneumon/o	_____
cyan/o	_____	pulmon/o	_____
epiglott/o	_____	py/o	_____
hydr/o	_____	rhin/o	_____
laryng/o	_____	sinus/o	_____
lob/o	_____	spir/o	_____
mediastin/o	_____	tel/o	_____
nas/o	_____	thorac/o	_____
or/o	_____	tonsill/o	_____
orth/o	_____	trache/o	_____
ox/o	_____		

Continued on following page

SUFFIXES

Suffix	Meaning	Suffix	Meaning
-algia	_____	-pnea	_____
-capnia	_____	-ptysis	_____
-centesis	_____	-rrhea	_____
-dynia	_____	-scopy	_____
-ectasis	_____	-sphyxia	_____
-ectomy	_____	-stenosis	_____
-lysis	_____	-stomy	_____
-osmia	_____	-thorax	_____
-oxia	_____	-tomy	_____
-phonia	_____	-trophy	_____
-plasty	_____		

PREFIXES

Prefix	Meaning	Prefix	Meaning
a-, an-	_____	hyper-	_____
brady-	_____	hypo-	_____
dys-	_____	para-	_____
em-	_____	per-	_____
eu-	_____	re-	_____
ex-	_____	tachy-	_____

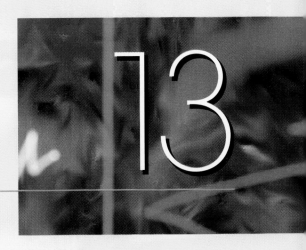

CHAPTER

Blood System

This chapter is divided into the following sections

In this chapter you will

- Identify terms relating to the composition, formation, and function of blood;
- Differentiate among the different types of blood groups;
- Identify terms related to blood clotting;
- Build words and recognize combining forms used in the blood system;
- Describe various pathological conditions affecting blood;
- Differentiate among various laboratory tests, clinical procedures, and abbreviations used in connection with the blood system; and
- Apply your new knowledge to understanding medical terms in their proper contexts, such as medical reports and records.

465

I. Introduction

The primary function of blood is to maintain a constant environment for the other living tissues of the body. Blood transports foods, gases, and wastes to and from the cells of the body. Food, digested in the stomach and small intestine, passes into the bloodstream through the lining cells of the small intestine. Blood then carries these nutrients to all body cells. Oxygen enters the body through the air sacs of the lungs. Blood cells then transport the oxygen to cells throughout the body. Blood also helps to remove the waste products released by cells. It carries gaseous waste (such as carbon dioxide) to the lungs to be exhaled. It carries solid waste, such as urea, to the kidneys to be expelled in the urine.

Chemical messengers called hormones are also carried by the blood from their sites of secretion in glands, such as the thyroid or pituitary, to distant sites where they regulate growth, reproduction, and energy production. These hormones will be discussed later in the endocrine chapter.

Finally, blood contains proteins and white blood cells that fight infection, and platelets (thrombocytes) that help the blood to clot.

II. Composition and Formation of Blood

Blood is composed of **cells,** or formed elements, suspended in a clear, straw-colored liquid called **plasma.** The cells constitute 45 per cent of the blood volume and include **erythrocytes** (red blood cells), **leukocytes** (white blood cells), and **platelets,** or **thrombocytes** (clotting cells). The remaining 55 per cent of blood is plasma, a solution of water, proteins, sugar, salts, hormones, and vitamins.

Cells

Most blood cells originate in the marrow cavity of bones. Both the red blood cells that carry oxygen and the white blood cells that fight infection arise from the same immature cells called **stem cells (hemocytoblasts).** Under the influence of proteins found in the bloodstream and bone marrow, the primitive stem cells change their size and shape and assume a specialized, or **differentiated,** form. In this process, the cells change in size from large (immature cells) to small (mature forms) and the cell nucleus shrinks (in red cells, the nucleus actually disappears). Figure 13–1 illustrates these changes in the formation of blood cells. Use Figure 13–1 only as a reference as you learn about the names of mature blood cells and their earlier forms. Don't try to memorize this intimidating chart!

Erythrocytes

As a red blood cell matures (from primitive erythroblast to normoblast to reticulocyte and finally to erythrocyte), it loses its nucleus and the cell assumes the shape of a disk. This shape (a depressed or hollow surface on each side of the cell, resembling a cough drop with a thin central portion) allows for a large surface area on the erythrocyte so that absorption and release of gases (oxygen and carbon dioxide) can take place. Red cells contain the unique protein **hemoglobin,** which consists of an iron-containing pigment called **heme** and a protein part called **globin.** Hemoglobin in the erythrocyte enables the cell to carry oxygen. The combination of oxygen and hemoglobin (oxyhemoglobin) produces the bright red color of blood.

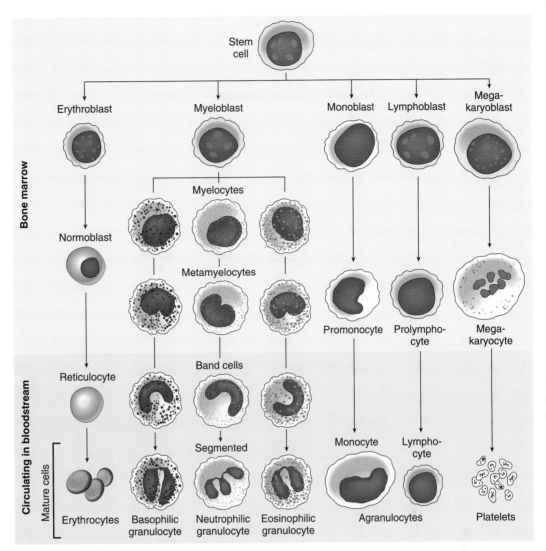

Figure 13-1

Stages in blood cell development (hematopoiesis). Notice that the suffix-blast is used to indicate immature forms of all cells. Band cells are identical to segmented granulocytes except that the nucleus is U-shaped and its lobes are connected by a band rather than by a thin thread, as are segmented forms.

Erythrocytes originate in the bone marrow. A hormone called **erythropoietin** (secreted by the kidney) stimulates their production (-*poiesis* means formation). Erythrocytes live and fulfill their role of transporting gases for about 120 days in the bloodstream. After this time, cells (called **macrophages**) in the spleen, liver, and bone marrow destroy the worn-out erythrocytes. Two to ten million red cells are destroyed each second, but because they are constantly replaced, the number of circulating cells remains constant (4–6 million per cu mm).

Macrophages breakdown erythrocytes and the hemoglobin within them into their heme and globin (protein) portions. The heme releases iron and decomposes into a dark green pigment called **bilirubin.** The iron in hemoglobin is reutilized to form new red cells or is stored in the spleen, liver, or bone marrow. Bilirubin is excreted into the bile by the liver, and from the bile it enters the small intestine where it can be

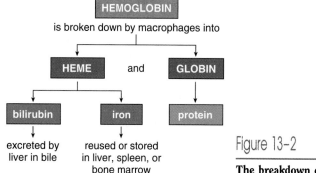

Figure 13-2

The breakdown of hemoglobin.

excreted in the stool. The green color then turns brown in the stool. Figure 13–2 reviews the sequence of events in hemoglobin breakdown.

Leukocytes

White blood cells (7000–9000 cells per cu mm) are less numerous than erythrocytes, but there are five different types of mature leukocytes. Figure 13–1 shows these five mature types of white blood cells: three granulocytic leukocytes (basophil, neutrophil, and eosinophil) and two agranulocytic leukocytes (monocyte and lymphocyte).

The **granulocytes,** also known as **polymorphonuclear leukocytes,** are the most numerous (about 60 per cent). Each is different and has a specialized function. **Basophils** contain dark-staining cytoplasmic granules that stain with a basic (alkaline) dye. The granules contain heparin (an anticlotting substance) and histamine (a chemical that is released in allergic responses). **Eosinophils** contain granules that stain with a red acidic dye called eosin. These granulocytes increase in numbers in allergic responses and are thought to engulf substances that trigger the allergies. **Neutrophils** contain granules that are neutral; that is, they do not stain intensely with either dye. Neutrophils are **phagocytes (phag/o** means to eat or swallow) that accumulate at sites of infection, where they ingest and destroy bacteria. Figure 13–3 shows phagocytosis by a neutrophil.

Granulocytes and their precursor cells are considered part of the **myeloid** (derived from bone marrow) line of cells. Their growth and proliferation in the bone marrow are stimulated by specific proteins called **colony-stimulating factors (CSFs). G-CSF** (granulocyte CSF), **GM-CSF** (granulocyte macrophage CSF), interleukin-1, and interleukin-3 have been produced commercially and are administered to promote or restore myeloid proliferation in cancer patients. Erythropoietin, like the colony-stimulating factors, is produced by recombinant DNA techniques and it stimulates red blood cell production.

Although all granulocytes are **polymorphonuclear** (they have multilobed nuclei), the term **polymorphonuclear leukocyte (poly)** is used most often to describe the **neutrophil,** which is the most numerous of the granulocytes.

Agranulocytes are **mononuclear** (containing one large nucleus) leukocytes that do not have dark-staining granules in their cytoplasm. These are the **lymphocytes** and **monocytes** (see Fig. 13–1). Lymphocytes arise in lymph nodes and circulate both in the bloodstream and in the parallel circulating system, the lymphatic system. They will be discussed in greater detail in Chapter 14, Lymphatic and Immune Systems.

Lymphocytes play an important role in the **immune** response that protects the body against infection. They can directly attack foreign matter and, in addition, make

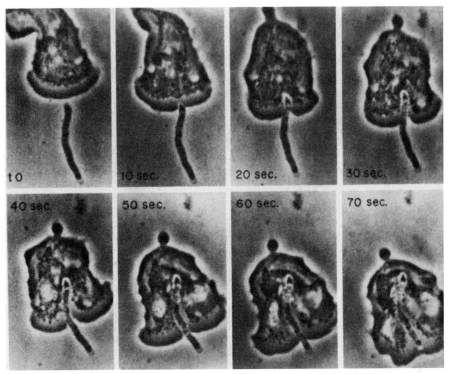

Figure 13-3

Phagocytosis (ingestion) of a bacterium by a neutrophil. (From Hirsch JG: Cinemicrophotographic observations of granule lysis in polymorphonuclear leucocytes during phagocytosis. J Exp Med 1962;116:827; by copyright permission of Rockefeller University Press.)

antibodies, which neutralize and destroy foreign **antigens** (bacteria and viruses). Monocytes are phagocytic cells that also fight disease. They move from the bloodstream into tissues (then they are called **macrophages**) and dispose of dead and dying cells and other tissue debris by phagocytosis.

Table 13–1 reviews the different types of leukocytes, their numbers in the blood, and their function.

Table 13-1. LEUKOCYTES

Leukocyte	Percentage in Blood	Function
GRANULOCYTE		
Basophil	0–1	Contains heparin (prevents blood from clotting) and histamine (involved in allergic responses)
Eosinophil	1–4	Phagocytic cell involved in allergic reactions
Neutrophil	50–70	Phagocytic cell that accumulates at sites of infection
AGRANULOCYTE		
Lymphocyte	20–40	Controls the immune response; makes antibodies to destroy antigens
Monocyte	3–8	Phagocytic cell that becomes a macrophage and digests bacteria and tissue debris

Platelets

Platelets, or thrombocytes, are formed in the red bone marrow from giant multinucleated cells called **megakaryocytes** (see Fig. 13–1). Tiny fragments of the megakaryocyte break off from the cell to form platelets. The main function of platelets is to help in the clotting of blood. The specific terms related to blood clotting will be discussed in a later section of this chapter.

Plasma

Plasma is the liquid part of the blood and consists of water, dissolved proteins, sugar, wastes, salts, hormones, and other substances. The four major plasma proteins are **albumin, globulin, fibrinogen,** and **prothrombin** (the last two proteins are clotting proteins).

Albumin maintains the proper proportion (and concentration) of water in the blood. Because albumin cannot pass easily through capillary walls, it remains in the blood and carries smaller molecules bound to its surface. It attracts water from the tissues back into the bloodstream and thus opposes the water's tendency to leave the blood and leak out into tissue spaces. **Edema** (swelling) results when too much fluid from blood "leaks" out into tissues. This happens in a mild form when a person ingests too much salt (water is retained in the blood and seeps out into tissues) and in a severe form when a person is burned in a fire. In this situation albumin escapes from capillaries as a result of the burn injury. Then water cannot be held in the blood; it escapes through the skin and blood volume drops.

The **globulin** portion of plasma contains antibodies that destroy foreign substances called antigens. There are three different kinds of globulins in plasma. They are **alpha, beta,** and **gamma,** and they can be separated by the process of **electrophoresis.** Plasma is placed in a special solution and an electric current is passed through the solution. The different protein molecules in the plasma separate out as they migrate at different speeds to the source of the electricity. Specific gamma globulins called **immunoglobulins** are capable of acting as antibodies. Examples of immunoglobulin antibodies are

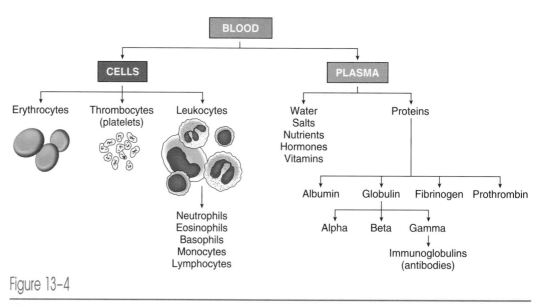

Figure 13–4

The composition of blood.

IgG (found in high concentration in the plasma) and **IgA** (found in breast milk, saliva, tears, and respiratory mucus). Other immunoglobulins are **IgM, IgD,** and **IgE.**

Plasmapheresis (-apheresis means to remove) is the process of separating plasma from the formed elements in the blood. This separation is mechanical, not electrical, as electrophoresis is. In plasmapheresis, the entire blood sample is spun in a centrifuge machine, and the plasma, being lighter in weight than the blood cells, moves to the top of the sample.

Figure 13–4 reviews the composition of blood.

III. Blood Groups

Transfusions of "whole blood" (cells and plasma) are used to replace blood lost after injury, during surgery, or in severe shock. A patient who is severely anemic and needs only red blood cells, will receive a transfusion of packed red cells (whole blood with most of the plasma removed). Transfusions cannot occur between any two people at random. Human blood falls into four main groups called A, B, AB, and O, and there are harmful effects of transfusing blood from a donor of one blood group into a recipient who has blood of another blood group.

Each of the blood groups has a specific combination of factors (**antigens** and **antibodies**) that are inherited. These antigen and antibody factors of the various blood types are:

Type A, containing **A antigen** and **anti-B antibody**
Type B, containing **B antigen** and **anti-A antibody**
Type AB, containing **A and B antigens** and **no anti-A or anti-B antibodies**
Type O, containing **no A or B antigens** and **both anti-A and anti-B antibodies**

The problem in transfusing blood from a type A donor into a type B recipient is that A antigens (from the A donor) will react adversely with the anti-A antibodies in the recipient's type B bloodstream. The adverse reaction is called **agglutination,** or clumping of the recipient's blood. The agglutination is fatal to the recipient because it stops the flow of blood. Similar problems can occur in other transfusions if the donor's antigens are incompatible with the recipient's antibodies.

People with type O blood are known as universal donors because their blood contains neither A nor B antigens. The anti-A and anti-B antibodies in O blood do not have an effect in the recipient because the antibodies are diluted in the recipient's bloodstream. Those with type AB blood are known as universal recipients because their blood contains neither anti-A nor anti-B antibodies, so that neither the A nor the B group antigens will cause agglutination in their blood.

Besides A and B antigens, there are many other antigens located on the surface of red blood cells. One of these is called the **Rh factor** (named because it was first found in the blood of a rhesus monkey). The term Rh-positive refers to a person who is born with the Rh antigen on her or his red blood cells. An Rh-negative person does not have the Rh antigen. There are no anti-Rh antibodies normally present in the blood of an Rh-positive or an Rh-negative person. However, if Rh-positive blood is transfused into an Rh-negative person, the recipient will begin to develop antibodies that would agglutinate any Rh-positive blood if another transfusion were to occur subsequently.

The same reactions occur during pregnancy if the fetus of an Rh-negative woman happens to be Rh-positive. This situation is described in Chapter 4 as an example of an antigen-antibody reaction.

Table 13-2. BLOOD GROUPS

Type	Percentage in Population	Red Cell Antigens	Plasma Antibodies
A	41	A	Anti-B
B	10	B	Anti-A
AB	4	A and B	Neither anti-A nor anti-B
O	45	Neither A nor B	Anti-A and anti-B
Rh positive	85	Rh factor	No anti-Rh
Rh negative	15	No Rh factor	Anti-Rh (occurs if an Rh-negative person is given Rh-positive blood)

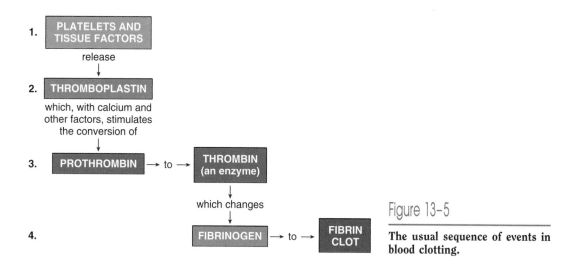

1. **PLATELETS AND TISSUE FACTORS**

release

2. **THROMBOPLASTIN**

which, with calcium and other factors, stimulates the conversion of

3. **PROTHROMBIN** → to → **THROMBIN (an enzyme)**

which changes

4. **FIBRINOGEN** → to → **FIBRIN CLOT**

Figure 13-5

The usual sequence of events in blood clotting.

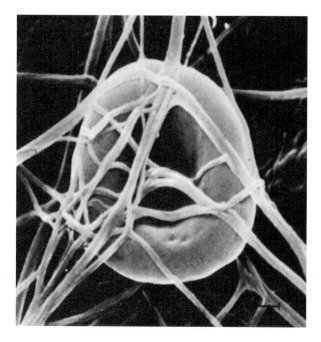

Figure 13-6

A red blood cell enmeshed in threads of fibrin. (From Page J, et al: Blood: The River of Life. Washington, DC, U.S. News Books, 1981, p 79.)

Table 13–2 shows the blood group types, their frequency of occurrence in the population, and their antigens and antibodies.

IV. Blood Clotting

Blood clotting, or **coagulation,** is a complicated process involving many different substances and chemical reactions. The final result (usually taking less than 15 minutes) is the formation of a **fibrin clot** from the plasma protein **fibrinogen.** Platelets are important in beginning the process following injury to tissues or blood vessels. The platelets clump, or aggregate, at the site of injury, releasing a protein, **thromboplastin,** which in combination with **calcium** and the sequential release of clotting factors (I–V and VII–XIII) promotes the formation of a fibrin clot. One of the clotting factors is a protein known as clotting factor VIII. It is missing in people who are born with hemophilia. Figure 13–5 reviews the basic sequence of events in the clotting process.

The fibrin threads form the clot by trapping red blood cells and platelets and plasma (Fig. 13–6 shows a red blood cell trapped by fibrin threads). Then the clot retracts into a tight ball, leaving behind a clear fluid called **serum.** Normally, clots (thrombi) do not form in blood vessels unless the vessel is damaged or the flow of blood is impeded. Anticoagulant substances in the bloodstream inhibit blood clotting, so thrombi and emboli (floating clots) do not form. **Heparin,** produced by tissue cells (especially liver cells), is an example of an anticoagulant. Other drugs (such as dicumarol) are given to patients with thromboembolic diseases to prevent the formation of clots.

V. Vocabulary

This list will help you review many of the new terms introduced in the text. Short definitions will reinforce your understanding of the terms. See Section XII of this chapter for help in pronouncing the more difficult terms.

agglutination   Clumping of recipient's blood cells when incompatible bloods are mixed.

albumin   Protein found in blood; maintains the proper amount of water in the blood. Also called **serum albumin.**

antibodies   Protein substances whose formation by lymphocytes is stimulated by the presence of antigens in the body. An antibody then helps to neutralize or inactivate the antigen that stimulated its formation.

antigens   Foreign materials that stimulate the production of an antibody. Naturally occurring antigens are the blood type factors A and B that are present at birth in some individuals.

basophil   White blood cell with large, dark, basic-staining granules.

bilirubin	Dark green pigment produced from hemoglobin when red blood cells are destroyed. Bilirubin is concentrated in bile by the liver and excreted in the feces.
coagulation	The process of blood clotting.
colony-stimulating factors	Proteins that stimulate the growth and proliferation of white blood cells (granulocytes).
corpuscle	Little body—refers to a blood cell.
differentiation	Change in structure and function of a cell as it matures; specialization.
electrophoresis	Method of separating substances (such as proteins) by electrical charge.
eosinophil	White blood cell with dense, reddish granules; associated with allergic reactions.
erythrocyte	A red blood cell. There are about 5 million in a speck of blood the size of a pinhead.
erythropoietin	A hormone secreted by the kidney that stimulates bone marrow to make red blood cells.
fibrin	Protein threads that form the basis of a blood clot.
fibrinogen	Plasma protein that is converted to fibrin in the clotting process.
formed elements	The cellular elements in blood.
globin	The protein part of hemoglobin.
globulin	Plasma protein is separated by electrophoresis into alpha, beta, and gamma globulins.
granulocytes	White blood cells with granules: eosinophils, neutrophils, and basophils.
heme	Iron-containing nonprotein portion of the hemoglobin molecule.
hemoglobin	Blood protein found in red blood cells; carries oxygen.
heparin	An anticoagulant produced by liver cells and found in blood and tissues.
immune reaction	Process by which an antibody neutralizes or inactivates an antigen.
immunoglobulin	A protein (globulin) with antibody activity; examples are IgG, IgM, IgA, IgE, IgD. Immun/o means protection.

leukocyte	A white blood cell.
lymphocyte	White blood cell (agranulocyte) that produces antibodies.
macrophages	Monocytes that have migrated from the blood to tissue spaces. They are large phagocytes that destroy red blood cells at the end of their 120-day life span. They also engulf foreign material in body tissues.
megakaryocyte	Platelet precursor formed in the bone marrow.
monocyte	A phagocytic white blood cell (agranulocyte) formed in bone marrow. Monocytes become macrophages as they leave the blood and enter body tissues.
myeloid	Derived from (-oid) bone marrow cells.
neutrophil	White blood cell (granulocyte) formed in bone marrow; a phagocyte with neutral-staining granules; also called a **polymorphonuclear leukocyte,** or **"poly."**
plasma	Liquid portion of blood; contains water, proteins, salts, nutrients, hormones, and vitamins.
plasmapheresis	Process of using a centrifuge to separate (-apheresis) or remove the formed elements from the blood plasma. Formed elements are retransfused into the donor, and fresh-frozen plasma is used to replace withdrawn plasma. The procedure may be done to collect plasma for analysis or therapy.
platelet	Smallest formed element in the blood; a thrombocyte.
prothrombin	Plasma protein; converted to thrombin in the clotting process.
reticulocyte	Developing red blood cell with a network of granules in its cytoplasm.
Rh factor	An antigen normally found on red blood cells of Rh-positive individuals.
serum	Plasma minus clotting proteins and cells.
stem cell	A cell in bone marrow that gives rise to different types of blood cells.
thrombin	Enzyme that helps convert fibrinogen to fibrin during coagulation.
thrombocyte	Platelet.
thromboplastin	A clotting factor that, in combination with calcium, promotes the formation of the fibrin clot.

VI. Combining Forms, Suffixes, and Terminology

Write the meanings of the medical terms in the spaces provided.

Combining Forms

Combining Form	Meaning	Terminology	Meaning
agglutin/o	clumping, sticking together	agglutination _____ *-ation means process.*	
baso/o	base (*alkaline, the opposite of acid*)	basophil _____ *-phil means attraction to.*	
chrom/o	color	hypochromia _____ *Reduction in the hemoglobin in red blood cells.*	
coagul/o	clotting	anticoagulant _____	
cyt/o	cell	cytology _____	
eosin/o	red, dawn, rosy	eosinophil _____	
erythr/o	red	erythrocytopenia _____ *-penia means deficiency.*	
granul/o	granules	granulocyte _____	
hem/o	blood	hemolysis _____ *Destruction of red blood cells. See hemolytic anemia, page 480, Section VII, Pathological Conditions.*	
hemat/o	blood	hematocrit _____ *-crit means to separate. The hematocrit gives the percentage of red blood cells in a volume of blood. See page 485, Section VIII, under Laboratory Tests.*	
hemoglobin/o	hemoglobin	hemoglobinopathy _____	

is/o	same, equal	anisocytosis _____

This term refers to an abnormality of red blood cells; they are of unequal (anis/o) size; -cytosis means a slight increase in numbers of cells.

kary/o	nucleus	megakaryocyte _____

leuk/o	white	leukocytopenia _____

Can be shortened to leukopenia.

mon/o	one, single	monocyte _____

The cell has a single, rather than a multilobed, nucleus.

morph/o	shape, form	morphology _____

myel/o	bone marrow	myeloblast _____

-blast indicates an immature cell.

neutr/o	neutral (neither base nor acid)	neutropenia _____

This term refers to neutrophils.

nucle/o	nucleus	mononuclear _____
		polymorphonuclear _____

phag/o	eat, swallow	phagocyte _____

poikil/o	varied, irregular	poikilocytosis _____

Irregularity in the shape of red blood cells. Poikilocytosis occurs in certain types of anemia.

sider/o	iron	sideropenia _____

spher/o	globe, round	spherocytosis _____

In this condition, the erythrocyte has a round shape, making the cell very fragile and easily able to be destroyed.

thromb/o	clot	thrombocytopenia _____

Suffixes

Suffix	Meaning	Terminology	Meaning
-apheresis	removal, carry away	plasmapheresis _____	

A centrifuge is used to spin blood in order to separate or remove the plasma from the other parts of blood.

leukapheresis _____

plateletpheresis _____

Note that the a of apheresis is dropped in this term. Platelets are removed from the donor's blood (and used in a patient), and the remainder of the blood is retransfused into the donor.

-blast	immature, embryonic	monoblast _____	

erythroblast _____

-cytosis	abnormal condition of cells (slight increase in cell numbers)	macrocytosis _____	

This term refers to red blood cells (macrocytes) that are larger (macro-) than normal size.

microcytosis _____

This term refers to red blood cells that are smaller (micro-) than normal size. Table 13–3 reviews terms related to abnormalities of red blood cell morphology.

Table 13-3. ABNORMALITIES OF RED BLOOD CELL MORPHOLOGY

Abnormality	Description
Anisocytosis	Cells are **unequal** in size
Hypo**chrom**ia	**Color** of cells is reduced (less hemoglobin)
Macrocytosis	Cells are **large**
Microcytosis	Cells are **small**
Poikilocytosis	Cells are **irregularly shaped**
Spherocytosis	Cells are **rounded**

-emia	blood condition	leukemia _____
		See page 482, Section VII, Pathological Conditions.
-globin	protein	hemoglobin _____
-globulin	protein	gamma globulin _____
-lytic	pertaining to destruction	thrombolytic therapy _____
-oid	resembling, derived from	myeloid _____
-osis	abnormal condition	thrombosis _____
-penia	deficiency	granulocytopenia _____
		pancytopenia _____
-phage	eat, swallow	macrophage _____
-philia	attraction for (an increase in cell numbers)	eosinophilia _____
		neutrophilia _____
-phoresis	carrying, transmission	electrophoresis _____
-poiesis	formation	hematopoiesis _____
		erythropoiesis _____
		Erythropoietin is produced by the kidney to stimulate red blood cell formation.
		myelopoiesis _____
-stasis	stop, control	hemostasis _____

VII. Pathological Conditions

Any abnormal or pathological condition of the blood is generally referred to as a blood **dyscrasia** (disease). The blood dyscrasias discussed in this section are organized in the following manner: diseases of red blood cells, disorders of blood clotting, diseases of white blood cells, and bone marrow disease.

Diseases of Red Blood Cells

anemia

Deficiency in erythrocytes or hemoglobin.

The most common type of anemia is **iron-deficiency anemia;** it is caused by a lack of iron, which is required for hemoglobin production (Fig. 13–7). Other types of anemia include:

1. aplastic anemia

Failure of blood cell production due to aplasia (absence of development, formation) **of bone marrow cells.**

The cause of most cases of aplastic anemia is unknown (idiopathic), but some cases have been linked to benzene exposure and to antibiotics such as chloramphenicol. **Pancytopenia** occurs as stem cells fail to produce leukocytes, platelets, and erythrocytes. Blood transfusions prolong life until the marrow resumes its normal functioning, and antibiotics are used to control infections. Bone marrow transplants (see Section VIII, under Clinical Procedures) have been successful as therapy.

2. hemolytic anemia

Reduction in red cells due to excessive destruction.

One example of hemolytic anemia is **congenital spherocytic anemia** (also called **hereditary spherocytosis**). Instead of their normal biconcave shape, erythrocytes are spheroidal. This shape makes them very fragile and easily able to be destroyed (hemolysis), which leads to anemia. The spherocytosis causes increased numbers of reticulocytes in the circulating blood as the bone marrow attempts to compensate for the hemolysis of mature erythrocytes. The excessive hemolysis leads to jaundice because of accumulation of bilirubin in the circulating bloodstream. Because cells in the spleen destroy red cells, the spleen may be removed with helpful results. In some cases, hemolytic anemia is due to production of **autoimmune** antibodies that destroy red cells. Figure 13–8 shows the altered shape of erythrocytes in hereditary spherocytosis.

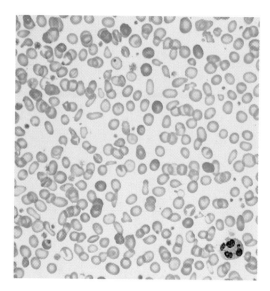

Figure 13–7

Iron-deficiency anemia. Note the small red blood cells containing a narrow rim of hemoglobin at the periphery. These cells are hypochromic and microcytic. Notice that some scattered cells are fully hemoglobinized. These were derived from a recent blood transfusion given to the patient. (Courtesy of Dr. Robert W. McKenna, Department of Pathology, University of Texas Southwestern Medical School, Dallas, TX; from Kumar V, Cotran RS, Robbins SL: Basic Pathology, 6th ed. Philadelphia, WB Saunders, 1997, p 354.)

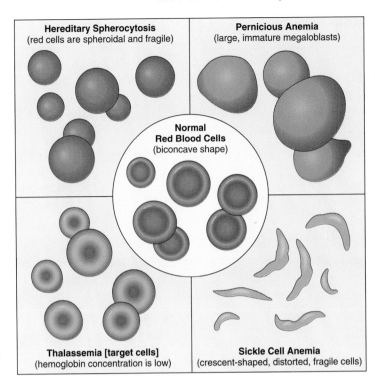

Figure 13–8

Normal red blood cells and
several types of anemia.

3. pernicious anemia

Lack of mature erythrocytes owing to inability to absorb vitamin B$_{12}$ into the body. (Pernicious means ruinous or hurtful.)

Vitamin B$_{12}$ is necessary for the proper development and maturation of erythrocytes. Although vitamin B$_{12}$ is a common constituent of food matter (liver, kidney, sardines, egg yolks, oysters), it cannot be absorbed into the bloodstream without the aid of a special substance called **intrinsic factor** that is normally found in gastric juice. Individuals with pernicious anemia lack this factor in their gastric juice, and the result is unsuccessful maturation of red blood cells, with an excess of large, immature, and poorly functioning cells **(megaloblasts)** in the circulation. Treatment is administration of vitamin B$_{12}$ for life. Figure 13–8 illustrates megaloblasts in pernicious anemia.

4. sickle cell anemia

A hereditary condition characterized by abnormal shape of erythrocytes and by hemolysis.

The crescent, or sickle, shape of the erythrocyte is caused by an abnormal type of hemoglobin (hemoglobin S) in the red cell (see Fig. 13–8). The distorted, fragile erythrocytes are poorly oxygenated and clump together, blocking blood vessels, leading to thrombosis and infarction (dead tissue). Symptoms include arthralgias, acute attacks of abdominal pain, and ulcerations of the extremities. The genetic defect (presence of the hemoglobin S gene) is particularly prevalent in black persons of African or African-American ancestry and appears with different degrees of severity, depending on the inheritance of one or two genes for the trait.

5. thalassemia

An inherited defect in the ability to produce hemoglobin, usually seen in persons of Mediterranean (*thalassa* is a Greek word meaning sea) **background.**

This condition presents in varying forms and degrees of severity (the most severe form is called **Cooley's anemia**), usually leads to hypochromic anemia (diminished hemoglobin content in red cells) (see Fig. 13–8).

hemochromatosis	**Excessive deposits of iron throughout the body.**

Hepatomegaly occurs and the skin is pigmented, so that it has a bronze hue; diabetes can occur and cardiac failure commonly develops. The condition is usually seen in men over 40 years of age.

polycythemia vera	**General increase in red blood cells (erythremia).**

Blood consistency is viscous (sticky) because of greatly increased numbers of erythrocytes. The bone marrow is hyperplastic, and leukocytosis and thrombocytosis accompany the increase in red blood cells. Treatment consists of reduction of red cell volume to normal levels by phlebotomy (removal of blood from a vein) and by suppressing production with myelotoxic drugs.

Disorders of Blood Clotting

hemophilia	**Excessive bleeding caused by a congenital** (hereditary) **lack of one of the protein substances (factor VIII) necessary for blood clotting.**

Although the platelet count of a hemophiliac patient is normal, there is a marked deficiency in a plasma clotting factor (factor VIII), which results in a very prolonged coagulation time. Treatment consists of administration of the deficient factor.

purpura	**Multiple pinpoint hemorrhages and accumulation of blood under the skin.**

Purpura means purple, and in this bleeding condition, hemorrhages into the skin and mucous membranes produce red-purple discoloration of the skin. The bleeding is caused by a fall in the number of platelets (thrombocytopenia). The cause of the disorder may be immunological, meaning the body produces an antiplatelet factor that harms its own platelets. **Idiopathic thrombocytopenic purpura** is a condition in which a patient makes an antibody that destroys his or her own platelets. Bleeding time is prolonged and the cause is unknown. Splenectomy (the spleen is the site of platelet destruction) and drug therapy with corticosteroids to discourage antibody synthesis are methods of treatment. Purpura is also seen in any other condition associated with a low platelet count, such as leukemia and drug reactions.

Diseases of White Blood Cells

leukemia	**An increase in cancerous white blood cells.**

This is a disease of the bone marrow in which malignant leukocytes fill the marrow and bloodstream. There are several types of leukemia, determined according to the particular leukocyte involved. The terms **acute** and **chronic** are used to refer to a large number of immature (in acute forms) or mature, differentiated (in chronic forms) leukocytes in the blood.

Acute leukemias have several common clinical characteristics: abrupt, stormy onset of symptoms, fatigue, fever and bleeding, bone pain and tenderness, lymphadenopathy, splenomegaly and hepatomegaly, and CNS symptoms, such as headache, vomiting, and paralysis. Four types of leukemia are:

acute myelogenous (myelocytic) leukemia (AML) — Immature granulocytes (myeloblasts) predominate. Platelets and erythrocytes are diminished because of infiltration and replacement of the bone marrow by large numbers of myeloblasts (Fig. 13–9A).

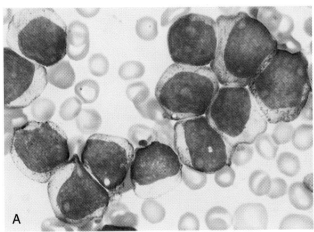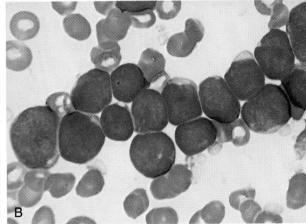

Figure 13-9

Acute leukemia. (A) Acute myeloblastic leukemia. Myeloblasts (immature granulocytes) predominate. AML affects primarily adults. The majority of patients achieve remission with intensive chemotherapy, but relapse is common. Bone marrow transplantation may be a curative therapy. **(B) Acute lymphoblastic leukemia.** Lymphoblasts (immature lymphocytes) predominate. ALL is a disease of children and young adults. Most children are cured with chemotherapy. (Courtesy of Dr. Robert W. McKenna, Department of Pathology, University of Texas Southwestern Medical School, Dallas, TX; from Kumar V, Cotran RS, Robbins SL: Basic Pathology, 6th ed. Philadelphia, WB Saunders, 1997, p 375.)

acute lymphocytic leukemia (ALL) — Immature lymphocytes (lymphoblasts) predominate. This form is seen most often in children and adolescents; onset is sudden (Figure 13–9B).

chronic myelogenous (myelocytic) leukemia (CML) — Both mature and immature granulocytes are present in the marrow and bloodstream. This is a slowly progressive illness with which patients may live for many years without encountering life-threatening problems.

chronic lymphocytic leukemia (CLL) — Abnormal numbers of relatively mature lymphocytes predominate in the marrow, lymph nodes, and spleen. This form of leukemia usually occurs in the elderly and follows a slowly progressive course.

All forms of leukemia are treated with chemotherapy, using drugs that prevent cell division and selectively injure rapidly dividing cells. Effective treatment can lead to a **remission** (disappearance of signs of disease). **Relapse** occurs when leukemia cells reappear in the blood and bone marrow, necessitating further treatment.

Transplantation of normal bone marrow from closely related donors is successful in restoring normal bone marrow function in some patients with acute leukemia. This procedure is performed following high-dose chemotherapy, which is administered to eliminate the leukemic cells.

granulocytosis

Abnormal increase in granulocytes in the blood.

An increase in granulocytes in the blood may occur in response to infection or inflammation of any type. **Eosinophilia** is an increase in eosinophilic granulocytes, which is seen in certain allergic conditions, such as asthma, or in parasitic infections (tapeworm, pinworm). **Basophilia** is an increase in basophilic granulocytes seen in certain types of leukemia.

mononucleosis	**An infectious disease evidenced by increased numbers of lymphocytes and enlarged cervical lymph nodes.**

This disease is caused by the Epstein-Barr virus (EBV). Lymphadenitis is present, with fever, fatigue, asthenia (weakness), and pharyngitis. Atypical lymphocytes are present in the blood, liver (hepatomegaly), and spleen (splenomegaly).

Mononucleosis is usually transmitted by direct oral contact (salivary exchange during kissing) and affects primarily young adults. No treatment is necessary for EBV infections. Antibiotics are not effective for self-limited viral illnesses. Rest during the period of acute symptoms and slow return to normal activities is advised.

Diseases of Bone Marrow Cells

multiple myeloma	**Malignant tumor of bone marrow.**

This is a progressive tumor of antibody-producing cells (called **plasma cells**). The malignant cells invade the bone marrow and destroy bony structures. The tumors cause overproduction of immunoglobulins and **Bence Jones protein,** an immunoglobulin fragment found in urine. Often, the condition leads to osteolytic lesions, hypercalcemia, anemia, renal damage, and increased susceptibility to infection. Treatment is with analgesics, radiotherapy, **palliative** (relieving, not curing) doses of chemotherapy, and special orthopedic supports.

VIII. Laboratory Tests, Clinical Procedures, and Abbreviations

Laboratory Tests

antiglobulin test (Coombs test)	Demonstrates whether the patient's erythrocytes are coated with antibody and is useful in determining the presence of antibodies in infants of Rh− women or in patients with autoimmune hemolytic anemia.
bleeding time	The time it takes for a small puncture wound to stop bleeding. Normal time is 8 minutes or less. Bleeding time is prolonged with use of aspirin and in platelet disorders such as thrombocytopenia. There are several testing methods, but the most widely used is the Simplate (an incision is made while constant pressure is applied using a sphygmomanometer).
complete blood count (CBC)	This usually includes the following studies: red blood cell count, white blood cell count (with differential), platelet count, hemoglobin test, hematocrit, and red cell indices—MCH, MCV, MCHC (see Abbreviations). These routine tests are performed by automatic machines.
coagulation (clotting) time	Time required for venous blood to clot in a test tube. Normal time is less than 15 minutes.

erythrocyte sedimentation rate (sed rate or ESR)	Speed at which erythrocytes settle out of plasma. Venous blood is collected, anticoagulant is added, and the blood is placed in a tube in a vertical position. The distance that the erythrocytes fall in a given period of time is the sedimentation rate. The rate is altered in disease conditions, such as infections, joint inflammation, and tumor, that increase the immunoglobulin content of the blood.
hematocrit (Hct)	Percentage of erythrocytes in a volume of blood. A sample of blood is spun in a centrifuge so that the erythrocytes fall to the bottom of the sample.
hemoglobin test (Hb, Hgb)	Total amount of hemoglobin in a sample of peripheral blood.
partial thromboplastin time	Measures the presence of factors that act at early points in the coagulation pathway. This test is used to follow patients taking certain blood thinners (anticoagulants).
platelet count	Number of platelets per cubic millimeter. Platelets normally average between 200,000 and 400,000 per cu mm.
prothrombin time	This is a test of the ability of blood to clot. It measures the time elapsed between the addition of calcium to a plasma sample and the appearance of a visible clot. The test is also used to follow patients taking certain blood thinners (anticoagulants).
red blood cell count (RBC)	Number of erythrocytes per cubic millimeter of blood. The normal number is 4–6 million per cu mm.
red blood cell morphology	A stained blood smear is examined to determine the shape or form of individual red cells. The presence of anisocytosis, poikilocytosis, sickle cells, and hypochromia can be noted.
white blood cell count (WBC)	This is the number of leukocytes per cubic millimeter. Automatic counting devices can record the numbers within seconds. Leukocytes normally average between 5000 and 10,000 per cu mm.
white blood cell differential	This test determines the numbers of different types of leukocytes (immature and mature forms). The cells are stained and counted under a microscope by a technician. A minimum of 100 cells is counted, and the percentages of neutrophils, lymphocytes, monocytes, basophils, and eosinophils are given. The term "left shift" is used to describe a condition in which there is an increase in immature neutrophils and a decrease in mature forms in the blood.

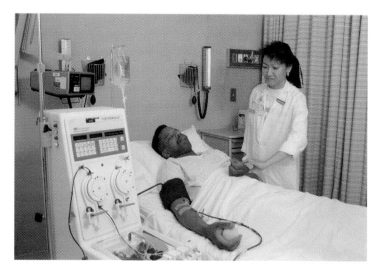

Figure 13–10

Leukapheresis. This machine is an automated blood cell separator that removes large numbers of white blood cells and returns red cells, platelets, and plasma to the individual. (From Black JM, Matassarin-Jacobs E: Medical-Surgical Nursing, 5th ed. Philadelphia, WB Saunders, 1997, p 1491.)

Clinical Procedures

apheresis

Separation of blood into its parts. It is performed to remove toxic substances or autoantibodies from the blood or to harvest blood cells. Leukapheresis, plateletpheresis, and plasmapheresis are examples (Fig. 13–10).

blood transfusion

In this procedure, whole blood or cells are taken from a donor, and after appropriate testing to ensure a close match of red cell or platelet type, the whole blood or cells are infused into a patient. Also prior to transfusion, tests are performed to ensure that the specimen is free of hepatitis and the acquired immunodeficiency syndrome (AIDS) virus. **Autologous transfusion** is the collection and later reinfusion of a patient's own (auto- means self) blood or blood components.

bone marrow biopsy

A needle is introduced into the bone marrow cavity, and a small amount of marrow is aspirated and examined under a microscope. This procedure is helpful in the diagnosis of blood disorders such as anemia, cytopenias, and leukemia.

bone marrow transplant

Bone marrow cells from a donor whose tissue and blood cells closely match those of the recipient are infused into a patient with leukemia or aplastic anemia. First the patient is given total-body irradiation or aggressive chemotherapy to kill all diseased cells and much of the normal bone marrow. The donor's marrow is then intravenously infused into the patient, and it repopulates the patient's marrow space with normal cells. Problems encountered subsequently may be serious infection, **graft versus host disease** (immune reaction of the donor's cells to the recipient's), and relapse of the original disease (such as leukemia) despite the treatment (Fig. 13–11).

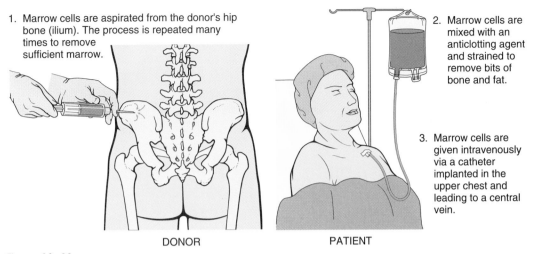

1. Marrow cells are aspirated from the donor's hip bone (ilium). The process is repeated many times to remove sufficient marrow.

2. Marrow cells are mixed with an anticlotting agent and strained to remove bits of bone and fat.

3. Marrow cells are given intravenously via a catheter implanted in the upper chest and leading to a central vein.

DONOR   PATIENT

Figure 13–11

Bone marrow transplantation. This is an **allogeneic** (all/o means other, different) **transplant** in which a relative or unrelated person having a close HLA (human leukocyte antigen) type is the donor. It has a high rate of morbidity (causing disease) and mortality (causing death) because of complications of incompatibility such as GVHD (graft versus host disease). In an **autologous transplant,** bone marrow is removed from the patient during a remission phase and given back to the patient after intensive chemotherapy (drug treatment). In a **stem cell transplant,** stem cells are harvested (removed) from the peripheral blood of the patient and then reinfused into the bloodstream when necessary.

ABBREVIATIONS

ABO	three main blood types	**GVHD**	graft versus host disease
ALL	acute lymphocytic leukemia	**Hct**	hematocrit
AML	acute myelogenous leukemia	**Hb, Hgb**	hemoglobin
baso	basophils	**HLA**	human leukocyte antigen
BMT	bone marrow transplant	**IgA, IgD, IgE, IgG, IgM**	immunoglobulins
CBC	complete blood count		
CLL	chronic lymphocytic leukemia	**lymphs**	lymphocytes
CML	chronic myelogenous leukemia	**MCH**	mean corpuscular hemoglobin, average amount of hemoglobin per cell
DIC	disseminated intravascular coagulation	**MCHC**	mean corpuscular hemoglobin concentration, average concentration of hemoglobin in a single red cell. When MCHC is low, the cell is hypochromic.
diff.	differential count (white blood cells)		
EBV	Epstein-Barr virus, the cause of mononucleosis	**MCV**	mean corpuscular volume, average volume or size of a single red blood cell. When MCV is high, the cells are macrocytic, and when low, the cells are microcytic.
eos	eosinophils		
Epo	erythropoietin		
ESR	erythrocyte sedimentation rate	**mono**	monocyte
G-CSF	granulocyte colony-stimulating factor	**poly, PMN, PMNL**	polymorphonuclear leukocyte
GM-CSF	granulocyte macrophage colony-stimulating factor	**PT**	prothrombin time

PTT	partial thromboplastin time	**SMAC**	Sequential Multiple Analyzer Computer, an automated chemistry system that determines substances in serum
RBC	red blood cell (red blood cell count)	**WBC**	white blood cell (white blood cell count)
sed rate	erythrocyte sedimentation rate		
segs	segmented, mature white blood cells		

IX. Practical Applications

Answers to the questions are on page 498 after Answers to Exercises.

Normal Laboratory Values

WBC 5000–10,000/cu mm
Differential:
   Segs (polys)   54–62%
   Lymphs   20–40%
   Eos   1–3%
   Baso   0–1%
   Mono   3–7%

RBC (M) 4.5–6.0 million
      (F) 4.0–5.5 million
Hct (M) 40–50%
      (F) 37–47%
Hgb (M) 14–16 gm/dL
      (F) 12–14 gm/dL
Platelets 200,000–400,000/cu mm

Three Short Cases

1. A 65-year-old Swedish lady visits her physician complaining of shortness of breath and swollen ankles. Lab tests reveal that her hematocrit is 18.0 and her hemoglobin 5.8. Her blood smear shows megaloblasts and her blood level of vitamin B_{12} is very low. What is a likely diagnosis?
   (A) aplastic anemia
   (B) hemochromatosis
   (C) pernicious anemia

2. A 22-year-old college student visits the clinic with a fever and complaining of a sore throat. Blood tests show a WBC of 28,000 with 95% myeloblasts (polys are 5%). Platelet count is 15,000, hemoglobin is 10, hematocrit is 22.5. What is your diagnosis?
   (A) chronic lymphocytic leukemia
   (B) acute myelogenous leukemia
   (C) thalassemia

3. A 35-year-old female goes to her physician complaining of spots on her legs and bleeding gums. On examination, she has minute purple spots covering her legs and evidence of dried blood in her mouth. Her CBC shows hemoglobin 14, hematocrit 42, WBC 5000 with normal differential, platelet count 4000 (with megakaryocytes in bone marrow). What is your diagnosis?
   (A) sickle cell anemia
   (B) hemolytic anemia
   (C) idiopathic thrombocytopenic purpura

Multiple Myeloma

Multiple myeloma is a neoplastic proliferation of plasma cells. The clinical manifestations of the disease result from the effects of the myeloma tumor cell mass in the bone marrow as well as from the myeloma proteins produced by the malignant cells. The effects of the tumor cell mass include lytic skeletal lesions, hypercalcemia, anemia, leukopenia, and thrombocytopenia. Clinical features related to the myeloma proteins include hyperviscosity [excessive stickiness], coagulopathy, and renal insufficiency [tubules get plugged with protein material].

X. Exercises

Remember to check your answers carefully with those given in Section XI, Answers to Exercises.

A. *Match the following cells with their meanings as given below.*

eosinophil   lymphocyte   monocyte
stem cell   platelet   neutrophil
basophil   erythrocyte

1. white blood cell (agranulocyte) formed in lymph tissue; it is a phagocyte and the precursor of a

   macrophage _____

2. thrombocyte or cell that helps blood clot _____

3. cell in the bone marrow that gives rise to different types of blood cells _____

4. leukocyte formed in lymph tissue; produces antibodies _____

5. leukocyte with dense, reddish granules having an affinity for red acid dye; associated with allergic

   reactions _____

6. red blood cell _____

7. leukocyte (polymorphonuclear granulocyte) formed in the bone marrow and having neutral-straining granules _____

8. leukocyte (granulocyte) whose granules have an affinity for basic dye; releases histamine and

   heparin _____

B. Give the meanings of the following terms that relate to blood cells.

1. corpuscle _____

2. granulocyte _____

3. mononuclear _____

4. polymorphonuclear _____

5. agranulocyte _____

6. erythroblast _____

7. megakaryocyte _____

8. macrophage _____

9. hemoglobin _____

10. myeloid _____

11. reticulocyte _____

12. myeloblast _____

C. Give the medical terms for the following descriptions.

1. liquid portion of blood _____

2. dark green pigment produced from hemoglobin when red blood cells are destroyed

   _____

3. iron-containing nonprotein part of hemoglobin _____

4. protein in plasma; can be separated into alpha, beta, and gamma types _____

5. hormone secreted by the kidneys to stimulate bone marrow to produce red blood cells

   _____

6. foreign material that stimulates the production of an antibody _____

7. plasma protein that maintains the proper amount of water in the blood _____

8. proteins made by lymphocytes in response to antigens in the blood _____

D. Give short answers for the following.

1. Name four plasma proteins. _____

2. What is the Rh factor? _____

3. What is agglutination? _____

4. A person with type A blood has _____ antigens and _____ antibodies in his or her blood.

5. A person with type B blood has _____ antigens and _____ antibodies in her or his blood.

6. A person with type O blood has _____ antigens and _____ antibodies in her or his blood.

7. A person with type AB blood has _____ antigens and _____ antibodies in her or his blood.

8. Can you transfuse blood from a type A donor into a type B recipient? _____

   Why? _____

9. Can you transfuse blood from a type AB donor into a type O recipient? _____

   Why? _____

10. What is electrophoresis? _____

11. What is immunoglobulin? _____

12. What is differentiation? _____

13. What is plasmapheresis? _____

E. Match the following terms related to clotting with their meanings as given below.

coagulation   heparin   prothrombin
serum   thrombin   fibrin
fibrinogen   thromboplastin

1. an anticoagulant substance produced by liver cells and found in the bloodstream and tissues

   _____

2. protein threads that form the basis of a blood clot _____

3. a plasma protein that is converted to thrombin in the clotting process _____

4. plasma minus clotting proteins and cells _____

5. a clotting factor that, in combination with calcium, promotes the clotting process _____

6. a plasma protein that is converted to fibrin in the clotting process _____

7. the process of clotting _____

8. an enzyme that helps convert fibrinogen to fibrin _____

F. Divide the following terms into component parts and give meanings of the complete terms.

1. anticoagulant _____

2. hemoglobinopathy _____

3. cytology _____

4. leukocytopenia _____

5. morphology _____

6. megakaryocyte _____

7. sideropenia _____

8. phagocyte _____

9. myeloblast _____

10. plateletpheresis _____

11. monoblast _____

12. myelopoiesis _____

13. hemostasis _____

14. thrombolytic _____

15. hematopoiesis _____

G. *Match the following terms concerning red blood cells with their meanings as given below.*

hematocrit	erythropoiesis	hemoglobin
hemolysis	polycythemia vera	anisocytosis
erythrocytopenia	poikilocytosis	macrocytosis
hypochromia	spherocytosis	microcytosis

1. irregularity in the shape of red blood cells _____

2. oxygen-containing protein in red blood cells _____

3. formation of red blood cells _____

4. deficiency in numbers of red blood cells _____

5. destruction of red blood cells _____

6. reduction of hemoglobin in red blood cells _____

7. variation in size of red blood cells _____

8. abnormal numbers of round, rather than normally biconcave-shaped, red blood cells

_____

9. increase in number of small red blood cells _____

10. general increase in numbers of red blood cells; erythremia _____

11. increase in numbers of large red blood cells _____

12. separation of blood so that the percentage of red blood cells in relation to the volume of a blood

sample is measured _____

H. *Describe the problem in each of the following forms of anemia.*

1. iron-deficiency anemia _____

2. pernicious anemia _____

3. sickle cell anemia _____

4. aplastic anemia _____

5. thalassemia _____

I. *Give the meanings of the following blood dyscrasias.*

1. idiopathic thrombocytopenic purpura _____

2. granulocytosis _____

3. hemophilia _____

4. hemochromatosis _____

5. multiple myeloma _____

6. mononucleosis _____

J. *Match the term in column I with its meaning in column II. Write the letter of the meaning in the space provided.*

Column I

1. relapse _____

2. remission _____

3. palliative _____

4. Bence Jones protein _____

5. purpura _____

6. pancytopenia _____

7. apheresis _____

8. eosinophilia _____

Column II

A. deficiency of all blood cells
B. immunoglobulin fragment found in the urine of patients with multiple myeloma
C. increase in numbers of granulocytes; seen in allergic conditions
D. relieving, but not curing
E. symptoms of the disease return
F. multiple pinpoint hemorrhages with accumulation of blood under the skin
G. symptoms of the disease disappear
H. separation of blood into its parts

K. Match the following laboratory test or clinical procedure with its description.

coagulation time   hematocrit   bleeding time
red blood cell morphology   erythrocyte sedimentation rate   bone marrow transplant
bone marrow biopsy   antiglobulin Coombs test   red blood cell count
autologous transfusion   white blood cell differential   platelet count

1. stained blood smear is examined to determine the shape (form) of individual red blood cells

   _____

2. measures the percentage of red blood cells in a volume of blood _____

3. determines the number of clotting cells per cubic millimeter _____

4. ability of venous blood to clot in a test tube _____

5. measures the speed at which erythrocytes settle out of plasma _____

6. determines the numbers of different types of white blood cells (immature and mature forms)

   _____

7. determines the presence of antibodies in infants of Rh-negative women or in patients with

   autoimmune hemolytic anemia _____

8. bone marrow cells from a donor are infused into a patient with leukemia or aplastic anemia

   _____

9. time it takes for a small puncture wound to stop bleeding _____

10. needle is introduced into the bone marrow cavity; small amount of marrow is aspirated and then

    examined under a microscope _____

11. gives the number of erythrocytes per cubic millimeter of blood _____

12. blood is collected from and later reinfused into the same patient _____

L. Give the meanings of the following abbreviations and then select from the sentences that follow the best association for each.

Column I

1. Hgb _____ ____

2. GVHD _____ ____

3. ALL _____ ____

4. PTT _____ ____

5. CML _____ ____

6. G-CSFs _____ ____

7. IgA, IgE, IgD _____ ____

8. CLL _____ ____

9. Hct _____ ____

10. AML _____ ____

Column II

A. This is a blood protein that helps transport oxygen to body tissues.

B. A malignant condition of white blood cells in which immature granulocytes predominate; normal bone marrow is replaced by myeloblasts.

C. A malignant condition of white blood cells in which immature lymphocytes predominate; children are affected and onset is sudden.

D. This test is used to follow patients who are taking certain anticoagulants.

E. This is the percentage of erythrocytes in a volume of blood.

F. A malignant condition of white blood cells in which both mature and immature granulocytes are present; a slowly progressive illness.

G. This is an immune reaction by a recipient's cells to a donor's cells; a possible outcome of a bone marrow transplant.

H. These proteins contain antibodies; they are gamma globulins.

I. A malignant condition of white blood cells in which relatively mature lymphocytes predominate in lymph nodes, spleen, and bone marrow; usually seen in elderly patients.

J. These are proteins that stimulate the formation and proliferation of white blood cells.

M. Select the terms that best complete the meanings of the sentences.

1. Gary, a 1-year-old African-American baby, was failing to gain weight normally. He seemed pale and without energy. His blood tests showed a decreased hemoglobin (5.0) and decreased hematocrit (16.5). After a blood smear revealed abnormally shaped red cells, the physician told Gary's mother that her son had **(iron-deficiency anemia, hemophilia, sickle cell anemia).**

2. While in the hospital, Mr. Klein was told he had an elevated **(red blood cell, white blood cell, platelet)** count with a "left shift." This was information that confirmed his diagnosis of a systemic infection.

3. While taking Coumadin, a blood thinner, Mr. Ratzan's physician made sure to check his **(prothrombin time, hematocrit, sed rate).**

4. When they checked Babette's blood type during her prenatal examination, she was **(B⁺, O⁺, AB⁻).** Her physician told her that she and her baby might have the condition of **(Rh incompatibility, multiple myeloma, pernicious anemia).**

5. Bobby was diagnosed at a very early age with a bleeding disorder called **(hemophilia, thalassemia, eosinophilia).** He needed factor VIII regularly, especially after even the slightest traumatic injury.

6. Bill was a 9-year-old boy who suddenly noticed many black and blue marks all over his legs. He had a fever and was tired all the time. The physician did a blood test that revealed pancytopenia. A bone marrow biopsy confirmed the diagnosis of **(acute lymphocytic leukemia, polycythemia vera, aplastic anemia).**

7. Suzy and her friends had been staying up late for weeks, cramming for exams. She developed a sore throat, fatigue, and swollen lymph nodes in her neck. Dr. Smith did a blood test, and the results showed lymphocytosis and antibodies to EBV in the bloodstream. His diagnosis was **(leukapheresis, lymphocytopenia, mononucleosis).**

XI. Answers to Exercises

A

1. monocyte
2. platelet
3. stem cell (hemocytoblast)
4. lymphocyte
5. eosinophil
6. erythrocyte
7. neutrophil
8. basophil

B

1. blood cell (little body)
2. white blood cell with dense, dark-staining granules (neutrophil, basophil, and eosinophil)
3. pertaining to (having) one (prominent) nucleus (monocytes and lymphocytes are mononuclear leukocytes)
4. pertaining to (having) a many-shaped nucleus (neutrophils are polymorphonuclear leukocytes)
5. white blood cell without dense, dark-staining granules in its cytoplasm (monocyte and lymphocyte)
6. immature red blood cell
7. forerunner (precursor) of platelets (formed in the bone marrow)
8. large phagocytes formed from monocytes and found in tissues; they destroy wornout red blood cells and engulf foreign material
9. blood protein found in red blood cells; enables the erythrocyte to carry oxygen
10. derived from bone marrow cells
11. immature, developing red blood cell with a network of granules in its cytoplasm
12. immature bone marrow cell that is the forerunner of granulocytes

C

1. plasma
2. bilirubin
3. heme
4. globulin
5. erythropoietin
6. antigen
7. albumin
8. antibodies

D

1. albumin, globulin, fibrinogen, and prothrombin
2. an antigen normally found on red blood cells of Rh-positive individuals
3. clumping of recipient's blood cells when incompatible bloods are mixed
4. A; anti-B
5. B; anti-A
6. no A or B; anti-A and anti-B
7. A and B; no anti-A and no anti-B
8. no; the A antigens will agglutinate with the anti-A antibodies in the B person's bloodstream
9. no; the A and B antigens will agglutinate with the anti-A and anti-B antibodies in the O person's bloodstream
10. a method of separating substances (such as proteins) by electrical charge
11. a type of gamma globulin (blood protein) that contains antibodies
12. change in the structure and function (specialization) of a cell as it matures
13. the process of using a centrifuge to separate or remove blood cells from plasma.

E

1. heparin
2. fibrin
3. prothrombin
4. serum
5. thromboplastin
6. fibrinogen
7. coagulation
8. thrombin

Continued on following page

F

1. anti/coagul/ant—a substance that prevents clotting
2. hemoglobin/o/pathy—disease (abnormality) of hemoglobin
3. cyt/o/logy—study of cells
4. leuk/o/cyt/o/penia—deficiency of white (blood) cells
5. morph/o/logy—study of the shape or form (of cells)
6. mega/kary/o/cyte—cell with a large (mega-) nucleus (kary); platelet precursor
7. sider/o/penia—deficiency of iron
8. phag/o/cyte—cell that eats or swallows other cells
9. myel/o/blast—immature bone marrow cell (gives rise to granulocytes)
10. platelet/pheresis—separation of platelets from the rest of the blood
11. mon/o/blast—immature monocyte
12. myel/o/poiesis—formation of bone marrow cells
13. hem/o/stasis—controlling or stopping the flow of blood
14. thromb/o/lytic—pertaining to destruction of clots
15. hemat/o/poiesis—formation of blood

G

1. poikilocytosis
2. hemoglobin
3. erythropoiesis
4. erythrocytopenia
5. hemolysis
6. hypochromia
7. anisocytosis
8. spherocytosis
9. microcytosis
10. polycythemia vera
11. macrocytosis
12. hematocrit

H

1. lack of iron leading to insufficient hemoglobin production
2. lack of mature erythrocytes due to inability to absorb vitamin B_{12} into the bloodstream (gastric juice lacks a factor that helps absorb B_{12})
3. abnormal shape (cresent-shape) of erythrocytes caused by an abnormal type of hemoglobin (hereditary disorder)
4. lack of all types of blood cells due to lack of development of bone marrow cells
5. defect in the ability to produce hemoglobin, leading to hypochromia

I

1. multiple pinpoint hemorrhages due to a deficiency of platelets (patient makes an antibody that destroys her or his own platelets); cause unknown (idiopathic)
2. abnormal condition of excess numbers of granulocytes (eosinophilia and basophilia)
3. excessive bleeding caused by a lack (hereditary and congenital) of one of the protein factors necessary for clotting
4. excessive deposits of iron in tissues of the body
5. malignant tumor of bone marrow
   (antibody-producing plasma cells are produced in large numbers)
6. acute infectious disease involving increased numbers of atypical lymphocytes; caused by an EBV infection

J

1. E
2. G
3. D
4. B
5. F
6. A
7. H
8. C

K

1. red blood cell morphology
2. hematocrit
3. platelet count
4. coagulation time
5. erythrocyte sedimentation rate
6. white blood cell differential
7. antiglobulin (Coombs) test
8. bone marrow transplant
9. bleeding time
10. bone marrow biopsy
11. red blood cell count
12. autologous transfusion

L

1. hemoglobin. A
2. graft versus host disease. G
3. acute lymphocytic leukemia. C
4. partial thromboplastin time. D
5. chronic myelogenous (myelocytic) leukemia. F
6. granulocyte colony-stimulating factors. J
7. immunoglobulins. H
8. chronic lymphocytic leukemia. I
9. hematocrit. E
10. acute myelogenous (myelocytic) leukemia. B

M

1. sickle cell anemia
2. white blood cell
3. prothrombin time
4. AB⁻; Rh incompatibility
5. hemophilia
6. aplastic anemia
7. mononucleosis

Answers to Practical Applications

1. C
2. B
3. C

XII. Pronunciation of Terms

Pronunciation Guide

ā as in āpe	ă as in ăpple
ē as in ēven	ĕ as in ĕvery
ī as in īce	ĭ as in ĭnterest
ō as in ōpen	ŏ as in pŏt
ū as in ūnit	ŭ as in ŭnder

To test your understanding of the terminology in this chapter, write the meaning of each term in the space provided. In addition, you may wish to cover the terms and write them by looking at your definitions. Make sure your spelling is correct. The page number after each term indicates where it is defined or used in the text so you can easily check your responses.

Vocabulary and Terminology

Term	Pronunciation	Meaning
agglutination (473)	ă-gloo-tĭ-NĀ-shŭn	
albumin (473)	ăl-BŪ-mĭn	
anisocytosis (477)	ăn-ī-sō-sī-TŌ-sĭs	
antibody (473)	ĂN-tĭ-bŏd-ē	
anticoagulant (476)	ăn-tĭ-cō-ĂG-ū-lănt	
antigen (473)	ĂN-tĭ-jĕn	
basophil (473)	BĀ-sō-fĭl	
bilirubin (474)	bĭl-ĭ-ROO-bĭn	
coagulation (474)	kō-ăg-ū-LĀ-shŭn	
corpuscle (474)	KŎR-pŭs'l	
cytology (476)	sī-TŎL-ō-jē	
differentiation (474)	dĭf-ĕr-ĕn-shē-Ā-shŭn	
electrophoresis (474)	ē-lĕk-trō-fō-RĒ-sis	
eosinophil (474)	ē-ō-SĬN-ō-fĭl	
eosinophilia (479)	ē-ō-sĭn-ō-FĬL-ē-ă	
erythroblast (478)	ĕ-RĬTH-rō-blăst	
erythrocytopenia (476)	ĕ-rĭth-rō-sī-tō-PĒ-nē-ă	
erythropoiesis (479)	ĕ-rĭth-rō-poy-Ē-sĭs	
erythropoietin (474)	ĕ-rĭth-rō-PŌ-ĕ-tĭn	
fibrin (474)	FĪ-brĭn	
fibrinogen (474)	fī-BRĬN-ō-jĕn	

gamma globulin (479)	GĂ-mă GLŎB-ū-lĭn	_____
globulin (474)	GLŎB-ū-lĭn	_____
granulocyte (474)	GRĂN-ū-lō-sīt	_____
granulocytopenia (479)	grăn-ū-lō-sī-tō-PĒ-nē-ă	_____
hemoglobin (474)	HĒ-mō-glō-bĭn	_____
hemoglobinopathy (476)	hē-mō-glō-bĭn-ŎP-ă-thē	_____
hemolysis (476)	hē-MŎL-ĭ-sĭs	_____
hemostasis (479)	hē-mŏ-STĀ-sĭs	_____
heparin (474)	HĔP-ă-rĭn	_____
hypochromia (476)	hī-pō-KRŌ-mē-ă	_____
immunoglobulin (474)	ĭm-ū-nō-GLŎB-ū-lĭn	_____
leukapheresis (478)	loo-kă-fĕ-RĒ-sĭs	_____
leukocytopenia (477)	loo-kō-sī-tō-PĒ-nē-ă	_____
lymphocyte (475)	LĬM-fō-sīt	_____
macrocytosis (478)	măk-rō-sī-TŌ-sĭs	_____
macrophage (475)	MĂK-rō-făj	_____
megakaryocyte (475)	mĕg-ă-KĀR-ē-ō-sīt	_____
microcytosis (478)	mī-krō-sī-TŌ-sĭs	_____
monoblast (478)	MŎN-ō-blăst	_____
monocyte (475)	MŎN-ō-sīt	_____
mononuclear (477)	mŏn-ō-NŪ-klē-ăr	_____
morphology (477)	mŏr-FŎL-ō-jē	_____
myeloblast (477)	MĪ-ĕ-lō-blăst	_____
myeloid (479)	MĪ-ĕ-loyd	_____
myelopoiesis (479)	mī-ĕ-lō-poy-Ē-sĭs	_____
neutropenia (477)	nū-trō-PĔ-nē-ă	_____
neutrophil (475)	NŪ-trō-fĭl	_____
neutrophilia (479)	nū-trō-FĬL-ē-ă	_____
pancytopenia (479)	păn-sī-tō-PĒ-nē-ă	_____

phagocyte (477)	FĂG-ō-sīt	_____
plasma (475)	PLĂZ-mă	_____
plasmapheresis (475)	plăz-mă-fĕ-RĒ-sĭs	_____
plateletpheresis (478)	plăt-lĕt-fĕ-RĒ-sĭs	_____
poikilocytosis (477)	poy-kĭ-lō-sī-TŌ-sĭs	_____
polymorphonuclear (477)	pŏl-ē-mŏr-fō-NŪ-klē-ăr	_____
prothrombin (475)	prō-THRŎM-bĭn	_____
reticulocyte (475)	rĕ-TĬK-ū-lō-sīt	_____
serum (475)	SĚ-rŭm	_____
sideropenia (477)	sĭd-ĕr-ō-PĒ-nē-ă	_____
spherocytosis (477)	sphĕr-ō-sī-TŌ-sĭs	_____
stem cell (475)	stĕm sĕl	_____
thrombin (475)	THRŎM-bĭn	_____
thrombocyte (475)	THRŎM-bō-sīt	_____
thrombolytic therapy (479)	thrŏm-bō-LĬ-tĭk THĚR-ă-pē	_____
thromboplastin (475)	thrŏm-bō-PLĂS-tĭn	_____
thrombosis (479)	thrŏm-BŌ-sĭs	_____

Pathological Conditions, Laboratory Tests, and Clinical Procedures

Term	Pronunciation	Meaning
acute lymphocytic leukemia (483)	ă-KŪT lĭm-fō-SĬ-tĭk loo-KĒ-mē-ă	_____
acute myelogenous leukemia (482)	ă-KŪT mī-ĕ-LŎJ-ĕ-nŭs loo-KĒ-mē-ă	_____
antiglobulin test (484)	ăn-tē-GLŎB-ū-lĭn tĕst	_____
apheresis (486)	ă-fĕ-RĒ-sĭs	_____
aplastic anemia (480)	ā-PLĂS-tĭk ă-NĒ-mē-ă	_____
autologous transfusion (486)	ăw-TŎL-ō-gŭs trăns-FŪ-zhŭn	_____
bleeding time (484)	BLĒ-dĭng tīm	_____
blood transfusion (486)	blŭd trăns-FŪ-zhŭn	_____

bone marrow biopsy (486)	bōn MĂ-rō BĪ-ŏp-sē	_____
bone marrow transplant (486)	bōn MĂ-rō TRĂNS-plănt	_____
chronic lymphocytic leukemia (483)	KRŎ-nĭk lĭm-fō-SĬ-tĭk loo-KĒ-mē-ă	_____
chronic myelogenous leukemia (483)	KRŎ-nĭk mī-ĕ-LŎJ-ĕ-nŭs loo-KĒ-mē-ă	_____
coagulation time (484)	kō-ăg-ū-LĀ-shŭn tīm	_____
dyscrasia (480)	dĭs-KRĀ-zē-ă	_____
erythrocyte sedimentation rate (485)	ĕ-RĬTH-rō-sīt sĕd-ĕ-mĕn-TĀ-shŭn rāt	_____
granulocytosis (483)	grăn-ū-lō-sī-TŌ-sis	_____
hematocrit (485)	hē-MĂT-ō-krĭt	_____
hemochromatosis (482)	hē-mō-krō-mă-TŌ-sĭs	_____
hemoglobin test (485)	HĒ-mō-glō-bĭn tĕst	_____
hemolytic anemia (480)	hē-mō-LĬ-tĭk ă-NĒ-mē-ă	_____
hemophilia (482)	hē-mō-FĬL-ē-ă	_____
mononucleosis (484)	mŏ-nō-nū-klē-Ō-sĭs	_____
multiple myeloma (484)	MŬL-tĭ-p'l mī-ĕ-LŌ-mă	_____
palliative (484)	PĂL-ē-ă-tĭv	_____
partial thromboplastin time (485)	PĂR-shŭl thrŏm-bō-PLĂS-tĭn tīm	_____
pernicious anemia (481)	pĕr-NĬSH-ŭs ă-NĒ-mē-ă	_____
polycythemia vera (482)	pŏl-ē-sī-THĒ-mē-ă VĔR-ă	_____
prothrombin time (485)	prō-THRŎM-bĭn tīm	_____
purpura (482)	PŬR-pū-ră	_____
relapse (483)	RĒ-lăps	_____
remission (483)	rē-MĬSH-ŭn	_____
sickle cell anemia (481)	SĬK'l sĕl ă-NĒ-mē-ă	_____
thalassemia (481)	thāl-ă-SĒ-mē-ă	_____

XIII. Review Sheet

Write the meanings of the word parts in the spaces provided. Check your answers with the information in the chapter or in the glossary (Medical Terms—English) at the end of the book.

COMBINING FORMS

Combining Form	Meaning	Combining Form	Meaning
agglutin/o		kary/o	
bas/o		leuk/o	
chrom/o		mon/o	
coagul/o		morph/o	
cyt/o		myel/o	
eosin/o		neutr/o	
erythr/o		nucle/o	
granul/o		phag/o	
hem/o		poikil/o	
hemat/o		sider/o	
hemoglobin/o		spher/o	
is/o		thromb/o	

Continued on following page

SUFFIXES

Suffix	Meaning	Suffix	Meaning
-apheresis	_____	-penia	_____
-blast	_____	-phage	_____
-cytosis	_____	-philia	_____
-emia	_____	-phoresis	_____
-globin	_____	-plasia	_____
-globulin	_____	-poiesis	_____
-lytic	_____	-stasis	_____
-oid	_____		

PREFIXES

Prefix	Meaning	Prefix	Meaning
a-, an-	_____	micro-	_____
anti-	_____	mono-	_____
hypo-	_____	pan-	_____
macro-	_____	poly-	_____
mega-	_____		

CHAPTER

Lymphatic and Immune Systems

This chapter is divided into the following sections

In this chapter you will

- Identify the structures and analyze terms related to the lymphatic system;
- Learn terms that describe basic elements of the immune system;
- Recognize terms that describe various pathological conditions affecting the lymphatic and immune systems;
- Identify laboratory tests, clinical procedures, and abbreviations that are pertinent to the lymphatic and immune systems; and
- Apply your new knowledge to understanding medical terms in their proper contexts, such as medical reports and records.

I. Introduction

Lymph is a clear, watery fluid (the term lymph comes from the Latin, meaning clear spring water) that surrounds body cells and flows in a system of lymph vessels that extends throughout the body.

Lymph differs from blood, but it has a close relationship with the blood systems. Lymph fluid does not contain erythrocytes or platelets, but it is rich in two types of white blood cells (leukocytes): lymphocytes and monocytes. The liquid part of lymph is similar to blood plasma in that it contains water, salts, sugar, and wastes of metabolism such as urea and creatinine, but it differs in that it contains less protein. Lymph actually originates from the blood. It is the fluid that filters out of tiny blood vessels into the spaces between cells. This fluid that surrounds body cells is called **interstitial fluid.** Interstitial fluid passes continuously into specialized thin-walled vessels called **lymph capillaries,** which are found coursing through tissue spaces (Fig. 14–1). The fluid in the lymph capillaries, now called **lymph** instead of interstitial fluid, passes through larger lymphatic vessels and through deposits of lymph tissues (called **lymph nodes**), finally to reach large lymph vessels in the upper chest. Lymph enters these large lymphatic vessels, which then empty into the bloodstream. Figure 14–2 illustrates the relationship between the blood and the lymphatic systems.

There are several functions of the lymphatic system. One is to act as a drainage system to transport needed proteins and fluid that have leaked out of the blood capillaries (and into the interstitial fluid) back to the bloodstream via the veins. In addition, the lymphatic vessels in the intestines absorb lipids (fats) from the small intestine and transport them to the bloodstream.

Another function of the lymphatic system is related to the **immune system:** the defense of the body against foreign organisms such as bacteria and viruses. Lymphocytes and monocytes, originating in lymph nodes and organs such as the spleen and thymus gland, protect the body by producing antibodies, by mounting a chemical attack on foreign cells, or by phagocytosis (engulfing and destroying foreign matter).

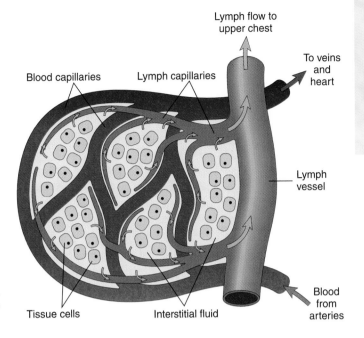

Figure 14-1

Interstitial fluid and lymph capillaries.

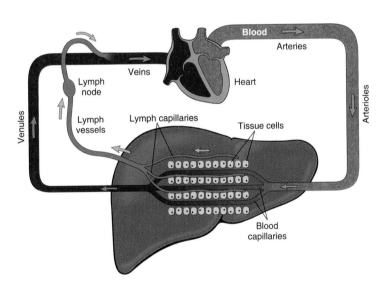

Figure 14-2

Relationship between the circulatory systems of blood and lymph.

II. Lymphatic System

Anatomy

Label Figure 14–3A as you read the following paragraphs.

Lymph capillaries [1] begin at the spaces around cells throughout the body. Like blood capillaries, they are thin-walled tubes. Lymph capillaries carry lymph from the tissue spaces to larger **lymph vessels** [2]. Lymph vessels have thicker walls than those of lymph capillaries and, like veins, contain valves so that lymph flows in only one direction, toward the thoracic cavity. Collections of stationary lymph tissue, called **lymph nodes** [3], are located along the path of the lymph vessels. These masses of lymph tissue are surrounded by a fibrous, connective tissue capsule (Fig. 14–4).

The function of lymph nodes is not only to produce lymph cells (lymphocytes) but also to filter lymph and trap substances from inflammatory and cancerous lesions. Special cells, called **macrophages,** are located in lymph nodes (as well as in the spleen, liver, lungs, brain, and spinal cord), and they can phagocytose foreign substances. When bacteria are present in lymph nodes that drain a particular area of the body, the nodes become swollen with collections of cells and their engulfed debris and become tender. Lymph nodes also fight disease when specialized lymphocytes **(B-cell lymphocytes),** present in the nodes, produce antibodies. Other lymphocytes **(T-cell lymphocytes)** attack bacteria and foreign cells by accurately recognizing a cell surface protein as foreign, attaching to the cells, poking holes in them, and injecting toxic chemicals into the cells.

Label the major sites of lymph node concentration on Figure 14–3. These are the **cervical** [4], **axillary** (armpit) [5], **mediastinal** [6], and **inguinal** (groin) [7] regions of the body. Remember that the **tonsils** are masses of lymph tissue in the throat near the mouth (oropharynx) and the **adenoids** are enlarged lymph tissue in the part of the throat near the nasal passages (nasopharynx).

Lymph vessels all lead toward the thoracic cavity and empty into two large ducts in the upper chest. These are the **right lymphatic duct** [8] and the **thoracic duct** [9]. The thoracic duct drains the lower body and the left side of the head, whereas the right lymphatic duct drains the right side of the head and chest (a much smaller area) (Fig. 14–3B). Both ducts carry the lymph into **large veins** [10] in the neck where lymph then merges with the blood system.

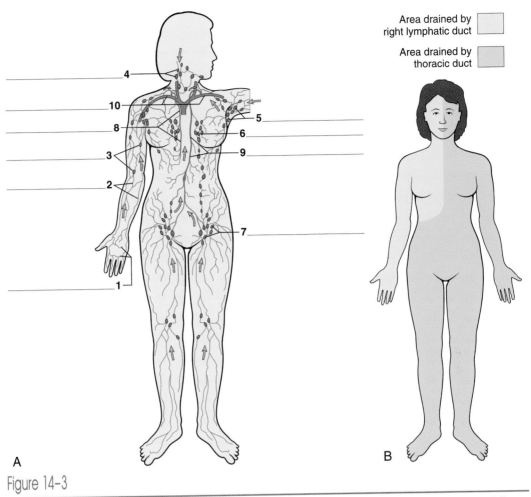

Area drained by
right lymphatic duct

Area drained by
thoracic duct

A

B

Figure 14-3

Lymphatic system. (A) Label the figure according to the descriptions in the text. **(B)** Note the different regions of the body drained by the right lymphatic duct and the thoracic duct.

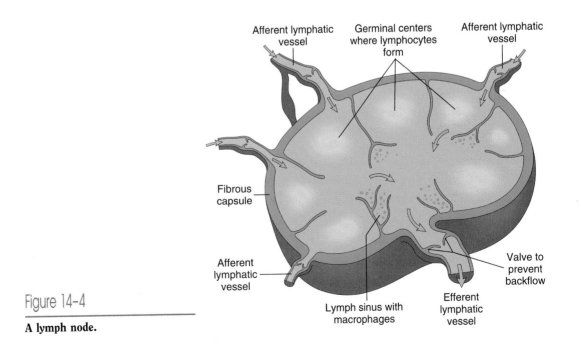

Afferent lymphatic
vessel

Germinal centers
where lymphocytes
form

Afferent lymphatic
vessel

Fibrous
capsule

Afferent
lymphatic
vessel

Lymph sinus with
macrophages

Efferent
lymphatic
vessel

Valve to
prevent
backflow

Figure 14-4

A lymph node.

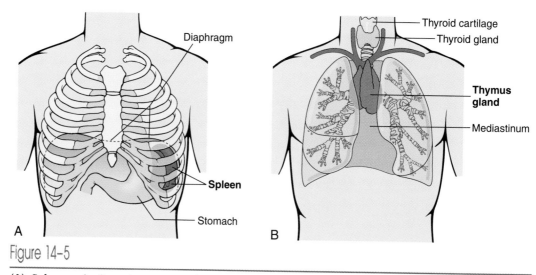

Figure 14-5

(A) Spleen and adjacent structures. **(B) Thymus gland** in its location in the mediastinum between the lungs.

Spleen and Thymus Gland

The spleen and the thymus gland are organs composed of lymph tissue.

The **spleen** (Fig. 14–5A) is located in the left upper quadrant of the abdomen, adjacent to the stomach. Although the spleen is not essential to life, it has several important functions:

1. Destruction of old erythrocytes by macrophages. Because of hemolytic activity in the spleen, bilirubin is formed there and added to the bloodstream.
2. Filtration of microorganisms and other foreign material from the blood.
3. Activation of lymphocytes as it filters out antigens from the blood. Activated B-cell lymphocytes produce antibodies.
4. Storage of blood, especially erythrocytes and platelets. A large number of platelets collect in the splenic blood pool.

The spleen is an organ that is easily and frequently injured, A sharp blow or injury to the upper abdomen (as from the impact of a car's steering wheel) may cause rupture of the spleen. Massive hemorrhage can occur when the spleen is ruptured, and immediate surgical removal (splenectomy) may be necessary. After splenectomy, the liver, bone marrow, and lymph nodes take over the functions of the spleen.

The **thymus gland** (Fig. 14–5B) is a lymphatic organ located in the upper mediastinum between the lungs. During fetal life and childhood it is quite large, but it becomes smaller with age. The thymus gland is composed of nests of lymphoid cells resting on a connective tissue stroma. It plays an important role in the body's ability to protect itself from disease (immunity), especially in fetal life and the early years of growth. It is known that a thymectomy (removal of the thymus gland) performed in an animal during the first weeks of life impairs the ability of the animal to make antibodies and to produce immune cells that fight against foreign antigens such as bacteria and viruses.

III. Immune System

The immune system is the body's special defense response against foreign organisms. This system includes the **lymphoid organs** (lymph nodes, spleen, and thymus gland) and their products (**lymphocytes** and **antibodies**) and **macrophages** (phagocytes that are found in the blood, brain, liver, lymph nodes, and spleen).

Immunity is the body's ability to resist foreign organisms and toxins (poisons) that damage tissues and organs. **Natural immunity** is a **genetic predisposition** present in the body at birth, it is not dependent on a specific immune response or a previous contact with an infectious agent. When bacteria enter the body, natural immunity protects the body as **phagocytes** such as neutrophils (white blood cells) migrate to the site of infection and ingest the bacteria. They release proteins that attract other immune cells and cause localized inflammation. Cells called **macrophages** move in to clear away the dead cells and debris as the infection subsides. Other cells, known as **natural killer (NK) cells** are lymphocytes that destroy tumor cells and virally infected cells.

Besides possessing natural immunity, a person may **acquire immunity.** In this way, the body develops powerful, specific immunity (such as antibodies and cells) against invading antigens. **Acquired active immunity** occurs in several ways. First, **having a disease** causes the production of antibodies that fight against foreign organisms and then remain in the body to protect against further infection. Next, receiving a **vaccination** containing a modified pathogen or toxin stimulates lymphocytes to produce antibodies without having undergone an attack of the disease. Finally, immunity can also be acquired through the transfer of immune cells (lymphocytes or bone marrow cells) from a donor, as in a bone marrow transplant, which stimulates the growth of immune cells in the bone marrow of the recipient.

When immediate protection is needed, **acquired passive immunity** is administered. In this case, the patient receives immune serum (antiserum) containing antibodies produced in another animal. Examples are **antitoxins** given in cases of poisonous snake bites and rabies infections. Injections of **gamma globulin,** which contain antibodies, also provide protection against disease or lessen its severity. Newborns receive passive acquired immunity as **maternal antibodies** pass through the placenta or in breast milk after birth. Figure 14–6 reviews the various types of immunity.

The immune response involves two major disease fighters: **B-cell lymphocytes** and **T-cell lymphocytes.** B cells are involved in **humoral immunity.** They produce antibodies in response to specific antigens. B cells originate from bone marrow stem cells. When a B cell is confronted with a specific type of antigen, it transforms into an antibody-producing cell called a **plasma cell.** Plasma cells produce antibodies called

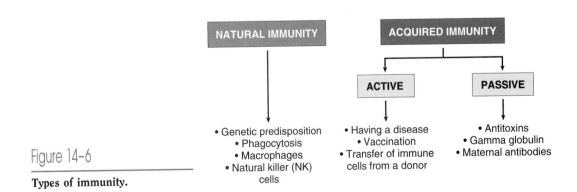

Figure 14-6

Types of immunity.

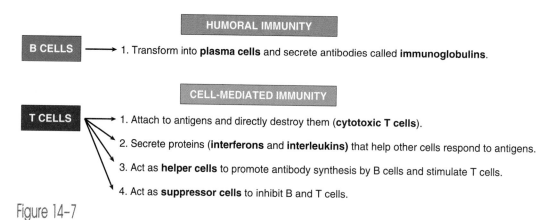

Figure 14-7

Functions of B-cell (humoral immunity) and T-cell lymphocytes (cell-mediated immunity).

immunoglobulins, such as **IgA, IgD, IgE, IgG,** and **IgM.** Immunoglobulins travel to the site of an infection to react with and neutralize antigens. IgG, the most abundant immunoglobulin, crosses the placenta to provide immunity for newborns. IgE is important in causing allergic reactions and fighting parasitic infections.

T-cell lymphocytes are involved in **cell-mediated immunity.** They originate from stem cells in the bone marrow and are processed in the thymus gland where they are acted on by thymic hormones. When a T cell encounters an antigen, the T cell multiplies rapidly to produce cells that destroy the antigen (bacteria, viruses, and cancer cells). T cells also react to transplanted tissues and skin grafts.

Some T cells are **cytotoxic cells (T8 cells)** that act directly on antigens to destroy them. Others produce proteins called **cytokines (interferons** and **interleukins)** that aid other cells in antigen destruction. One special class of T cells called **helper cells (T4 cells)** promotes antibody production by B cells and stimulates T cells. **Suppressor cells** inhibit the activity of B and T cells. Disease may occur when the normal ratio of helper to suppressor cells (normally 2:1) is altered. For example, in AIDS (acquired immunodeficiency syndrome) the number of helper (T4) cells is diminished. Figure 14–7 summarizes the functions of T- and B-cell lymphocytes.

Another important cell of the immune system is a **dendritic cell.** This cell, derived from monocytes, specializes in recognizing and digesting foreign antigens such as proteins and carbohydrates. The antigens are then presented on the surface of the dendritic cell and this stimulates a B- and T-cell response that destroys the antigen. Immunity can be transferred by exposing dendritic cells in culture to an antigen (tumor protein) and then infusing the cells into a patient. The antigen-sensitive dendritic cells are then able to stimulate the patient's B and T cells to attack the antigen-presenting dendritic cells. Clinical experiments that test treating cancer and AIDS with sensitized dendritic cells are under way.

IV. Vocabulary

This list will help you review many of the new terms introduced in the text. Short definitions will reinforce your understanding of the terms. See Section XI of this chapter for help in pronouncing the more difficult terms.

acquired immunity	Formation of antibodies and lymphocytes after exposure to an antigen.
adenoids	Masses of lymph tissue in the nasopharynx.
antibodies	Proteins, produced by plasma cells, that destroy antigens.
axillary nodes	Lymph nodes in the armpit (under arm).
B cells	Lymphocytes that transform into plasma cells and secrete antibodies. The B refers to the bursa of Fabricius, an organ in birds in which B-cell differentiation and growth were first noted to occur.
cell-mediated immunity	An immune response involving T-cell lymphocytes; antigens are destroyed by direct action of cells.
cervical nodes	Lymph nodes in the neck region.
cytotoxic cells	T-cell lymphocytes that directly kill foreign cells; also called **T8 cells.**
dendritic cells	Antigen-presenting cells derived from monocytes.
helper cells	T cells that aid B cells in recognizing antigens and stimulating antibody production; also called **T4 cells.**
humoral immunity	Immune response in which B cells transform into plasma cells and secrete antibodies.
immune response or immunity	The body's capacity to resist all types of organisms and toxins that can damage tissue and organs.
immunoglobulins	Antibodies (gamma globulins) such as IgA, IgE, IgG, IgM, and IgD that are secreted by plasma cells in humoral immunity.
inguinal nodes	Lymph nodes in the groin region (area where the legs join the trunk of the body).
interferons	Antiviral proteins secreted by T cells; they also stimulate macrophages to ingest bacteria.
interleukins	Proteins that stimulate the growth of B- or T-cell lymphocytes and activate specific components of the immune response.
interstitial fluid	Fluid in the spaces between cells. This fluid becomes lymph when it enters lymph capillaries.

lymph	Fluid found within lymphatic vessels and collected from tissues throughout the body.
lymph capillaries	The tiniest lymphatic vessels.
lymphoid organs	Lymph nodes, spleen, and thymus gland.
lymph nodes	Stationary lymph tissue along lymph vessels.
lymph vessels	Carriers of lymph throughout the body; lymph vessels empty lymph into veins in the upper part of the chest.
macrophage	A large phagocyte found in lymph nodes and other tissues of the body.
mediastinal nodes	Lymph nodes in the area between the lungs in the thoracic (chest) cavity.
natural immunity	A person's own genetic ability to fight off disease.
natural killer (NK) cells	Cells of lymphocyte origin that have the ability to recognize and destroy foreign cells (viruses and tumor cells) without prior sensitization.
plasma cell	A cell that secretes an antibody and originates from B-cell lymphocytes.
right lymphatic duct	A large lymph vessel in the chest that receives lymph from the upper right part of the body.
spleen	An organ near the stomach that produces, stores, and eliminates blood cells.
suppressor cells	T-cell lymphocytes that inhibit the activity of B- and T-cell lymphocytes.
T cells	Lymphocytes formed in the thymus gland; they act directly on antigens to destroy them or produce chemicals such as interferons and interleukins that are toxic to antigens.
thoracic duct	Large lymph vessel in the chest that receives lymph from below the diaphragm and from the left side of the body above the diaphragm; it empties the lymph into veins in the upper chest.
thymus gland	Organ in the mediastinum that produces T-cell lymphocytes and aids in the immune response.
tonsils	Masses of lymph tissue in the back of the oropharynx.
toxin	A poison; a protein produced by certain bacteria, animals, and plants.
vaccination	Introduction of altered antigens (viruses or bacteria) to produce an immune response and protection against disease. The term comes from the Latin *vacca,* meaning cow, and was used when the first inoculations were given with organisms that caused the mild disease cow pox to produce immunity to smallpox.

V. Combining Forms, Prefixes, and Terminology

Write the meanings of the medical terms in the spaces provided.

| Combining Forms | | | |
Combining Form	Meaning	Terminology	Meaning
immun/o	protection	autoimmune diseases _____	

Examples are rheumatoid arthritis and lupus erythematosus. These are chronic, disabling diseases caused by the abnormal production of antibodies to normal body tissues. Symptoms are inflammation of joints, skin rash, and fever. Glucocorticoid drugs (prednisone) and other immunosuppressants are effective as treatment.

immunoglobulin _____

immunosuppression _____

This may occur because of exposure to drugs (corticosteroids) or as the result of disease (AIDS and cancer).

lymph/o	lymph	lymphopoiesis _____	

lymphedema _____

Interstitial fluid collects within the spaces between cells secondary to obstruction of lymph vessels and nodes.

lymphocytopenia _____

lymphocytosis _____

lymphoid _____

-oid means resembling or derived from. Lymphoid organs include lymph nodes, spleen, and thymus gland.

lymphaden/o	lymph node (gland)	lymphadenopathy _____	
		lymphadenitis _____	
splen/o	spleen	splenomegaly _____	
		splenectomy _____	
		hypersplenism _____	

A syndrome marked by splenomegaly and often associated with blood cell destruction, anemia, leukopenia, and thrombocytopenia.

thym/o	thymus gland	thymoma _____
		thymectomy _____
tox/o	poison	toxic _____

| **Prefix** | | | |
Prefix	**Meaning**	**Terminology**	**Meaning**
ana-	backward, away from	anaphylaxis _____	

-phylaxis means protection. This is an exaggerated or unusual hypersensitivity to foreign proteins or other substances. Vasodilation and a decrease in blood pressure can be life threatening.

| inter- | between | interstitial fluid _____ | |

-stitial means pertaining to standing or positioned.

VI. Disorders of the Lymphatic and Immune Systems

Immunodeficiency

acquired immunodeficiency syndrome (AIDS)

Syndrome associated with suppression of the immune system and marked by opportunistic infections, secondary neoplasms, and neurological problems.

This syndrome is caused by the **human immunodeficiency virus (HIV).** HIV destroys T-cell helper lymphocytes (also called **CD4+ cells)** and thus disrupts the cell-mediated immune response. Infectious diseases associated with AIDS are opportunistic infections because HIV lowers resistance and allows infection by bacteria and parasites that are easily otherwise contained by normal defenses. Table 14–1 lists many of these opportunistic infections.

Malignancies associated with AIDS are **Kaposi sarcoma** (a cancer arising from the lining cells of capillaries, which produce bluish-red skin nodules) and **lymphoma** (cancer of lymph nodes).

Persons exposed to HIV and who have antibodies in their blood against HIV are **HIV-positive.** HIV is found in blood, semen, vaginal and cervical secretions, saliva, and other body fluids (breast milk, urine, and cerebrospinal fluid). Transmission of HIV may occur by three routes: sexual contact, blood inoculation (sharing of contaminated needles, accidental needle sticks, contact with contaminated blood or blood products), and passage of the virus from infected mothers to their newborns. Table 14–2 summarizes the common routes of transmission of HIV.

HIV-infected patients may remain asymptomatic for as many as 10 years. Symptoms associated with HIV are lymphadenopathy, neurological disease, oral thrush (fungal infection), night sweats, fatigue, and evidence of opportunistic infections.

Drugs that are used to treat AIDS are inhibitors of the viral enzyme called **reverse transcriptase (RT).** After invading the CD4+ lymphocyte, HIV releases

Table 14-1. OPPORTUNISTIC INFECTIONS WITH AIDS

Infection	Description
Candidiasis	Yeast-like fungus *(Candida)* normally present in the mouth, skin, intestinal tract, and vagina overgrows, causing infections of the mouth (thrush), respiratory tract, and skin.
Cryptococcus (Crypto)	Yeast-like fungus *(Cryptococcus)* causes lung, brain, and blood infections. Pathogen is found in pigeon droppings, nesting places, air, water, and soil.
Cryptosporidiosis	One-celled parasitic *(Cryptosporidium)* infection of the gastrointestinal tract and brain and spinal cord. Organism is commonly found in farm animals.
Cytomegalovirus (CMV)	Virus causes enteritis and retinitis (inflammation of the retina at the back of the eye). Found in saliva, semen, cervical secretions, urine, feces, blood, and breast milk, but usually causes disease only when the immune system is compromised.
Herpes simplex	Viral infection causes small blisters on the skin of the lips or nose or on the genitals.
Histoplasmosis (Histo)	Fungal infection due to inhalation of dust contaminated with *Histoplasma capsulatum;* causes fever, chills, and lung infection. Pathogen is found in bird and bat droppings.
Mycobacterium avium-intracellulare (MAI)	Bacterial disease with fever, malaise, night sweats, anorexia, diarrhea, weight loss, and lung and blood infections.
Pneumocystis carinii pneumonia (PCP)	One-celled organism causes lung infection, with fever, cough, chest pain, and sputum production. Pathogen is found in air, water, and soil and is carried by animals. It is treated with trimethoprim and sulfamethoxazole (Bactrim), a combination of antibiotics, or with pentamidine. Aerosolized pentamidine, which is inhaled, can prevent recurrence of PCP.
Toxoplasmosis (Toxo)	Parasitic infection involving the central nervous system (CNS) and causing fever, chills, visual disturbances, confusion, hemiparesis (sight paralysis in one-half of the body), and seizures. Pathogen is acquired by eating uncooked lamb or pork, unpasteurized dairy products, raw eggs, or vegetables.
Tuberculosis (TB)	Bacterial disease *(Mycobacterium tuberculosis)* involving the lungs. Symptoms are fever, loss of weight, anorexia, and low energy.

Table 14-2. COMMON ROUTES OF TRANSMISSION

Route	People Affected
Receptive anal intercourse	Men and women
Receptive vaginal intercourse	Women
Sharing of needles and equipment (users of IV drugs)	Men and women
Contaminated blood (hemophiliacs)	Men and women
From mother *in utero*	Neonates

RT to help it grow and multiply inside the cell. Examples of **RT inhibitors (RTIs)** are zidovudine (Retrovir) and lamivudine (Epivir). A second, newer class of anti-HIV drugs are inhibitors of the viral protease (proteolytic) enzyme. HIV needs protease at a later stage than it needs RT to make viral parts that will spread throughout the body. Combinations of **protease inhibitors** and RT inhibitors have greatly increased the effectiveness of anti-HIV therapy, and in many cases have abolished evidence of the presence of the viral infection in affected people.

Hypersensitivity

allergy

Abnormal hypersensitivity acquired by exposure to an antigen; all/o means other.

Allergic reactions occur when a person is exposed to a sensitizing agent **(allergen),** and the immune response that follows on reexposure to the allergen is damaging to the body. These reactions can vary from allergic rhinitis or hay fever (caused by pollen or animal dander) to systemic **anaphylaxis (ana-** means backward, **-phylaxis** means protection), in which an extraordinary hypersensitivity reaction occurs throughout the body, leading to hypotension, shock, respiratory distress, and edema of the larynx.

Anaphylaxis can be life threatening, but the patient usually survives if the airways are kept open and she or he is treated immediately with epinephrine (Adrenalin) and antihistamines.

Other allergies include asthma (pollens, dust, molds), urticaria, or hives (foods, drugs), and atopic dermatitis (soaps, cosmetics, chemicals). **Atopic** means related to atopy, a hypersensitivity or allergic state arising from an inherited predisposition. A person who is atopic is prone to allergies.

Malignancies

lymphoma

Malignant tumor of lymph nodes and lymph tissue.

There are many forms of lymphoma, varying according to the particular cell type and its degree of differentiation. Some examples are:

Hodgkin disease — Malignant tumor of lymph tissue in the spleen and lymph nodes. This disease is characterized by lymphadenopathy (lymph nodes enlarge), splenomegaly, fever, weakness, and loss of weight and appetite. The diagnosis is often made by identifying a malignant cell (Reed-Sternberg cell) in the lymph nodes (Fig. 14–8). If disease is localized, the treatment of choice is

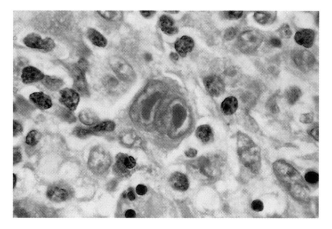

Figure 14-8

Hodgkin disease. Notice the binucleate **Reed-Sternberg cell** in the center of the slide. It is found in lymph nodes and is surrounded by lymphocytes. (Courtesy of Dr. Robert W. McKenna, Department of Pathology, University of Texas Southwestern Medical School, Dallas, TX; from Kumar V, Cotran RS, Robbins SL: Basic Pathology, 6th ed. Philadelphia, WB Saunders, 1997, p 370.)

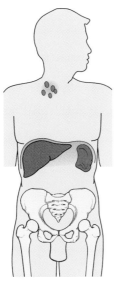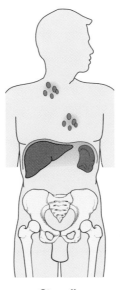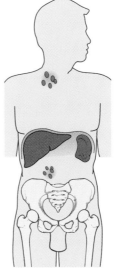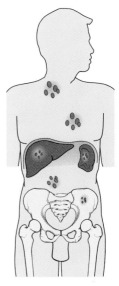

| **Stage I** | **Stage II** | **Stage III** | **Stage IV** |
| Involvement of single lymph node or group of nodes | Involvement of two or more sites on same side of diaphragm | Disease on both sides of diaphragm. May include spleen or localized extranodal disease | Widespread extralymphatic involvement (liver, bone marrow, lung, skin) |

Figure 14-9

Staging of Hodgkin disease involves assessing the extent of spread of the disease. Lymph node biopsies, laparotomy with liver and lymph node biopsies, and splenectomy may be necessary for staging.

radiotherapy (using high-dose radiation). If the disease is more widespread, chemotherapy is given alone or in combination with radiotherapy. There is a very high probability of cure with available treatments. Figure 14–9 illustrates staging of Hodgkin disease.

Non-Hodgkin lymphoma — Types of this disease include **lymphocytic lymphoma** (composed of lymphocytes) and **histiocytic lymphoma** (composed of large lymphocytes that resemble histiocytes or large macrophages). Chemotherapy and radiation are used to cure and stop the progress of this disease.

multiple myeloma

Malignant tumor of bone marrow cells.

This is a tumor composed of plasma cells (antibody-producing B-cell lymphocytes) associated with high levels of one of the specific immunoglobulins, usually IgG. **Waldenstrom macroglobulinemia** is another tumor of malignant B-cell lymphocytes. This disease involves B cells that produce large quantities of IgM (a globulin of high molecular weight). Increased IgM concentration impairs the passage of blood through capillaries in the brain and eyes, causing a hyperviscosity syndrome (thickening of the blood).

thymoma

Malignant tumor of the thymus gland.

Some symptoms of thymoma are cough, dyspnea, dysphagia, fever, chest pain, weight loss, and anorexia. Often, the tumor is associated with other disorders, such as myasthenia gravis and cytopenias.

Surgery is the principal method of treating thymoma; postoperative radiation therapy is used for patients with evidence of spread of the tumor.

STUDY SECTION

Practice spelling each term and know its meaning.

allergen	A substance capable of causing a specific hypersensitivity in the body; a type of antigen.
anaphylaxis	An exaggerated or unusual hypersensitivity to foreign protein or other substance.
atopy	A hypersensitive or allergic state involving an inherited predisposition. From the Greek word *atopia,* which means strangeness.
CD4+ lymphocytes	Helper T cells that carry the CD4+ protein antigen on their surface. HIV binds to CD4+ and infects and kills T cells bearing this protein.
Hodgkin disease	A malignant tumor of lymph tissue in spleen and lymph nodes; Hodgkin lymphoma.
human immunodeficiency virus	The virus (retrovirus) that causes AIDS; HIV.
Kaposi sarcoma	A malignant (cancerous) condition associated with AIDS; arises from the lining of capillaries and appears as bluish-red skin nodules.
opportunistic infections	Infectious diseases associated with AIDS; they occur because AIDS lowers the body's resistance and allows infection by bacteria and parasites that normally are easily contained.
protease inhibitor	A drug that treats AIDS by blocking the production of protease, a proteolytic enzyme that helps to create new viral pieces for HIV.
retrovirus	An RNA virus that makes copies of itself by using the host cell's DNA; this is in reverse (retro-) fashion because the regular method is for DNA to copy itself onto RNA. A retrovirus (like HIV) carries an enzyme, called **reverse transcriptase,** that enables it to reproduce within the host cell.
reverse transcriptase inhibitor	A drug that treats AIDS by blocking reverse transcriptase, an enzyme needed to make copies of the HIV virus.

VII. Laboratory Tests, Clinical Procedures, and Abbreviations

Laboratory Tests

ELISA
Enzyme-linked immunosorbent assay. This test is used to screen blood for antibody to AIDS virus. A positive result indicates probable exposure to the virus and possibly that the virus is in the blood. Since false-positive results can occur with this test, a back-up test (Western blot) is used to confirm positive findings.

Western blot
This test detects the presence of AIDS virus antibodies in serum.

CT scan
Computed tomography (x-ray views in a transverse plane) is used to diagnose abnormalities of lymphoid organs, such as lymph nodes, spleen, and thymus gland.

immunoelectrophoresis
A test that separates human immunoglobulins (IgM, IgG, IgE, IgA, IgD). It detects the presence of abnormal levels of antibodies in patients with conditions such as multiple myeloma and Waldenstrom macroglobulinemia.

ABBREVIATIONS

AIDS	acquired immunodeficiency syndrome	**KS**	Kaposi sarcoma
CD4+	protein on T-cell helper lymphocyte that is infected with HIV in AIDS	**MAI**	*Mycobacterium avium-intracellulare* (causes bacterial disease seen in AIDS patients)
CMV	cytomegalovirus (causes opportunistic AIDS-related infection)	**NK cells**	natural killer cells; lymphocytes that react against virally infected cells and tumor cells
Crypto	cryptococcus (causes opportunistic AIDS-related infection)	**PCP**	*Pneumocystis carinii* pneumonia (opportunistic AIDS-related infection)
ELISA	enzyme-linked immunosorbent assay (test for presence of antibodies to AIDS virus in serum)	**RTIs**	reverse transcriptase inhibitors; for example, zidovudine (Retrovir) and lamivudine (Epivir)
HD	Hodgkin disease		
Histo	histoplasmosis (fungal infection seen in AIDS patients)	**T4**	T-cell lymphocyte that is destroyed by the AIDS virus; helper T cells
HIV	human immunodeficiency virus (causes AIDS)	**T8**	T-cell lymphocyte (cytotoxic or killer cell)
HSV	herpes simplex virus	**Toxo**	toxoplasmosis (parasitic infection associated with AIDS)
IgA, IgD, IgE, IgG, IgM	immunoglobulins		

VIII. Practical Applications

Answers to the questions are on page (528) after Answers to Exercises.

Medical Terminology in Sentences

1. In addition to the opportunistic infections and malignancies that typically characterize AIDS, pathology of the central nervous system (CNS) occurs with some regularity. Specifically, CNS tumors, encephalitis, meningitis, progressive leukoencephalopathy, and myelitis have been reported in patients with HIV infection. Cases of dementia and delirium [clouding of consciousness] have also been reported as psychiatric complications.

2. Protease inhibitors interrupt HIV replication, blocking an enzyme called protase. When protease is blocked, HIV cannot infect new cells. Protease inhibitors can reduce HIV in the blood and increase CD4 cell counts. Examples of protease inhibitors are indinavir (Crixivan) and nelfinavir (Viracept).

3. Lymph nodes that are nontender and rock-hard are suspicious for metastatic carcinoma.

4. Infectious mononucleosis and Hodgkin disease are more common in young adults, whereas non-Hodgkin lymphoma and chronic lymphocytic leukemia are more common in middle-aged and elderly people.

5. Oral candidiasis (thrush) presenting without a history of recent antibiotic therapy, chemotherapy, or immunosuppression often indicates the possibility of HIV infection.

Questions

1. What parts of the body are commonly affected by the AIDS virus?
   (A) kidney and urinary bladder
   (B) brain and spinal cord
   (C) pancreas and thyroid glands

2. Which CNS condition is often seen in AIDS patients?
   (A) inflammation of the brain and membranes around the brain
   (B) fluid collection in the brain
   (C) disc impinging on the spinal cord

3. Aside from delirium, what other psychiatric complication has been reported in AIDS patients?
   (A) loss of intellectual abilities
   (B) feelings of persecution
   (C) fears such as claustrophobia and agoraphobia

4. Protease is a (an)
   (A) antiviral enzyme
   (B) enzyme that helps HIV infect new cells
   (C) reverse transcriptase inhibitor

5. CD4 T-cell counts can be increased by
   (A) high levels of HIV in the blood
   (B) protease inhibitors
   (C) lymphocyte inhibiting agents

6. Metastatic carcinoma means that
   (A) the tumor has spread to a secondary location
   (B) lymph nodes are not usually affected
   (C) tumor is localized

7. Hodgkin disease
   (A) commonly affects elderly people
   (B) is a type of lymphoma affecting young adults
   (C) is an infectious disease

8. What condition may indicate an AIDS virus infection?
   (A) high blood sugar
   (B) oral leukoplakia
   (C) fungal infection of the mouth

IX. Exercises

Remember to check your answers carefully with those given in Section X, Answers to Exercises.

A. Name the structure or fluid based on its meaning below.

1. stationary lymph tissue along the path of lymph vessels all over the body _____

2. large lymph vessel in the chest that drains lymph from the lower part and left side of the body

   above the diaphragm _____

3. organ near the stomach that produces, stores, and eliminates blood cells _____

4. masses of lymph tissue in the nasopharynx _____

5. organ in the mediastinum that produces T-cell lymphocytes and helps in the immune response

   _____

6. tiniest lymph vessels _____

7. large lymph vessel in the chest that drains lymph from the upper right part of the body

   _____

8. fluid that lies between cells and becomes lymph as it enters lymph capillaries

   _____

B. Give the locations of the following lymph nodes.

1. inguinal nodes _____

2. axillary nodes _____

3. cervical nodes _____

4. mediastinal nodes _____

C. Circle the correct answer in each sentence.

1. An immune response in which B cells transform into plasma cells and secrete antibodies is known as (cell-mediated immunity, humoral immunity).

2. Lymphocytes, formed in the thymus gland, that act on antigens are (B cells, T cells, macrophages).

3. An immune response in which T cells destroy antigens is called (cell-mediated immunity, humoral immunity).

4. Lymphocytes that transform into plasma cells and secrete antibodies are called (B cells, T cells, macrophages).

D. Match the following cell names with their meanings as given below.

helper cell   plasma cell   suppressor cell
macrophage   dendritic cell   natural killer (NK) cell

1. cell that originates from a B-cell lymphocyte and secretes antibodies _____

2. large phagocyte found in lymph nodes and other tissues of the body _____

3. T cell that aids B cells in recognizing antigens; also called a T4 cell _____

4. A cell of lymphocyte origin that can recognize and destroy foreign cells without prior sensitization

_____

5. T cell that inhibits the activity of B-cell lymphocytes _____

6. Antigen-presenting cell derived from a monocyte _____

E. Match the following terms in column I with their descriptions in column II.

Column I

1. immunoglobulins _____

2. toxins _____

3. helper cells _____

4. suppressor cells _____

5. cytotoxic cells _____

6. plasma cells _____

7. interferons _____

Column II

A. antibodies—IgA, IgE, IgG, IgM, IgD
B. T-cell lymphocytes—stimulate antibody production; T4 cells
C. poisons (antigens)
D. T-cell lymphocytes that inhibit the activity of B-cell lymphocytes
E. antiviral proteins secreted by T cells
F. transformed B cells that secrete antibodies
G. T-cell lymphocytes; T8 cells

F. Build medical terms.

1. removal of the spleen _____

2. enlargement of the spleen _____

3. formation of lymph _____

4. tumor of the thymus gland _____

5. inflammation of lymph glands (nodes) _____

6. deficiency of lymph cells _____

7. pertaining to poison _____

8. disease of lymph glands (nodes) _____

G. Match the following terms with their meanings below.

thymectomy   lymphedema   anaphylaxis
lymphoid organs   hypersplenism   AIDS
allergen   Hodgkin disease

1. syndrome marked by enlargement of the spleen and associated with anemia, leukopenia, and

   anemia _____

2. an extraordinary hypersensitivity to a foreign protein; marked by hypotension, shock, and respira-

   tory distress _____

3. an antigen capable of causing allergy (hypersensitivity) _____

4. disorder in which the immune system is suppressed by exposure to HIV _____

5. removal of a mediastinal organ _____

6. malignant tumor of lymph nodes and spleen marked by the presence of Reed-Sternberg cells in

   lymph nodes _____

7. tissue that produces lymphocytes—spleen, thymus, tonsils, and adenoids _____

8. swelling of tissues due to interstitial fluid accumulation _____

H. Match the following terms or abbreviations related to AIDS with their meanings below.

opportunistic infections   protease inhibitor   Kaposi sarcoma
HIV   ELISA   T4 helper lymphocytes
Western blot   PCP   RT inhibitor

1. a cancerous condition associated with AIDS (bluish-red skin nodules appear)

   _____

2. human immunodeficiency virus; the retrovirus that causes AIDS _____

3. white blood cells that are destroyed by the AIDS virus _____

4. pneumonia (*Pneumocystis carinii* pneumonia) that occurs in AIDS patients

   _____

5. group of infectious diseases associated with AIDS _____

6. test used to screen blood for antibody to AIDS virus _____

7. test used to detect the antibody to the AIDS virus in the blood _____

8. drug used to treat AIDS by blocking the growth of the AIDS virus _____

9. drug used to treat AIDS by blocking the production of a proteolytic enzyme

_____

I. Complete the following terms according to their definitions. Pay close attention to the proper spelling of each term.

1. chronic, disabling diseases caused by abnormal production of antibodies to normal tissue:

   auto _____ diseases

2. a hypersensitivity or allergic state with an inherited predisposition: a _____

3. a malignant tumor of lymph nodes; histiocytic and lymphocytic are types of this disease:

   non-_____

4. fluid that lies between cells throughout the body: inter _____ fluid

5. formation of lymphocytes or lymphoid tissue: lympho _____

6. chronic swelling of a part of the body due to collection of fluid between tissues secondary to

   obstruction of lymph vessels and nodes: lymph _____

7. an unusual or exaggerated allergic reaction to a foreign protein: ana _____

8. introduction of altered antigens to produce an immune response and protection from disease:

   vac _____

9. test that separates human immunoglobins: immuno _____

J. Select the correct term to complete each sentence.

1. Mr. Blake had been HIV-positive for 5 years before he developed (**PCP, thymoma, multiple myeloma**) and was diagnosed with (**Hodgkin disease, non-Hodgkin lymphoma, AIDS**).

2. Mary developed rhinitis, rhinorrhea, and red eyes every spring when pollen was prevalent. She consulted her doctor about her bad (**hypersplenism, allergies, lymphadenitis**).

3. Paul felt some marble-sized lumps in his left groin. His doctor told him that he had an infection in his foot and had developed secondary (**axillary, cervical, inguinal**) lymphadenopathy.

4. Mr. Jones was referred to a dermatologist and an oncologist when his primary physician noticed purple spots on his arms and legs. Because he had AIDS, his physician was worried about (**Kaposi sarcoma, splenomegaly, thrombocytopenic purpura**).

X. Answers to Exercises

A

1. lymph nodes
2. thoracic duct
3. spleen
4. adenoids
5. thymus gland
6. lymph capillaries
7. right lymphatic duct
8. interstitial fluid

B

1. groin region
2. armpit region
3. neck (of the body) region
4. space between the lungs in the chest

C

1. humoral immunity
2. T cells
3. cell-mediated immunity
4. B cells

D

1. plasma cell
2. macrophage
3. helper cell
4. natural killer (NK) cell
5. suppressor cell
6. dendritic cell

E

1. A
2. C
3. B
4. D
5. G
6. F
7. E

F

1. splenectomy
2. splenomegaly
3. lymphopoiesis
4. thymoma
5. lymphadenitis
6. lymphocytopenia
7. toxic
8. lymphadenopathy

G

1. hypersplenism
2. anaphylaxis
3. allergen
4. AIDS
5. thymectomy
6. Hodgkin disease
7. lymphoid organs
8. lymphedema

H

1. Kaposi sarcoma
2. HIV
3. T4 helper lymphocytes
4. PCP
5. opportunistic infections
6. ELISA (enzyme-linked immunosorbent assay)
7. Western blot
8. RT inhibitor
9. protease inhibitor

I

1. autoimmune
2. atopy
3. non-Hodgkin lymphoma
4. interstitial
5. lymphopoiesis
6. lymphedema
7. anaphylaxis
8. vaccination
9. immunoelectrophoresis

J

1. PCP; AIDS
2. allergies
3. inguinal
4. Kaposi sarcoma

Answers to Practical Applications

1. B
2. A
3. A
4. B
5. B
6. A
7. B
8. C

XI. Pronunciation of Terms

Pronunciation Guide

ā as in āpe   ă as in ăpple
ē as in ēven   ĕ as in ĕvery
ī as in īce   ĭ as in ĭnterest
ō as in ōpen   ŏ as in pŏt
ū as in ūnit   ŭ as in ŭnder

To test your understanding of the terminology in this chapter, write the meaning of each term in the space provided. In addition, you may wish to cover the terms and write them by looking at your definitions. Make sure your spelling is correct. The page number after each term indicates where it is defined or used in the text so you can easily check your responses.

Vocabulary and Terminology

Term	Pronunciation	Meaning
acquired immunity (513)	ă-KWĪ-erd ĭ-MŪ-nĭ-tē	
acquired immunodeficiency syndrome (516)	ă-KWĪ-ĕrd ĭm-ū-nō-dĕ-FĬSH-ĕn-sē SĬN-drōm	
adenoids (513)	ĂD-ĕ-noydz	
allergen (520)	ĂL-ĕr-jĕn	
allergy (518)	ĂL-ĕr-jē	
anaphylaxis (518)	ăn-ă-fă-LĂK-sĭs	
antibodies (513)	ĂN-tĭ-bŏ-dēz	
atopy (520)	ĂT-ō-pē	
autoimmune diseases (515)	āw-tō-ĭ-MŪN dĭ-ZĒZ-ez	
axillary nodes (513)	ĂKS-ĭ-lăr-ē nōdz	
cell-mediated immunity (513)	sĕl-MĒ-dē-ā-tĕd ĭ-MŪ-nĭ-tē	
cervical nodes (513)	SĔR-vĭ-k'l nōdz	
cytotoxic cells (513)	sī-tō-TŎK-sĭk sĕlz	
dendritic cells (513)	dĕn-DRĬ-tik sĕlz	
Hodgkin disease (518)	HŎJ-kĭn dĭ-ZĒZ	
human immunodeficiency virus (520)	HŪ-măn ĭm-ū-nō-dĕ-FĬSH-ĕn-sē VĪ-rŭs	
humoral immunity (513)	HŪ-mŏr-ăl ĭ-MŪ-nĭ-tē	

hypersensitivity (518)   hī-pĕr-sĕn-sĭ-TĬV-ĭ-tē   _____

hypersplenism (515)   hī-pĕr-SPLĔN-ĭzm   _____

immune response (513)   ĭ-MŪN rĕ-SPŎNS   _____

immunoelectrophoresis (521)   ĭm-ū-nō-ē-lĕk-trō-phŏr-Ē-sĭs   _____

immunoglobulins (513)   ĭm-ū-nō-GLŎB-ū-lĭnz   _____

immunosuppression (515)   ĭm-ū-nō-sū-PRĔ-shun   _____

inguinal nodes (513)   ĬNG-gwĭ-năl nōdz   _____

interferons (513)   ĭn-tĕr-FĔR-ŏnz   _____

interleukins (513)   ĭn-tĕr-LOO-kĭnz   _____

interstitial fluid (513)   ĭn-tĕr-STĬSH-ăl FLOO-ĭd   _____

Kaposi sarcoma (520)   KĂ-pō-sē (kă-Pōs-sē) săr-KŌ-mă   _____

lymph (514)   lĭmf   _____

lymphadenitis (515)   lĭm-FĂH-dĕ-nī-tĭs   _____

lymphadenopathy (515)   lĭm-făd-ĕ-NŎP-ăh-thē   _____

lymph capillaries (514)   lĭmf KĂP-ĭ-lă-rēz   _____

lymphedema (515)   lĭmf-ĕ-DĒ-mă   _____

lymph nodes (514)   lĭmf nōdz   _____

lymphocytes (506)   LĬM-fō-sītz   _____

lymphocytosis (515)   lĭm-fō-sī-TŌ-sĭs   _____

lymphocytopenia (515)   lĭm-fō-sī-tō-PĒ-nē-ă   _____

lymphoid organs (514)   LĬM-foid ŎR-gănz   _____

lymphoma (518)   lĭm-FŌ-mă   _____

lymphopoiesis (515)   lĭm-fō-poy-Ē-sĭs   _____

lymph vessels (514)   lĭmf VĔS-ĕlz   _____

macrophage (514)   MĂK-rō-făj   _____

mediastinal nodes (514)   mē-dē-ăs-TĪ-năl nōdz   _____

natural immunity (514)   NĂ-tū-răl ĭm-MŪ-nĭ-tē   _____

non-Hodgkin lymphoma (519)	nŏn-HŎJ-kĭn lĭm-FŌ-mă	_____
opportunistic infections (520)	ŏp-pŏr-tū-NĬS-tĭk ĭn-FĔK-shŭnz	_____
plasma cell (514)	PLĂZ-mă sĕl	_____
protease inhibitor (520)	PRŌ-tē-ās ĭn-HĬB-ĭ-tor	_____
retrovirus (520)	rĕ-trō-VĪ-rŭs	_____
reverse transcriptase inhibitor (520)	rē-VĔRS trănz-SCRĬP-tās ĭn-HĬB-ĭ-tŏr	_____
right lymphatic duct (514)	rīt lĭm-FĂ-tĭk dŭkt	_____
spleen (514)	splēn	_____
splenectomy (515)	splĕ-NĔK-tō-mē	_____
splenomegaly (515)	splĕ-nō-MĔG-ă-lē	_____
thoracic duct (514)	thō-RĂ-sĭk dŭkt	_____
thymectomy (516)	thī-MĔK-tō-mē	_____
thymoma (516)	thī-MŌ-mă	_____
thymus gland (514)	THĪ-mŭs glănd	_____
tonsils (514)	TŎN-sĭlz	_____
toxic (516)	TŎK-sĭk	_____
toxins (514)	TŎK-sĭnz	_____
vaccination (514)	văk-sĭ-NĀ-shun	_____
Western blot (521)	WĔS-tĕrn blŏt	_____

XII. Review Sheet

Write the meaning of the word parts in the spaces provided. Check your answers with the information in the chapter or in the glossary (Medical Terms—English) at the end of the book.

COMBINING FORMS

Combining Form	Meaning	Combining Form	Meaning
axill/o	_____	lymphaden/o	_____
cervic/o	_____	splen/o	_____
immun/o	_____	thym/o	_____
inguin/o	_____	tox/o	_____
lymph/o	_____		

SUFFIXES

Suffix	Meaning	Suffix	Meaning
-cytosis	_____	-penia	_____
-edema	_____	-phylaxis	_____
-globulin	_____	-poiesis	_____
-megaly	_____	-stitial	_____
-oid	_____	-suppression	_____
-pathy	_____		

PREFIXES

Prefix	Meaning	Prefix	Meaning
ana-	_____	inter-	_____
auto-	_____	retro-	_____
hyper-	_____		

CHAPTER 15

Musculoskeletal System

This chapter is divided into the following sections

In this chapter you will

- Define terms relating to the structure and function of bones, joints, and muscles;
- Describe the process of bone formation and growth;
- Locate and name the major bones of the body;
- Analyze the combining forms, prefixes, and suffixes used to describe bones, joints, and muscles;
- Explain various musculoskeletal disease conditions and terms related to bone fractures;
- Identify important laboratory tests, clinical procedures, and abbreviations relating to the musculoskeletal system; and
- Apply your new knowledge to understanding medical terms in their proper contexts, such as medical reports and records.

I. Introduction

The musculoskeletal system includes the bones, muscles, and joints. All have important functions in the body. **Bones** provide the framework around which the body is constructed and protect and support internal organs. Bones also assist the body in movement because they are a point of attachment for muscles. The inner core of bones is composed of hematopoietic tissue (red bone marrow manufacturers blood cells), whereas other parts of bone are storage areas for minerals necessary for growth, such as calcium and phosphorus.

Joints are the places at which bones come together. Several different types of joints are found within the body. The type of joint found in any specific location is determined by the need for greater or lesser flexibility of movement.

Muscles, whether attached to bones or to internal organs and blood vessels, are responsible for movement. Internal movement involves the contraction and relaxation of muscles that are a part of viscera, and external movement is accomplished by the contraction and relaxation of muscles that are attached to the bones.

Physicians who treat bones and bone and joint diseases are **orthopedists.** Originally, orthopedics was a branch of medicine dealing with correcting deformities in children (**orth/o** means straight, **ped/o** means child). **Rheumatologists** are other physicians who also treat joint diseases. **Rheumat/o** means watery flow and relates to joint diseases because various forms of arthritis are marked by the collection of fluid in the joint spaces.

Osteopathic physicians (DOs) practice **osteopathy,** which is a separate school of medicine using diagnostic and therapeutic measures based on the belief that the body is capable of healing itself when bones are in proper position and adequate nutrition is provided. **Chiropractors (chir/o** means hand) are neither physicians nor osteopaths. They use physical means to manipulate the spinal column, believing that disease is caused by pressure on nerves.

II. Bones

A. Formation and Structure

Formation

Bones are complete organs composed chiefly of connective tissue called **osseous** (bony) **tissue** plus a rich supply of blood vessels and nerves. Osseous tissue consists of a combination of **osteocytes** (bone cells), dense connective tissue strands known as **collagen,** and intercellular **calcium salts.**

During fetal development, the bones of the fetus are composed of **cartilaginous tissue,** which resembles osseous tissue but is more flexible and less dense because of a lack of calcium salts in its intercellular spaces. As the embryo develops, the process of depositing calcium salts in the soft, cartilaginous tissue occurs and continues throughout the life of the individual after birth. The gradual replacement of cartilage and its intercellular substance by immature bone cells and calcium deposits is called **ossification** (bone formation).

Osteoblasts are the immature osteocytes that produce the bony tissue that replaces cartilage during ossification. **Osteoclasts** (**-clast** means to break) are large cells that function to reabsorb, or digest, bony tissue. Osteoclasts (also called **bone phagocytes**) digest bone tissue from the inner sides of bones and thus enlarge the inner bone cavity so that the bone does not become overly thick and heavy. When a bone breaks, osteoblasts lay down the mineral bone matter (calcium salts), and osteoclasts remove excess bone debris (smooth out the bone).

Osteoblasts and osteoclasts work together in all bones throughout life, tearing down (osteoclasts) and rebuilding (osteoblasts) bony tissue. This allows bone to respond to mechanical stresses placed upon it and thus enables it to be a living tissue, constantly rebuilding and renewing itself.

The formation of bone is dependent to a great extent on a proper supply of **calcium** and **phosphorus** to the bone tissue. These minerals must be taken into the body along with a sufficient amount of vitamin D. Vitamin D helps the passage of calcium through the lining of the small intestine and into the bloodstream. Once calcium and phosphorus are in the bones, osteoblastic activity produces an enzyme that causes the formation of calcium phosphate, a substance that gives bone its characteristic hard quality. It is the major calcium salt.

Not only are calcium and phosphorus part of the hard structure of bone tissue but calcium is also stored elsewhere in bones, and small quantities are present in the blood. If the proper amount of calcium is lacking in the blood, nerve fibers are unable to transmit impulses effectively to muscles, the heart muscle becomes weak, and muscles attached to bones undergo spasms.

The necessary level of calcium in the blood is maintained by the parathyroid gland, which secretes a hormone to release calcium from bone storage. An excess of the hormone (caused by tumor or another pathological process) will raise blood calcium at the expense of the bones, which become weakened by the loss of calcium.

Structure

There are 206 bones of various types in the body. **Long bones** are found in the thigh, lower leg, and upper and lower arm. These bones are very strong, are broad at the ends where they join with other bones, and have large surface areas for muscle attachment.

Short bones are found in the wrist and ankle and have small, irregular shapes. **Flat bones** are found covering soft body parts. These are the shoulder blades, ribs, and pelvic bones. **Sesamoid bones** are small, rounded bones resembling a grain of sesame in shape. They are found near joints, and they increase the efficiency of muscles near a particular joint. The kneecap is the largest example of a sesamoid bone.

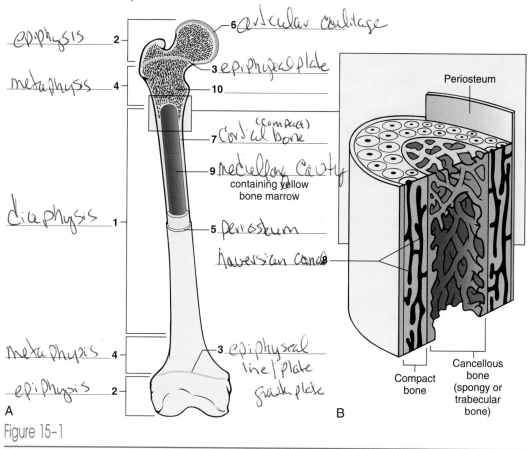

epiphysis — 2
metaphysis — 4
diaphysis — 1
metaphysis — 4
epiphysis — 2
A

6 articular cartilage
3 epiphyseal plate
10 _____
7 Cortical bone (compact)
9 medullary cavity
containing yellow
bone marrow
5 periosteum
haversian canals 8
3 epiphyseal
line/plate
growth plate

Periosteum
Compact bone
Cancellous bone (spongy or trabecular bone)
B

Figure 15-1

(A) Divisions of a long bone and interior bone structure. (B) Composition of compact (cortical) bone.

Figure 15–1A shows the anatomical divisions of a long bone such as the thigh bone or upper arm bone. Label the figure as you read the following.

The shaft, or middle region, of a long bone is called the **diaphysis** [1]. Each end of a long bone is called an **epiphysis** [2]. The **epiphyseal line** or **plate** [3] represents an area of cartilage tissue that is constantly being replaced by new bony tissue as the bone grows; it is also commonly known as the growth plate. Cartilage cells at the edges of the epiphyseal plate form new bone, and this is responsible for the lengthening of bones during childhood and adolescence. The plate calcifies and disappears when the bone has achieved its full growth. The **metaphysis** [4] is the flared portion of the bone; it lies between the epiphysis and the diaphysis. It is adjacent to the epiphysis plate.

The **periosteum** [5] is a strong, fibrous, vascular membrane that covers the surface of a long bone, except at the ends of the epiphyses. It has a large nerve supply, as well. Bones other than long bones are also covered by periosteum. Beneath the periosteum is the layer of osteoblasts, which deposit calcium phosphate in the bony tissue.

The ends of long bones and the surface of any bone that meets another bone to form a joint are covered with **articular cartilage** [6]. When two bones come together to form a joint, the bones themselves do not touch precisely. The articular cartilage that caps the end of one bone comes in contact with that of the other bone. Articular cartilage is a very smooth, strong, and slick tissue. It cushions a joint and allows it to move smoothly and efficiently. Unlike the cartilage of the epiphyseal plate, which disappears when a bone achieves its full growth, articular cartilage is present throughout life.

Compact (cortical) bone [7] is a layer of hard, dense bone that lies under the periosteum in all bones and chiefly around the diaphysis of long bones. Within the compact bone is a system of small canals containing blood vessels that bring oxygen and nutrients to the bone and remove waste products such as carbon dioxide. Figure 15–1B shows these channels, called **haversian canals** [8], in the compact bone. Compact bone is tunneled out in the central shaft of the long bones by a **medullary cavity** [9] that contains **yellow bone marrow.** Yellow bone marrow is composed chiefly of fat cells.

Cancellous bone [10], sometimes called **spongy** or **trabecular bone,** is much more porous and less dense than compact bone. The mineral matter in it is laid down in a series of separated bony fibers called a spongy latticework or **trabeculae.** It is found largely in the epiphyses and metaphyses of long bones, in the medullary cavity, and in the middle portion of most other bones of the body as well. Spaces in cancellous bone contain **red bone marrow.** This marrow, as opposed to yellow marrow, which is fatty tissue, is richly supplied with blood and consists of immature and mature blood cells in various stages of development.

In an adult, the ribs, pelvic bone, sternum (breastbone), and vertebrae, as well as the epiphyses of long bones, contain red bone marrow within cancellous tissue. The red marrow in the long bones is plentiful in young children but decreases through the years and is replaced by yellow marrow.

B. Processes and Depressions in Bones

Bone processes are enlarged areas that extend out from bones to serve as attachments for muscles and tendons. Label Figure 15–2A and B, which shows the shapes of some of the common bony processes:

Bone head [1]—rounded end of a bone separated from the body of the bone by a neck; usually covered by articular cartilage.
Trochanter [2]—large process on the femur for attachment of muscle.
Tubercle [3]—small, rounded process on many bones for attachment of tendons or muscles.
Tuberosity [4]—large, rounded process on many bones for attachment of muscles or tendons.
Condyle [5]—rounded, knuckle-like process at the joint; usually covered by articular cartilage.

Figure 15-2

(A) **Bone process on the femur** (thigh bone) **and (B) humerus** (upper arm bone). The bone neck separates the bone head from the rest of the bone. A fossa is a shallow depression or cavity in a bone. The fossa on the humerus is a space for the olecranon process on the lower arm bone (ulna) when the elbow is extended.

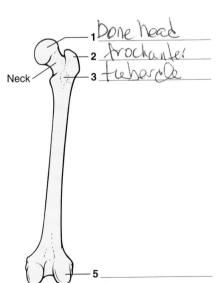

Neck

1 Bone head
2 Trochanter
3 tubercle

5

A   FEMUR (posterior view)

4 tuberosity
3 Condyle
tubercle

Olecranon (elbow) fossa
5 Condyle

B   HUMERUS (posterior view)

Bone depressions are the openings or hollow regions in a bone that help to join one bone to another and that serve as passageways for blood vessels and nerves. The names of some common depressions in bone are:

Fossa—shallow cavity in or on a bone.
Foramen—opening for blood vessels and nerves.
Fissure—a narrow, deep, slit-like opening.
Sinus—a hollow cavity within a bone.

C. Cranial Bones

The bones of the skull, or cranium, protect the brain and structures related to it, such as the sense organs. Muscles for controlling head movements and chewing motions are connected to the cranial bones. The cranial bones join each other at joints called **sutures.**

The cranial bones of a newborn child are not completely joined. There are gaps of unossified tissue in the skull at birth. These are called soft spots, or **fontanelles** (little fountains). The pulse of blood vessels can be felt under the skin in those areas.

Figure 15–3 illustrates the bones of the cranium. Label them as you read the following descriptions:

Frontal bone [1]—forms the forehead and the roof of the bony sockets that contain the eyes.
Parietal bone [2]—there are two parietal bones (one on each side of the skull) that form the roof and upper part of the sides of the cranium.
Temporal bone [3]—two temporal bones form the lower sides and base of the cranium. Each bone encloses an ear and contains a fossa for joining with the mandible (lower jaw bone). The **temporomandibular joint (TMJ)** is the area of connection between the temporal and mandibular bones. The **mastoid process** is a round (**mast/o** means breast) process of the temporal bone behind the ear. The **styloid process** (**styl/o** means pole or stake) projects downward from the temporal bone.
Occipital bone [4]—forms the back and base of the skull and joins the parietal and temporal bones, forming a suture. The inferior portion of the occipital bone has an opening called the **foramen magnum** through which the spinal cord passes (Fig. 15–4).
Sphenoid bone [5]—this bat-shaped bone extends behind the eyes and forms part of the base of the skull. Because it joins with the frontal, occipital, and ethmoid bones, it serves as an anchor to hold those skull bones together (**sphen/o** means wedge). The **sella turcica** (meaning Turkish saddle) is a depression in the sphenoid bone in which the pituitary gland is located (see Fig. 15–4).
Ethmoid bone [6]—this thin, delicate bone is composed primarily of spongy, cancellous bone. It supports the nasal cavity and forms part of the orbits of the eyes (**ethm/o** means sieve).

Study Figure 15–4, which shows these cranial bones as viewed looking downward at the floor of the cranial cavity.

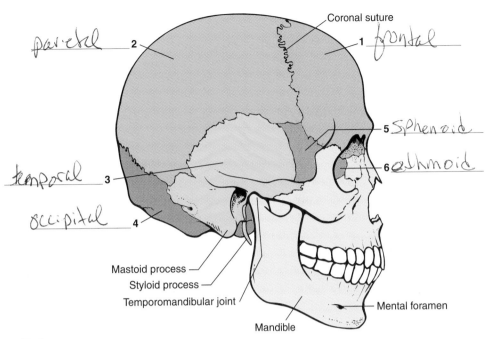

Figure 15-3

Cranial bones, lateral view. The **mental** (ment/o means chin) **foramen** is the opening in the mandible that allows blood vessels and nerves to enter and leave. The **coronal suture** is the connection across the skull between the two parietal bones and the frontal bone.

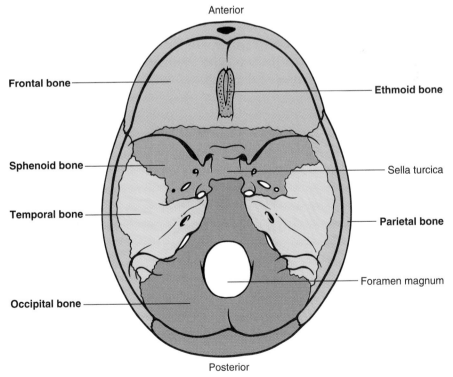

Figure 15-4

Cranial bones, looking downward at the floor of the cranial cavity.

D. Facial Bones

All the facial bones, except one, are joined together by sutures, so that they are immovable. The mandible (lower jaw bone) is the only facial bone capable of movement. This ability is necessary for activities such as mastication (chewing) and speaking.

Figure 15–5 shows the facial bones; label it as you read the following descriptions of the facial bones:

Nasal bones [1]—two slender nasal (**nas/o** means nose) bones support the bridge of the nose. They join with the frontal bone superiorly and form part of the nasal septum.

Lacrimal bones [2]—two paired lacrimal (**lacrim/o** means tear) bones are located at the corner of each eye. These thin, small bones contain fossae for the lacrimal gland (tear gland) and canals for the passage of the lacrimal duct.

Maxillary bones [3]—two large bones compose the massive upper jaw bones **(maxillae).** They are joined by a suture in the median plane. If the two bones do not come together normally before birth, the condition known as **cleft palate** results.

Mandibular bone [4]—this is the lower jaw bone **(mandible).** Both the maxilla and the mandible contain the sockets called alveoli in which the teeth are embedded. The mandible joins the skull at the region of the temporal bone, forming the temporomandibular joint (TMJ) on either side of the skull.

Zygomatic bones [5]—two bones, one on each side of the face, form the high portion of the cheek.

Vomer [6]—this thin, single, flat bone forms the lower portion of the nasal septum.

Sinuses, or air cavities, are located in specific places within the cranial and facial bones to lighten the skull and warm and moisten air as it passes through. Figure 15–6 shows the sinuses of the skull.

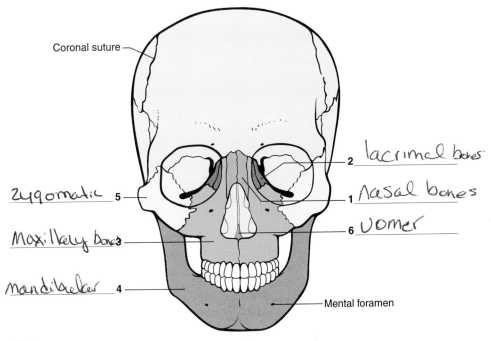

Coronal suture

2 lacrimal bones
1 Nasal bones
6 Vomer

zygomatic 5

Maxillary bones 3

mandibular 4

Mental foramen

Figure 15-5

Facial bones.

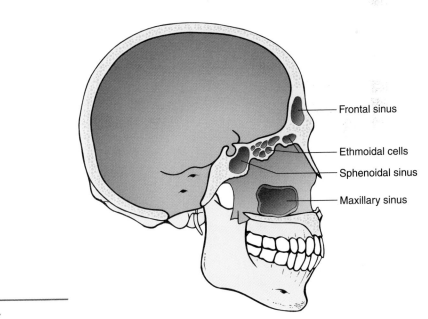

Frontal sinus

Ethmoidal cells

Sphenoidal sinus

Maxillary sinus

Figure 15-6

Sinuses of the skull.

E. Vertebral Column and Structure of Vertebrae

The **vertebral**, or **spinal**, **column** is composed of 26 bone segments, called vertebrae, that are arranged in five divisions from the base of the skull to the tailbone. The bones are separated by pads of cartilage called intervertebral discs (disks).

Figure 15–7 illustrates these divisions of the vertebral column.

The first 7 bones of the vertebral column, forming the bony aspect of the neck are the **cervical (C1–C7) vertebrae.** These vertebrae do not articulate (join) with the ribs.

The second set of 12 vertebrae are known as the **thoracic (T1–T12) vertebrae.** These vertebrae articulate with the 12 pairs of ribs.

The third set of 5 vertebral bones are the **lumbar (L1–L5) vertebrae.** They are the strongest and largest of the back bones. Like the cervical vertebrae, these bones do not articulate with the ribs.

The **sacrum** is a slightly curved, triangularly shaped bone. At birth it is composed of 5 separate segments (sacral bones); these gradually become fused in the young child.

The **coccyx** is the tailbone, and it, too, is a fused bone, having been formed from 4 small coccygeal bones.

Figure 15–8A illustrates the general structure of a vertebra. Although the individual vertebrae in the separate regions of the spinal column are all slightly different in structure, they do have several parts in common.

A vertebra is composed of an inner, thick, round portion called the **vertebral body** [1]. Between the body of one vertebra and the bodies of the vertebrae lying beneath and above are **intervertebral cartilaginous discs** (disks), which help to provide flexibility and cushion most shocks to the vertebral column.

The **vertebral arch** [2] is the posterior part of the vertebra, and it consists of a **spinous process** [3], a **transverse process** [4], and **lamina** [5]. The **neural canal** [6] is the space between the vertebral body and the vertebral arch through which the spinal cord passes. Figure 15–8B shows a lateral view of several vertebrae. Note the location of the spinal cord running through the neural canal.

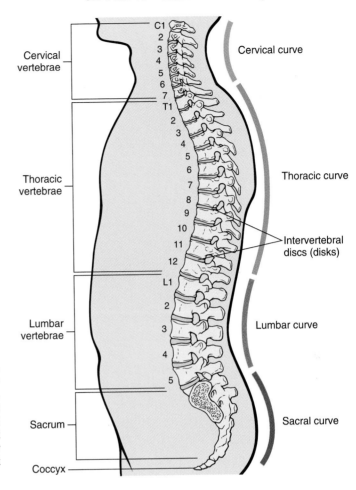

Figure 15-7

Vertebral column. Notice the four curves of the vertebral column. The sacral and thoracic curvatures are present at birth. The cervical curvature develops when an infant holds its head erect. The lumbar curvature develops as an infant begins to stand and walk.

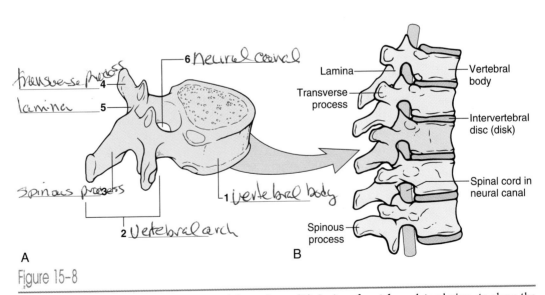

A   B

Figure 15-8

(A) General structure of a vertebra, viewed from above. **(B) Series of vertebrae,** lateral view, to show the position of the spinal cord behind the vertebral bodies and intervertebral discs.

F. Bones of the Thorax, Pelvis, and Extremities

Label Figure 15–9 as you read the following descriptions of the bones of the thorax (chest cavity), pelvis (hip bone), and extremities (arms and legs):

Bones of the Thorax

Clavicle [1]—collar bone; a slender bone, one on each side of the body, connecting the breastbone to each shoulder blade.

Scapula [2]—shoulder blade; two flat, triangular bones, one on each dorsal side of the thorax. The extension of the scapula that joins with the clavicle to form a joint above the shoulder is called the **acromion** (**acr/o** means extremity, **om/o** means shoulder). The joint formed by these two bones is known as the acromio-clavicular joint. Figure 15–10 shows a posterior view of the scapula.

Sternum [3]—breastbone; a flat bone extending down the midline of the chest. The uppermost part of the sternum articulates on the sides with the clavicle and ribs, and the lower, narrower portion is attached to the diaphragm and abdominal muscles. The lower portion of the sternum is called the **xiphoid process** (**xiph/o** means sword).

Ribs [4]—there are 12 pairs of ribs. The first 7 pairs join the sternum anteriorly through cartilaginous attachments called **costal cartilages.** Ribs 1–7 are called **true ribs.** They join with the sternum anteriorly and with the vertebral column in the back. Ribs 8–10 are called **false ribs.** They join with the vertebral column in the back but join the 7th rib anteriorly instead of attaching to the sternum. Ribs 11 and 12 are the **floating ribs** because they are completely free at their anterior extremity. Figure 15–10 shows a posterior view of the rib cage.

Bones of the Arm and Hand

These are described as if the patient is in the anatomical position—palms forward.

Humerus [5]—upper arm bone; the large head of the humerus is rounded and joins with the glenoid fossa of the scapula to form the shoulder joint (see Fig. 15–10).

Ulna [6]—medial lower arm bone; the proximal bony process of the ulna at the elbow is called the **olecranon** (elbow bone). The olecranon is the bony point of the elbow when the elbow is bent.

Radius [7]—lateral lower arm bone (in line with the thumb).

Carpals [8]—wrist bones; there are two rows of 4 bones in the wrist.

Metacarpals [9]—there are 5 radiating bones in the fingers. These are the bones of the palm of the hand.

Phalanges [10] (singular: **phalanx**)—finger bones; each finger (except the thumb) has 3 phalanges: a proximal, middle, and distal phalanx. The thumb has only 2 phalanges: a proximal and a distal phalanx.

Bones of the Pelvis

Pelvic girdle (pelvis) [11]—hip bone. This collection of bones supports the trunk of the body and articulates with the thigh bone to form the hip joint. The adult pelvic bone is composed of 3 pairs of fused bones: the ilium, ischium, and pubis, which articulate posteriorly with the sacrum of the vertebral column.

Figure 15-9

Bones of the thorax, pelvis, and extremities.

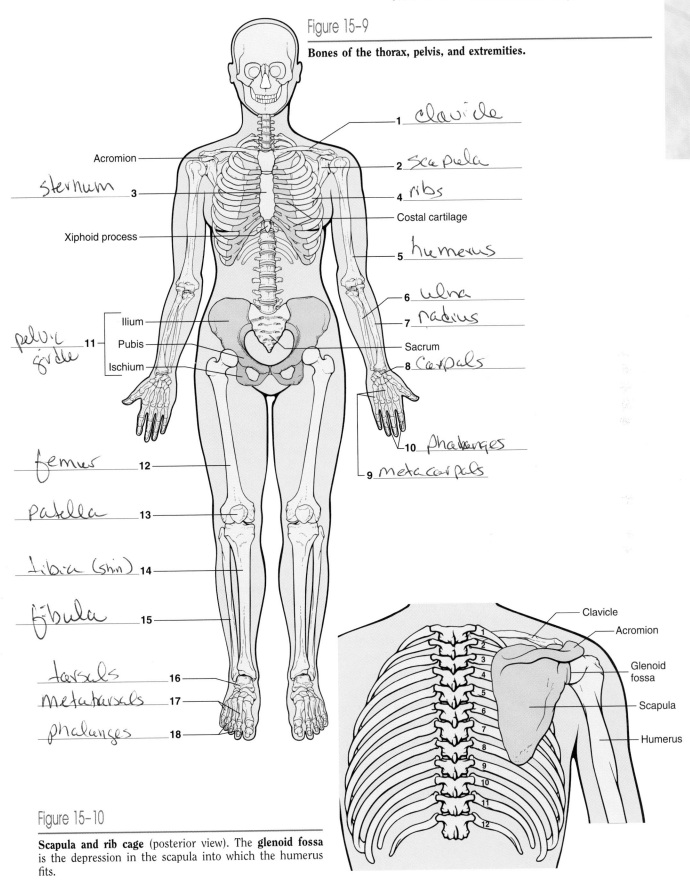

Acromion

sternum 3

Xiphoid process

Ilium
pelvic girdle   11   Pubis
Ischium

1 clavicle
2 scapula
4 ribs
Costal cartilage
5 humerus
6 ulna
7 radius
Sacrum
8 carpals

10 phalanges
9 metacarpals

femur   12

patella   13

tibia (shin) 14

fibula   15

tarsals   16
metatarsals   17
phalanges   18

Figure 15-10

Scapula and rib cage (posterior view). The **glenoid fossa** is the depression in the scapula into which the humerus fits.

Clavicle
Acromion
Glenoid fossa
Scapula
Humerus

The **ilium** is the uppermost and largest portion. Dorsally, the two parts of the ilium do not meet. Rather, they join the sacrum on either side to form the sacroiliac joints. The connection between the iliac bones and the sacrum is very firm, and very little motion occurs at these joints. The superior part of the ilium is known as the **iliac crest.** It is filled with red bone marrow and serves as an attachment for abdominal wall muscles.

The **ischium** (**isch/o** means back) is the posterior part of the pelvis. The ischium and the muscles attached to it are what you sit on.

The **pubis** is the anterior part and the two pubes join by way of a cartilaginous disc. This area is called the **pubic symphysis.** Like the sacroiliac joints, this area is quite rigid.

The region within the ring of bone formed by the pelvic girdle is called the **pelvic cavity.** The rectum, sigmoid colon, bladder, and female reproductive organs lie within the pelvic cavity and are protected by the rigid architecture of the pelvic girdle.

Bones of the Leg and Foot

Femur [12]—thigh bone; this is the longest bone in the body. At its proximal end it has a rounded head that fits into a depression, or socket, in the pelvis. This socket is called the **acetabulum.** The acetabulum was named because of its resemblance to a rounded cup the Romans used for vinegar (acetum). The head of the femur and the acetabulum form the "ball and socket" joint otherwise known as the hip joint.

Patella [13]—kneecap; this is a small, flat bone that lies in front of the articulation between the femur and one of the lower leg bones called the tibia. It is a sesamoid bone surrounded by protective tendons and held in place by muscle attachments.

Tibia [14]—largest of 2 bones of the lower leg; the tibia runs under the skin in the front part of the leg. It joins with the femur at the patella, and at its distal end (ankle) forms a flare that is the bony prominence (medial **malleolus**) at the inside of the ankle. The tibia is commonly called the **shin bone.**

Fibula [15]—smaller of 2 lower leg bones; this thin bone, well hidden under the leg muscles, runs parallel to the tibia. At its distal part, it forms a flare, which is the bony prominence (lateral **malleolus**) on the outside of the ankle. The tibia, fibula, and **talus** (the first of the tarsal bones) come together to form the **ankle joint.**

Tarsals [16]—bones of the hind part of the foot; these are 7 short bones that resemble the carpal bones of the wrist but are larger. The **calcaneus** is the largest of these bones and is also called the **heel bone** (Fig. 15–11). The **talus** is one of three bones that form the ankle joint.

Metatarsals [17]—bones of the midfoot; there are 5 metatarsal bones, which are similar to the metacarpals of the hand. Each leads to the phalanges of the toes.

Phalanges of the toes [18]—bones of the forefoot; similar to the hand, there are 2 phalanges in the big toe and 3 in each of the other toes.

Figure 15–11 illustrates the bones of the foot.

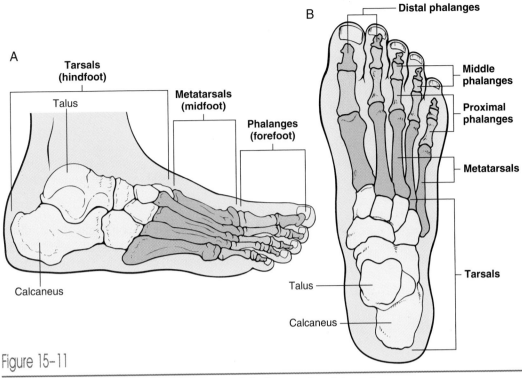

Figure 15-11

(A) Bones of the foot, lateral view. **(B) Bones of the foot,** as viewed from above.

G. Vocabulary

This list will help you review many of the new terms introduced in the text. Short definitions will reinforce your understanding of the terms. See Section IX of this chapter for help in pronouncing the more difficult terms.

acetabulum	Rounded depression, or socket, in the pelvic bone where the femur (thigh bone) joins the pelvis, forming the hip joint.
acromion	Outward extension of the shoulder bone forming the point of the shoulder. It overlies the shoulder joint and articulates with the clavicle.
articular cartilage	Thin layer of cartilage occurring at the ends of long bones and covering any part of any bone that comes together with another bone to form a joint.
calcium	One of the mineral constituents of bone. Calcium phosphate is the major calcium salt in bones.
cancellous bone	Spongy, porous, trabecular bone.
cartilaginous tissue (cartilage)	Flexible, rubbery connective tissue. It is found on joint surfaces throughout life and in the immature skeleton at the epiphyseal growth plate.
collagen	Dense connective tissue strands found in bone.
compact bone	Hard, dense bone tissue.

condyle   Knuckle-like process at the end of a bone near the joint.

cranial bones   Skull bones: ethmoid, frontal, occipital, parietal, sphenoid, and temporal.

diaphysis   Shaft, or midportion, of a long bone.

disc (disk)   Flat, round, plate-like structure. An intervertebral disc is a fibrocartilaginous substance between two vertebrae.

epiphyseal plate   Cartilaginous area at the ends of long bones where lengthwise growth takes place.

epiphysis   Each end of a long bone; the area beyond the epiphyseal plate.

facial bones   Bones of the face: lacrimal, mandible, maxillae, nasal, vomer, and zygomatic.

fissure   Narrow, slit-like opening between bones.

fontanelle   Soft spot (incomplete bone formation) between the skull bones of an infant.

foramen   Opening or passage in bones where blood vessels, nerves, or both enter and leave. The **foramen magnum** is the opening of the occipital bone through which the spinal cord passes.

fossa   Shallow cavity in a bone.

haversian canals   Minute spaces filled with blood vessels; found in compact bone.

malleolus   Round process on both sides of the ankle joint. The lateral malleolus is part of the fibula, and the medial malleolus is part of the tibia.

mastoid process   Round projection on the temporal bone behind the ear.

medullary cavity   Central, hollowed-out area in the shaft of a long bone.

metaphysis   The flared portion of a long bone, lying between the diaphysis (shaft) and the epiphyseal plate (meta- means between).

olecranon   Large process on the proximal end of the ulna; the point of the flexed elbow.

osseous tissue   Bone tissue.

ossification   Process of bone formation.

osteoblast   Bone cell that helps form bone tissue.

osteoclast   Bone cell that absorbs and removes unwanted bone tissue.

periosteum   Membrane surrounding bones; rich in blood vessels and nerve tissue.

phosphorus	Mineral substance found in bones in combination with calcium.
pubic symphysis	Area of confluence (coming together) of the two pubic bones. They are joined (sym- means together, -physis means to grow) by a fibrocartilaginous disc.
red bone marrow	Found in cancellous bone; site of hematopoiesis.
ribs	These 24 elongated, curved bones form the bony wall of the chest. True ribs are the first 7 pairs; false ribs are pairs 8–10; floating ribs are pairs 11 and 12.
sinus	Cavity within a bone.
styloid process	Pole-like process on the temporal bone.
trabeculae	Supporting bundles of bony fibers in cancellous (spongy) bone.
trochanter	Large process below the neck of the femur; attachment site for muscles and tendons.
tubercle	Small, rounded process on a bone; attachment site for muscles and tendons.
tuberosity	Large, rounded process on a bone; attachment site for muscles and tendons.
vertebra	An individual back bone composed of the vertebral body, vertebral arch, spinous process, transverse process, lamina, and neural canal.
xiphoid process	Lower, narrow portion of the sternum.
yellow bone marrow	Fatty tissue found in the diaphyses of long bones.

H. Combining Forms and Suffixes

These are divided into two groups: general terms and terms related to specific bones. Write the meanings of the medical terms in the spaces provided.

GENERAL TERMS Combining Forms			
Combining Forms	Meaning	Terminology	Meaning
calc/o	calcium	hypercalcemia _____	
	calci/o	decalcification _____	
		de- means less or lack of; -fication is the process of making.	

kyph/o	humpback (posterior curvature in the thoracic region)	kyphosis _____ *The term (from the Greek) means hill or mountain, indicating a hump on the back. A person's height is reduced, and kyphosis may lead to pressure on the spinal cord or peripheral nerves.*
lamin/o	lamina (part of the vertebral arch)	laminectomy _____ *An operation often performed to relieve the symptoms of compression of the spinal cord or spinal nerve roots.*
lord/o	curve, swayback (anterior curvature in the lumbar region)	lordosis _____ *This term is used to describe the normal anterior curvature of the spinal column in the lumbar region. An excessive, abnormal anterior curvature, or swayback, condition is known as hyperlordosis. The word lordosis is derived from Greek, describing a person leaning backward in a lordly fashion.*
lumb/o	loins, lower back	lumbar _____ lumbosacral _____ lumbodynia _____ *Also called lumbago.*
myel/o	bone marrow	myelopoiesis _____
orth/o	straight	orthopedic _____ *Ped/o means child.*
oste/o	bone	osteitis _____ osteodystrophy _____ osteogenesis _____ *Osteogenesis imperfecta is an inherited congenital anomaly marked by brittle bones and multiple fractures; also called brittle bone disease.*
scoli/o	crooked, bent (lateral curvature)	scoliosis _____ *The spinal column is bent abnormally to the side. Scoliosis is the most common spinal deformity in adolescent girls (Fig. 15–12).*
spondyl/o (used to make words about conditions of the structure)	vertebra	spondylitis _____ spondylosis _____ *This term indicates degeneration of the intervertebral discs (disks) in the cervical, thoracic, and lumbar regions. Symptoms include pain and restriction of movement.*

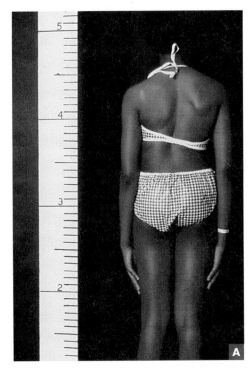

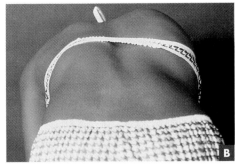

Figure 15-12

Moderate thoracic idiopathic adolescent scoliosis. (A) Notice the scapular asymmetry in the upright position. This results from rotation of the spine and attached rib cage. **(B)** Bending forward reveals a mild rib hump deformity. (From Zitelli B, Davis H: Atlas of Pediatric Physical Diagnosis, 3rd ed. St. Louis, Mosby-Wolfe, 1997.)

vertebr/o (used to describe the structure)   vertebra   vertebral _____

Suffixes			
Suffix	**Meaning**	**Terminology**	**Meaning**
-blast	embryonic or immature cell	osteoblast _____	
-clast	to break	osteoclast _____ *This cell breaks down bone to remove bone tissue.*	
-listhesis	slipping	spondylolisthesis _____ *(spŏn-dĭ-lō-lĭs-THĒ-sĭs), the forward slipping (subluxation) of a vertebra over a lower vertebra.*	
-malacia	softening	osteomalacia _____ *A condition in which vitamin D deficiency leads to decalcification of bones; known as rickets in children.*	
-physis	to grow	epiphysis _____ pubic symphysis _____	

-porosis	pore, passage	osteoporosis _____
		Loss of bony tissue and decreased mass of bone. See page (556), Section II (I), Pathological Conditions and Fractures.
-tome	instrument to cut	osteotome _____
		This surgical chisel is designed to cut bone.

TERMS RELATED TO SPECIFIC BONES
Combining Forms

Combining Forms	Meaning	Terminology	Meaning
acetabul/o	acetabulum (hip socket)	acetabular _____	
calcane/o	calcaneus (heel bone)	calcaneal _____	
		The calcaneus is one of the tarsal (hindfoot) bones.	
carp/o	carpals (wrist bones)	carpal _____	
clavicul/o	clavicle (collar bone)	supraclavicular _____	
		supra- means above.	
cost/o	ribs (true ribs, false ribs, and floating ribs)	subcostal _____	
		chondrocostal _____	
		Cartilage that is attached to the ribs.	
crani/o	cranium (skull bones)	craniotomy _____	
		craniotome _____	
femor/o	femur (thigh bone)	femoral _____	
fibul/o	fibula (smaller lower leg bone)	fibular _____	
		See perone/o.	
humer/o	humerus (upper arm bone)	humeral _____	
ili/o	ilium (upper part of the pelvic bone)	iliac _____	
isch/o	ischium (posterior part of the pelvic bone)	ischial _____	

malleol/o	malleolus (process on each side of the ankle)	malleolar _____ *The medial malleolus is at the lower end of the tibia, and the lateral malleolus is at the lower end of the fibula.*
mandibul/o	mandible (lower jaw bone)	mandibular _____
maxill/o	maxilla (upper jaw bone)	maxillary _____
metacarp/o	metacarpals (hand bones)	metacarpectomy _____
metatars/o	metatarsals (foot bones)	metatarsalgia _____
olecran/o	olecranon (elbow)	olecranal _____
patell/o	patella (kneecap)	subpatellar _____
pelv/i	pelvis (hip bone)	pelvimetry _____
perone/o	fibula	peroneal _____
phalang/o	phalanges (finger bones)	phalangeal _____
pub/o	pubis (anterior part of the pelvic bone)	pubic _____
radi/o	radius (lower arm bone—thumb side)	radial _____
scapul/o	scapula (shoulder bone)	scapular _____
stern/o	sternum (breast bone)	sternal _____
tars/o	tarsals (bones of the hindfoot)	tarsectomy _____
tibi/o	tibia (shin bone)	tibial _____
uln/o	ulna (lower arm bone—little finger side)	ulnar _____

I. Pathological Conditions and Fractures

Ewing sarcoma

Malignant bone tumor.

Pain and swelling are common, with the tumor sometimes involving the entire shaft (medullary cavity) of a long bone. This tumor usually occurs at an early age (5–15 years old), and radiotherapy with chemotherapy represents the best chance for cure (60–70 per cent of patients are cured before metastases occur).

exostosis

Bony growth arising from the surface of bone (ex- means out, -ostosis means condition of bone).

Osteochondromas (composed of cartilage and bone) are **exostoses** and are usually found on the metaphyses of long bones near the epiphyseal plates.

A **bunion** is a swelling of the metatarsophalangeal joint near the base of the big toe and is accompanied by the build-up of soft tissue and underlying bone.

fracture

Sudden breaking of a bone.

A **closed fracture** means that a bone is broken but there is no open wound in the skin, whereas an **open** (compound) **fracture** means a bone is broken and there is an open wound in the skin. A **pathological fracture** is caused by disease of the bone or change in the tissue surrounding the bone, making it weak. A tumor in a bone, for instance, can make a bone weak and lead to a pathological fracture. **Crepitus** is the crackling sound produced when ends of bones rub each other or rub against roughened cartilage.

Some examples of fractures (Fig. 15–13) are:

Colles fracture — occurs near the wrist joint at the lower end of the radius.

comminuted fracture — bone is splintered or crushed into several pieces. A simple fracture means that a bone breaks in only one place and is therefore not comminuted.

compression fracture — bone is compressed; often occurs in vertebrae.

greenstick fracture — bone is partially broken and partially bent on the opposite side, as when a green stick breaks; occurs in children.

impacted fracture — fracture in which one fragment is driven firmly into the other.

Treatment of fractures involves **reduction,** which is the restoration of the bone to its normal position. A **closed reduction** is manipulative reduction without a surgical incision; in an **open reduction,** an incision is made into the fracture site. A **cast** (solid mold of the body part) is applied to fractures to immobilize the injured bone.

osteogenic sarcoma

Malignant tumor arising from bone (osteosarcoma).

This is the most common type of malignant bone tumor. Osteoblasts multiply without control and form large bony tumors, especially at the ends of long bones (half the lesions are located just below or just above the knee) (Fig. 15–14). Metastasis takes place through the bloodstream and often occurs to the lungs. Surgical resection followed by chemotherapy improves the survival rate.

Malignant tumors from other parts of the body (breast, prostate, lung, and kidney) may metastasize (spread) to bones; they are called **metastatic bone lesions.**

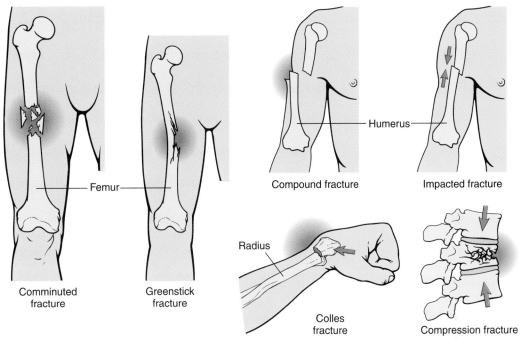

Femur — Comminuted fracture

Greenstick fracture

Humerus — Compound fracture

Impacted fracture

Radius — Colles fracture

Compression fracture

Figure 15-13

Types of fractures.

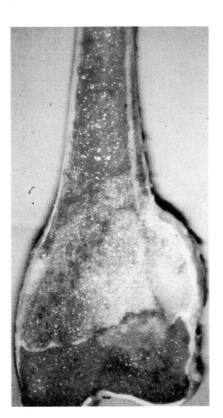

Figure 15-14

Osteosarcoma. The tumor has grown through the cortex of the bone and elevated the periosteum. (From Kumar V, Cotran RS, Robbins SL: Basic Pathology, 6th ed. Philadelphia, WB Saunders, 1997.)

osteomalacia

Softening of bone, with inadequate amounts of mineral (calcium) in the bone.

Osteomalacia occurs primarily as a disease of infancy and childhood and is then known as **rickets.** Bones fail to receive adequate amounts of calcium and phosphorus, and they become soft, bend easily, and become deformed.

Vitamin D is usually deficient in the diet, and this prevents calcium and phosphorus from being absorbed into the bloodstream from the intestines. Vitamin D is formed by the action of sunlight on certain compounds (such as cholesterol) in the skin; thus, rickets is more common in large, smoky cities during the winter months.

Treatment most often consists of administration of large daily doses of vitamin D and an increase in dietary intake of calcium and phosphorus.

osteomyelitis

Inflammation of the bone and bone marrow secondary to infection.

Bacteria enter the body through a wound and spread to the bone. Children are most often affected, and the infection usually occurs in the long bones of the legs and arms. Adults can be affected too, usually as the result of an open fracture.

The lesion begins as an inflammation with pus collection. Pus tends to spread down the medullary cavity and outward to the periosteum. Antibiotic therapy corrects the condition if the infection is treated quickly. If treatment is delayed, an **abscess** can form. An abscess is a walled-off area of infection that can be difficult or impossible to penetrate with antibiotics. Surgical drainage of an abscess is usually necessary.

osteoporosis

Decrease in bone density (mass); thinning and weakening of bone.

This condition is also called **osteopenia** because the interior of bones is diminished in structure, as if the steel skeleton of a building had rusted and been worn down (Fig. 15–15). Osteoporosis commonly occurs in older women as a consequence of estrogen deficiency with menopause. Lack of estrogen promotes excessive bone resorption (osteoclast activity) and less bone deposition. Weakened bones are subject to fractures (as in the hip); loss of height and kyphosis occur as vertebrae collapse (Fig. 15–16).

Estrogen replacement therapy and increased intake of calcium may be helpful for some patients. A weight-bearing daily exercise program is also important.

Osteoporosis can occur with atrophy caused by disuse, as in a limb that is in a cast, in the legs of a paraplegic, or in a bedridden patient. It may also occur in men as part of the aging process and in patients who have been given corticosteroid (hormones made by the adrenal gland and used to treat inflammatory conditions) therapy.

talipes

Congenital abnormality of the hindfoot (involving the talus).

Several varieties of talipes are known. They are thought to result from congenital anomalies, abnormal positioning of the fetus, or both while in the womb. The most common form is **talipes equinovarus** (equin/o means horse), or **clubfoot.** In this congenital deformity, the patient cannot stand with the sole of the foot flat on the ground. The defect can be corrected by orthopedic splinting in the early months of infancy or, if that fails, by surgery.

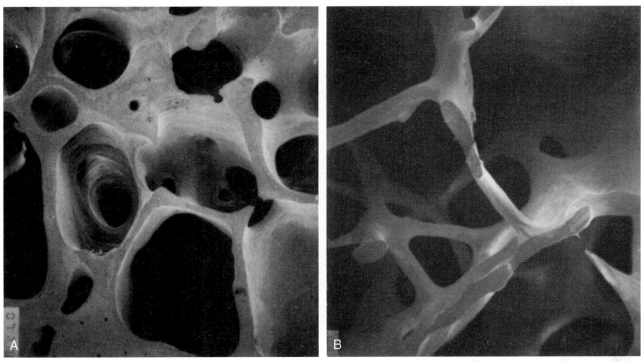

Figure 15–15

Scanning electromicrograph of (A) normal bone and **(B) bone with osteoporosis.** Notice the thinning and wide separation of the trabeculae in the osteoporotic bone. (From Dempster DW, Shane E, Horbert W, et al: A simple method for correlative light and scanning electron microscopy of human iliac crest bone biopsies: qualitative observations in normal and osteoporotic subjects. J Bone Miner Res 1986;1:15.)

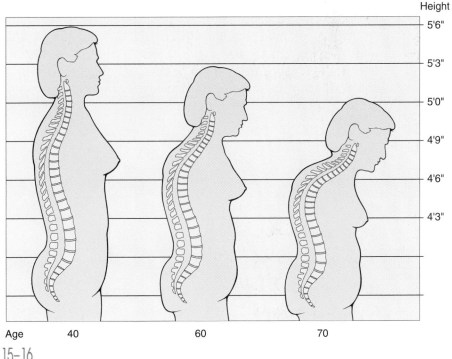

Figure 15–16

Kyphosis. Loss of bone mass due to osteoporosis produces posterior curvature of the spine in the thoracic region. A normal spine is shown at 40 years of age, and osteoporotic changes are illustrated at 60 and at 70 years of age. The changes in the spine can cause a loss of as much as 6 to 9 inches in height.

III. Joints

A. Types of Joints

A joint (articulation) is a coming together of two or more bones. Some joints are immovable, such as the **suture joints** between the skull bones. Other joints, such as those between the vertebrae, are partially movable. Most joints, however, allow considerable movement. These freely movable joints are called **synovial joints.** Examples of synovial joints are the ball-and-socket type (the hip and shoulder joints) and the hinge type (elbow, knee, and ankle joints). Label the structures in Figure 15–17 as you read the following description of a synovial joint:

The bones in a synovial joint are surrounded by a **joint capsule** [1] composed of fibrous tissue. **Ligaments** (thickened fibrous bands of connective tissue) anchor one bone to another and thereby add considerable strength to the joint capsule in critical areas. Bones at the joint are covered with a smooth surface called the **articular cartilage** [2]. The **synovial membrane** [3] lies under the joint capsule and lines the **synovial cavity** [4] between the bones. The synovial cavity is filled with a special lubricating fluid produced by the synovial membrane. This **synovial fluid** contains water and nutrients that nourish as well as lubricate the joints so that friction on the articular cartilage is minimal.

B. Bursae

Bursae (singular: **bursa**) are closed sacs of synovial fluid lined with a synovial membrane and are located near but not within a joint. Bursae are present wherever two types of tissue are closely opposed and need to slide past one another with as little friction as possible. Bursae serve as layers of lubrication between the tissues. Common sites of bursae are between **tendons** (connective tissue that connects a muscle to bone) and bones, between **ligaments** (connective tissue binding bone to bone) and bones, and between skin and bones in areas where bony anatomy is prominent.

Some common locations of bursae are at the elbow joint (olecranon bursa), knee joint (patellar bursa), and shoulder joint (subacromial bursa). Figure 15–18A shows a lateral view of the knee joint with bursae. Figure 15–18B is a frontal view of the knee showing ligaments that provide stability for the joint.

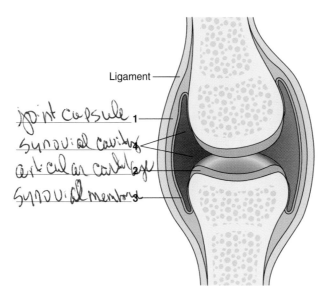

Ligament

Figure 15–17

Structure of a synovial joint.

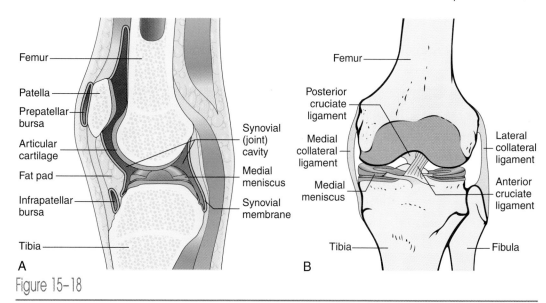

Figure 15-18

(A) Sagittal section of the knee showing bursae and other structures. A **meniscus** (pl., menisci) is a crescent-shaped piece of cartilage that acts as a protective cushion in a synovial joint such as the knee. A "torn cartilage" in the knee is a damaged meniscus and is frequently repaired with arthroscopic surgery. **(B) Frontal section of the knee.** Notice the **anterior cruciate ligament (ACL),** which may be damaged ("torn ligament") with knee injury. Repair of the ACL can require extensive surgery and may involve months of physical therapy for return of normal function.

C. Vocabulary

This list will help you review many of the new terms introduced in this text. Short definitions will reinforce your understanding of the terms. See Section IX of this chapter for help in pronouncing the more difficult terms.

articulation	Joint.
bursa (plural: **bursae)**	Sac of fluid near a joint; promotes smooth sliding of one tissue against another.
ligament	Connective tissue binding bones to other bones; supports, strengthens, and stabilizes the joint.
suture joint	Type of joint in which apposed surfaces are closely united.
synovial cavity	Space between bones at a synovial joint; contains synovial fluid produced by the synovial membrane.
synovial fluid	Viscous (sticky) fluid within the synovial cavity. Synovial fluid is similar in viscosity to egg white; this accounts for the origin of the term (syn- means like, ov/o means egg).
synovial joint	A freely movable joint.
synovial membrane	Membrane lining the synovial cavity; it produces synovial fluid.
tendon	Connective tissue that binds muscles to bones.

D. Combining Forms and Suffixes

Write the meanings of the medical terms in the spaces provided.

Combining Forms

Combining Form	Meaning	Terminology	Meaning

ankyl/o   crooked, bent, stiff

ankylosis _____

*A fusion of bones across a joint space by either bony tissue (**bony ankylosis**) or growth of fibrous tissue (**fibrous ankylosis**). This immobility and stiffening of the joint most often occurs in rheumatoid arthritis.*

arthr/o   joint

arthroplasty _____

Replacement arthroplasty is the replacement of one or both bone ends by a prosthesis (artificial part) of metal or plastic.

arthrotomy _____

hemarthrosis _____

hydrarthrosis _____

Synovial fluid collects abnormally in the joint.

periarthritis _____

articul/o   joint   articular cartilage _____

burs/o   bursa   bursitis _____

Causes (etiology) may be related to stress placed on the bursa or diseases such as gout or rheumatoid arthritis. The bursa becomes inflamed and movement is limited and painful. Intrabursal injection of corticosteroids as well as rest and splinting of the limb are helpful in treatment.

chondr/o   cartilage

achondroplasia _____

This is an inherited condition in which the bones of the arms and legs fail to grow to normal size owing to a defect in cartilage and bone formation. Dwarfism occurs, with short limbs and a normal-sized head and trunk.

chondroma _____

chondromalacia _____

Chondromalacia patellae *is a softening and roughening of the articular cartilaginous surface of the kneecap, resulting in pain, a grating sensation, and mechanical "catching" behind the patella.*

ligament/o	ligament	ligamentous _____	
rheumat/o	watery flow	rheumatologist _____	

Various forms of arthritis are marked by collection of fluid in joint spaces.

synov/o	synovial membrane	synovitis _____	
ten/o	tendon	tenorrhaphy _____	
		tenosynovitis _____	

synov/o here refers to the sheath (covering) around the tendon.

tendin/o	tendon	tendinitis _____	

Suffixes			
Suffix	**Meaning**	**Terminology**	**Meaning**
-desis	to bind, tie together	arthrodesis _____	

Bones are fused across the joint space by surgery (artificial ankylosis). This operation is performed when a joint is very painful, unstable, or chronically infected.

-stenosis	narrowing	spinal stenosis _____	

Narrowing of the neural canal or nerve root canals in the lumbar spine. Symptoms (pain, paresthesias, urinary retention, incontinence) come from compression of the cauda equina (nerves that spread out from the lower end of the spinal cord like a horse's tail).

E. Pathological Conditions

arthritis **Inflammation of joints.**

Some of the more common forms are:

1. ankylosing spondylitis **Chronic, progressive arthritis with stiffening of joints, primarily of the spine.**

Bilateral sclerosis (hardening) of the sacroiliac joints is a diagnostic sign. Joint changes are similar to those seen in rheumatoid arthritis, and the condition can respond to corticosteroids and anti-inflammatory drugs.

2. gouty arthritis **Inflammation of joints caused by excessive uric acid in the body.**

A defect in the metabolism of uric acid causes too much of it to accumulate in blood **(hyperuricemia)**, joints, and soft tissues near joints. The uric acid crystals (salts) destroy the articular cartilage and damage the synovial membrane. A joint chiefly affected is the big toe; hence, the condition is often called **podagra** (pod/o means foot, -agra means excessive pain). Treatment consists of drugs to lower uric acid production (allopurinol) and to prevent inflammation (colchicine and indomethacin) and a special diet that avoids foods that are rich in uric acid, such as red meats, red wines, and fermented cheeses.

3. osteoarthritis

Progressive, degenerative joint disease characterized by loss of articular cartilage and hypertrophy of bone (formation of osteophytes, or bone spurs) at articular surfaces.

This condition, also known as **degenerative joint disease,** occurs mainly in the hips and knees of older individuals and is marked by a narrowing of the joint space (due to loss of cartilage). Treatment consists of aspirin and other analgesics to reduce inflammation and pain and physical therapy to loosen impaired joints. Figure 15–19 compares a normal joint with those that have changes characteristic of osteoarthritis and rheumatoid arthritis.

End-stage osteoarthritis is the most common reason for joint replacement surgery (total joint arthroplasty).

4. rheumatoid arthritis

A chronic disease in which joints become inflamed and painful. It is believed to be caused by an immune (autoimmune) reaction against joint tissues, particularly against the synovial membrane.

The small joints of the hands and feet are affected first and larger joints later. Women are more commonly afflicted than men. Synovial membranes become inflamed and thickened, damaging the articular cartilage and preventing easy movement (see Fig. 15–19). Sometimes fibrous tissue forms and calcifies, creating a bony **ankylosis** (union) at the joint and preventing any movement at all. Swollen, painful joints accompanied by **pyrexia** (fever) are symptoms.

Diagnosis is by a blood test that shows the presence of the rheumatoid factor (an antibody) and x-rays revealing changes around the affected joints. Treatment consists of heat applications and drugs (aspirin, gold compounds, and corticosteroids) to reduce inflammation and pain.

bunion

Abnormal swelling of the medial aspect of the joint between the big toe and the first metatarsal bone.

A bursa often develops over the site, and chronic irritation from ill-fitting shoes can cause a build-up of soft tissue and underlying bone. Bunionectomy may be indicated if other measures (changing shoes and use of anti-inflammatory agents) fail.

carpal tunnel syndrome (CTS)

Compression (by a wrist ligament) of the median nerve as it passes between the ligament and the bones and tendons of the wrist (the carpal tunnel) (Fig. 15–20).

This condition most often affects middle-aged women, and pain and burning sensations occur in the fingers and hand, sometimes extending to the elbow. Symptoms most often affect the index (2nd) and long fingers, although the thumb and radial half of the ring (4th) finger may also be symptomatic. Excessive wrist movement, arthritis, hypertrophy of bone, and swelling of the wrist can produce CTS.

Treatment is splinting the wrist to immobilize it, use of anti-inflammatory medications, and injection of cortisone into the carpal tunnel. If these measures fail, surgical release of the carpal ligament can be helpful.

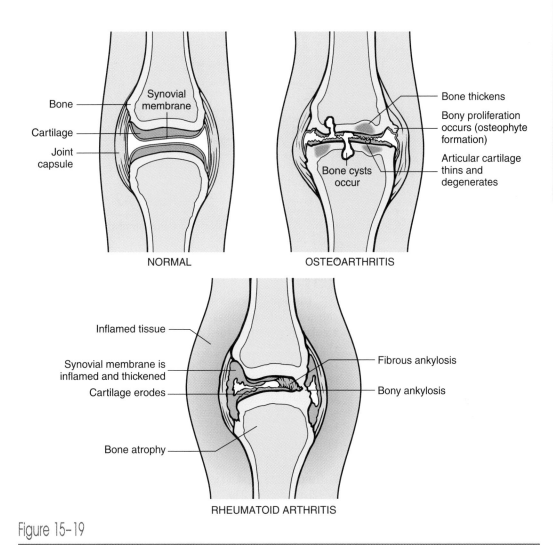

Figure 15-19

Changes in a joint with **osteoarthritis (OA)** and **rheumatoid arthritis (RA).**

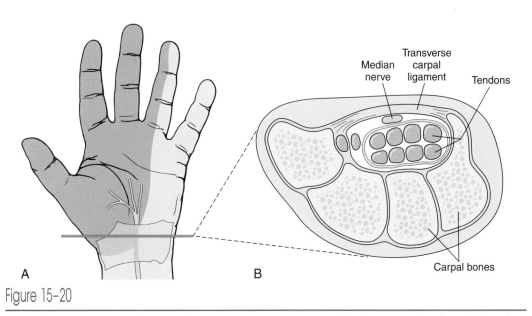

Figure 15-20

Carpal tunnel syndrome (CTS). (A) The median nerve's sensory distribution in the thumb, first three fingers, and palm. **(B)** Cross section of a right hand at the level indicated in (A). Note the position of the median nerve between the carpal ligament and the tendons and carpal bones.

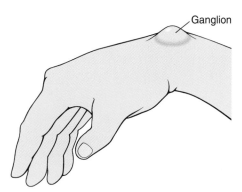

Ganglion

Figure 15-21

Ganglion of the wrist.

dislocation	**Displacement of a bone from its joint.**

Dislocated bones do not articulate with each other. The most common cause of dislocations is trauma. Some examples of dislocations are **acromioclavicular dislocation** (disruption of the articulation between the acromion and clavicle, also known as a shoulder separation); **shoulder dislocation** (disruption of articulation between the head of the humerus and the glenoid fossa of the scapula); **hip dislocation** (disruption of articulation between the head of the femur and the acetabulum of the pelvis).

Treatment of dislocations involves **reduction,** which is restoration of the bones to their normal positions. A **subluxation** is a partial or incomplete dislocation.

ganglion	**A fluid-filled cyst arising from the joint capsule or a tendon in the wrist** (Fig. 15–21).

herniation of an intervertebral disc (disk)	**Abnormal protrusion of a fibrocartilaginous intervertebral disc into the neural canal or spinal nerves.**

This condition is commonly referred to as **slipped disc.** Pain is experienced as the protruded disc (Fig. 15–22) presses on spinal nerves or on the spinal cord. Low-back pain and **sciatica** (pain radiating down the leg) are symptoms when the disc protrudes in the lumbar spine. Neck pain and burning pain radiating down an arm are characteristic of a herniated disc in the

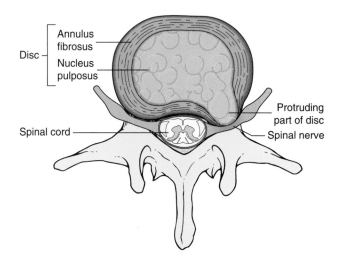

Disc — Annulus fibrosus

Nucleus pulposus

Spinal cord

Protruding part of disc

Spinal nerve

Figure 15-22

Protrusion of an intervertebral disc (looking down on a vertebra). Note how the inner portion (nucleus pulposus) of the disc herniates and presses on the spinal nerve.

cervical spine. Bed rest, physical therapy, and drugs for pain help in initial treatment. In patients with chronic or recurrent disc herniation, **laminectomy** (surgical removal of a portion of the vertebral arch to allow visualization of the protruded disc) and dissection (removal of all or part of the protruding disc) may be advised. Spinal fusion of the two vertebrae may be necessary as well. Endoscopic discectomy is a new technique of removing the disc by inserting a tube through the skin and aspirating the disc through the tube. Chemonucleolysis is injection of a disc-dissolving enzyme (such as chymopapain) into the center of a herniated disc in an effort to relieve pressure on the compressed nerve or spinal cord.

Lyme disease

A recurrent disorder marked by severe arthritis, myalgia, malaise, and neurologic and cardiac symptoms.

Also known as **Lyme arthritis,** the cause of the condition is a spirochete (bacterium) that is carried by a tick. It was first reported in Old Lyme, Connecticut, and is now found throughout the eastern coast of the United States. It is treated with antibiotics.

sprain

Trauma to a joint with pain, swelling, and injury to ligaments.

Sprains may also involve damage to blood vessels, muscles, tendons, and nerves. A **strain** is a less serious injury involving the overstretching of muscle. Application of ice, elevation of the joint, and application of a gentle compressive wrap are immediate measures to relieve pain and minimize swelling due to sprains.

systemic lupus erythematosus (SLE)

Chronic inflammatory disease involving joints, skin, kidneys, nervous system, heart, and lungs.

This condition affects connective tissue (specifically a protein component called **collagen**) in tendons, ligaments, bones, and cartilage all over the body. Typically, there is a red, scaly rash on the face over the nose and cheeks (Fig. 15–23). Patients, usually women, experience joint pain (polyarthralgia), pyrexia (fever), and malaise. SLE is believed to be an autoimmune disease that can be diagnosed by the presence of abnormal antibodies in the bloodstream and characteristic white blood cells called LE cells. Treatment involves giving corticosteroids, hormones made by the adrenal gland that are used to treat inflammatory conditions.

The name lupus (meaning wolf) has been used since the 13th century because physicians thought the shape and color of the skin lesions resembled the bite of a wolf.

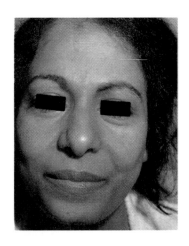

Figure 15–23

Butterfly rash that may accompany systemic lupus erythematosus. (From Lookingbill DP, Marks JG: Principles of Dermatology, 2nd ed. Philadelphia, WB Saunders, 1993.)

IV. Muscles

A. Types of Muscles

There are three types of muscles in the body. Label Figure 15–24 as you read the following descriptions of the various types of muscles:

Striated muscles [1], also called **voluntary** or **skeletal muscles,** are the muscle fibers that move all bones as well as the face and eyes. Through the central and peripheral nervous system, we have conscious control over these muscles. Striated muscle fibers (cells) have a pattern of dark and light bands, or fibrils, in their cytoplasm. Fibrous tissue that envelops and separates muscles is called **fascia,** which contains the muscle's blood, lymph, and nerve supply.

Smooth muscles [2], also called **involuntary** or **visceral muscles,** are those muscle fibers that move internal organs such as the digestive tract, blood vessels, and secretory ducts leading from glands. These muscles are controlled by the autonomic nervous system. They are called smooth because they have no dark and light fibrils in their cytoplasm. Skeletal muscle fibers are arranged in bundles, whereas smooth muscle forms sheets of fibers as it wraps around tubes and vessels.

Cardiac muscle [3] is striated in appearance but is like smooth muscle in its action. Its movement cannot be consciously controlled. The fibers of cardiac muscle are branching fibers and are found in the heart.

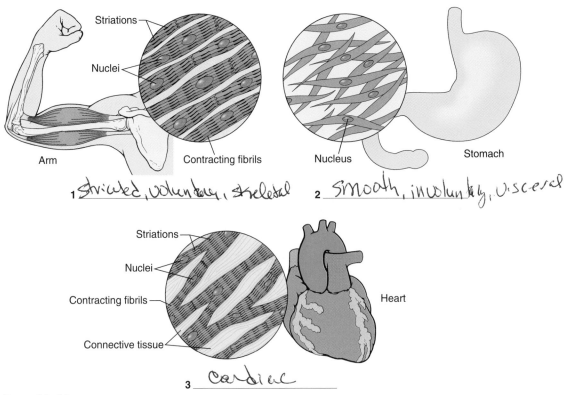

1 _Striated, voluntary, skeletal_ 2 _Smooth, involuntary, visceral_

3 _Cardiac_

Figure 15–24

Types of muscles.

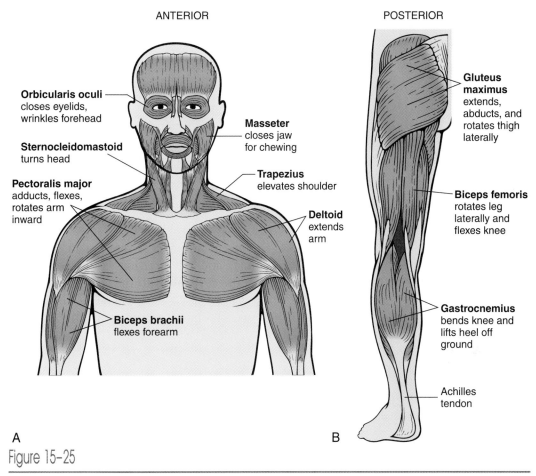

ANTERIOR

POSTERIOR

Orbicularis oculi
closes eyelids,
wrinkles forehead

Sternocleidomastoid
turns head

Pectoralis major
adducts, flexes,
rotates arm
inward

Biceps brachii
flexes forearm

Masseter
closes jaw
for chewing

Trapezius
elevates shoulder

Deltoid
extends
arm

**Gluteus
maximus**
extends,
abducts, and
rotates thigh
laterally

Biceps femoris
rotates leg
laterally and
flexes knee

Gastrocnemius
bends knee and
lifts heel off
ground

Achilles
tendon

A

B

Figure 15-25

(A) Selected muscles of the head, neck, torso, and arm and their functions. (B) Selected muscles of the posterior aspect of the leg and their functions.

B. Actions of Skeletal Muscles

Skeletal (striated) muscles (over 600 in the human body) are the muscles that move bones. Figure 15–25 shows some skeletal muscles of the head, neck, and torso and muscles of the posterior aspect of the leg. When a muscle contracts, one of the bones to which it is joined remains virtually stationary as a result of other muscles that hold it in place. The point of attachment of the muscle to the stationary bone is called the **origin (beginning)** of that muscle. However, when the muscle contracts, another bone to which it is attached does move. The point of junction of the muscle to the bone that moves is called the **insertion** of the muscle. The origin of a muscle lies proximal in the skeleton, whereas its insertion lies distal.

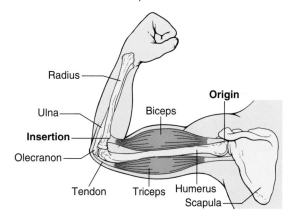

Figure 15-26

Origin and insertion of the biceps in the upper arm. Note also the origin of the triceps at the humerus and scapula and the insertion at the olecranon of the ulna.

Figure 15–26 shows the biceps and triceps muscles in the upper arm. One origin of the biceps is at the scapula, and its insertion is at the radius. Tendons are the connective tissue bands that connect muscles to the bones.

Muscles can perform a variety of actions. Some of the terms used to describe those actions are listed here with a short description of the specific type of movement performed (Fig. 15–27):

Action	Meaning
flexion	Decreasing the angle between two bones; bending a limb.
extension	Increasing the angle between two bones; straightening out a limb.
abduction	Movement away from the midline of the body.
adduction	Movement toward the midline of the body.
rotation	Circular movement around an axis.
dorsiflexion	Decreasing the angle of the ankle joint so that the foot bends backward (upward). This is the opposite movement of stepping on the gas when driving a car.
plantar flexion	The motion that extends the foot downward toward the ground as when pointing the toes or stepping on the gas. Plant/o means sole of the foot.
supination	As applied to the hand, the act of turning the palm forward, or up.
pronation	As applied to the hand, the act of turning the palm backward, or down.

Your medical dictionary has a complete list of the muscles of the body, with a description of their origins, insertions, and various actions.

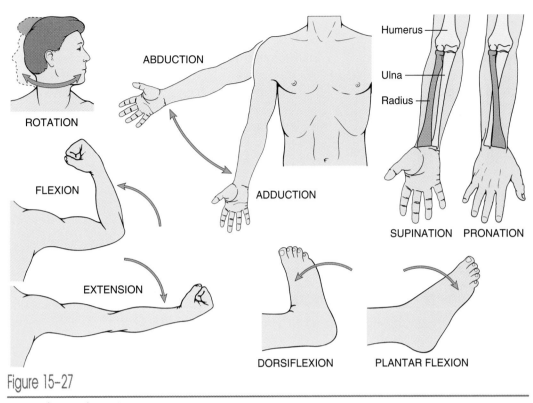

Figure 15-27

Types of muscular actions.

C. Vocabulary

This list will help you review many of the new terms introduced in the text. Short definitions will reinforce your understanding of the terms. See Section IX of this chapter for help in pronouncing the more difficult terms.

abduction	Movement away from the midline of the body.
adduction	Movement toward the midline of the body.
dorsiflexion	Backward (upward) bending of the foot.
extension	Straightening of a flexed limb.
fascia	Fibrous membrane separating and enveloping muscles.
flexion	Bending.
insertion of a muscle	Connection of the muscle to a bone that moves.
origin of a muscle	Connection of the muscle to a stationary bone.
plantar flexion	Bending the sole of the foot downward toward the ground.

pronation	Turning the palm backward.
rotation	Circular movement around a central point.
skeletal muscle	Muscle connected to bones; voluntary or striated muscle.
smooth muscle	Muscle connected to internal organs; involuntary or visceral muscle.
striated muscle	Skeletal muscle.
supination	Turning the palm forward.
visceral muscle	Smooth muscle.

D. Combining Forms, Suffixes, and Prefixes

Write the meanings of the medical terms in the spaces provided.

Combining Forms

Combining Form	Meaning	Terminology	Meaning
fasci/o	fascia (forms sheaths enveloping muscles)	fasciectomy _____	
fibr/o	fibrous connective tissue	fibromyalgia _____	
		*Chronic pain and stiffness in muscles and fibrous tissue, especially of the back, shoulders, neck, hips, and knees. Fatigue is a common complaint. The condition has previously been called **fibrositis or rheumatism.***	
leiomy/o	smooth (visceral) muscle that lines the walls of internal organs	leiomyoma _____	
		leiomyosarcoma _____	
my/o	muscle	myalgia _____	
		electromyography _____	
		myopathy _____	

myocardi/o	heart muscle	myocardial _____	
myos/o	muscle	myositis _____	
plant/o	sole of the foot	plantar flexion _____	
rhabdomy/o	skeletal (striated) muscle connected to bones	rhabdomyoma _____	
		rhabdomyosarcoma _____	

Suffixes			
Suffix	**Meaning**	**Terminology**	**Meaning**
-asthenia	lack of strength	myasthenia gravis _____	
		Muscles lose strength because of a failure in transmission of the nervous impulse from the nerve to the muscle cell.	
-trophy	development, nourishment	atrophy _____	
		Decrease in size of an organ or tissue.	
		hypertrophy _____	
		Increase in size of an organ or tissue.	
		amyotrophic _____	
		*In **amyotrophic lateral sclerosis** (Lou Gehrig disease), muscles are affected (paralysis occurs) by degeneration of nerves in the spinal cord and lower region of the brain.*	

Prefixes			
Prefix	**Meaning**	**Terminology**	**Meaning**
ab-	away from	abduction _____	
		duct/o means to lead.	
ad-	toward	adduction _____	
dorsi-	back	dorsiflexion _____	
poly-	many, much	polymyalgia _____	

E. Pathological Conditions

muscular dystrophy	**A group of inherited diseases characterized by progressive weakness and degeneration of muscle fibers without involvement of the nervous system.**

Duchenne dystrophy is the most common form. Muscles enlarge **(pseudo-hypertrophy)** as fat replaces functional muscle cells that have degenerated and atrophied. Onset of muscle weakness occurs soon after birth, and diagnosis can be made by muscle biopsy and electromyography.

polymyositis	**Chronic inflammatory myopathy.**

This condition is marked by symmetrical muscle weakness and pain, often accompanied by a rash around the eyes, face, and limbs. Evidence that polymyositis is an autoimmune disorder is growing stronger, and some patients recover completely with immunosuppressive therapy.

V. Laboratory Tests, Clinical Procedures, and Abbreviations

Laboratory Tests

antinuclear antibody test (ANA)	A sample of plasma is tested for the presence of antibodies that are found in patients with systemic lupus erythematosus.
erythrocyte sedimentation rate (ESR)	This test measures the rate at which erythrocytes fall to the bottom of a test tube. Elevated sedimentation rates are associated with inflammatory disorders such as rheumatoid arthritis.
rheumatoid factor test	A sample of blood is tested for the presence of the rheumatoid factor (an antibody found in the serum of patients with rheumatoid arthritis).
serum calcium (Ca)	Measurement of the amount of calcium in blood (serum).
serum creatine phosphokinase (CPK)	Creatine phosphokinase is an enzyme normally present in skeletal and cardiac muscle. Elevated serum CPK levels are found in muscular dystrophy, myocardial infarction, and skeletal muscle disorders.
serum phosphorus (P)	Measurement of the amount of phosphorus in a sample of serum.
uric acid test	This test measures the amount of uric acid in a sample of blood. High values are associated with gouty arthritis.

Clinical Procedures

arthrocentesis	Surgical puncture of the joint space with a needle. Synovial fluid is removed for analysis.
arthrography	Process of taking x-ray pictures of a joint after injection of opaque contrast material.

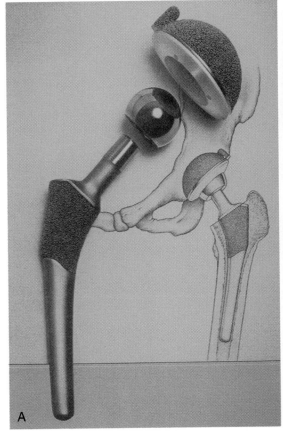
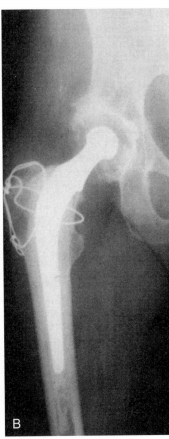

Figure 15-28

(A) Acetabular and femoral components of a total hip arthroplasty. (B) Radiograph showing a hip after a **Charnley total hip arthroplasty.** (*A* from Jebson LR, Coons DD: Total Hip Arthroplasty. Surg Technol October 1998; *B* from Petty W: Total Joint Replacement. Philadelphia, WB Saunders, 1991.)

arthroplasty

Surgical repair of a joint. Total hip arthroplasty is replacement of the femoral head and acetabulum with prostheses that are cemented into the bone (Fig. 15-28).

arthroscopy

Visual examination of the inside of a joint with an endoscope. Small surgical instruments are passed into the joint to remove and repair damaged tissue. Arthroscopy is used primarily to visualize the knee, ankle, and shoulder (Fig. 15-29).

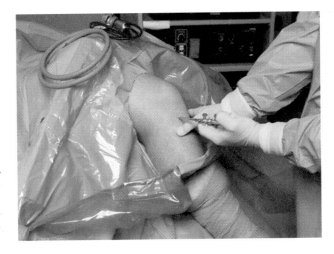

Figure 15-29

Arthroscopy of the knee. An arthroscope is used in the diagnosis of pathological changes. (From Lewis SM, Collier IC, Heitkemper MM: Medical-Surgerical Nursing: Assessment and Management of Clinical Problems, 4th ed. St. Louis, Mosby, 1996.)

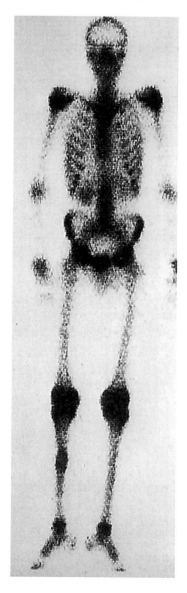

Figure 15-30

A technetium-99m bone scan of a skeleton showing an area of increased radioactive uptake on the right tibia that indicates a bone tumor. (From Walter JB: An Introduction to the Principles of Disease, 3rd ed. Philadelphia, WB Saunders, 1992.)

bone scan

A radioactive phosphate substance is injected intravenously, and uptake of the substance in bone is measured by a special scanning device. Areas that take up excessive amounts of radioactive substance may contain tumors, infection, inflammation, stress fractures or other destructive changes (Fig. 15-30).

dual-energy x-ray absorptiometry

X-rays are taken of bones in the spinal column, pelvis, and wrist, and a machine (an x-ray detector) measures how well the rays penetrate the bones. This is a test of bone density and is used to diagnose osteoporosis.

electromyography (EMG)

The process of recording the strength of muscle contraction as a result of electrical stimulation.

muscle biopsy

Removal of muscle tissue for microscopic examination.

ABBREVIATIONS

ACL	anterior cruciate ligament	L1–L5	lumbar vertebrae
ANA	antinuclear antibody	LE cell	lupus erythematosus cell
C1–C7	cervical vertebrae	Ortho.	orthopedics, orthopaedics
Ca	calcium	P	phosphorus
CPK	creatine phosphokinase	RA	rheumatoid arthritis
CTS	carpal tunnel syndrome	RF	rheumatoid factor
DEXA	dual-energy x-ray absorptiometry; a test of bone density	ROM	range of motion
DTR	deep tendon reflexes	sed rate	erythrocyte sedimentation rate
EMG	electromyography	SLE	systemic lupus erythematosus
ESR	erythrocyte sedimentation rate	T1–T12	thoracic vertebrae
IM	intramuscular	TMJ	temporomandibular joint

VI. Practical Applications

This section contains an actual medical report using terms that you have studied in this and previous chapters. Explanations of more difficult terms are added in brackets. Answers are on page (590) after Answers to Exercises.

Skeletal Memorial Hospital—Department of Radiology

PA [posteroanterior] and lateral chest: The heart is enlarged in its transverse diameter. The lungs are fully expanded and free of active disease.

Thoracic spine shows a scoliosis of the upper thoracic spine convex to the left. There is 50 per cent wedge compression fracture of T6 and slight wedge compression fracture of T5. There is also anterior wedge compression fracture of T12.

Lumbar spine shows 90 per cent compression fractures of L1 and L3 with 30 per cent compression fractures L2 and L5. All bones are markedly osteoporotic. There is calcification within the aortic arch. There are gallstones in the right upper quadrant. The findings in the spine are most compatible with osteoporotic compression fractures. During the procedure, the patient had a sickable* episode and fell, striking her head. A skull series, done at no cost to the patient, shows no evidence of bony fracture. The pineal gland is calcified and has a midline location. The sella turcica is normal.

---

* This word was incorrectly transcribed. The correct term is syncopal.

Operating Schedule—Skeletal Memorial Hospital

Match the operation in column I with an accompanying diagnosis or reason for surgery in column II.

Column I—Operations

1. Excision, osteochondroma, R calcaneous _____

2. TMJ arthroscopy with probable arthrotomy _____

3. L4–5 laminectomy and discectomy _____

4. Arthroscopy, left knee _____

5. Open reduction, malleolar fracture _____

6. R occipital craniotomy with tumor resection _____

7. Excision, distal end right clavicle, with prob. acrominoplasty _____

8. Acetabuloplasty with open reduction hip _____

Column II—Diagnoses

A. fracture of the ankle
B. patellar ligament injury
C. neoplastic lesion in brain
D. exostosis on heel bone
E. pelvic fracture
F. pain and malocclusion of jaw bones
G. lower back pain radiating down one leg
H. pain in shoulder joint with bone tumor evident on x-ray

VII. Exercises

Remember to check your answers carefully with those given in Section VIII, Answers to Exercises.

A. *Complete the following sentences.*

1. Bones are composed of bony connective tissue called _____ tissue.

2. Bone cells are called _____.

3. The bones of a fetus are composed mainly of _____.

4. During bone development, immature bone cells called _____ produce bony tissue.

5. Large bone cells called _____ digest bone tissue to shape the bone and smooth it out.

6. Two mineral substances necessary for proper development of bones are _____

and _____ .

7. A round, small bone resembling a sesame seed in shape and covering the knee joint is called a

(an) _____ bone.

8. The shaft of a long bone is called the _____ .

9. The ends of a long bone are called the _____ .

10. The cartilaginous area at the end of a long bone where growth takes place is called the

_____ .

11. Red bone marrow is found in spongy or _____ bone.

12. Yellow bone marrow is composed of _____ tissue.

13. The strong membrane surrounding the surface of a bone is the _____ .

14. Hard, dense bone tissue lying under the periosteum is _____ .

15. A series of canals containing blood vessels lie within the outer dense tissue of bone and are called

the _____ canals.

16. A thin layer of cartilage surrounding the ends of bones at the joints is _____ .

17. The _____ is a central, hollowed-out area in the shaft of long bones.

18. A physician who treats bones and bone diseases is called a (an) _____ .

19. A person who uses his or her hands to manipulate the spinal column (in the belief that diseases

are caused by pressure on spinal nerves) is a (an) _____ .

20. A doctor who treats patients based on the belief that the body can be healed when bones are in

proper position and adequate nutrition is provided in a (an) _____ .

B. Give a short description of each term.

1. metaphysis _____

2. sinus _____

3. tubercle _____

4. condyle _____

5. fossa _____

6. tuberosity _____

7. trochanter _____

8. foramen _____

9. fissure _____

10. bone head _____

C. Match the following cranial and facial bones with their meanings as given below.

mandible   nasal bone   maxilla   vomer
ethmoid bone   temporal bone   parietal bone   lacrimal bones
zygomatic bone   occipital bone   sphenoid bone   frontal bone

1. forms the roof and upper side parts of the skull _____

2. delicate bone, composed of spongy, cancellous tissue; supports the nasal cavity and orbits of the

   eye _____

3. forms the back and base of the skull _____

4. forms the forehead _____

5. bat-shaped bone extending behind the eyes to form the base of the skull _____

6. bone near the ear and connecting to the lower jaw _____

7. cheek bone _____

8. bone that supports the bridge of the nose _____

9. thin, flat bone forming the lower portion of the nasal septum _____

10. lower jaw bone _____

11. upper jaw bone _____

12. two paired bones, one located at the corner of each eye _____

D. Name the five divisions of the spinal column.

1. _____   4. _____

2. _____   5. _____

3. _____

E. *Identify the following parts associated with a vertebra.*

1. space through which the spinal cord passes _____

2. piece of cartilage between each vertebra _____

3. posterior part of a vertebra _____

4. anterior part of a vertebra _____

F. *Give the medical names of the following bones.*

1. shoulder blade _____

2. upper arm bone _____

3. breastbone _____

4. thigh bone _____

5. finger bones _____

6. hand bones _____

7. medial lower arm bone _____

8. lateral lower arm bone _____

9. collar bone _____

10. wrist bones _____

11. backbone _____

12. kneecap _____

13. shin bone (larger of two lower leg bones)

_____

14. smaller of two lower leg bones _____

15. three parts of the hip bone are: _____

_____, and _____

16. midfoot bones _____

G. *Give the meanings of the following terms associated with bones.*

1. foramen magnum _____

2. calcaneus _____

3. acromion _____

4. xiphoid processs _____

5. lamina _____

6. malleolus _____

7. acetabulum _____

8. pubic symphysis _____

9. olecranon _____

10. fontanelle _____

11. mastoid process _____

12. styloid process _____

H. Give the meanings of the following terms.

1. osteogenesis _____

2. hypercalcemia _____

3. spondylosis _____

4. epiphyseal _____

5. decalcification _____

6. ossification _____

7. osteitis _____

8. costoclavicular _____

I. Build medical terms.

1. pertaining to the shoulder bone _____

2. instrument to cut the skull _____

3. pertaining to the upper arm bone _____

4. pertaining to below the knee cap _____

5. softening of cartilage _____

6. pertaining to a toe bone _____

7. removal of hand bones _____

8. pertaining to the shin bone _____

9. pertaining to the heel bone _____

10. poor bone development _____

11. removal of the lamina of the vertebral arch _____

12. pertaining to the sacrum and ilium _____

J. Give medical terms for the following.

1. formation of bone marrow _____

2. clubfoot _____

3. humpback _____

4. high levels of calcium in the blood _____

5. benign tumors arising from the bone surface _____

6. brittle bone disease _____

7. lateral curvature of the spine _____

8. abnormal anterior curvature of the spine _____

9. forward slipping (subluxation) of a vertebra over a lower vertebra _____

10. pain in the lumbar spine; lumbago _____

K. Match the term in column I with its description in column II. Write the letter of the description in the space provided.

Column I

1. greenstick fracture _____

2. closed fracture _____

3. comminuted fracture _____

4. compound (open) fracture _____

5. Colles fracture _____

6. cast _____

7. open reduction _____

8. closed reduction _____

9. impacted fracture _____

10. compression fracture _____

Column II

A. fracture of the lower end of the radius at the wrist
B. break in bone with wound in the skin
C. one side of the bone is fractured; the other side is bent
D. bone is put in proper place without incision of skin
E. mold of the bone applied to fractures to immobilize the injured bone
F. bone is broken by pressure from another bone; often in vertebrae
G. bone is splintered or crushed
H. bone is put in proper place after incision through the skin
I. bone is broken and one end is wedged into the interior of the adjoining bone
J. break in the bone without an open skin wound

L. Give the meanings of the following terms.

1. osteoporosis _____

2. osteomyelitis _____

3. osteogenic sarcoma _____

4. crepitus _____

5. osteomalacia _____

6. abscess _____

7. osteopenia _____

8. Ewing sarcoma _____

9. metastatic bone lesion _____

M. Complete the following sentences.

1. A joint in which apposed bones are closely united as in the skull bones is called a (an)

_____.

2. Connective tissue that binds muscles to bones is a (an) _____.

3. Another term for a joint is a (an) _____.

4. Connective tissue that binds bones to other bones is a (an) _____.

5. Fluid found near a joint is called _____.

6. The membrane that lines the joint cavity is the _____.

7. A sac of fluid near a joint is a (an) _____.

8. Smooth cartilage that surrounds the surface of bones at joints is _____.

9. Surgical repair of a joint is called _____.

10. Inflammation surrounding a joint is known as _____.

N. Complete the following terms based on the definitions provided.

1. inflammation of a tendon: _____ itis

2. tumor (benign) of cartilage: _____ oma

3. tumor (malignant) of cartilage: _____ oma

4. incision of a joint: arthr _____

5. softening of cartilage: chondro _____

6. abnormal condition of blood in the joint: _____ osis

7. inflammation of a sac of fluid near the joint: _____ itis

8. a doctor who specializes in treatment of joint disorders: _____ logist

9. abnormal condition of a crooked, stiffened, immobile joint: _____ osis

10. suture of a tendon: ten _____

O. Select from the following terms to name the abnormal conditions below.

systemic lupus erythematosus	achondroplasia	ankylosing spondylitis
gouty arthritis	rheumatoid arthritis	bunion
tenosynovitis	osteoarthritis	carpal tunnel syndrome
dislocation	ganglion	Lyme disease

1. an inherited condition in which the bones of the arms and the legs fail to grow normally because of a defect in cartilage and bone formation; type of dwarfish _____

2. degenerative joint disease; chronic inflammation of bones and joints _____

3. inflammation of joints caused by excessive uric acid in the body (hyperuricemia) _____

4. chronic joint disease; inflamed and painful joints owing to autoimmune reaction against normal joint tissue, and synovial membranes become swollen and thickened _____

5. tick-borne bacterium causes this condition marked by arthritis, myalgia, malaise, and neurological and cardiac symptoms _____

6. abnormal swelling of a metatarsophalangeal joint _____

7. cystic mass arising from a tendon in the wrist _____

8. chronic, progressive arthritis with stiffening of joints, especially of the spine (vertebrae)

_____

9. chronic inflammatory disease affecting not only the joints but also the skin (red rash on the face), kidneys, heart, and lungs _____

10. inflammation of a tendon sheath _____

11. compression of the median nerve in the wrist as it passes through an area between a ligament and tendons, bones, and connective tissue _____

12. displacement of a bone from its joint _____

P. Give the meanings of the following terms.

1. subluxation _____

2. arthrodesis _____

3. pyrexia _____

4. podagra _____

5. sciatica _____

6. herniation of an intervertebral disc _____

7. laminectomy _____

8. sprain _____

9. strain _____

10. hyperuricemia _____

Q. Select the term that best fits the definition given.

1. fibrous membrane separating and enveloping muscles: (fascia, flexion)

2. movement away from the midline of the body: (abduction, adduction)

3. connection of the muscle to a stationary bone: (insertion, origin) of the muscle

4. connection of the muscle to a bone that moves: (insertion, origin) of the muscle

5. muscle that is connected to internal organs; involuntary muscle: (skeletal, visceral) muscle

6. muscle that is connected to bones; voluntary muscle: (skeletal, visceral) muscle

7. pain of many muscles: (myositis, polymyalgia)

8. pertaining to heart muscle: (myocardial, myasthenia)

9. process of recording electricity within muscles: (muscle biopsy, electromyography)

10. increase in development (size) of an organ or tissue: (hypertrophy, atrophy)

R. Match the term for muscle action with its meaning. Write the letter of the meaning in the space provided.

Column I

1. extension _____

2. rotation _____

3. flexion _____

4. adduction _____

5. supination _____

6. abduction _____

7. pronation _____

8. dorsiflexion _____

9. plantar flexion _____

Column II

A. movement away from the midline
B. turning the palm backward
C. turning the palm forward
D. straightening out a limb
E. bending the sole of the foot downward
F. circular movement around an axis
G. bending a limb
H. movement toward the midline
I. backward (upward) bending of the foot

S. Give the meanings of the following abnormal conditions affecting muscles.

1. leiomyosarcoma _____

2. rhabdomyoma _____

3. polymyositis _____

4. fibromyalgia _____

5. muscular dystrophy _____

6. myasthenia gravis _____

7. amyotrophic lateral sclerosis _____

T. Match the term in column I with its meaning in column II. Write the letter of the answer in the space provided.

Column I

1. antinuclear antibody test   _____

2. serum creatine phosphokinase   _____

3. uric acid test   _____

4. rheumatoid factor test   _____

5. bone scan   _____

6. muscle biopsy   _____

7. arthroscopy   _____

8. acetylcholine   _____

9. phosphorus   _____

10. arthrography   _____

Column II

A. radioactive substance is injected and traced in tissue
B. chemical found in myoneural space
C. test for presence of an antibody found in the serum of patients with rheumatoid arthritis
D. substance necessary for proper bone development
E. visual examination of a joint
F. test tells if patient has gouty arthritis
G. test tells if patient has systemic lupus erythematosus
H. removal of tissue for microscopic examination
I. process of taking x-ray pictures of a joint
J. elevated levels of this enzyme are found in muscular disorders

U. Select the term that best completes the meaning of the sentence.

1. Selma, a 40-year-old secretary, had been complaining of wrist pain with tingling sensations in her fingers for months. Dr. Ayres diagnosed her condition as **(osteomyelitis, rheumatoid arthritis, carpal tunnel syndrome).**

2. Daisy tripped while playing tennis and landed on her hand. She had excruciating pain and a **(Ewing, Colles, pathological)** fracture that required casting.

3. In her 50s, Estee started hunching over more and more. Her doctor realized that she was developing **(gouty arthritis, osteoarthritis, osteoporosis)** and prescribed calcium pills and exercise.

4. Paul had a skiing accident and tore ligaments in his knee. Dr. Miller recommended **(electromyography, hypertrophy, arthroscopic surgery)** to repair the ligaments.

5. For several months after her first pregnancy Else noticed a red rash on her face and cheeks. Her joints were giving her pain and she had a slight fever. Her ANA was elevated and her doctor suspected that she had **(SLE, polymyositis, muscular dystrophy).**

V. Give meanings for the following abbreviations and then select the letter from the sentences that follow that is the best association for each.

Column I

1. ROM _____ ____

2. DEXA _____ ____

3. TMJ _____ ____

4. EMG _____ ____

5. ACL _____ ____

6. SLE _____ ____

7. C1–C5 _____ ____

8. T1–T12 _____ ____

Column II

A. This is the connection between the lower jaw bone and a bone of the skull.

B. This is a band of fibrous tissue connecting bones in the knee.

C. These are bones of the spinal column in the chest region.

D. This is a test of strength of electrical transmission within muscle.

E. This autoimmune disease affects joints, skin, and other body tissues.

F. This measurement in degrees of a circle assesses the extent a joint can be flexed or extended.

G. These are bones of the spinal column in the neck region.

H. This is a test of bone density as an assessment of osteoporosis.

VIII. Answers to Exercises

A

1. osseous
2. osteocytes
3. cartilage
4. osteoblasts
5. osteoclasts
6. calcium and phosphorus
7. sesamoid
8. diaphysis
9. epiphyses
10. epiphyseal plate
11. cancellous or trabecular
12. fat
13. periosteum
14. compact bone
15. haversian
16. articular cartilage
17. medullary cavity
18. orthopedist
19. chiropractor
20. osteopath

B

1. flared portion of a long bone that lies between the diaphysis and the epiphyseal plate
2. hollow cavity within the bone
3. small, rounded process for attachment of tendons or muscles
4. rounded, knuckle-like process at the joint
5. shallow cavity in or on a bone
6. large, rounded process for attachment of muscles or tendons
7. large process on the femur for attachment of muscles
8. opening in a bone for blood vessels and nerves
9. narrow, deep, slit-like opening
10. rounded end of a bone separated from the rest of the bone by a neck

C

1. parietal bone
2. ethmoid bone
3. occipital bone
4. frontal bone
5. sphenoid bone
6. temporal bone
7. zygomatic bone
8. nasal bone
9. vomer
10. mandible
11. maxilla
12. lacrimal bones

D

1. cervical
2. thoracic
3. lumbar
4. sacral
5. coccygeal

Continued on following page

E

1. neural canal
2. intervertebral disc (disk)
3. vertebral arch
4. vertebral body

F

1. scapula
2. humerus
3. sternum
4. femur
5. phalanges
6. metacarpals
7. ulna
8. radius
9. clavicle
10. carpals
11. vertebral column
12. patella
13. tibia
14. fibula
15. ilium, ischium, pubis
16. metatarsals

G

1. opening of the occipital bone through which the spinal cord passes
2. heel bone; largest of the tarsal bones
3. extension of the scapula
4. lower portion of the sternum
5. portion of the vertebral arch
6. the bulge on either side of the ankle joint; the lower end of the fibula is the
   lateral malleolus, and the lower end of the tibia is the medial malleolus
7. depression in the hip bone into which the femur fits
8. area of fusion of the two pubis bones, at the midline
9. bony process at the proximal end of the ulna; elbow joint
10. soft spot between the bones of the skull in an infant
11. round process on the temporal bone behind the ear
12. pole-like process projecting downward from the temporal bone

H

1. formation of bone; osteogenesis imperfecta is known as brittle bone disease
2. excessive calcium in the blood
3. abnormal condition of the vertebrae; degenerative changes in the spine
4. pertaining to the epiphysis
5. removal of calcium from bones
6. formation of bone
7. inflammation of bone; osteitis deformans
   or Paget disease causes deformed bones such as bowed legs
8. pertaining to the ribs and clavicle

I

1. scapular
2. craniotome
3. humeral
4. subpatellar
5. chondromalacia
6. phalangeal
7. metacarpectomy
8. tibial
9. calcaneal
10. osteodystrophy
11. laminectomy
12. sacroiliac

J

1. myelopoiesis
2. talipes
3. kyphosis
4. hypercalcemia
5. exostoses
6. osteogenesis imperfecta
7. scoliosis
8. lordosis
9. spondylolisthesis
10. lumbodynia

K

1. C
2. J
3. G
4. B
5. A
6. E
7. H
8. D
9. I
10. F

L

1. increased porosity in bone; decrease in bone density
2. inflammation of bone and bone marrow
3. cancerous tumor of bone; osteoblasts multiply at the ends of long bones
4. crackling sensation as broken bones move against each other
5. softening of bones; rickets in children due to loss of calcium in bones
6. collection of pus
7. deficiency of bone; occurs in osteoporosis
8. malignant tumor of bone, often
   involving the entire shaft of a long bone
9. malignant tumor that has spread to bone from the breast, lung, kidney, or prostate gland

M

1. suture joint; a synovial joint is a freely movable joint
2. tendon
3. articulation
4. ligament
5. synovial fluid
6. synovial membrane
7. bursa
8. articular cartilage
9. arthroplasty
10. periarthritis

N

1. tendinitis
2. chondroma
3. chondrosarcoma
4. arthrotomy
5. chondromalacia
6. hemarthrosis
7. bursitis
8. rheumatologist
9. ankylosis
10. tenorrhaphy

O

1. achondroplasia
2. osteoarthritis
3. gouty arthritis
4. rheumatoid arthritis
5. Lyme disease
6. bunion
7. ganglion
8. ankylosing spondylitis
9. systemic lupus erythematosus
10. tenosynovitis
11. carpal tunnel syndrome
12. dislocation

P

1. partial or incomplete displacement of a bone from the joint
2. surgical fixation of a joint (binding it together by fusing the joint surfaces)
3. fever; increase in body temperature
4. pain in a big toe from gouty arthritis
5. pain radiating from the back to the leg (along the sciatic nerve); most
commonly caused by a protruding intervertebral disc
6. protrusion of a disc into the neural canal or the spinal nerves
7. removal of a portion of the vertebral arch (lamina) to relieve pressure from a protruding intervertebral disc
8. trauma to a joint with pain, swelling, and injury to ligaments
9. overstretching of a muscle
10. high levels of uric acid in the bloodstream; a symptom of gouty arthritis

Q

1. fascia
2. abduction
3. origin of the muscle
4. insertion of the muscle
5. visceral muscle
6. skeletal muscle
7. polymyalgia
8. myocardial
9. electromyography
10. hypertrophy

R

1. D
2. F
3. G
4. H
5. C
6. A
7. B
8. I
9. E

S

1. malignant tumor of smooth (involuntary, visceral) muscle
2. benign tumor of striated (voluntary, skeletal) muscle
3. inflammation of many muscles; polymyositis rheumatica is a chronic inflammatory condition causing muscle weakness and pain
4. pain of muscle and fibrous tissue (especially of the back); also called fibrositis or rheumatism
5. group of inherited muscular diseases marked by progressive weakness and degeneration of muscles without nerve involvement
6. loss of strength of muscles (often with
paralysis) owing to a defect at the space between the nerve and the muscle cell
7. muscles degenerate (paralysis occurs) owing to degeneration of nerves in the spinal cord and lower region of the brain; Lou Gehrig disease

T

1. G
2. J
3. F
4. C
5. A
6. H
7. E
8. B
9. D
10. I

Continued on following page

U

1. carpal tunnel syndrome
2. Colles
3. osteoporosis

4. arthroscopic surgery
5. SLE

V

1. range of motion. F
2. dual-energy x-ray absorptiometry. H
3. temporomandibular joint. A
4. electromyography. D

5. anterior cruciate ligament. B
6. systemic lupus erythematosus. E
7. 1st cervical vertebra to 5th cervical vertebra. G

8. 1st thoracic vertebra to 12th thoracic vertebra. C

Answers to Practical Applications

1. D
2. F
3. G

4. B
5. A
6. C

7. H
8. E

IX. Pronunciation of Terms

Pronunciation Guide

ā as in āpe
ē as in ēven
ī as in īce
ō as in ōpen
ū as in ūnit

ă as in ăpple
ĕ as in ĕvery
ĭ as in ĭnterest
ŏ as in pŏt
ŭ as in ŭnder

To test your understanding of the terminology in this chapter, write the meaning of each term in the space provided. In addition, you may wish to cover the terms and write them by looking at your definitions. Make sure your spelling is correct. The page number after each term indicates where it is defined or used in the text so you can easily check your responses.

Terms Related to Bones

Term	Pronunciation	Meaning
acetabulum (547)	ăs-ĕ-TĂB-ū-lŭm	
acromion (547)	ă-KRŌ-mē-ŏn	
articular cartilage (547)	ăr-TĬK-ū-lăr KĂR-tĭ-lăj	
calcaneal (552)	kăl-KĀ-nē-ăl	
calcaneus (552)	kăl-KĀ-nē-ŭs	
calcium (547)	KĂL-sē-ŭm	
cancellous bone (547)	KĂN-sĕ-lŭs bōn	
carpals (552)	KĂR-pălz	
cartilage (547)	KĂR-tĭ-lĭj	

cervical vertebrae (542)	SĔR-vĭ-kăl VĔR-tĕ-brā	_____
chondrocostal (552)	kŏn-drō-KŎS-tăl	_____
clavicle (552)	KLĂV-ĭ-k'l	_____
coccyx (542)	KŎK-sĭks	_____
Colles fracture (554)	KŎL-ēz FRĂK-shŭr	_____
comminuted fracture (554)	KŎM-ĭ-nūt-ĕd FRĂK-shŭr	_____
compact bone (547)	KŎM-păkt bōn	_____
condyle (548)	KŎN-dīl	_____
cranial bones (548)	KRĀ-nē-ăl bōnz	_____
craniotome (552)	KRĀ-nē-ō-tōm	_____
craniotomy (552)	krā-nē-ŎT-ō-mē	_____
crepitus (554)	KRĔP-ĭ-tŭs	_____
decalcification (549)	dē-kăl-sĭ-fĭ-KĀ-shŭn	_____
diaphysis (548)	dī-ĂF-ĭ-sĭs	_____
epiphyseal plate (548)	ĕp-ĭ-FĬZ-ē-ăl plāt	_____
epiphysis (548)	ĕ-PĬF-ĭ-sĭs	_____
ethmoid bone (538)	ĔTH-moyd bōn	_____
Ewing sarcoma (554)	Ū-ĭng săr-kō-mă	_____
exostosis (554)	ĕk-sŏs-TŌ-sĭs	_____
facial bones (548)	FĀ-shăl bōnz	_____
femoral (552)	FĔM-ŏr-ăl	_____
femur (552)	FĒ-mŭr	_____
fibula (552)	FĬB-ū-lă	_____
fibular (552)	FĬB-ū-lăr	_____
fissure (548)	FĬSH-ŭr	_____
fontanelle (548)	fŏn-tă-NĔL	_____
foramen (548)	fō-RĀ-mĕn	_____
fossa (548)	FŎS-ă	_____

frontal bone (538)	FRŎN-tăl bōn	
haversian canals (548)	hă-VĔR-shăn kă-NĂLZ	
humeral (552)	HŪ-mĕr-ăl	
humerus (552)	HŪ-mĕr-ŭs	
hypercalcemia (549)	hī-pĕr-kăl-SĒ-mē-ă	
iliac (552)	ĬL-ē-ăk	
ilium (552)	ĬL-ē-ŭm	
impacted fracture (554)	ĭm-PĂK-tĕd FRĂK-shŭr	
ischial (552)	ĬSH-ē-ăl or Ĭs-kē-ăl	
ischium (552)	ĬSH-ē-ŭm or Ĭs-kē-um	
kyphosis (550)	kī-FŌ-sĭs	
lacrimal bones (540)	LĂ-krĭ-măl bōnz	
lamina (542)	LĂM-ĭ-nă	
laminectomy (550)	lăm-ĭ-NĔK-tō-mē	
lordosis (549)	lŏr-DŌ-sĭs	
lumbar vertebrae (542)	LŬM-băr VĔR-tĕ-brā	
lumbodynia (550)	lŭm-bō-DĬN-ē-ă	
lumbosacral (550)	lŭm-bō-SĀ-krăl	
malleolar (553)	mă-LĒ-ō-lăr	
malleolus (548)	măl-LĒ-ō-lŭs	
mandible (553)	MĂN-dĭ-b'l	
mandibular (553)	măn-DĬB-ū-lăr	
mastoid process (548)	MĂs-toyd PRŌ-sĕs	
medullary cavity (548)	MĔD-ū-lăr-ē KĂ-vĭ-tē	
metacarpals (553)	mĕt-ă-KĂR-pălz	
metacarpectomy (553)	mĕt-ă-kăr-PĔK-tō-mē	
metaphysis (548)	mĕ-TĂ-fĭ-sĭs	
metatarsalgia (553)	mĕt-ă-tăr-SĂL-jă	
metatarsals (553)	mĕt-ă-TĂR-sălz	

myelopoiesis (550)	mī-ĕ-lō-poy-Ē-sĭs	_____
nasal bone (540)	NĀ-zăl bōn	_____
occipital bone (538)	ŏk-SĬP-ĭ-tăl bōn	_____
olecranal (553)	ō-LĔK-ră-năl	_____
olecranon (548)	ō-LĔK-ră-nŏn	_____
orthopedic (550)	ŏr-thō-PĒ-dĭk	_____
osseous tissue (548)	ŎS-ē-ŭs TĬSH-ū	_____
ossification (548)	ŏs-ĭ-fĭ-KĀ-shŭn	_____
osteitis (550)	ŏs-tē-Ī-tĭs	_____
osteoblast (548)	ŎS-tē-ō-blăst	_____
osteoclast (548)	ŎS-tē-ō-klăst	_____
osteodystrophy (550)	ŏs-tē-ō-DĬS-trō-fē	_____
osteogenesis imperfecta (550)	ŏs-tē-ō-JĔN-ĕ-sĭs ĭm-pĕr-FĔK-tă	_____
osteogenic sarcoma (554)	ŏs-tē-ō-JĔN-ĭk săr-KŌ-mă	_____
osteomalacia (551)	ŏs-tē-ō-mă-LĀ-shă	_____
osteomyelitis (556)	ŏs-tē-ō-mī-ĕ-LĪ-tĭs	_____
osteoporosis (556)	ŏs-tē-ō-pŏr-Ō-sĭs	_____
osteotome (552)	ŎS-tē-ō-tōm	_____
parietal bones (538)	pă-RĪ-ĭ-tăl bōnz	_____
patella (546)	pă-TĔL-ă	_____
pelvimetry (553)	pĕl-VĬM-ĕ-trē	_____
periosteum (548)	pĕ-rē-ŎS-tē-um	_____
peroneal (553)	pĕr-ō-NĒ-ăl	_____
phalangeal (553)	fă-lăn-JĒ-ăl	_____
phalanges (553)	fă-LĂN-jēz	_____
phosphorus (549)	FŎS-fō-rŭs	_____
pubic symphysis (549)	PŪ-bĭk SĬM-fĭ-sĭs	_____

pubis (553) PŪ-bĭs _____

radial (553) RĀ-dē-ăl _____

radius (553) RĀ-dē-ŭs _____

reduction (554) rĕ-DŬK-shŭn _____

ribs (549) rĭbz _____

sacral vertebrae (542) SĀ-krăl VĔR-tĕ-brā _____

scapula (553) SKĂP-ū-lă _____

scapular (553) SKĂP-ŭ-lăr _____

scoliosis (550) skō-lē-Ō-sĭs _____

sinus (549) SĪ-nŭs _____

sphenoid bone (538) SFĔ-noyd bōn _____

spondylitis (550) spŏn-dĭ-LĪ-tĭs _____

spondylolisthesis (551) spŏn-dĭ-lō-lĭs-THĒ-sĭs _____

spondylosis (550) spŏn-dĭ-LŌ-sĭs _____

sternum (553) STĔR-nŭm _____

styloid process (549) STĪ-loyd PRŌ-sĕs _____

subcostal (552) sŭb-KŎS-tăl _____

subpatellar (553) sŭb-pă-TĔL-lăr _____

supraclavicular (552) sŭ-pră-klă-VĬK-ū-lăr _____

talipes (556) TĂL-ĭ-pĕz _____

tarsals (553) TĂR-sălz _____

tarsectomy (553) tăr-SĔK-tō-mē _____

temporal bones (538) TĔM-pōr-ăl bōnz _____

thoracic vertebrae (542) thō-RĂS-ĭk VĔR-tĕ-brā _____

tibia (553) TĬB-ē-ă _____

tibial (553) TĬB-ē-ăl _____

trabeculae (549) tră-BĔK-ū-lē _____

trochanter (549) trō-KĂN-tĕr _____

tubercle (549)	TŪ-bĕr-k'l	
tuberosity (549)	tū-bĕ-RŎS-ĭ-tē	
ulna (553)	ŬL-nă	
ulnar (553)	ŬL-năr	
vomer (540)	VŌ-mĕr	
xiphoid process (549)	ZĬF-oyd PRŌ-sĕs	
zygomatic bones (540)	zī-gō-MĂ-tĭk bōnz	

Terms Related to Joints and Muscles

Term	**Pronunciation**	**Meaning**
abduction (571)	ăb-DŬK-shŭn	
achondroplasia (560)	ā-kŏn-drō-PLĀ-zē-ă	
adduction (571)	ă-DŬK-shŭn	
amyotrophic lateral sclerosis (571)	ā-mī-ō-TRŌ-fĭk LĂT-ĕr-ăl sklĕ-RŌ-sĭs	
ankylosing spondylitis (561)	ăng-kĭ-LŌ-sĭng spŏn-dĭ-LĪ-tĭs	
ankylosis (560)	ăng-kĭ-LŌ-sĭs	
arthrocentesis (572)	ăr-thrō-sĕn-TĒ-sĭs	
arthrodesis (561)	ăr-thrō-DĒ-sĭs	
arthrography (572)	ăr-THRŎG-ră-fē	
arthroplasty (560)	ĂR-thrō-plăs-tē	
arthroscopy (573)	ăr-THRŎS-kō-pē	
arthrotomy (560)	ăr-THRŌT-ō-mē	
articular cartilage (560)	ăr-TĬK-ū-lăr KĂR-tĭ-lĭj	
articulation (559)	ăr-tĭk-ū-LĀ-shŭn	
atrophy (571)	ĂT-rō-fē	
bunion (562)	BŬN-yŭn	
bursa (plural: bursae) (559)	BĔR-să (BĔR-sē)	

bursitis (560)	bŭr-SĪ-tis	_____
carpal tunnel syndrome (562)	KĂR-păl TŬN-nĕl SĬN-drōm	_____
chondroma (560)	kŏn-DRŌ-mă	_____
chondromalacia (560)	kŏn-drō-mă-LĀ-shă	_____
dislocation (564)	dĭs-lō-KĀ-shŭn	_____
dorsiflexion (571)	dŏr-sē-FLĔK-shŭn	_____
electromyography (574)	ē-lĕk-trō-mī-ŎG-ră-fē	_____
extension (569)	ĕk-STĔN-shŭn	_____
fascia (569)	FĂSH-ē-ă	_____
fasciectomy (570)	făsh-ē-ĔK-tō-mē	_____
fibromyalgia (570)	fī-brō-mī-ĂL-jă	_____
flexion (569)	FLĔK-shŭn	_____
ganglion (564)	GĂNG-lē-ŏn	_____
gouty arthritis (561)	GŎW-tē ăr-THRĪ-tĭs	_____
hemarthrosis (560)	hĕm-ăr-THRŌ-sĭs	_____
hydrarthrosis (560)	hī-drăr-THRŌ-sĭs	_____
hypertrophy (571)	hī-PĔR-trō-fē	_____
hyperuricemia (561)	hī-pĕr-ŭr-ĭ-SĒ-mē-ă	_____
leiomyoma (570)	lī-ō-mī-Ō-mă	_____
leiomyosarcoma (570)	lī-ō-mī-ō-săr-KŌ-mă	_____
ligament (559)	LĬG-ă-mĕnt	_____
ligamentous (561)	lĭg-ă-MĔN-tŭs	_____
Lyme disease (565)	līm dĭ-ZĒZ	_____
muscular dystrophy (572)	MŬS-kū-lăr DĬs-trō-fē	_____
myalgia (570)	mī-ĂL-jă	_____
myopathy (570)	mī-ŎP-ă-thē	_____
myositis (571)	mī-ō-SĪ-tĭs	_____

osteoarthritis (562)   ŏs-tē-ō-ăr-THRĪ-tĭs   _____

plantar flexion (569)   PLĂN-tăr FLĔK-shun   _____

podagra (562)   pō-DĂG-ră   _____

polymyalgia (571)   pŏl-ē-mĭ-ĂL-jă   _____

polymyositis (572)   pŏl-ē-mī-ō-SĪ-tĭs   _____

pronation (570)   prō-NĀ-shŭn   _____

pyrexia (562)   pī-RĔK-sē-ă   _____

rhabdomyoma (571)   răb-dō-mī-Ō-mă   _____

rhabdomyosarcoma (571)   răb-dō-mī-ō-săr-KŌ-mă   _____

rheumatoid arthritis (562)   ROO-mă-toyd ăr-THRĪ-tĭs   _____

rheumatologist (561)   roo-mă-TŎL-ō-jĭst   _____

rotation (570)   rō-TĀ-shŭn   _____

sprain (565)   sprān   _____

strain (565)   strān   _____

striated muscle (570)   STRĪ-ā-tĕd MŬS-el   _____

subluxation (564)   sŭb-lŭk-SĀ-shŭn   _____

supination (570)   sū-pĭ-NĀ-shŭn   _____

suture joint (559)   SŪ-chŭr joint   _____

synovial fluid (559)   sī-NŌ-vē-ăl FLOO-ĭd   _____

synovial joint (559)   sī-NŌ-vē-ăl joint   _____

synovial membrane (559)   sī-NŌ-vē-ăl MĔM-brān   _____

synovitis (561)   sī-nō-VĪ-tĭs   _____

systemic lupus   sĭs-TĔM-ĭk LŪ-pŭs   _____
  erythematosus (565)   ĕ-rĭ-thē-mă-TŌ-sŭs   _____

tendinitis (561)   tĕn-dĭ-NĪ-tĭs   _____

tendon (559)   TĔN-dŭn   _____

tenorrhaphy (561)   tĕn-ŎR-ă-fē   _____

tenosynovitis (561)   tĕn-ō-sī-nō-VĪ-tĭs   _____

visceral muscle (570)   VĬS-ĕr-ăl MŬS-ĕl   _____

X. Review Sheet

Write the meanings of the word parts in the spaces provided. Check your answers with the information in the chapter or in the glossary (Medical Terms—English) at the end of the book.

COMBINING FORMS

Combining Form	Meaning	Combining Form	Meaning
acetabul/o		ili/o	
ankyl/o		isch/o	
arthr/o		kyph/o	
articul/o		lamin/o	
burs/o		leiomy/o	
calc/o		ligament/o	
calcane/o		lord/o	
calci/o		lumb/o	
carp/o		malleol/o	
cervic/o		mandibul/o	
chondr/o		maxill/o	
clavicul/o		metacarp/o	
coccyg/o		metatars/o	
cost/o		my/o	
crani/o		myel/o	
fasci/o		myocardi/o	
femor/o		myos/o	
fibr/o		olecran/o	
fibul/o		orth/o	
humer/o		oste/o	

patell/o	_____	scapul/o	_____
ped/o	_____	scoli/o	_____
pelv/i	_____	spondyl/o	_____
perone/o	_____	stern/o	_____
phalang/o	_____	synov/o	_____
plant/o	_____	tars/o	_____
pub/o	_____	ten/o	_____
radi/o	_____	tendin/o	_____
rhabdomy/o	_____	thorac/o	_____
rheumat/o	_____	tibi/o	_____
sacr/o	_____	uln/o	_____
sarc/o	_____	vertebr/o	_____

SUFFIXES

Suffix	Meaning	Suffix	Meaning
-algia	_____	-penia	_____
-asthenia	_____	-physis	_____
-blast	_____	-plasty	_____
-clast	_____	-porosis	_____
-desis	_____	-stenosis	_____
-emia	_____	-tome	_____
-listhesis	_____	-trophy	_____
-malacia	_____		

Continued on following page

PREFIXES

Prefix	Meaning	Prefix	Meaning
a-, an-	_____	hyper-	_____
ab-	_____	meta-	_____
ad-	_____	peri-	_____
dia-	_____	poly-	_____
dorsi-	_____	sub-	_____
epi-	_____	supra-	_____
exo-	_____	sym-	_____

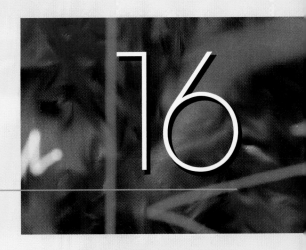

CHAPTER 16

Skin

This chapter is divided into the following sections
- I. Introduction
- II. Structure of the Skin
- III. Accessory Organs of the Skin
- IV. Vocabulary
- V. Combining Forms and Suffixes
- VI. Lesions, Symptoms, Abnormal Conditions, and Skin Neoplasms
- VII. Laboratory Tests, Clinical Procedures, and Abbreviations
- VIII. Practical Applications
- IX. Exercises
- X. Answers to Exercises
- XI. Pronunciation of Terms
- XII. Review Sheet

In this chapter you will
- Identify the layers of the skin and the accessory structures associated with the skin;
- Build medical words using the combining forms that are related to the specialty of dermatology;
- Describe lesions, symptoms, and pathological conditions that relate to the skin;
- Identify laboratory tests, clinical procedures, and abbreviations that pertain to the skin; and
- Apply your new knowledge to understanding medical terms in their proper contexts, such as medical reports and records.

I. Introduction

The skin and its accessory organs (hair, nails, and glands) are known as the **integumentary system** of the body. Integument means covering, and the skin (weighing 8–10 pounds over an area of 22 square feet in an average adult) is the outer covering for the body. It is, however, more than a simple body covering. This complex system of specialized tissues contains glands that secrete several types of fluids, nerves that carry impulses, and blood vessels that aid in the regulation of the body temperature. The following paragraphs review the many important functions of the skin.

First, as a protective membrane over the entire body, the skin guards the deeper tissues of the body against excessive loss of water, salts, and heat and against invasion of pathogens and their toxins. Secretions from the skin are slightly acidic in nature, and this contributes to the skin's ability to prevent bacterial invasion.

Second, the skin contains two types of glands that produce important secretions. These glands under the skin are the **sebaceous** and the **sweat glands.** The sebaceous glands produce an oily secretion called **sebum,** and the sweat glands produce a watery secretion called **sweat.** Sebum and sweat are carried to the outer edges of the skin by ducts and excreted from the skin through openings, or pores. Sebum helps to lubricate the surface of the skin, and sweat helps to cool the body as it evaporates from the skin surface.

Third, nerve fibers located under the skin act as receptors for sensations such as pain, temperature, pressure, and touch. Thus, the adjustment of an individual to her or his environment is dependent on the sensory messages relayed to the brain and spinal cord by the sensitive nerve endings in the skin.

Fourth, several different tissues in the skin aid in maintaining the body temperature (thermoregulation). Nerve fibers coordinate thermoregulation by carrying messages to the skin from heat centers in the brain that are sensitive to increases and decreases in body temperature. Impulses from these fibers cause blood vessels to dilate to bring blood to the surface and cause sweat glands to produce the watery secretion that carries heat away.

II. Structure of the Skin

Figure 16–1A shows the three layers of the skin. Label these layers from the outer surface inward.

Epidermis [1]—a thin, cellular membrane layer.
Dermis [2]—dense, fibrous, connective tissue layer.
Subcutaneous tissue [3]—thick, fat-containing tissue.

Epidermis

The empidermis is the outermost, totally cellular layer of the skin. It is composed of **squamous epithelium.** Epithelium is the covering of both the internal and the external surfaces of the body. Squamous epithelial cells are flat and scale-like. In the outer layer of the skin, these cells are arranged in several layers **(strata)** and are therefore called **stratified squamous epithelium.**

The epidermis lacks blood vessels, lymphatic vessels, and connective tissue (elastic fibers, cartilage, fat) and is therefore dependent on the deeper dermis (also called corium) layer and its rich network of capillaries for nourishment. In fact, oxygen and

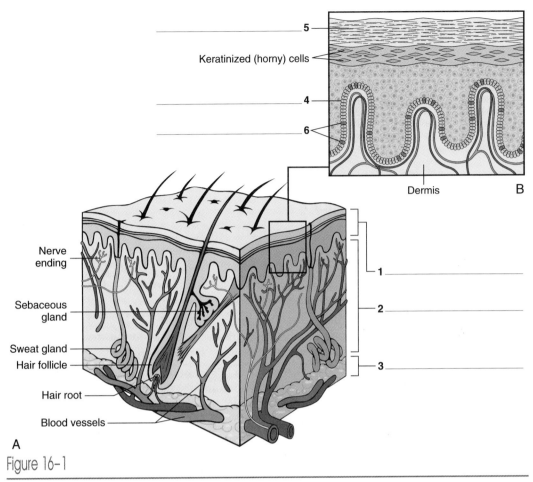

Figure 16-1

The skin. (A) Three layers of the skin. (B) Epidermis.

nutrients seep out of the capillaries in the dermis, pass through tissue fluid, and supply nourishment to the deeper layers of the epidermis.

Figure 16–1B illustrates the multilayered cells of the epidermis. The deepest layer is called the **basal layer** [4]. The cells in the basal layer are constantly growing and multiplying and give rise to all the other cells in the epidermis. As the basal layer cells divide, they are pushed upward and away from the blood supply of the dermal layer by a steady stream of younger cells. In their movement toward the most superficial layer of the epidermis, called the **stratum corneum** [5], the cells flatten, shrink, lose their nuclei, and die, becoming filled with a hard protein material called **keratin.** The cells are then called **horny cells,** reflecting their composition of keratin. Finally, within 3–4 weeks after beginning as a basal cell in the deepest part of the epidermis, the keratinized cell is sloughed off from the surface of the skin. The epidermis is thus constantly renewing itself, cells dying at the same rate at which they are replaced.

The basal layer of the epidermis contains special cells called **melanocytes** [6]. Melanocytes form and contain a black pigment called **melanin** that is transferred to other epidermal cells and gives color to the skin. The number of melanocytes in all races is the same but the amount of melanin within each cell accounts for the color differences among the races. Individuals with darker skin possess more melanin within the melanocytes, not a greater number of melanocytes. The presence of melanin in the epidermis is vital for protection against the harmful effects of ultraviolet radiation, which can manifest themselves as skin cancer. Individuals who are incapable of forming melanin at all are called **albino** (meaning white). Skin and hair are white. Their eyes are red because in the absence of pigment, the tiny blood vessels are visible in the iris (normally pigmented portion) of the eye.

Melanin production increases with exposure to strong ultraviolet light, and this creates a suntan, which is a protective response. When the melanin cannot absorb all the ultraviolet rays, the skin becomes sunburned and inflamed (redness, swelling, and pain). Over a period of years, excessive exposure to sun can tend to cause wrinkles and even cancer of the skin. Because dark-skinned people have more melanin, they have fewer wrinkles and they are less likely to develop skin cancer.

Dermis (Corium)

The dermis layer, directly below the epidermis is composed of blood and lymph vessels and nerve fibers, as well as the accessory organs of the skin, which are the hair follicles, sweat glands, and sebaceous glands. To support the elaborate system of nerves, vessels, and glands, the dermis contains connective tissue cells and fibers that account for the extensibility and elasticity of the skin.

The dermis is composed of interwoven elastic and **collagen** fibers. Collagen (**colla** means glue) is a fibrous protein material found in bone, cartilage, tendons, and ligaments, as well as in the skin. It is tough and resistant but also flexible. In the infant, collagen is loose and delicate, and it becomes harder as the body ages. During pregnancy, overstretching of a woman's skin may break the elastic collagen fibers and stretch the collagen resulting in linear markings called striae or stretch marks. Collagen fibers support and protect the blood and nerve networks that pass through the dermis. Collagen diseases affect connective tissues of the body. Examples of these connective tissue collagen disorders are systemic lupus erythematosus and scleroderma (see Section VI, under Abnormal Conditions).

Subcutaneous Layer

The subcutaneous layer of the skin is another connective tissue layer; it specializes in the formation of fat. **Lipocytes** (fat cells) are predominant in the subcutaneous layer, and they manufacture and store large quantities of fat. Obviously, areas of the body and individuals vary as far as fat deposition is concerned. Functionally, this layer of the skin is important in protection of the deeper tissues of the body and as a heat insulator.

III. Accessory Organs of the Skin

Hair

A hair fiber is composed of a tightly fused meshwork of horny cells filled with the hard protein called **keratin.** Hair growth is similar to the growth of the epidermal layer of the skin. Deep-lying cells in the hair root (see Fig. 16–1) produce horny cells that move upward through the **hair follicles** (shafts or sacs that hold the hair fibers). Melanocytes are located at the root of the hair follicle, and they support the melanin pigment for the horny cells of the hair fiber. Hair turns gray when the melanocytes stop producing melanin.

Of the 5 million hairs on the body, about 100,000 are on the head. They grow about ½ inch (1.3 cm) a month, and cutting the hair has no effect on its rate of growth.

Nails

Nails are hard, keratin plates covering the dorsal surface of the last bone of each toe and finger. They are composed of horny cells that are cemented together tightly and can extend indefinitely unless cut or broken. A nail grows in thickness and length as a result of division of cells in the region of the nail root, which is at the base (proximal portion) of the nail plate.

Most nails grown about 1 mm a week, which means that fingernails may regrow in 3–5 months. Toenails grow more slowly than fingernails; it takes 12–18 months for toenails to be replaced completely.

The **lunula** is a semilunar (half-moon), white region at the base of the nail plate, and it is generally found in the thumbnail of most people and in varying degrees in other fingers. Air mixed in with keratin and cells rich in nuclei give the lunula its whitish color. The **cuticle,** a narrow band of epidermis (layer of keratin), is at the base and sides of the nail plate. The **paronychium** is the soft tissue surrounding the nail border. Figure 16–2A illustrates the anatomic structure of a nail.

Nail growth and appearance commonly alter during systemic disease. For example, grooves in nails may occur with high fevers and serious illness, and spoon nails (flattening of the nail plate) occur in iron deficiency anemia. Onycholysis (onych/o = nail) is the loosening of the nail plate with separation from the nail bed. It may occur with infection of the nail (Fig. 16–2B).

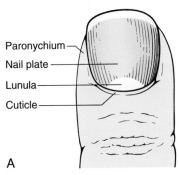

Paronychium
Nail plate
Lunula
Cuticle

A

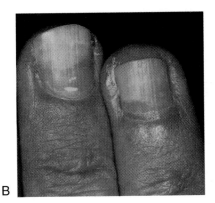

B

Figure 16-2

(A) Anatomical structure of a nail. (B) Onycholysis. Infection or trauma to the nail may be the cause of the loosening of the nail from its plate. (B from Seidel HM: Mosby's Guide to Physical Examination, 4th ed. St. Louis, CV Mosby, 1998.)

Glands

Sebaceous Glands

Sebaceous glands are located in the dermal layer of the skin over the entire body, with the exception of the palms (hands) and soles (feet). They secrete an oily substance called **sebum.** Sebum, containing lipids, lubricates the skin and minimizes water loss. Sebaceous glands are closely associated with hair follicles, and their ducts open into the hair follicle through which the sebum is released. Figure 16–1 shows the relationship of the sebaceous gland to the hair follicle. The sebaceous glands are influenced by sex hormones, which cause them to hypertrophy at puberty and atrophy in old age. Overproduction of sebum during puberty contributes to blackhead (comedo) formation and acne in some individuals.

Sweat Glands

Sweat glands are tiny, coiled glands found on almost all body surfaces (about 2 million in the body). They are most numerous in the palm of the hand (3000 glands per sq in) and on the sole of the foot. Figure 16–1 illustrates how the coiled sweat gland originates deep in the dermis and straightens out to extend up through the epidermis. The tiny opening on the surface is called a **pore.**

Sweat, or perspiration, is almost pure water, with dissolved materials such as salt making up less than 1 per cent of the total composition. It is colorless and odorless. The odor produced when sweat accumulates on the skin is due to the action of bacteria on the sweat.

Sweat cools the body as it evaporates into the air. Perspiration is controlled by the sympathetic nervous system, whose nerve fibers are activated by the heart regulatory center in the hypothalamic region of the brain, which stimulates sweating.

A special variety of sweat gland, active only from puberty onward and larger than the ordinary kind, is concentrated in a few areas of the body near the reproductive organs and in the armpits. These glands secrete an odorless sweat, but it contains certain substances that are easily broken down by bacteria on the skin. The breakdown products are responsible for the characteristic human body odor. The milk-producing mammary gland is another type of modified sweat gland; it secretes milk after the birth of a child.

IV. Vocabulary

This list will help you review many of the new terms introduced in the text. Short definitions will reinforce your understanding of the terms. See Section XI of this chapter for help in pronouncing the more difficult terms.

albino	A person with skin deficient in pigment.
basal layer	The deepest region of the epidermis; it gives rise to all the epidermal cells.
collagen	Structural protein found in the skin and connective tissue.
cuticle	Band of epidermis at the base and sides of the nail plate.
dermis	The middle layer of the skin; also called corium.
epidermis	The outermost layer of the skin.
epithelium	Layer of skin cells forming the outer and inner surfaces of the body.
hair follicle	The sac or tube within which each hair grows.
horny cell	A keratin-filled cell in the epidermis.
integumentary system	The skin and its accessory structures such as hair and nails.
keratin	A hard protein material found in the epidermis, hair, and nails. Keratin means horn and is commonly found in the horns of animals.
lipocyte	A fat cell.
lunula	The half-moon–shaped, white area at the base of a nail.
melanin	A pigment that gives the skin color. It is formed by melanocytes in the epidermis.
sebaceous gland	An oil-secreting gland in the dermis that is associated with hair follicles.
sebum	An oily substance secreted by sebaceous glands.
squamous epithelium	Flat, scale-like cells composing the epidermis.
stratified	Arranged in layers.

stratum (plural: **strata**)   A layer (of cells).

stratum corneum   The outermost layer of the epidermis, which consists of flattened, keratinized (horny) cells.

subcutaneous tissue   The innermost layer of the skin, containing fat tissue.

V. Combining Forms and Suffixes

Write the meanings of the medical terms in the spaces provided.

Combining Forms			
Combining Form	Meaning	Terminology	Meaning
adip/o	fat (see **lip/o** and **steat/o**)	adipose _____	
albin/o	white	albinism _____	

Table 16–1 lists combining forms for colors and examples of terms using those combining forms.

Table 16-1. COLORS

Combining Form	Meaning	Terminology
albin/o	white	*albin*ism
anthrac/o	black (as coal)	*anthrac*osis
chlor/o	green	*chlor*ophyll
cirrh/o	tawny yellow	*cirrh*osis
cyan/o	blue	*cyan*osis
eosin/o	rosy	*eosin*ophil
erythr/o	red	*erythr*ocyte
jaund/o	yellow	*jaund*ice
leuk/o	white	*leuk*oderma
lute/o	yellow	corpus *lute*um
melan/o	black	*melan*ocyte
poli/o	gray	*poli*omyelitis
xanth/o	yellow	*xanth*oma

caus/o	burn, burning	causalgia _____
		Intensely unpleasant burning sensation in skin and muscles when there is damage to nerves.
cauter/o	heat, burn	electrocautery _____
		A knife used during surgery to burn through tissue. It is very effective in minimizing blood loss.
cutane/o	skin (see **derm/o**)	subcutaneous _____
derm/o **dermat/o**	skin	epidermis _____
		dermatitis _____
		Atopic dermatitis is of unknown cause; it is marked by itching and scratching. In 70 per cent of cases, there is a family history of the condition. Atopy is an allergic reaction for which there is a genetic predisposition.
		dermatoplasty _____
		dermatologist _____
		dermabrasion _____
		Abrasion means a scraping away. This is a surgical procedure performed to remove acne scars, tatoos, or fine wrinkles.
		epidermolysis _____
		Loosening of the epidermis with the development of large blisters; occurs after injury.
diaphor/o	profuse sweating (see **hidr/o**)	diaphoresis _____
erythem/o **erythemat/o**	redness	erythema _____
		Flushing; widespread redness of the skin.
		erythematous _____
hidr/o	sweat	anhidrosis _____
		Do not confuse hidr/o with hydr/o (water)!
ichthy/o	scaly, dry (fish-like)	ichthyosis _____
		A hereditary condition in which the skin is dry, rough, and scaly because of a defect in keratinization. Ichthyosis can also be acquired, appearing with malignancies such as lymphomas and multiple myeloma.

kerat/o	hard, horny tissue	keratosis _____ *See page 618, Section VI, under Skin Neoplasms.*
leuk/o	white	leukoplakia _____ *-plakia means plaques.*
lip/o	fat	lipoma _____ liposuction _____ *Removal of subcutaneous fat tissue through a tube that is introduced into the fatty area via a small incision. The fat is aspirated (suctioned) out.*
melan/o	black	melanocyte _____ melanoma _____ *This is a malignant skin tumor. See page 618, Section VI, under Skin Neoplasms.*
myc/o	fungus (fungi include yeasts, molds, and mushrooms)	dermatomycosis _____ *An example is ringworm (athlete's foot)*
onych/o	nail (see **ungu/o**)	onycholysis _____ *Separation of the nail plate from the nail bed in fungal infections or after trauma.* onychomycosis _____ *The nails become white, opaque, thick, and brittle.* paronychia _____ *par- means near or beside. Paronychia is the inflammation and swelling of the soft tissue around the nail and is associated with torn cuticles or ingrown nails.*
phyt/o	plant	dermatophytosis _____ *Examples are fungal infections of the hands and feet.*

pil/o	hair (see **trich/o**), hair follicle	pilosebaceous _____	

sebace/o means a gland that secretes sebum.

seb/o	sebum (oily secretion from sebaceous glands)

seborrhea _____

Excessive secretion from sebaceous glands. **Seborrheic dermatitis is commonly known as dandruff.**

squam/o	scale-like

squamous epithelium _____

Cells are flat and scale-like.

steat/o	fat

steatoma _____

A cystic collection of sebum (fatty material) that forms in a sebaceous gland and can become infected; **sebaceous cyst.**

trich/o	hair

trichomycosis _____

ungu/o	nail

subungual _____

xanth/o	yellow

xanthoma _____

Nodules develop under the skin owing to excess lipid deposits. Usually associated with a high cholesterol level. Plaques that appear on the eyelids of elderly people are called xanthelasmas (-elasma means a flat plate).

xer/o	dry

xeroderma _____

-derma means skin. This is a mild form of ichthyosis.

Suffixes

Suffix	Meaning	Terminology	Meaning
-derma	skin	pyoderma _____	
		leukoderma _____	

VI. Lesions, Symptoms, Abnormal Conditions, and Skin Neoplasms

Cutaneous Lesions

A **lesion** is an area of damaged tissue, caused by disease or trauma. The following terms describe common skin lesions, which are illustrated in Figure 16–3.

cyst	**A thick-walled, closed sac or pouch containing fluid or semisolid material.**
	Examples of cysts are the **pilonidal cyst,** which is found over the sacral area of the back in the midline and contains hairs (**pil/o** means hair, **nid/o** means nest); and the **sebaceous cyst,** which is a collection of yellowish, cheesy sebum commonly found on the scalp, vulva, and scrotum.
fissure	**A groove or crack-like sore.**
	An anal fissure is a break in the skin lining and anal canal.
macule	**A discolored (often reddened) flat lesion.**
	Freckles, tattoo marks, and flat moles are examples.

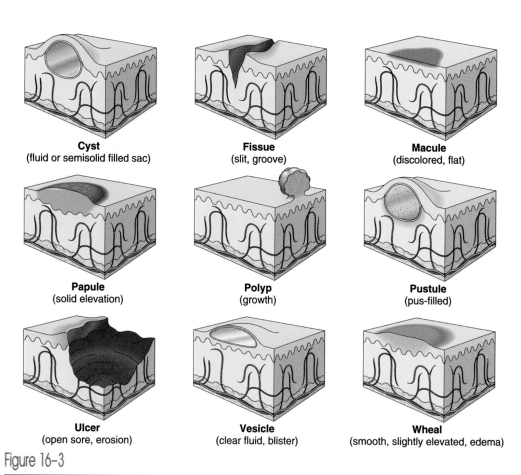

Cyst
(fluid or semisolid filled sac)

Fissue
(slit, groove)

Macule
(discolored, flat)

Papule
(solid elevation)

Polyp
(growth)

Pustule
(pus-filled)

Ulcer
(open sore, erosion)

Vesicle
(clear fluid, blister)

Wheal
(smooth, slightly elevated, edema)

Figure 16-3

Cutaneous lesions.

Figure 16-4

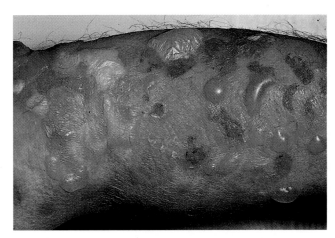

Bullae (large blisters) in pemphigus (a chronic skin disorder in older individuals). The pemphigoid (pemphix means blister) bullae occur as the entire thickness of the epidermis detaches from its foundation. (From Kumar V, Cotran RS, Robbins SL: Basic Pathology, 6th ed. Philadelphia, WB Saunders, 1997.)

papule

A small (less than 1 cm in diameter), solid elevation of the skin.

Pimples are examples of papules. A larger, solid elevation is a **nodule.**

polyp

A mushroom-like growth extending on a stalk from the surface of mucous membrane.

Polyps are commonly found in the nose and sinuses, urinary bladder, and uterus.

pustule

A small elevation of the skin containing pus.

A pustule is a small **abscess** on the skin.

ulcer

An open sore or erosion of the skin or mucous membrane.

Decubitus ulcers (bedsores) are caused by pressure that results from lying in one position (**decubitus** means lying down). Ulcers usually involve loss of tissue substance and pus formation.

vesicle

A small collection of clear fluid (serum); blister.

Vesicles are found in burns, allergies, and dermatitis. **Bullae** (singular: **bulla**) are large vesicles (Fig. 16–4).

wheal

A smooth, slightly elevated, edematous (swollen) area that is redder or paler than the surrounding skin.

Wheals may be circumscribed, as in a mosquito bite, or may involve a wide area, as in allergic reactions. Wheals are often accompanied by itching and are seen in hives, anaphylaxis, and insect bites.

Symptoms

alopecia

Absence of hair from areas where it normally grows.

Alopecia, or baldness, may be hereditary (usual progressive loss of scalp hair in men); or it may be due to disease, injury, or treatment (chemotherapy) or may occur in old age. **Alopecia areata** is an idiopathic condition in which hair falls out in patches.

ecchymosis (plural: **ecchymoses**)	**Bluish-black mark (macule) on the skin; black-and-blue mark.**

Ecchymoses (ec- means out, chym/o means to pour) are caused by hemorrhages into the skin from injury or spontaneous leaking of blood from vessels. |
| **petechia** (plural: **petechiae**) | **A small, pinpoint hemorrhage.**

Petechiae are smaller versions of ecchymoses. |
| **pruritus** | **Itching.**

Pruritus is associated with most forms of dermatitis and with other conditions as well. It arises as a result of stimulation of nerves in the skin by enzymes released in allergic reactions or by irritation caused by substances in the blood or by foreign bodies. |
| **purpura** | **Merging ecchymoses and petechiae over any part of the body.** |
| **urticaria (hives)** | **An acute allergic reaction in which red, round wheals develop on the skin.**

Pruritus may be intense, and the cause is commonly allergy to foods (such as shellfish or strawberries). Localized edema (swelling) occurs as well. |
| **vitiligo** (vĭt-ĭl-Ī-gō) | **Loss of pigment (depigmentation) in areas of the skin (milk-white patches).**

Also known as **leukoderma** (Fig. 16–5). There is an increased association of vitiligo with certain autoimmune conditions such as thyroiditis, hyperthyroidism, and diabetes mellitus. |

Abnormal Conditions

acne	**Papular and pustular eruption of the skin.**

Acne vulgaris (**vulgaris** means ordinary) is caused by the buildup of sebum and keratin in the pores of the skin. A **blackhead** or **comedo** (plural: **comedones**) is a sebum plug partially blocking the pore (Fig. 16–6). If the pore becomes completely blocked, a **whitehead** forms. Bacteria in the skin break down the sebum, producing inflammation in the surrounding tissue. Papules, pustules, and cysts can thus form. Treatment consists of long-term antibiotic use and medications to dry the skin. Benzoyl peroxide and tretinoin (Retin-A) are medications used to prevent comedo formation; isotretinoin (Accutane) is used in severe cystic acne. |
| **burns** | **Injury to tissues caused by heat contact.**

Examples are dry heat (fire), moist heat (steam or liquid), chemicals, lightning, electricity, and radiation. Burns are usually as follows:
first-degree burns — superficial epidermal lesions, erythema, hyperesthesia, and no blisters. Sunburn is an example.
second-degree burns (partial-thickness burn injury) — epidermal and dermal lesions, erythema, blisters, and hyperesthesia (Fig. 16–7A).
third-degree burns (full-thickness burn injury) — epidermis and dermis are destroyed (necrosis of skin), and subcutaneous layer is damaged leaving charred, white tissue (Fig. 16–7B). |

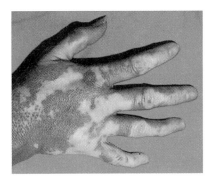

Figure 16-5

Vitiligo on the hand (Latin: *vitium* meaning a blemish). Epidermal melanocytes are completely lost in depigmented areas through an autoimmune process. (From Jarvis C: Physical Examination and Health Assessment, 2nd ed. Philadelphia, WB Saunders, 1996.)

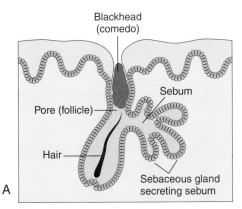

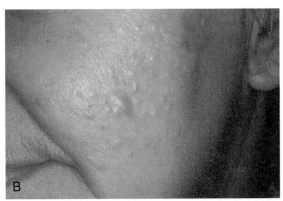

Figure 16-6

(A) Formation of a blackhead (comedo) in a dilated pore filled with sebum, bacteria, and pigment. (B) Acne. (B from Callen JP, Greer KE, Hood AF, et al: Color Atlas of Dermatology. Philadelphia, WB Saunders, 1993.)

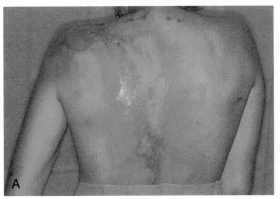

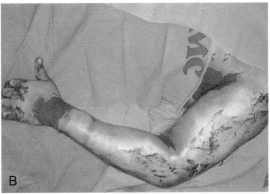

Figure 16-7

Burns. (A) Second-degree burn injury. Wound sensation is painful and very sensitive to touch and air currents. **(B) Third-degree burn** showing variable color (deep-red, white, black and brown). The wound itself is insensate (does not respond to pinprick sensation). (From Black JM, Matassarin-Jacobs E: Medical-Surgical Nursing, 5th ed. Philadelphia, WB Saunders, 1997.)

eczema

Inflammatory skin disease with erythematous, papulovesicular lesions.

This chronic or acute dermatitis is often accompanied by pruritus and may occur without any obvious cause. It is a common allergic reaction in children and also occurs in adults. Allergy may be to foods, dust, or pollens. Treatment depends on the cause but usually includes the use of corticosteroids.

exanthematous viral diseases

Rash (exanthem) of the skin due to a viral infection.

Examples are **rubella** (German measles), **rubeola** (measles), and **varicella** (chickenpox).

gangrene

Death of tissue associated with loss of blood supply.

In this condition, ischemia resulting from injury, inflammation, frostbite, diseases such as diabetes, or arteriosclerosis can lead to necrosis of tissue followed by bacterial invasion and putrefaction (proteins are decomposed by bacteria).

impetigo

Bacterial inflammatory skin disease characterized by vesicles, pustules, and crusted-over lesions.

This is a contagious **pyoderma** (**py/o** means pus) and is usually caused by staphylococci or streptococci. Systemic use of antibiotics and proper cleansing of lesions are effective treatments.

psoriasis

Chronic, recurrent dermatosis marked by itchy, scaly, red patches covered by silvery gray scales (Fig. 16–8).

Psoriasis commonly forms on the forearms, knees, legs, and scalp. It is neither infectious nor contagious but is caused by an increased rate of growth of the basal layer of the epidermis. The cause is unknown, but the condition runs in families and may be brought on by anxiety. Treatment is palliative (relieving but not curing) and includes topical lubricants, keratolytics, and steroids. PUVA (psoralen-ultraviolet A) light therapy is also used.

scabies

A contagious, parasitic infection of the skin with intense pruritus.

Scabies (from *scabere,* meaning to scratch) is often spread through sexual contact, and commonly affected areas are the penis, groin, nipples, and skin between the fingers. Treatment is topical medicated cream to destroy the scabies mites (tiny parasites).

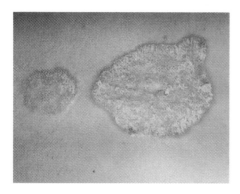

Figure 16-8

Psoriasis. Scaly erythematous patch, with silvery scales on top. (From Jarvis C: Physical Examination and Health Assessment, 2nd ed. Philadelphia, WB Saunders, 1996.)

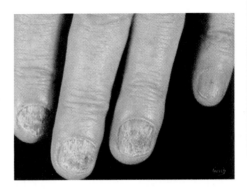

Figure 16-9

Tinea unguium. Fungal infection of the nail causes the distal nail plate to turn yellow or white. Hyperkeratotic debris accumulates, causing the nail to separate from the nail bed (onycholysis). (Courtesy of the American Academy of Dermatology and Institute for Dermatologic Communication and Education, Evanston, IL. From Seidel HM: Mosby's Guide to Physical Examination, 4th ed. St. Louis, CV Mosby, 1998.)

scleroderma	**A chronic progressive disease of the skin with hardening and shrinking of connective tissue.**

Fibrous scar tissue infiltrates the skin and the heart, lungs, kidneys, and esophagus may be affected as well. Skin is thick, hard, and rigid, and pigmented patches may occur. The cause is not known. Palliative treatment consists of drugs, such as immunosuppressives and anti-inflammatory agents, and physical therapy.

systemic lupus erythematosus (SLE)	**Chronic inflammatory disease of collagen in the skin, of joints, and of internal organs.**

Lupus (meaning wolf-like; physicians thought the shape and color of the skin lesions resembled the bite of a wolf) produces a characteristic "butterfly" pattern of redness over the cheeks and nose. In more severe cases, the extent of erythema increases and all exposed areas of the skin may be involved. Primarily a disease of females, lupus is an autoimmune condition. High levels of antibodies are found in the patient's blood. Corticosteroids and immunosuppressive drugs are used to control symptoms.

SLE should be differentiated from chronic **discoid lupus erythematosus (DLE),** which is a milder, scaling, plaque-like, superficial eruption of the skin confined to the face, scalp, ears, chest, arms, and back. The reddish patches heal and leave scars.

tinea	**Infection of the skin caused by a fungus.**

Tinea, or **ringworm,** so called because the infection is in a ring-like pattern, is highly contagious and causes severe pruritus. Examples are **tinea pedis** (athlete's foot), which affects the skin between the toes, **tinea capitis** (on the scalp), **tinea barbae** affecting the skin under a beard), and **tinea unguium** (affecting the nails) (Fig. 16–9). Treatment is with antifungal agents. The word *tinea* is from Latin and means a worm.

Skin Neoplasms

Benign Neoplasms

callus	**Increased growth of cells in the horny layer of the epidermis due to pressure or friction.**

The feet and the hands are common sites. A **corn** is a type of callus that develops a hard core (a whitish, corn-like central kernel).

keloid	**Hypertrophied, thickened scar that occurs after trauma or surgical incision.**

Keloids occur because of excessive collagen formation in the skin during connective tissue repair. The term comes from the Greek *kelis,* meaning a blemish.

A normal scar left by a healed wound is called a **cicatrix** (SĬK-ă-trĭx).

keratosis	**Thickened area of the epidermis.**

Some keratoses are red and are due to excessive exposure to light **(actinic keratosis)**. **Seborrheic keratoses** are yellow or brown and are also called **senile warts.** Both types occur in middle age and old age.

leukoplakia	**White, thickened patches on mucous membrane tissue of the tongue or cheek.**

This is a precancerous lesion. It is common in smokers and may be caused by chronic inflammation.

nevus (plural: nevi)	**Pigmented lesion of the skin.**

Nevi include dilated blood vessels (telangiectasis) radiating out from a point (vascular spiders), hemangiomas, and moles. Many are present at birth, but some are acquired.

Dysplastic nevi (Fig. 16–10A) are moles that do not form properly and may progress to form a type of skin cancer called melanoma (see **malignant melanoma).**

verruca	**Epidermal growth caused by a virus (wart).**

Plantar warts (verrucae) occur on the soles of the feet, juvenile warts occur on the hands and face of children, and venereal warts occur on the genitals and around the anus. Warts may be removed by use of acids, electrocautery, or freezing with liquid nitrogen (cryosurgery). If the virus remains in the skin, the wart can regrow.

Cancerous Lesions

basal cell carcinoma	**Malignant tumor of the basal cell layer of the epidermis.**

This is the most frequent type of skin cancer. It is a slow-growing tumor that usually occurs on the upper half of the face, near the nose. It almost never metastasizes.

Kaposi sarcoma	**Malignant, vascular, neoplastic growth characterized by cutaneous nodules usually on the lower extremities.**

Nodules range in color from deep pink to dark blue and purple. The condition is associated with acquired immunodeficiency syndrome (AIDS).

malignant melanoma	**Cancerous growth composed of melanocytes.**

This malignancy is attributed to the intense exposure to sunlight that many people experience. Melanoma usually begins as a mottled, light brown to black, flat macule with irregular borders (Fig. 16–10B). The lesions may turn shades of red, blue, and white and may crust on the surface and bleed. Melanomas often arise in preexisting moles (dysplastic nevi) and frequently appear on the upper back, lower legs, head, and neck.

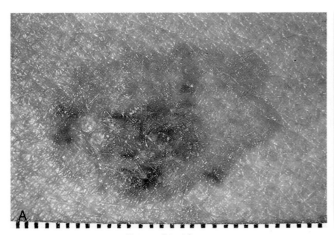
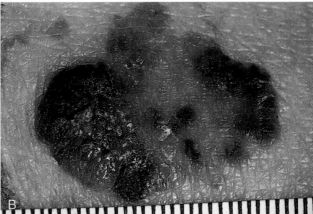

Figure 16-10

(A) **Dysplastic nevus.** The nevus has an irregular contour, variegated color, and a typical center of darker pigment with a "pebbly" surface. (B) **Malignant melanoma.** The most important clinical sign is a change in the color of a pigmented lesion. Melanomas show variations in pigmentation, appearing in shades of black, brown, red, dark blue, and gray. (From Kumar V, Cotran RS, Robbins SL: Basic Pathology, 6th ed. Philadelphia, WB Saunders, 1997.)

Biopsy is required to diagnose melanoma, and prognosis following excision is determined by the depth of invasion through the skin layers. On this basis melanomas have been classified levels I to V. Level I indicates that the growth is confined to the epidermis, and levels IV and V represent penetration to the lower levels of the dermis and subcutaneous layer (Fig. 16–11).

Melanomas often metastasize to the lung, liver, and brain. Treatment includes excision of the tumor, regional lymphadenectomy, chemotherapy/immunotherapy, or radiotherapy to prevent metastasis.

squamous cell carcinoma **Malignant tumor of the squamous epithelial cells of the epidermis.**

This tumor may grow in places other than the skin, wherever squamous epithelium is found (mouth, larynx, bladder, esophagus, and so forth). It may arise from actinic (sun-related) keratoses and metastasize to lymph nodes. Treatment is surgical excision or radiotherapy.

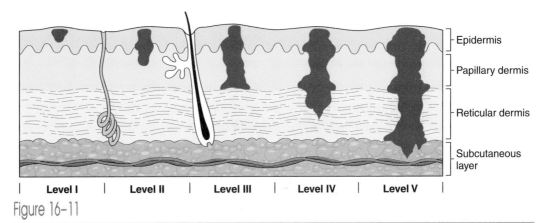

Figure 16-11

Staging of melanoma by depth of invasion (Clark levels). A progressively worse prognosis is associated with increasing invasion of the dermis and subcutaneous layers of the skin.

VII. Laboratory Tests, Clinical Procedures, and Abbreviations

Laboratory Tests

bacterial analyses

Samples of **purulent** (pus-filled) material or **exudate** (fluid that accumulates in a space or passes out of tissues) are sent to the laboratory for examination to determine what type of bacteria are present.

fungal tests

Scrapings from skin lesions are placed on a growth medium for several weeks and then examined microscopically for evidence of fungal growth.

Clinical Procedures

cryosurgery

Tissue is destroyed by the application of intensely cold liquid nitrogen.

Mohs surgery

Thin layers of a malignant growth are removed, and each is examined under the microscope; also called **microscopically controlled surgery.**

skin biopsy

Skin lesions, such as pigmented nevi, chronic dermatoses, or any lesion in which there is the possibility of present or future malignant change, are removed and sent to the pathology laboratory for examination. A **punch biopsy** (used to obtain tissue in cases in which complete excision is not feasible) involves the use of a surgical instrument that removes a core of tissue by rotation of its sharp, circular edge. In a **shave biopsy,** tissue is excised using a cut parallel to the surface of the surrounding skin.

skin testing for allergy or disease

The **patch test** is performed by applying to the skin a small piece of gauze or filter paper on which has been placed a suspected allergy-causing substance. If the area becomes reddened or swollen, the result is considered positive. The **scratch test** involves making several scratches in the skin and inserting a very minute amount of test material in the scratches. The test is considered negative if no reaction occurs. **Intradermal tests** are performed by injection of a reactive substance between layers of the skin and observation of the skin for a subsequent reaction. This test is used for the detection of sensitivity to infectious agents such as tuberculosis (**Mantoux tests, PPD test**) or diphtheria (**Schick test**). Strong reactions indicate ongoing infection.

ABBREVIATIONS

bx	biopsy	**PUVA**	psoralen–ultraviolet A light therapy
Derm.	dermatology	**SLE**	systemic lupus erythematosus
DLE	discoid lupus erythematosus	**subcu, subq**	subcutaneous
PPD	purified protein derivative		

VIII. Practical Applications

This section contains actual medical reports using terms that you have studied in this and previous chapters. Explanations of more difficult terms are added in brackets. Answers to the questions are on page 630 after Answers to Exercises.

Disease Descriptions

1. **Candidiasis** [*Candida* is a yeast-like fungus]: This fungus is normally found on mucous membranes, skin, and vaginal mucosa. Under certain circumstances (excessive warmth; administration of birth control pills, antibiotics, and corticosteroids; debilitated states; infancy), it can change to a pathogen and cause localized or generalized mucocutaneous disease. Examples are paronychial lesions, lesions in areas of the body where rubbing opposed surfaces is common (groin, perianal, axillary, inframammary, and interdigital), thrush (white plaques attached to oral or vaginal mucous membranes), and vulvovaginitis.

2. **Cellulitis:** This is a common nonsuppurative infection of connective tissue with severe inflammation of the dermal and subcutaneous layers of the skin. Cellulitis appears on an extremity as a reddish-brown area of edematous skin. A surgical wound, puncture, skin ulcer, or patch of dermatitis is the usual means of entry for bacteria (most cases are caused by streptococci). Therapy entails rest, elevation, hot wet packs, and penicillin. Any cellulitis on the face should be given special attention because the infection may extend directly to the brain.

3. **Mycosis fungoides:** This is a rare, chronic skin condition caused by the infiltration of malignant lymphocytes. Contrary to its name (myc/o = fungus), it is not caused by a fungus but was formerly thought to be of fungal origin. It is characterized by generalized erythroderma and large, reddish, raised tumors that spread and ulcerate. In some cases, the malignant cells may involve lymph nodes and other organs. Treatment with topical nitrogen mustard and radiation can be effective in controlling the disease.

Write Up: Physical Examination of the Skin

A wide variety of lesions are seen on the face, shoulders, and back. The predominant lesions are pustules on an inflammatory base. Many pustules are confluent [running together] over the chin and forehead. Comedones are present on the face, especially along the nasolabial folds. Inflammatory papules are present on the lower cheeks and chin. Large abscesses and ulcerated cysts are present over the upper shoulder area. Numerous scars are present over the face and upper back.

Continued on following page

Questions on the Case Report

1. In this skin condition, the dominant damage to tissue involves:
   (A) discolored flat lesions
   (B) grooves or crack-like sores
   (C) small elevations containing pus

2. Comedones are:
   (A) sebum plugs partially blocking skin pores
   (B) contagious, infectious plugs of sebum
   (C) small, pinpoint hemorrhages

3. Papules are also known as:
   (A) purpura
   (B) pimples
   (C) freckles

4. In the scapular region, lesions are:
   (A) large pigmented areas
   (B) numerous collections of blisters
   (C) large collections of sacs containing pus with erosion of skin

5. A hypertrophied scar (cicatrix) is known also as a:
   (A) wheal
   (B) keloid
   (C) polyp

6. What is your diagnosis of this skin condition, based on the physical examination?
   (A) acne vulgaris
   (B) leukoplakia
   (C) scabies

IX. Exercises

Remember to check your answers carefully with those given in Section X, Answers to Exercises.

A. *Select from the following terms to complete the sentences below.*

dermis	sebum	cuticle
melanin	basal layer	stratum corneum
keratin	lunula	lipocyte
collagen		

1. A fat cell is a (an) _____.

2. The half-moon–shaped white area at the base of a nail is the _____.

3. A structural protein found in skin and connective tissue is _____.

4. A black pigment found in the epidermis is _____.

5. The deepest region of the epidermis is the _____.

6. The outermost layer of the epidermis, which consists of flattened, keratinized cells, is the

_____.

7. An oily substance secreted by sebaceous glands is _____.

8. The middle layer of the skin is the _____.

9. A hard, protein material found in epidermis, hair, and nails is _____.

10. A band of epidermis at the base and sides of the nail plate is the _____.

B. Complete the following terms based on their meanings as given below.

1. The outermost layer of skin: epi _____

2. Profuse sweating: dia _____

3. Excessive secretion from sebaceous glands: sebo _____

4. Inflammation and swelling of soft tissue around a nail: par _____

5. Fungal infections of hands and feet: dermato _____

6. Burning sensation (pain) in skin: caus _____

C. Match the term in column I with the descriptive meanings in column II. Write the letter of the answer in the space provided.

Column I

1. squamous epithelium _____

2. sebaceous gland _____

3. albinism _____

4. electrocautery _____

5. subcutaneous tissue _____

6. collagen _____

7. dermis _____

8. melanocyte _____

9. erythema _____

10. dermabrasion _____

Column II

A. middle, connective tissue layer of skin
B. surgical procedure to scrape away tissue
C. flat, scale-like cells
D. connective tissue protein
E. pigment deficiency of the skin
F. contains a dark pigment
G. widespread redness of skin
H. contains lipocytes
 I. oil-producing organ
 J. a knife is used to burn through tissue

D. Build medical terms based on the definitions and word parts given.

1. surgical repair of the skin: dermato _____

2. pertaining to under the skin: sub _____

3. abnormal condition of lack of sweat: an _____

4. abnormal condition of proliferation of horny, keratinized cells: kerat _____

5. abnormal condition of dry, scaly skin: _____osis

6. loosening of the epidermis: epidermo _____

7. yellow tumor (nodule under the skin): _____oma

8. pertaining to under the nail: sub _____

9. abnormal condition of fungus in the hair: _____mycosis

10. abnormal condition of nail fungus: onycho _____

E. Give the meanings for the following combining forms.

1. melan/o _____

2. adip/o _____

3. squam/o _____

4. xanth/o _____

5. myc/o _____

6. onych/o _____

7. pil/o _____

8. xer/o _____

9. steat/o _____

10. trich/o _____

11. erythem/o _____

12. albin/o _____

13. ichthy/o _____

14. hist/o _____

15. ungu/o _____

16. cauter/o _____

F. Match the cutaneous lesion with its meaning below.

polyp   wheal   macule
papule   ulcer   cyst
vesicle   fissure   nodule
pustule

1. circumscribed collection of clear fluid (blister) _____

2. smooth, slightly elevated edematous area _____

3. discolored, flat lesion (freckle) _____

4. a groove or crack-like sore _____

5. a mushroom-like growth extending from the surface of a mucous membrane _____

6. circumscribed collection of pus (small abscess) _____

7. a closed sac containing fluid or semisolid material _____

8. open sore or erosion of the skin _____

9. solid elevation of the skin (pimple) _____

10. larger than 1-cm, solid elevation of the skin _____

G. Give the medical terms for the following.

1. baldness _____

2. purplish, macular patch caused by hemorrhages into the skin _____

3. itching _____

4. acute allergic reaction in which red, round wheals develop on the skin _____

5. loss of pigment in areas of the skin _____

6. merging ecchymoses over the body _____

7. blackhead _____

8. small, pinpoint hemorrhages _____

H. Match the pathological skin condition with its description below.

impetigo   tinea   squamous cell carcinoma
psoriasis   scleroderma   acne vulgaris
gangrene   malignant melanoma   decubitus ulcer
eczema   basal cell carinoma   systemic lupus erythematosus

1. malignant neoplasm originating in scale-like cells of the epidermis _____

2. buildup of sebum and keratin in pores of the skin leading to papular and pustular eruptions

_____

3. fungal skin infection _____

4. chronic disease marked by hardening and shrinking of connective tissue in the skin

_____

5. bedsore _____

6. necrosis of skin tissue resulting from ischemia _____

7. chronic or acute inflammatory skin disease with erythematous, pustular, or papular lesions

_____

8. widespread inflammatory disease of the joints and collagen of the skin with "butterfly" rash on

the face _____

9. cancerous tumor composed of melanocytes _____

10. chronic, recurrent dermatosis marked by silvery-gray scales covering red patches on the skin

_____

11. malignant neoplasm originating in the basal layer of the epidermis _____

12. contagious, infectious pyoderma _____

I. Select the term that best fits the definition given.

1. contagious parasitic infection with intense pruritus: (scleroderma, scabies)

2. measles: (rubella, rubeola)

3. chickenpox: (varicella, eczema)

4. thickened cicatrix (scar): (tinea, keloid)

5. white patches on mucous membrane of tongue or cheek: (leukoplakia, albinism)

6. characterized by a rash: (gangrene, exanthematous)

7. thickening of epidermis related to sunlight exposure: (actinic keratosis, callus)

8. small, pinpoint hemorrhages: (psoriasis, petechiae)

9. large blisters: (bullae, purpura)

10. colored pigmentation of skin (mole): (nevus, verruca)

11. sac of fluid and hair over sacral region: (ecchymosis, pilonidal cyst)

12. acute allergic reaction in which hives develop: (vitiligo, urticaria)

J. Describe the following types of burns.

1. second-degree burn _____

2. first-degree burn _____

3. third-degree burn _____

K. Match the following medical terms with their more common meanings below.

pruritus   seborrheic dermatitis   alopecia
decubitus ulcer   comedones   vesicles
nevi   verrucae   tinea pedis
ecchymosis   urticaria   exanthem

1. blackheads _____   7. warts _____

2. moles _____   8. athlete's foot _____

3. baldness _____   9. "black-and-blue" mark _____

4. itching _____   10. dandruff _____

5. hives _____   11. blisters _____

6. bedsore _____   12. rash _____

L. What is wrong with the skin in the following conditions?

1. pyoderma _____

2. xeroderma _____

3. leukoderma _____

4. erythema _____

5. dermatomycosis _____

6. callus _____

7. keloid _____

8. purpura _____

9. telangiectasis _____

10. gangrene _____

M. Give short answers for the following.

1. Two skin tests for allergy are _____ and _____ .

2. The _____ test is an intradermal test for diphtheria.

3. The _____ test or _____ test is a test for tuberculosis.

4. Purulent means _____ .

5. A surgical procedure to core out a disc of skin for microscopic analysis is a (an) _____ .

6. The procedure in which thin layers of a malignant growth are removed and each is examined under the microscope is called _____ .

7. A type of skin cancer associated with AIDS and marked by dark blue-purple lesions over the skin is called _____ .

8. Moles that do not form properly and may progress to form melanomas are called _____ .

9. Removal of skin tissue using a cut parallel to the surface of the surrounding skin is called a (an) _____ .

10. Destruction of tissue by use of intensely cold temperatures is called _____ .

11. Scraping away skin to remove acne scars and fine wrinkles on the skin is called _____ .

12. Removal of subcutaneous fat tissue by aspiration is called _____ .

N. Circle the term that best completes the meaning of the sentence.

1. Since he'd been a teenager, Jim had had red, scaly patches on his elbows and the backs of his knees. Dr. Horn diagnosed Jim's dermatological condition as (**vitiligo, impetigo, psoriasis**) and prescribed a special cream.

2. Clarissa noticed a rash across the bridge of her nose and aching in her joints. She saw a rheumatologist who did some blood work and diagnosed her condition as (**rheumatoid arthritis, systemic lupus erythematosus, scleroderma**).

3. Bea had large, red patches all over her trunk and neck after eating shrimp. The doctor prescribed hydrocortisone cream to relieve her itching (**seborrhea, acne, urticaria**).

4. The poison ivy caused incredible (**pruritus, calluses, keratosis**) and Maggie was scratching her arms raw.

5. Kelly was fair-skinned with red hair. She had many benign nevi on her arms and legs, but Dr. Keefe was especially worried about one lesion with an irregular, raised border that he biopsied and found to be malignant (**melanoma, Kaposi sarcoma, pyoderma**).

X. Answers to Exercises

A

1. lipocyte	5. basal layer	9. keratin
2. lunula	6. stratum corneum	10. cuticle
3. collagen	7. sebum	
4. melanin	8. dermis	

B

1. epidermis	5. dermatophytosis
2. diaphoresis	or dermatomycosis (tinea)
3. seborrhea	6. causalgia
4. paronychia	

C

1. C	5. H	9. G
2. I	6. D	10. B
3. E	7. A	
4. J	8. F	

D

1. dermatoplasty	5. ichthyosis	9. trichomycosis
2. subcutaneous	6. epidermolysis	10. onychomycosis
3. anhidrosis	7. xanthoma	
4. keratosis	8. subungual	

E

1. black	7. hair	13. scaly, dry
2. fat	8. dry	14. tissue
3. scale-like	9. fat, sebum	15. nail
4. yellow	10. hair	16. heat, burn
5. fungus	11. redness	
6. nail	12. white	

Continued on following page

F

1. vesicle
2. wheal
3. macule
4. fissure
5. polyp
6. pustule
7. cyst
8. ulcer
9. papule
10. nodule

G

1. alopecia
2. ecchymosis
3. pruritus
4. urticaria
5. vitiligo
6. purpura
7. comedo
8. petechiae

H

1. squamous cell carcinoma
2. acne vulgaris
3. tinea
4. scleroderma
5. decubitus ulcer
6. gangrene
7. eczema
8. systemic lupus erythematosus
9. malignant melanoma
10. psoriasis
11. basal cell carcinoma
12. impetigo

I

1. scabies
2. rubeola
3. varicella
4. keloid
5. leukoplakia
6. exanthematous
7. actinic keratosis
8. petechiae
9. bullae
10. nevus
11. pilonidal cyst
12. urticaria

J

1. damage to the epidermis and dermis with blisters, erythema, and hyperesthesia
2. damage to the epidermis with erythema and hyperesthesia; no blisters
3. destruction of both epidermis and dermis and damage to subcutaneous layer

K

1. comedones
2. nevi
3. alopecia
4. pruritus
5. urticaria
6. decubitus ulcer
7. verrucae
8. tinea pedis
9. ecchymosis
10. seborrheic dermatitis
11. vesicles
12. exanthem

L

1. collections of pus in the skin
2. dry skin
3. white patches of skin (vitiligo)
4. redness of skin
5. abnormal condition of fungal infection in the skin
6. increased growth of epidermal horny-layer cells due to excess pressure or friction
7. thickened, hypertrophied scar tissue
8. merging ecchymoses (purple patches) under the skin
9. abnormal dilation (-ectasis) of tiny blood vessels (angi/o) under the skin (tel-means complete)
10. necrosis (death) of skin tissue

M

1. scratch; patch
2. Schick
3. Mantoux; PPD
4. pus-filled
5. punch biopsy
6. Mohs surgery
7. Kaposi sarcoma
8. dysplastic nevi
9. shave biopsy
10. cryosurgery
11. dermabrasion
12. liposuction

N

1. psoriasis
2. systemic lupus erythematosus
3. urticaria
4. pruritus
5. melanoma

Answers to Practical Applications

1. C
2. A
3. B
4. C
5. B
6. A

XI. Pronunciation of Terms

Pronunciation Guide

ā as in āpe   ă as in ăpple
ē as in ēven   ĕ as in ĕvery
ī as in īce   ĭ as in ĭnterest
ō as in ōpen   ŏ as in pŏt
ū as in ūnit   ŭ as in ŭnder

To test your understanding of the terminology in this chapter, write the meaning of each term in the space provided. In addition, you may wish to cover the terms and write them by looking at your definitions. Make sure your spelling is correct. The page number after each term indicates where it is defined or used in the text so you can easily check your responses.

Vocabulary, Combining Forms, and Suffixes

Term	Pronunciation	Meaning
adipose (608)	ĂD-ĭ-pōs	_____
albinism (608)	ĂL-bĭ-nĭzm	_____
albino (607)	ăl-BĪ-nō	_____
alopecia (613)	ăl-ō-PĒ-shē-ă	_____
anhidrosis (609)	ăn-hī-DRŌ-sĭs	_____
basal layer (607)	BĀ-săl LĀ-ĕr	_____
causalgia (609)	kăw-ZĂL-jă	_____
collagen (607)	KŎL-ă-jĕn	_____
cuticle (607)	KŪ-tĭ-k'l	_____
dermabrasion (609)	dĕrm-ă-BRĀ-zhŭn	_____
dermatologist (609)	dĕr-mă-TŎL-ō-jĭst	_____
dermatomycosis (610)	dĕr-mă-tō-mī-KŌ-sĭs	_____
dermatophytosis (610)	dĕr-mă-tō-fī-TŌ-sĭs	_____
dermatoplasty (609)	DĔR-mă-tō-plăs-tē	_____
dermis (607)	DĔR-mĭs	_____
diaphoresis (609)	dī-ă-fŏr-RĒ-sĭs	_____
electrocautery (609)	ĕ-lĕk-trō-KĂW-tĕr-ē	_____
epidermis (607)	ĕp-ĭ-DĔR-mĭs	_____
epidermolysis (609)	ĕp-ĭ-dĕr-MŎL-ĭ-sĭs	_____
epithelium (607)	ĕp-ĭ-THĒL-ē-ŭm	_____

erythema (609)	ĕr-ĭ-THĒ-mă	_____
erythematous (609)	ĕr-ĭ-THĒ-mă-tŭs	_____
hair follicle (607)	hār FŎL-ĭ-k'l	_____
ichthyosis (609)	ĭk-thē-Ō-sĭs	_____
integumentary system (607)	ĭn-tĕg-ū-MĔN-tăr-ē SĬS-tĕm	_____
keratin (607)	KĔR-ă-tĭn	_____
keratosis (610)	kĕr-ă-TŌ-sĭs	_____
leukoderma (611)	lū-kō-DĔR-mă	_____
leukoplakia (610)	lū-kō-PLĀ-kē-ă	_____
lipocyte (607)	LĬP-ō-sīt	_____
lipoma (610)	lī-PŌ-mă or lĭ-PŌ-mă	_____
liposuction (610)	lī-pō-SŬK-shun	_____
lunula (607)	LŪ-nū-lă	_____
melanin (607)	MĔL-ă-nĭn	_____
melanocyte (610)	mĕ-LĂN-ō-sīt	_____
melanoma (610)	mĕl-ă-NŌ-mă	_____
onycholysis (610)	ŏn-ĭ-kē-ŎL-ĭ-sĭs	_____
onychomycosis (610)	ŏn-ĭ-kō-mī-KŌ-sĭs	_____
paronychia (610)	păr-ō-NĬK-ē-ă	_____
pilosebaceous (611)	pī-lō-sĕ-BĀ-shŭs	_____
pyoderma (611)	pī-ō-DĔR-mă	_____
sebaceous gland (607)	sĕ-BĀ-shŭs glănd	_____
seborrhea (611)	sĕb-ō-RĒ-ă	_____
seborrheic dermatitis (611)	sĕb-ō-RĒ-ĭk dĕr-mă-TĪ-tĭs	_____
sebum (607)	SĒ-bŭm	_____
squamous epithelium (607)	SKWĀ-mŭs ĕp-ĭ-THĒ-lē-uˇm	_____
steatoma (611)	stē-ă-TŌ-mă	_____
stratified (607)	STRĂT-ĭ-fīd	_____

stratum (plural: strata) (608)	STRĂ-tŭm (STRă-tă)	_____
subcutaneous (609)	sŭb-kū-TĀ-nē-ŭs	_____
subungual (611)	sŭb-ŬNG-wăl	_____
trichomycosis (611)	trĭk-ō-mī-KŌ-sĭs	_____
xanthoma (611)	zăn-THŌ-mă	_____
xeroderma (611)	zē-rō-DĔR-mă	_____

Lesions, Symptoms, Abnormal Conditions, and Neoplasms; Laboratory Tests and Clinical Procedures

Term	Pronunciation	Meaning
acne (614)	ĂK-nē	_____
basal cell carcinoma (618)	BĀ-săl sĕl kăr-sĭ-NŌ-mă	_____
bulla (plural: bullae) (613)	BŬL-ă (BŬL-ē)	_____
callus (617)	KĂL-ŭs	_____
cicatrix (618)	SĬK-ă-trĭks	_____
comedo (plural: comedones) (614)	KŎM-ĕ-dō (kŏm-ĕ-DŌNZ)	_____
cyst (612)	sĭst	_____
decubitus ulcer (613)	dē-KŪ-bĭ-tŭs ŬL-sĕr	_____
ecchymosis (plural: ecchymoses) (614)	ĕk-ĭ-MŌ-sĭs (ĕk-ĭ-MŌ-sēz)	_____
eczema (616)	ĔK-zĕ-mă	_____
exanthematous viral disease (616)	ĕg-zăn-THĔM-ă-tŭs VĪ-răl dĭ-ZĒZ	_____
fissure (612)	FĬSH-ŭr	_____
fungal tests (620)	FŬNG-ăl tĕsts	_____
gangrene (616)	găng-GRĒN	_____
impetigo (616)	ĭm-pĕ-TĪ-gō	_____
Kaposi sarcoma (618)	KĂH-pō-sē săr-KŌ-mă	_____
keloid (618)	KĒ-lŏyd	_____

macule (612)	MĂK-ūl	
Mohs surgery (620)	mōz SŬR-jĕ-rē	
nevus (plural: nevi) (618)	NĒ-vŭs (NĒ-vī)	
papule (613)	PĂP-ūl	
petechia (plural: petechiae) (614)	pĕ-TĒ-kē-ă (pĕ-TĒ-kē-ī)	
pilonidal cyst (612)	pī-lō-NĪ-dăl sĭst	
polyp (613)	PŎL-ĭp	
pruritus (614)	pr͞oo-RĪ-tŭs	
psoriasis (616)	sō-RĪ-ă-sĭs	
purpura (614)	PĔR-pĕr-ă	
purulent (629)	PŪ-r͞oo-lĕnt	
pustule (613)	PŬS-tūl	
rubella (616)	r͞oo-BĔL-ă	
rubeola (616)	r͞oo-bē-Ō-lă	
scabies (616)	SKĀ-bēz	
scleroderma (617)	sklĕr-ō-DĔR-mă	
squamous cell carcinoma (619)	SKWĀ-mŭs sĕl kăr-sĭ-NŌ-mă	
systemic lupus erythematosus (617)	sĭs-TĔM-ĭk L͞OO-pŭs ĕr-ĭ-thē-mă-TŌ-sĭs	
tinea (617)	TĬN-ē-ă	
ulcer (613)	ŬL-sĕr	
urticaria (614)	ŭr-tĭ-KĀ-rē-ă	
varicella (616)	văr-ĭ-SĔL-ă	
verruca (plural: verrucae) (618)	vĕ-R͞OO-kă (vĕ-R͞OO-kē)	
vesicle (613)	VĔS-ĭ-k'l	
vitiligo (614)	vĭt-ĭl-Ī-gō	
wheal (613)	wēl	

XII. Review Sheet

Write the meanings of the word parts in the spaces provided and test yourself. Check your answers with the information in the chapter or in the glossary (Medical Terms—English) at the end of the book.

COMBINING FORMS

Combining Form	Meaning	Combining Form	Meaning
adip/o		lip/o	
albin/o		melan/o	
caus/o		myc/o	
cauter/o		onych/o	
cutane/o		phyt/o	
derm/o		pil/o	
dermat/o		py/o	
diaphor/o		seb/o	
erythem/o		sebace/o	
erythemat/o		squam/o	
hidr/o		steat/o	
hydr/o		trich/o	
ichthy/o		ungu/o	
kerat/o		xanth/o	
leuk/o		xer/o	

Continued on following page

SUFFIXES

Suffix	Meaning	Suffix	Meaning
-algia	_____	-osis	_____
-derma	_____	-ous	
-esis	_____	-plakia	_____
-lysis	_____	-plasty	_____
-ose	_____	-rrhea	_____

GIVE COMBINING FORMS FOR THE FOLLOWING (FIRST LETTERS ARE GIVEN).

fat	a_____	sweat	d_____
	l_____		h_____
	s_____	yellow	x_____
white	a_____	dry	x_____
	l_____	scaly, dry	i_____
skin	c_____	redness	e_____
	d_____		e_____
nail	o_____	hard, horny	k_____
	u_____	burn, burning	c_____
hair	p_____	black	m_____
	t_____	fungus	m_____
		plant	p_____

CHAPTER 17

Sense Organs: The Eye and the Ear

This chapter is divided into the following sections

In this chapter you will

- Identify locations and functions of the major parts of the eye and ear;
- Name the combining forms, prefixes, and suffixes most commonly used to describe these organs and their parts;
- Describe the pathological conditions that may affect the eye and ear;
- Identify clinical procedures that pertain to ophthalmology and otology; and
- Apply your new knowledge to understanding medical terms in their proper contexts, such as medical reports and records.

637

I. Introduction

In the previous chapter, we learned that the sensitive nerve endings in the dermis layer of the skin receive impulses from various stimuli applied to the external surfaces of the body. These nerve endings transmit electrical messages, initiated by the stimuli, to regions of the brain (cerebrum and thalamus) so that we can recognize sensations such as temperature, touch, pain, and pressure. In Chapter 10 (Nervous System), we learned that nerve cells that carry impulses from a sensory organ or sensory receptor area, such as the skin, taste buds, and **olfactory** regions (centers of smell in the nose), to the brain are called **afferent sensory neurons.**

The **eye** and the **ear** are sense organs, like the skin, taste buds, and olfactory regions. As such, they are receptors whose sensitive cells may be activated by a particular form of energy or stimulus in the external or internal environment. The sensitive cells in the eye and ear respond to the stimulus by initiating a series of nerve impulses along afferent sensory neurons that lead to the brain.

No matter what kind of stimulus is applied to a particular receptor, the sensation felt is determined by the regions in the brain that are connected to that receptor. Thus, mechanical injury that might stimulate receptor cells in the eye and ear would produce sensations of vision (flashes of light) and sound (ringing in the ears). Similarly, if one could make a nerve connection between the sensitive receptor cells of the ear and the area in the brain associated with sight, it would be possible to perceive, or "see," sounds.

Figure 17–1 recapitulates the general pattern of events when such stimuli as light and sound are applied to sense organs such as the eye and ear.

II. The Eye

A. Anatomy and Physiology

Label Figure 17–2 as you read the following:

Light rays enter the dark center of the eye, the **pupil** [1]. The **conjunctiva** [2] is a mucous membrane that lines the eyelids and coats the anterior portion of the eyeball over the white of the eye. The conjunctiva is clear and colorless except when blood vessels are dilated. Dust and smoke may cause the blood vessels to dilate and give the conjunctiva a reddish appearance, commonly known as bloodshot eyes.

Before entering the eye through the pupil, light must pass through the **cornea** [3]. The cornea is a fibrous, transparent tissue that extends over the pupil and colored portion of the eye. The function of the cornea is to bend, or **refract,** the rays of light, so that they are focused properly on the sensitive receptor cells in the posterior region of the eye. The cornea is avascular (has no blood vessels) but receives its nourishment from blood vessels near its junction with the white of the eye, the **sclera** [4]. Corneal

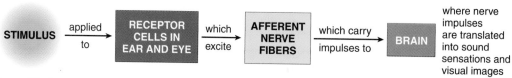

Figure 17–1

Pattern of events in the stimulation of a sense organ.

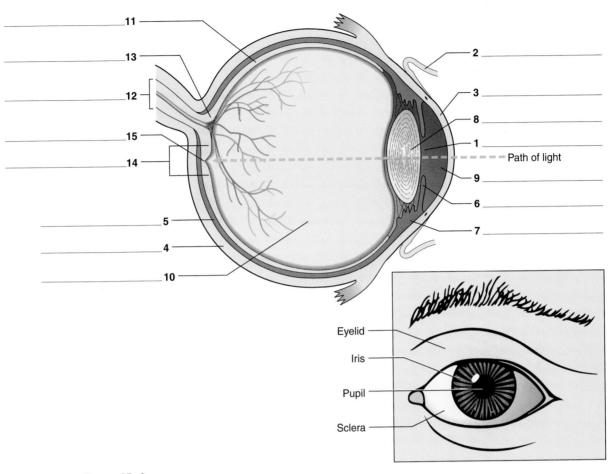

Path of light

Eyelid

Iris

Pupil

Sclera

Figure 17-2

The structure of the eye.

transplants for people with scarred or opaque corneas are successful because the cornea has no blood supply and antibodies responsible for rejection of foreign tissue do not reach it. The sclera is a tough, fibrous, supportive, connective tissue that extends from the cornea on the anterior surface of the eyeball to the optic nerve in the back of the eye.

The **choroid** [5] is a dark brown membrane inside the sclera. It contains many blood vessels that supply nutrients to the eye. The choroid is continuous with the pigment-containing **iris** [6] and the **ciliary body** [7] on the anterior surface of the eye.

The iris is the colored (it can appear blue, green, hazel, gray, or brown) portion of the eye that surrounds the pupil. Muscles of the iris constrict the pupil in bright light and dilate the pupil in dim light, thereby regulating the amount of light entering the eye. The inset in Figure 17–2 shows the iris and its relationship to the pupil.

The ciliary body, on each side of the **lens** [8], contains muscles that can adjust the shape and thickness of the lens. These changes in the shape of the lens aid in the **refraction** of light rays. The lens is thinned or flattened (for distant vision) and thickened (for close vision) by the muscles of the ciliary body. This refractive power of the lens is called **accommodation.**

Besides regulating the shape of the lens, the ciliary body also secretes a fluid called **aqueous humor,** which is found in the **anterior chamber** [9] of the eye. Aqueous

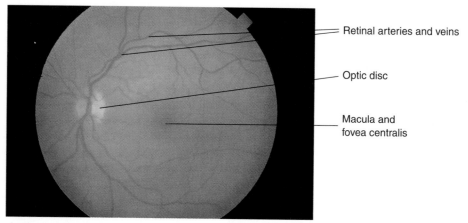

Figure 17-3

The posterior, inner part (fundus) of the eye, showing the retina as seen through an ophthalmoscope. (From Jarvis C: Physical Examination and Health Assessment, 2nd ed. Philadelphia, WB Saunders, 1996.)

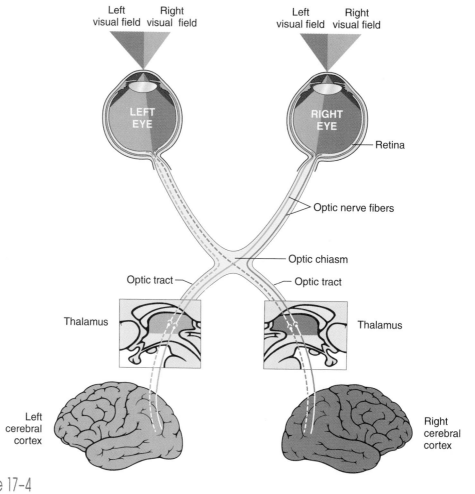

Figure 17-4

Visual pathway from the retina to the cerebral cortex (occipital lobe of the brain). Notice that one half of the visual field of each eye is projected to the other (contralateral) side of the brain.

humor maintains the shape of the anterior portion of the eye and nourishes the structures in that region. The fluid is constantly produced and leaves the eye through a canal that carries it into the bloodstream. Another cavity of the eye is the **vitreous chamber,** which is a large region behind the lens that is filled with a soft, jelly-like material, the **vitreous humor** [10]. Vitreous humor maintains the shape of the eyeball and is not constantly re-formed. Its escape from the eye can cause blindness. Both the aqueous and the vitreous humors function to further refract light rays.

The **retina** [11] is the thin, delicate, and sensitive nerve layer of the eye. As light energy, in the form of waves, travels through the eye, it is refracted (by the cornea, lens, and fluids), so that it focuses on sensitive receptor cells of the retina called the **rods** and **cones.** There are approximately 6.5 million cones and 120 million rods in the retina. The cones function in bright levels of light and are responsible for color and central vision. There are three types of cones, each type stimulated by one of the primary colors in light (red, green, or violet). Most cases of color blindness affect either the green or the red receptors, so that the two colors cannot be distinguished from each other. Rods function at reduced levels of light and are responsible for peripheral vision.

Light energy, when focused on the retina, causes a chemical change in the rods and cones, initiating nerve impulses that then travel from the eye to the brain via the **optic nerve** [12]. The region in the eye where the optic nerve meets the retina is called the **optic disc** [13]. Because there are no light receptor cells in the optic disc, it is known as the blind spot of the eye. The **macula** [14] is a small, oval, yellowish area to the side of the optic disc. It contains a central depression called the **fovea centralis** [15] that is composed largely of cones and is the location of the sharpest vision in the eye. If a portion of the fovea or macula is damaged, vision is reduced and central-vision blindness occurs. Figure 17–3 shows the retina of a normal eye as seen through an ophthalmoscope. The **fundus** of the eye is this posterior, inner part that is visualized through the ophthalmoscope.

Figure 17–4 illustrates the pathway of the light-stimulated nervous impulse from the sensitive cells of the retina to the visual region of the cerebral cortex in the brain. The rods and cones in the **retina** synapse (meet) with neurons that lead to the **optic nerve fibers.** As the optic nerve fibers travel into the brain, the fibers located more medially cross in an area called the **optic chiasm.** Nerve fibers from the right half of each retina (the purple lines in the figure) now form an **optic tract,** synapsing in the **thalamus** of the brain and ending in the right visual region of the **cerebral cortex.** Similarly, fibers from the left half of each retina (the orange lines in the figure) merge to form the optic tract and pass from the thalamus to the left region of the **cerebral cortex.** In the visual area of the cerebral cortex (the occipital lobe of the brain) the images (one from each eye) are fused, and a single visual sensation with a three-dimensional effect is experienced. This is called **binocular vision.**

Damage to nerve cells in the **right cerebral cortex** (such as that caused by a stroke) causes loss of vision in the left visual field. Similarly, damage in the **left cerebral cortex** causes loss of vision in the right visual field. This loss of vision in the contralateral (opposite side) visual field is called **hemianopsia** (**hemi-** means half, **an-** means without, **-opsia** means vision).

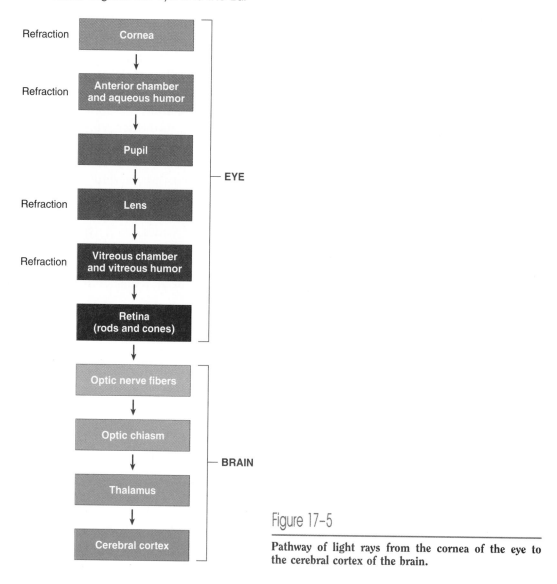

Figure 17-5

Pathway of light rays from the cornea of the eye to the cerebral cortex of the brain.

Figure 17-5 summarizes the pathway of light rays from the cornea to the inner visual region in the cerebral cortex of the brain.

B. Vocabulary

This list will help you review many of the new items introduced in the text. Short definitions will reinforce your understanding of the terms. See Section VII of this chapter for help in pronouncing the more difficult terms.

accommodation	The normal adjustment of the eye for seeing objects at various distances. The lens is made thinner or fatter by the ciliary body to bring an object into focus on the retina.
anterior chamber	The area behind the cornea and in front of the lens and iris. It contains aqueous humor.

aqueous humor Fluid produced by the ciliary body and found in the anterior and posterior chambers.

biconvex Having two sides that are rounded, elevated, and curved evenly, like part of a sphere. The lens of the eye is a biconvex body.

choroid layer The middle, vascular layer of the eye, between the retina and the sclera.

ciliary body The structure on each side of the lens that connects the choroid and the iris. It contains ciliary muscles, which control the shape of the lens, and it secretes aqueous humor.

cones Photosensitive receptor cells in the retina that transform light energy into a nerve impulse. Cones are responsible for color and central vision.

conjunctiva A delicate membrane lining the eyelids and covering the anterior eyeball.

cornea Fibrous transparent layer of clear tissue that extends over the anterior portion of the eyeball.

fovea centralis The tiny pit or depression in the retina that is the region of clearest vision.

fundus of the eye The posterior, inner part of the eye.

iris The colored portion of the eye.

lens A transparent, biconvex body behind the pupil of the eye. It bends light rays to bring them into focus on the retina.

macula A yellowish region on the retina lateral to and slightly below the optic disc; contains the fovea centralis.

optic chiasm The point at which the fibers of the optic nerve cross in the brain (**chiasm** means crossing).

optic disc (disk) The region at the back of the eye where the optic nerve meets the retina. It is the blind spot of the eye because it contains only nerve fibers and no rods or cones and is thus insensitive to light.

optic nerve The cranial nerve that carries impulses from the retina to the brain (cerebral cortex).

pupil The dark opening of the eye, surrounded by the iris, through which light rays pass.

refraction The bending of light rays by the cornea, lens, and fluids of the eye to bring the rays into focus on the retina. **Refract** means to break (-fract) back (re-).

retina	The light-sensitive nerve cell layer of the eye that contains receptor cells called rods and cones.
rods	Photosensitive receptor cells of the retina that are essential for vision in dim light and for peripheral vision.
sclera	The tough, white, outer coat of the eyeball.
vitreous humor	Soft, jelly-like material behind the lens; helps to maintain the shape of the eyeball.

C. Combining Forms, Suffixes, and Terminology: Structures and Fluids; Conditions

Write the meanings of the medical terms in the spaces provided.

STRUCTURES AND FLUIDS
Combining Forms

Combining Form	Meaning	Terminology	Meaning
aque/o	water	aqueous humor _____	
blephar/o	eyelid (see also **palpebr/o**)	blepharitis _____	
		blepharoptosis _____	
		blef-ă-rŏp-TŌ-sis. Also called ptosis. This condition may be caused by abnormalities of the eyelid muscle or by nerve damage.	
conjunctiv/o	conjunctiva	conjunctivitis _____	
		Commonly called pinkeye.	
cor/o	pupil (see also **pupill/o**)	anisocoria _____	
		anis/o means unequal. Anisocoria may be an indication of neurological injury or disease.	
corne/o	cornea (see also **kerat/o**)	corneal ulcer _____	
		From the Latin corneus meaning horny. Perhaps, as it protrudes outward, the cornea was thought to resemble the bud of a growing horn.	
cycl/o	ciliary body or muscle of the eye	cycloplegic _____	

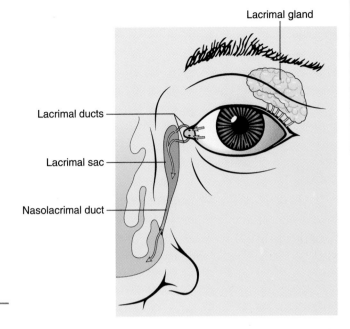

Figure 17-6

Lacrimal (tear) gland and ducts.

dacry/o	tears, tear duct (see also **lacrim/o**)	dacryoadenitis _____ *Figure 17-6 shows the lacrimal gland and lacrimal ducts.*
ir/o **irid/o**	iris (colored portion of the eye around the pupil)	iritis _____ iridic _____ iridectomy _____
kerat/o	cornea	keratitis _____ keratotomy _____ *In radial keratotomy, slit-like cuts are made in the cornea to flatten it for a correction of myopia (near-sightedness).*
lacrim/o	tears	lacrimal _____ lacrimation _____
ocul/o	eye	intraocular _____
ophthalm/o	eye	ophthalmologist _____ *A medical doctor who specializes in treating disorders of the eye.* ophthalmic _____ ophthalmoplegia _____

opt/o   eye, vision   optic _____
optic/o

                                        optometrist _____

                                        A nonmedical person who can examine eyes to determine vision
                                        problems and prescribe lenses (doctor of optometry; OD).

                                        optician _____

                                        A nonmedical person who grinds lenses and fits glasses but
                                        cannot prescribe lenses.

palpebr/o   eyelid   palpebral _____

papill/o   optic disc (disk);   papilledema _____
                   nipple-like
                                        -edema means swelling. This condition is associated with
                                        increased intracranial pressure and hyperemia (increased blood
                                        flow) in the region of the optic disc.

phac/o   lens of the eye   phacoemulsification _____
phak/o
                                        This is a technique of cataract extraction using ultrasonic
                                        vibrations to fragment (emulsify) the lens and aspirate it out of
                                        the eye.

                                        aphakia _____

                                        This may be congenital, but most often it is the result of
                                        extraction of a cataract (clouded lens).

pupill/o   pupil   pupillary _____

retin/o   retina   retinitis _____

                                        Retinitis pigmentosa *is a genetic disorder (pigmented scar forms*
                                        on the retina) that destroys retinal rods. Decreased vision and
                                        night blindness (nyctalopia) occur.

                                        hypertensive retinopathy _____

                                        Lesions, such as narrowed arterioles, microaneurysms,
                                        hemorrhages, and exudates (fluid leakage) are found on
                                        examination of the fundus.

scler/o   sclera (white of   corneoscleral _____
                   the eye)
                                        scleritis _____

uve/o   uvea; vascular   uveitis _____
                   layer of the eye
                   (iris, ciliary body,
                   and choroid)

vitre/o   glassy   vitreous humor _____

CONDITIONS
Combining Forms

Combining Form	Meaning	Terminology	Meaning
ambly/o	dull, dim	amblyopia	

-opia means vision. Amblyopia is a partial loss of sight and is also known as lazy eye. This is because it is associated with failure of the eyes to work together to focus on the same point.

dipl/o	double	diplopia	
glauc/o	gray	glaucoma	

-oma here means mass or collection of fluid (aqueous humor). The term comes from the dull gray-green gleam of the affected eye in advanced cases. See page 650, Section II (E), Pathological Conditions.

mi/o	smaller, less	miosis	

Contraction of the pupil. A **miotic** *is a drug (such as pilocarpine) that causes the pupil to contract.*

mydr/o	widen, enlarge	mydriasis	

Enlargement of pupils. Atropine and cocaine cause dilation, or enlargement, of pupils.

nyct/o	night	nyctalopia	

-opia means vision; -al comes from ala meaning blindness. Night blindness is poor vision at night, but good vision on bright days. Deficiency of vitamin A leads to nyctalopia.

phot/o	light	photophobia	

Sensitivity to light.

presby/o	old age	presbyopia	

See page 649, Section II (D), Errors of Refraction.

scot/o	darkness	scotoma	

An area of depressed vision surrounded by an area of normal vision; a blind spot. This can result from damage to the retina or the optic nerve.

xer/o	dry	xerophthalmia	

Suffixes			
Suffix	**Meaning**	**Terminology**	**Meaning**
-opia	vision	hyperopia _____	
		Hypermetropia (farsightedness). See Section II (D), Errors of Refraction.	
-opsia	vision	hemianopsia _____	
		Absence of vision in half of the visual field (space of vision of each eye). Stroke victims frequently have damage to the brain on one side of the visual cortex and experience hemianopsia (the visual loss is in the right or left visual field of both eyes).	
-tropia	to turn	esotropia _____	
		Inward (eso-) turning of an eye. **Exotropia** *is an outward turning of an eye. These are examples of* **strabismus** *(defect in eye muscles so that both eyes cannot be focused on the same point at the same time).*	

D. Errors of Refraction

astigmatism

Defective curvature of the cornea or lens of the eye.

This problem results from one or more abnormal curvatures of the cornea or lens. This causes light rays to be unevenly and not sharply focused on the retina, so that the image is distorted. A cylindrical lens placed in the proper position in front of the eye can correct this problem (Fig. 17–7A).

hyperopia (hypermetropia)

Farsightedness.

As Figure 17–7B illustrates, the eyeball in this condition is too short or the refractive power of the lens is too weak. Parallel rays of light tend to focus behind the retina, and this results in a blurred image. A convex lens (thicker in the middle than at the sides) bends the rays inward before they reach the cornea, and thus the rays can be focused properly on the retina.

myopia

Nearsightedness.

In myopia (**my-** comes from Greek *myein* meaning to shut, referring to the observation that myopic persons usually peer through half-closed eyelids), the eyeball is too long or the refractive power of the lens so strong that light rays do not properly focus on the retina. The image perceived is blurred because the light rays are focused in front of the retina. Concave glasses (thicker at the periphery than in the middle) correct this condition because the lenses spread the rays out before they reach the cornea, and thus they can be properly focused directly on the retina (Fig. 17–7C).

presbyopia

Impairment of vision due to old age.

With increasing age, loss of elasticity of the ciliary body impairs its ability to adjust the lens for accommodation to near vision. The lens of the eye cannot become fat to bend the rays coming from near objects (less than 20 feet). The light rays focus behind the retina, as in hyperopia. Therefore, a convex lens is needed to refract the rays coming from objects closer than 20 feet.

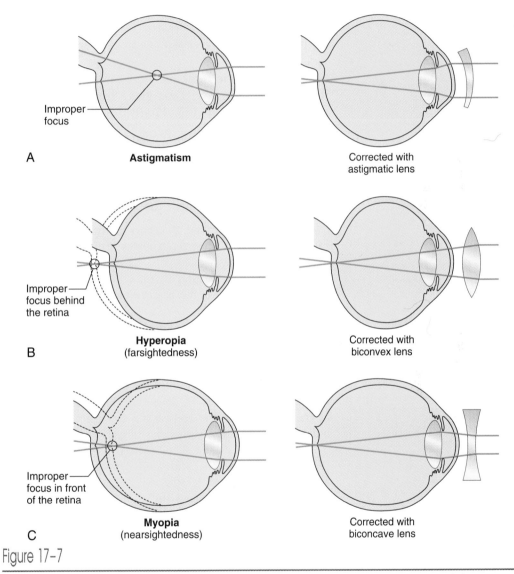

A   **Astigmatism**

Improper focus

Corrected with astigmatic lens

Improper focus behind the retina

B   **Hyperopia** (farsightedness)

Corrected with biconvex lens

Improper focus in front of the retina

C   **Myopia** (nearsightedness)

Corrected with biconcave lens

Figure 17-7

Errors of refraction. (A) Astigmatism and its correction. **(B)** Hyperopia and its correction. **(C)** Myopia and its correction. Dashed lines in B and C indicate the contour and size of the normal eye.

E. Pathological Conditions

cataract

Clouding of the lens, causing decreased vision (Fig. 17–8).

A cataract is a type of degenerative eye disease (protein in the lens aggregates and clouds vision) and is linked to the process of aging (senile cataracts). Some cataracts, however, are present at birth, and others occur with diabetes mellitus, ocular trauma, and prolonged high-dose corticosteroid administration. Vision appears blurred as the lens clouds over and becomes opaque. Lens cloudiness can be seen with an ophthalmoscope or the naked eye. Surgical removal of the lens and implantation of an artificial lens behind the iris are treatments for cataracts. If an intraocular lens cannot be inserted, the patient may wear eyeglasses or contact lenses to help refraction.

chalazion

Small, hard, cystic mass on the eyelid; formed as a result of chronic inflammation of a sebaceous gland (meibomian gland) along the margin of the eyelid (Fig. 17–9).

Chalazions (kă-LĀ-zē-ŏnz) often require incision and drainage.

diabetic retinopathy

Retinal effects of diabetes mellitus include microaneurysms, hemorrhages, dilation of retinal veins, and neovascularization (new blood vessels forming near the optic disc).

Edema (macular edema) occurs as fluid leaks from blood vessels into the retina and vision is blurred. **Exudates** (fluid leaking from the blood) appear in the retina as yellow-white spots. Laser photocoagulation and vitrectomy (see pages 654 and 656, Section II [F], Clinical Procedures) are helpful to patients in whom hemorrhaging has been severe.

glaucoma

Increased intraocular pressure results in damage to the retina and optic nerve.

Intraocular pressure is elevated because of the inability of aqueous humor to drain from the eye and enter the bloodstream. Normally, aqueous humor is formed by the ciliary body, flows into the anterior chamber, and leaves the eye at the angle where the cornea and iris meet. If fluid cannot leave, pressure builds up in the anterior chamber (Fig. 17–10).

Glaucoma is diagnosed by means of **tonometry** (see page 655, Section II [F], Clinical Procedures), with an instrument applied externally to the eye after administration of local anesthetic.

Administration of drugs (miotics) to lower intraocular pressure may prove effective in controlling the condition. Sometimes, laser therapy is used to tighten fibers in the ciliary body or to create a hole in the periphery of the iris, which allows aqueous humor to flow more easily to the anterior chamber and thus reduces intraocular pressure.

hordeolum (stye)

A localized, purulent, inflammatory staphylococcal infection of a sebaceous gland in the eyelid.

Hot compresses may help localize the infection and promote drainage. In some cases, surgical incision may be necessary. **Hordeolum** (hŏr-DĒ-ō-lŭm) means barley corn.

Figure 17-8

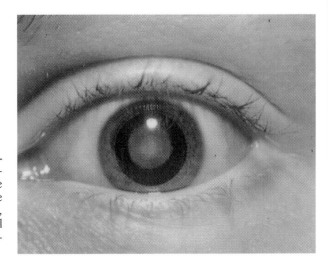

Cataract. The lens appears cloudy. (Courtesy of Ophthalmic Photography at the University of Michigan, W.K. Kellogg Eye Center, Ann Arbor, MI. From Black JM, Matassarin-Jacobs E: Medical-Surgical Nursing, 5th ed. Philadelphia, WB Saunders, 1997.)

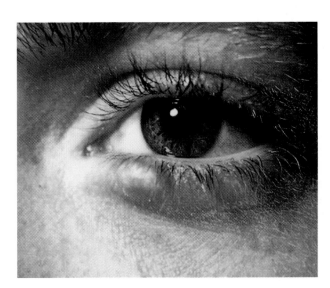

Figure 17-9

Chalazion. (Courtesy of Ophthalmic Photography at the University of Michigan, W.K. Kellogg Eye Center, Ann Arbor, MI. From Black JM, Matassarin-Jacobs E: Medical-Surgical Nursing, 5th ed. Philadelphia, WB Saunders, 1997.)

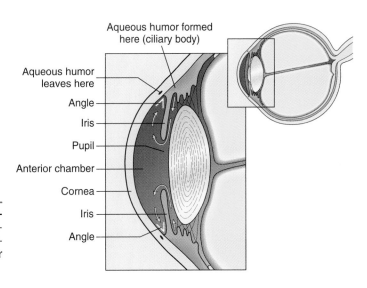

Figure 17-10

Glaucoma and circulation of aqueous humor. Circulation is impaired in glaucoma, so that aqueous fluid builds up in the anterior chamber.

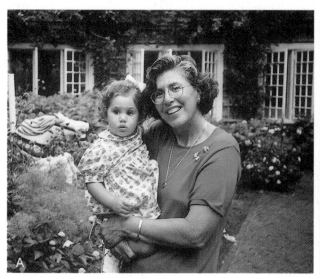
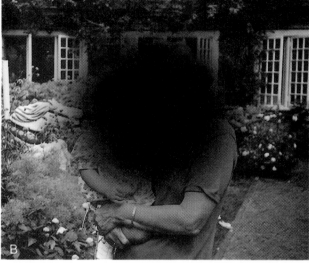

Figure 17-11

(A) Picture as seen with **normal vision. (B)** The same scene as it would appear to someone with **macular degeneration.** (Photograph shows the author with her granddaughter, Beatrix Bess (Bebe) Thompson, August 1999.)

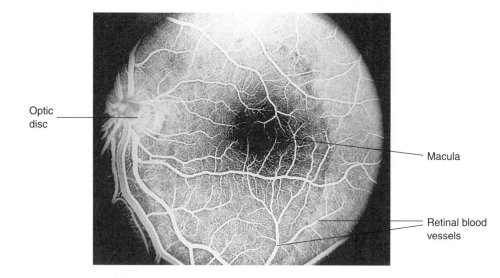

Optic disc

Macula

Retinal blood vessels

Figure 17-12

A normal fluorescein angiogram. (From Black JM, Matassarin-Jacobs E: Medical-Surgical Nursing, 5th ed. Philadelphia, WB Saunders, 1997.)

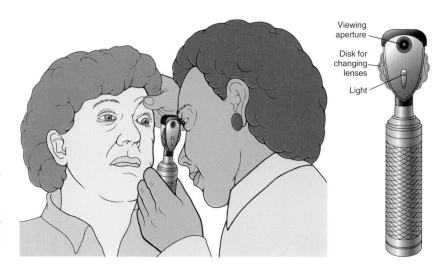

Viewing aperture

Disk for changing lenses

Light

Figure 17-13

Ophthalmoscopy. In addition to examining the cornea, lens, and vitreous humor for opacities (cloudiness), the examiner can see the blood vessels at the back of the eye (fundus) and note degenerative changes in the retina.

macular degeneration (age-related)	**Progressive damage to the macula of the retina.**

Age-related macular degeneration (ARMD) is one of the leading causes of blindness in the elderly. It causes severe loss of central vision (Fig. 17–11). Peripheral vision (using the part of the retina that is outside the macula region) is retained.

There are two forms of ARMD. The "dry" form (affecting about 85 per cent of patients) is marked by atrophy and degeneration of retinal cells. The "wet" form results from development of new (neovascular) and leaky (exudative) blood vessels close to the macula.

Early cases are often treated with lasers that may have the unfortunate side effect of destroying normal retinal cells as well as the damaged areas beneath them. Radiation therapy for the "wet" form is an experimental treatment. |
| **retinal detachment** | **Two layers of the retina separate from each other.**

Trauma to the eye, head injuries, bleeding, scarring from infection, or shrinkage of the vitreous humor can produce holes or tears in the retina and result in the separation of layers. Patients often see flashes of light and then later notice a shadow or "curtain" falling across the field of vision. Floaters are black spots indicating that bleeding has occurred as a result of detachment.

Photocoagulation (making pinpoint burns to form scar tissue and seal holes) and cryotherapy (creating a "freezer burn" that forms a scar and knits a tear together) are used to repair retinal tears. A **scleral buckle** (see page 656, Section II [F], Clinical Procedures) made of silicone may be sutured to the sclera directly over the detached portion of the retina to push the two retinal layers together. |
| **strabismus** | **Abnormal deviation of the eye.**

A failure of the eyes to look in the same direction because of weakness of a muscle controlling the position of one eye. Different forms of strabismus include **esotropia** (one eye turns inward; cross-eyed), **exotropia** (one eye turns outward; wall-eyed), and **hypertropia** (upward deviation of one eye). Treatment includes medications in the form of eyedrops, corrective lenses, eye exercises and patching of the normal eye, or surgery to restore muscle balance.

In children, strabismus may lead to **diplopia** and possibly **amblyopia** (partial loss of vision or lazy eye). Amblyopia is reversible until the retina is fully developed at about 7 years of age. |

F. Clinical Procedures

Diagnostic

fluorescein angiography	Fluorescein (a dye) is injected intravenously, and movement of blood is then observed by ophthalmoscopy to detect diabetic or hypertensive retinopathy and lesions in the macular area of the retina (Fig. 17–12).
ophthalmoscopy	This is a visual examination of the interior of the eye. The pupil is dilated so that the physician can see lesions of the cornea, lens, and retina (Fig. 17–13).

slit lamp ocular examination

The slit lamp (Fig. 17–14) is an instrument that permits examination of anterior ocular structures under microscopic magnification. Fluorescein dye is used to highlight corneal irregularities. Devices attached to a slit lamp expand the scope of the examination. For example, a **tonometer** (ton/o = tension) measures intraocular pressure, and a **gonioscope** (goni/o = angle) visualizes the anterior chamber angle (see Fig. 17–14).

visual acuity (clearness) test

A test of clarity of vision. The patient reads a chart (the standard is the Snellen eye chart) that contains black letters of gradually decreasing size (Fig. 17–15A). The chart is placed at a distance of 20 feet. Visual acuity is expressed as a ratio, such as 20/20. The first number is the distance the patient is standing from the chart. The second number is the distance at which a person with normal vision could have read the same line of the chart. If the best a person can see is the 20/200 line, this means that at 20 feet the patient can see what a person with normal vision can see at 200 feet.

visual field examination

This test measures the area within which objects may be seen when the eye is fixed, looking straight ahead without moving the head (Fig. 17–15B).

Treatment

cataract surgery

There are two general methods of removing a cataract: intracapsular and extracapsular. **Intracapsular extraction** is removal of the entire lens, including its capsule. **Extracapsular extraction** involves removal of most lens tissue, but the back part of the lens capsule is left in place. This can be performed by **aspiration-irrigation** (a hollow needle withdraws the lens material, and the anterior chamber of the eye is washed out) and **phacoemulsification** (ultrasonic vibration is used to break up portions of the lens, so that it can be aspirated through the ultrasonic probe). Some patients develop clouding of the back part of the lens capsule after extracapsular extraction and may need further treatment with an ophthalmic laser (neodymium-YAG or "cold" laser).

In most patients, an intraocular lens (IOL) is implanted at the same time the defective lens is removed.

enucleation

Removal of the entire eyeball. This surgery is necessary to treat tumors such as ocular melanoma (a malignant tumor arising from pigmented cells in the choroid layer of the eye).

keratoplasty

This procedure, also called **corneal transplant,** involves replacement of a section of a scarred or opaque cornea with normal, transparent cornea in an effort to restore vision (Fig. 17–16).

laser photocoagulation

Argon laser (high-energy light) beams are used to stimulate coagulation of tissue (blood vessels) in the interior of the eye. Photocoagulation is useful to treat diabetic retinopathy and age-related macular degeneration (blood vessels are sealed to prevent leakage, or abnormal growth of blood vessels is prevented). Laser is an acronym for light amplification by stimulated emission of radiation.

Figure 17–14

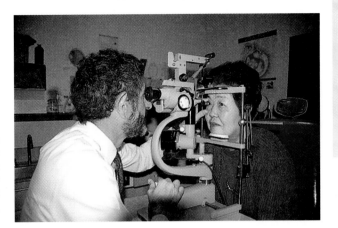

Slit-lamp examination measuring intraocular pressure by tonometry. (From Lewis SM, Collier IC, Heitkemper MM: Medical-Surgical Nursing: Assessment and Management of Clinical Problems, 4th ed. St. Louis, Mosby, 1996.)

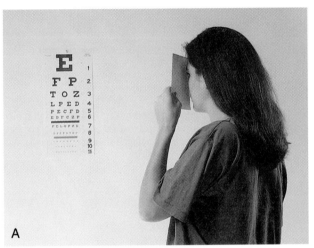

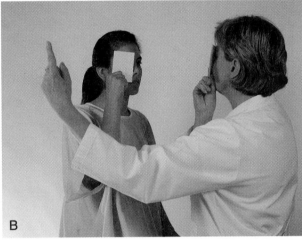

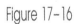

Figure 17–15

(A) The Snellen chart assesses visual acuity. **(B) Visual fields** are examined by comparing the patient's field of vision with that of the examiner's (assuming the examiner's is normal). (From Jarvis C: Physical Examination and Health Assessment, 2nd ed. Philadelphia, WB Saunders, 1996.)

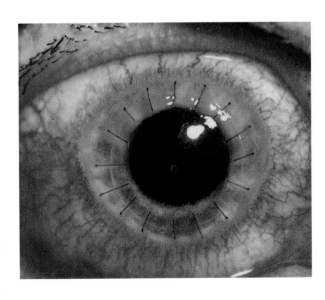

Figure 17–16

Clinical appearance of the eye after keratoplasty. (Courtesy of Ophthalmic Photography at the University of Michigan, W.K. Kellogg Eye Center, Ann Arbor, MI; from Black JM, Matassarin-Jacobs E: Medical-Surgical Nursing: Clinical Management for Continuity of Care, 5th ed. Philadelphia, WB Saunders, 1997.)

LASIK
This is a method of correcting myopia by using an eximer laser to remove corneal tissue (by sculpting it). The top layer of the cornea is lifted (a flap is made) and then a laser is used to sculpt the cornea. Once the refractive ablation is complete, the corneal flap is repositioned.

scleral buckle
Suture of a silicone band to the sclera directly over a detached portion of the retina. The band pushes the two parts of the retina against each other to bring together the two layers of a detached retina.

vitrectomy
Removal of the vitreous humor and its replacement with a clear solution. This is necessary when blood and scar tissue accumulate in the vitreous humor (a complication of diabetic retinopathy).

G. Abbreviations

ARMD	Age-related macular degeneration	**OU**	each eye (Latin, *oculus uterque*)
IOL	intraocular lens	**PERRLA**	pupils equal, round, reactive to light and accommodation
IOP	intraocular pressure		
LASIK	laser *in situ* keratomileusis	**PRK**	photorefractive keratectomy; a laser is used to reshape the cornea and correct errors of refraction such as myopia and astigmatism
OD	right eye (Latin, *oculus dexter*); doctor of optometry (optometrist)		
		VA	visual acuity
OS	left eye (Latin, *oculus sinister*)	**VF**	visual field

III. The Ear

A. Anatomy and Physiology

Sound waves are received by the outer ear, conducted to special receptor cells within the ear, and transmitted by those cells to nerve fibers that lead to the auditory region of the brain in the cerebral cortex. It is within the nerve fibers of the cerebral cortex that the sensations of sound are perceived.

Label Figure 17–17 as you read the following paragraphs describing the anatomy and physiology of the ear.

The ear can be divided into three separate regions—outer ear, middle ear, and inner ear. The outer and middle ears function in the conduction of sound waves through the ear, and the inner ear contains structures that receive the auditory waves and relay them to the brain.

Outer Ear

Sound waves enter the ear through the **pinna,** also called the **auricle** [1], which is the projecting part, or flap, of the ear. The **external auditory meatus (auditory canal)** [2] leads from the pinna and is lined with numerous glands that secrete a yellowish-brown, waxy substance called **cerumen.** Cerumen lubricates and protects the ear.

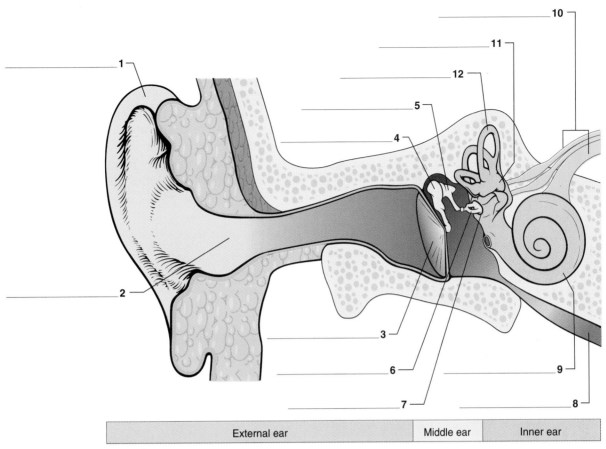

| External ear | Middle ear | Inner ear |

Figure 17-17

Anatomy of the ear.

Middle Ear

Sound waves travel through the auditory canal and strike a membrane between the outer and the middle ear. This is the **tympanic membrane,** or **eardrum** [3]. As the eardrum vibrates, it moves three small bones, or **ossicles,** that conduct the sound waves through the middle ear. These bones, in the order of their vibration, are the **malleus** [4], the **incus** [5], and the **stapes** [6]. As the stapes moves, it touches a membrane called the **oval window** [7], which separates the middle from the inner ear.

Before proceeding with the pathway of sound conduction and reception into the inner ear, an additional structure that affects the middle ear should be mentioned. The **auditory** or **eustachian tube** [8] is a canal leading from the middle ear to the pharynx. It is normally closed but opens upon swallowing. In an efficient way, this tube can prevent damage to the eardrum and shock to the middle and inner ears. Normally the pressure of air in the middle ear is equal to the pressure of air in the external environment. However, if you ascend in the atmosphere, as in flying in an airplane, climbing a high mountain, or riding a fast elevator, the atmospheric pressure, and that in the outer ear, drops, while the pressure in the middle ear remains the same—greater than that in the outer ear. This inequality of air pressure on the inside and outside of the eardrum forces the eardrum to bulge outward and eventually to burst. Swallowing opens the eustachian tube so that air can leave the middle ear and enter the throat until the atmospheric and middle ear pressures are balanced. The eardrum then relaxes, and the danger of its bursting is averted.

Inner Ear

Sound vibrations, having been transmitted by the movement of the eardrum to the bones of the middle ear, reach the inner ear via the fluctuations of the oval window that separates the middle and inner ears. The inner ear is also called the **labyrinth** because of its circular, maze-like structure. The part of the labyrinth that leads from the oval window is a bony, snail-shaped structure called the **cochlea** [9]. The cochlea contains special auditory liquids called **perilymph** and **endolymph** through which the vibrations travel. Also present in the cochlea is a sensitive auditory receptor area called the **organ of Corti.** In the organ of Corti, tiny hair cells receive vibrations from the auditory liquids and relay the sound waves to **auditory nerve fibers** [10], which end in the auditory center of the cerebral cortex, where these impulses are interpreted and "heard."

Study Figure 17–18, which is a schematic representation of the pathway of sound vibrations from the outer ear to the brain.

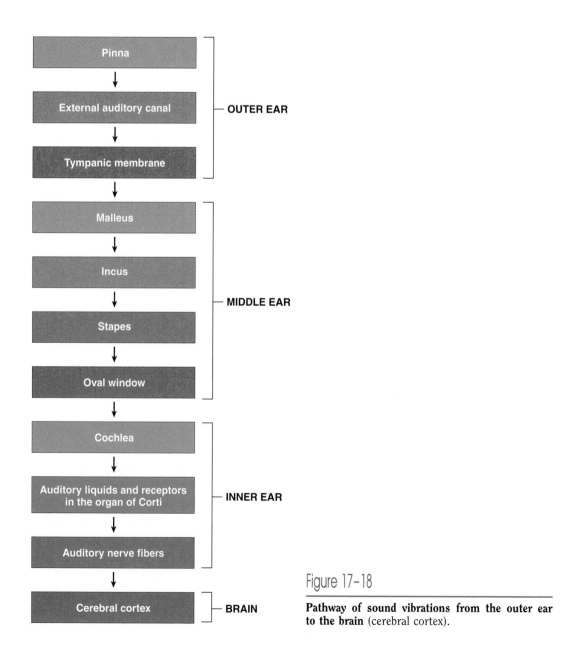

Figure 17-18

Pathway of sound vibrations from the outer ear to the brain (cerebral cortex).

The ear is an important organ of equilibrium (balance), as well as an organ for hearing. Refer back to Figure 17–17. The **vestibule** [11] connects the cochlea (for hearing) to three **semicircular canals** [12] for balance. The semicircular canals (containing two membranous sacs called the saccule and utricle) contain a fluid, endolymph, as well as sensitive hair cells. In an intricate manner, the fluid and hair cells fluctuate in response to the movement of the head. This sets up impulses in nerve fibers that lead to the brain. Messages are then sent to muscles in all parts of the body to assure that equilibrium is maintained.

B. Vocabulary

This list will help you review many of the new terms introduced in the text. Short definitions will reinforce your understanding of the terms. See Section VII of this chapter for help in pronouncing the more difficult terms.

auditory canal	The channel that leads from the pinna to the eardrum.
auditory meatus	Auditory canal.
auditory nerve fibers	These nerves carry impulses from the inner ear to the brain (cerebral cortex). This is the vestibulocochlear nerve (cranial nerve VIII).
auditory tube	Channel between the middle ear and the nasopharynx; **eustachian tube.**
auricle	The flap of the ear; the protruding part of the external ear, or **pinna.**
cerumen	A waxy substance secreted by the external ear; also called **ear wax.**
cochlea	A snail-shaped, spirally wound tube in the inner ear; contains hearing-sensitive receptor cells.
endolymph	Fluid within the labyrinth of the inner ear.
eustachian tube	Auditory tube.
incus	The second ossicle (bone) of the middle ear; incus means **anvil.**
labyrinth	The maze-like series of canals of the inner ear. This includes the cochlea, vestibule, and semicircular canals.
malleus	The first ossicle of the middle ear; malleus means hammer.
organ of Corti	A sensitive auditory receptor area found in the cochlea of the inner ear.
ossicle	Small bone of the ear; includes the malleus, incus, and stapes.
oval window	A membrane between the middle and the inner ears.

perilymph	Fluid contained in the labyrinth of the inner ear.
pinna	The auricle; flap of the ear.
semicircular canals	Passages in the inner ear associated with maintaining equilibrium.
stapes	The third ossicle of the middle ear. Stapes means stirrup.
tympanic membrane	A membrane between the outer and the middle ear; also called the **eardrum.**
vestibule	The central cavity of the labyrinth, connecting the semicircular canals and the cochlea. The vestibule contains two structures, the saccule and utricle, that help to maintain equilibrium.

C. Combining Forms, Suffixes, and Terminology

Write the meaning of the medical term in the space provided.

Combining Forms

Combining Form	Meaning	Terminology	Meaning
acous/o	hearing	acoustic _____	
audi/o	hearing, the sense of hearing	audiometer _____	
		audiogram _____	
audit/o	hearing	auditory _____	
aur/o **auricul/o**	ear (see also ot/o)	aural _____	
		postauricular _____	
cochle/o	cochlea	cochlear _____	
mastoid/o	mastoid process	mastoiditis _____	

The mastoid process is the posterior portion of the temporal bone that extends downward behind the external auditory meatus. Mastoiditis is usually caused by bacterial infection that spreads from the middle ear.

myring/o	eardrum, tympanic membrane (see also **tympan/o**)	myringotomy _____ myringitis _____
ossicul/o	ossicle	ossiculoplasty _____
ot/o	ear	otic _____ otomycosis _____ otopyorrhea _____ otolaryngologist _____
salping/o	eustachian tube, auditory tube	salpingopharyngeal _____ *In the context of female anatomy, salping/o means the fallopian tubes.*
staped/o	stapes (third bone of the middle ear)	stapedectomy _____ *After stapedectomy a prosthetic device is used to connect the incus and the oval window (Fig. 17–19). See otosclerosis, page 663.*

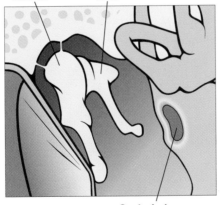

Malleus   Incus

A

Oval window
(stapes – separating the incus and
oval window – has been removed)

B

**Prosthesis
in place**

Figure 17-19

(A) Stapedectomy. Using microsurgical technique and a laser, the stapes bone is removed from the middle ear. **(B) A prosthetic device** (wire, Teflon, or metal) is placed onto the incus and attached to a hole in the oval window.

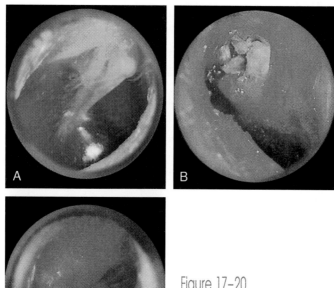

Figure 17–20

(A) Healthy tympanic membrane. (B) Tympanic membrane with cholesteatoma. (C) Tympanic membrane with acute otitis media. (A, B, and C from Barkauskas VH, et al: Health and Physical Assessment, 2nd ed. St. Louis, Mosby, 1998; courtesy of Richard A. Buckingham, Clinical Professor, Otolaryngology, Abraham Lincoln School of Medicine, University of Illinois, Chicago.)

tympan/o	eardrum, tympanic membrane	tympanoplasty _____ *Surgical reconstruction of the bones of the middle ear with reconnection of the eardrum to the oval window. Figure 17–20A shows a normal tympanic membrane (eardrum).*
vestibul/o	vestibule	vestibulocochlear _____

Suffixes			
Suffix	**Meaning**	**Terminology**	**Meaning**
-acusis or -cusis	hearing	hyperacusis _____ *Abnormally acute sensitivity to sounds.* presbycusis _____ *This type of nerve deafness occurs with the process of aging.*	
-otia	ear condition	macrotia _____ *Abnormally large ears; congenital anomaly.* microtia _____ *Abnormally small ears; congenital anomaly.*	

D. Abnormal and Pathological Conditions

acoustic neuroma

Benign tumor arising from the acoustic nerve (8th cranial nerve) in the brain.

This tumor causes tinnitus (ringing in the ears), vertigo (dizziness), and decreased hearing as its initial symptoms. Small tumors may be resected by microsurgical techniques or ablated (removed) by radiosurgery (using powerful and precise x-ray beams rather than a surgical incision).

cholesteatoma

Collection of skin cells and cholesterol in a sac within the middle ear.

These cyst-like masses produce a foul-smelling discharge and are most often the result of chronic otitis media. They are associated with perforations of the tympanic membrane (Fig. 17–20B).

deafness

Loss of the ability to hear.

Nerve deafness is caused by impairment of the cochlea or auditory (acoustic) nerve. Conduction deafness is caused by impairment of the middle ear ossicles and membranes that transmit sound waves into the cochlea.

Ménière disease

Disorder of the labyrinth of the inner ear marked by elevated endolymph pressure within the cochlea (cochlear hydrops) and semicircular canals (vestibular hydrops).

Symptoms are tinnitus, heightening sensitivity to loud sounds, progressive loss of hearing, headache, nausea, and vertigo. Attacks last minutes or continue for hours. The cause is unknown, and treatment is bed rest, sedation, and drugs to combat nausea and vertigo. Surgery may be necessary to relieve accumulation of fluid from the inner ear.

otitis media

Inflammation of the middle ear.

Acute otitis media is infection of the middle ear following an upper respiratory infection (URI). Pain and fever with redness and loss of mobility of the tympanic membrane are symptoms (Fig. 17–20C). As bacteria invade the middle ear, pus formation occurs **(suppurative otitis media).** It is treated with antibiotics, but if the condition becomes chronic, myringotomy may be required to ventilate the middle ear.

Serous otitis media is a noninfectious inflammation with accumulation of serous fluid. It often results from a dysfunctional or obstructed eustachian tube. Treatment includes myringotomy to aspirate fluid and tympanostomy tubes placed in the eardrum to allow ventilation of the middle ear.

otosclerosis

Hardening of the bony tissue of the labyrinth of the ear.

The result of this condition is that bone forms around the oval window and causes fixation or **ankylosis** (stiffening) of the stapes bone (ossicle). Conduction deafness occurs as the ossicles cannot pass on vibrations when sound enters the ear. Stapedectomy with replacement by a **prosthesis** (artificial part) is effective in restoring hearing (see Fig. 17–19). In order to perform this operation, the oval window must be **fenestrated** (opened) using a laser.

tinnitus

The sensation of noises (ringing, buzzing, whistling, booming) in the ears.

Caused by irritation of delicate hair cells in the inner ear, this disease symptom may be associated with presbycusis, Ménière disease, otosclerosis, chronic otitis, labyrinthitis, and other disorders. Tinnitus can be persistent and severe and can interfere with a patient's daily life. Treatment includes biofeedback to help the patient relax and exert control over stress and anxiety if these are contributing factors.

Tinnitus, a Latin-derived term, means tinkling.

vertigo

Sensation of irregular or whirling motion either of oneself or of external objects.

Vertigo can result from disease in the labyrinth of the inner ear or in the nerve that carries messages from the semicircular canals to the brain. Equilibrium and balance are affected, and nausea may occur as well.

E. Clinical Procedures

audiometry

An instrument (audiometer) delivers acoustic stimuli of specific frequencies to determine the patient's hearing for each frequency. Test results are plotted on a graph called an **audiogram.**

cochlear implant

A device allowing persons who are profoundly hearing impaired to understand speech. As a prosthetic replacement for the cochlea, it bypasses damaged cochlear hair cells and stimulates the auditory nerve. It consists of a microphone, speech processor, external transmitter, and implanted receiver. The receiver is implanted under the skin near the mastoid process above and behind the ear. It sends electrical signals to electrodes planted within the cochlea, which stimulate auditory nerves leading to the brain.

otoscopy

Visual examination of the ear with an otoscope (Fig. 17–21A).

pneumatic otoscopy

Visual examination of the external ear and tympanic membrane using air to change pressure in the external auditory canal. By increasing and decreasing the pressure in the external canal, the normal tympanic membrane should move in and out, respectively (Fig. 17–21B).

tuning fork tests

A vibration source (tuning fork) is placed on the mastoid process and then in front of the external auditory meatus to test bone and air conduction **(Rinne test).** The **Weber test** compares bone conduction in the two ears (a vibrating tuning fork is placed on the center of the forehead).

F. Abbreviations

AD	right ear (Latin, *auris dextra*)	**ENG**	electronystagmography; a test of the balance mechanism of the inner ear by assessing eye movements (nystagmus is rapidly twitching eye movement)
AS	left ear (Latin, *auris sinistra*)		
AU	both ears (Latin, *auris uterque*)	**ENT**	ears, nose, and throat
EENT	eyes, ears, nose, and throat	**PE tube**	polyethylene ventilating tube (placed in the eardrum)

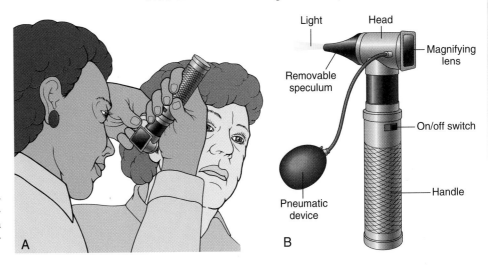

Figure 17-21

(A) Correct technique for otoscopy. (B) An otoscope with a pneumatic device for pneumatic otoscopy.

IV. Practical Applications

This section contains two listings of services and diagnoses and a medical report using terms that you have studied in this and previous chapters. Explanations of more difficult terms are added in brackets. Answers to the questions are on page 676 after Answers to Exercises.

Operating Schedule and Diagnoses: Eye and Ear Hospital

Match the operation in column I with a diagnosis in column II.

Operation—Column I

1. extracapsular cataract
   extraction with IOL; OS _____

2. blepharoplasty _____

3. scleral buckle _____

4. vitrectomy _____

5. radical mastoidectomy _____

6. keratoplasty _____

7. cochlear implant _____

8. argon laser photocoagulation
   of the macula _____

9. incision and drainage of
   hordeolum _____

Diagnosis—Column II

A. scarred and torn cornea
B. ptosis of eyelid skin
C. retinal detachment
D. diabetic retinopathy
E. macular degeneration
F. chronic stye
G. chronic infection of a bone
   behind the ear
H. severe deafness
I. senile cataract; left eye

Operative Report

Preoperative Diagnosis. Bilateral chronic serous otitis media adenotonsillitis.
Operation. Bilateral myringotomies and ventilation tube insertion; T and A.
Procedure. With the patient in the supine position and under general endotracheal anesthesia, inspection of AD was made under the operating microscope. The external canal was clear, tympanic membrane was divided. A purulent discharge appeared to be present. This drainage was suctioned out and the ear thoroughly lavaged [washed out]. A ventilating tube was put in place and otic drops were administered. Same procedure for AS.

The patient was placed in the Rose position [supine with the head over the table edge in full extension] and the adenoids removed with adenoid curettes and adenoid biopsy forceps. A nasopharyngeal sponge was put in place. The right tonsil was then grasped with tonsil forceps, dissected free, and removed with snare. Bleeding was controlled with suction cautery. The nasopharyngeal sponge was removed and no further bleeding noted. The patient tolerated the procedure well and left the OR in good condition.

V. Exercises

Remember to check your answers carefully with those given in Section VI, Answers to Exercises.

A. Match the structure of the eye with its description below. Write the letter of the description in the space provided.

Column I

1. pupil   _____

2. conjunctiva   _____

3. cornea   _____

4. sclera   _____

5. choroid   _____

6. iris   _____

7. ciliary body   _____

8. lens   _____

9. retina   _____

10. vitreous humor _____

Column II

A. contains sensitive cells called rods and cones that transform light energy into nerve impulses
B. contains muscles that control the shape of the lens and secretes aqueous humor
C. transparent structure behind the iris and in front of the vitreous humor; it refracts light rays onto the retina
D. jelly-like material behind the lens that helps to maintain the shape of the eyeball
E. dark center off the eye through which light rays enter
F. vascular layer of the eyeball that is continuous with the iris
G. delicate membrane lining the eyelids and covering the anterior eyeball
H. fibrous layer of clear tissue that extends over the anterior portion of the eyeball
I. colored portion of the eye; surrounds the pupil
J. tough, white, outer coat of the eye

B. Supply the terms that complete the following sentences.

1. The region at the back of the eye where the optic nerve meets the retina is the

   _____ .

2. The normal adjustment of the lens (becoming fatter or thinner) to bring an object into focus on

   the retina is called _____ .

3. A yellowish region on the retina lateral to the optic disc (disk) is the _____ .

4. The tiny pit or depression in the retina that is the region of clearest vision is the

   _____ .

5. The bending of light rays by the cornea, lens, and fluids of the eye is called _____ .

6. The point at which the fibers of the optic nerve cross in the brain is the _____ .

7. The photosensitive receptor cells in the retina that make the perception of color possible are the

   _____ .

8. The photosensitive receptor cells in the retina that make vision in dim light possible are the

   _____ .

9. The _____ is the area behind the cornea and in front of the lens and iris.
   It contains aqueous humor.

10. The posterior, inner part of the eye is the _____ .

C. Give the meanings of the following terms.

1. optic nerve _____

2. biconvex _____

3. anisocoria _____

4. cycloplegic _____

5. palpebral _____

6. mydriasis _____

7. miosis _____

8. papilledema _____

9. photophobia _____

10. scotoma _____

D. Complete the medical terms based on their meanings and the word parts given.

1. inflammation of an eyelid: _____ itis

2. inflammation of the conjunctiva: _____ itis

3. inflammation of a tear gland: _____ itis

4. inflammation of the iris: _____ itis

5. inflammation of the cornea: _____ itis

6. inflammation of the white of the eye: _____ itis

7. inflammation of the retina: _____ itis

8. prolapse of the eyelid: blephar _____

9. pertaining to tears: _____ al

10. pertaining to within the eye: intra _____

E. Match the following terms with their meanings as given below.

optician   xerophthalmia   corneal ulcer
ophthalmologist   uveitis   esotropia
optometrist   retinitis   exotropia
aphakia   hemianopsia   hypertropia

1. the fibrous layer of clear tissue over the front of the eyeball has a defect resulting from trauma or

   infection _____

2. inflammation of the vascular layer of the eye (iris, ciliary body, and choroid) _____

3. condition of dry eyes _____

4. absence of vision in half of the visual field _____

5. the eye abnormally turns outward _____

6. a medical doctor who treats diseases of the eyes _____

7. a nonmedical person who can examine eyes and prescribe glasses _____

8. a nonmedical person who grinds lenses and fits glasses _____

9. absence of the lens of the eye _____

10. the eye abnormally turns inward _____

F. Describe the following visual conditions.

1. amblyopia _____

2. hyperopia _____

3. presbyopia _____

4. myopia _____

5. nyctalopia _____

6. diplopia _____

7. astigmatism _____

G. Complete the following sentences.

1. In the myopic eye, light rays do not focus properly on the _____. Either

the eyeball is too _____ or the refractive power of the lens is too

_____, so that the image is blurred and comes to a focus in

_____ of the retina. The type of lens used to correct this refractive error is

called a _____ lens.

2. In the hyperopic eye, the eyeball is too _____ or the refractive power of

the lens too _____, so that the image is blurred and focused in

_____ of the retina. The type of lens used to correct this refractive error is

called a _____ lens.

3. A miotic is a drug that _____ the pupil of the eye.

4. A mydriatic is a drug that _____ the pupil of the eye.

H. Match the following abnormal conditions of the eye with their meanings as given below.

glaucoma   diabetic retinopathy   retinitis pigmentosa
cataract   strabismus   retinal detachment
chalazion   hordeolum (stye)   macular degeneration

1. retinal microaneurysms, hemorrhages, dilation of retinal veins, and neovascularization occur secondary to an abnormal endocrine condition _____

2. two layers of the retina separate from each other _____

3. abnormal deviations of the eye occur (esotropia and exotropia) _____

4. clouding of the lens causes decreased vision _____

5. loss of central vision caused by deterioration of the macula of the retina _____

6. a localized, purulent infection of a sebaceous gland in the eyelid _____

7. a small, hard, cystic mass on the eyelid; formed as a result of chronic inflammation of a sebaceous gland _____

8. increased intraocular pressure results in retinal and optic nerve damage _____

9. a pigmented scar forms on the retina and leads to nyctalopia; an inherited condition

_____

I. The picture shows how a patient with one of the following conditions would view the scene. What is the patient's condition?

1. glaucoma

2. cataract

3. stroke (hemianopsia)

4. age-related macular degeneration

J. Give the meaning of the following combining forms.

1. lacrim/o _____   3. kerat/o _____

2. dacry/o _____   4. corne/o _____

5. blephar/o _____

6. palpebr/o _____

7. cor/o _____

8. pupill/o _____

9. phac/o _____

10. phak/o _____

11. ocul/o _____

12. ophthalm/o _____

13. opt/o _____

14. scot/o _____

K. *Match the following clinical procedures with their meanings as given below.*

tonometry	ophthalmoscopy	LASIK
fluorescein angiography	visual acuity test	keratoplasty
visual field examination	slit lamp ocular examination	phacoemulsification
laser photocoagulation	vitrectomy	scleral buckle

1. ultrasonic vibrations break up the lens, and it is aspirated from the eye _____

2. test of clearness of vision _____

3. measurement of tension or pressure within the eye; glaucoma test _____

4. high-energy light radiation beams are used to stop retinal hemorrhaging

   _____

5. a laser removes corneal tissue (sculpts it) to correct myopia _____

6. intravenous injection of dye followed by examination of the eyes and blood vessels

   _____

7. suture of a silicone band to the sclera to correct retinal detachment _____

8. test to measure the area within which objects are seen when the eyes are looking straight ahead

   _____

9. removal (and replacement) of diseased fluid in the chamber behind the lens of the eye

   _____

10. visual examination of the interior of the eye after dilation of the pupil _____

11. use of an instrument for microscopic examination of parts of the eye _____

12. corneal transplant surgery _____

L. Give the meanings of the following abbreviations.

1. OU _____

2. VA _____

3. OD _____

4. OS _____

5. VF _____

6. IOL _____

7. IOP _____

8. PERRLA _____

M. Arrange the following terms in the correct order to indicate their sequence in the transmission of sound waves to the brain from the outer ear.

incus, tympanic membrane, pinna, cochlea, malleus, oval window,
external auditory canal, auditory liquids and receptors, stapes,
auditory nerve fibers, cerebral cortex

1. _____   7. _____

2. _____   8. _____

3. _____   9. _____

4. _____   10. _____

5. _____   11. _____

6. _____

N. Give the meanings of the following medical terms.

1. labyrinth _____

2. semicircular canals _____

3. auditory (eustachian) tube _____

4. stapes _____

5. organ of Corti _____

6. perilymph and endolymph _____

7. cerumen _____

8. vestibule _____

9. oval window _____

10. tympanic membrane _____

O. Complete the following terms based on their definitions.

1. instrument to examine the ear: _____ scope

2. removal of the third bone of the middle ear: _____ ectomy

3. pertaining to the auditory tube and throat: _____ pharyngeal

4. flow of pus from the ear: oto _____

5. instrument to measure hearing: _____ meter

6. incision of the eardrum: _____ tomy

7. surgical repair of the eardrum: _____ plasty

8. deafness due to old age: _____ cusis

9. small ear: micr _____

10. inflammation of the middle ear: ot _____ _____

P. Give the meanings of the following medical terms.

1. vertigo _____

2. Ménière disease _____

3. otosclerosis _____

4. tinnitus _____

5. labyrinthitis _____

6. cholesteatoma _____

7. suppurative otitis media _____

8. acoustic neuroma _____

9. mastoiditis _____

10. myringitis _____

Q. Give the meanings of the following abbreviations relating to otology.

1. AU _____

2. AS _____

3. AD _____

4. EENT _____

5. ENT _____

6. PE tube _____

R. Select the correct term to complete each sentence.

1. Dr. Jones specializes in pediatric ophthalmology. His examination of children with poor vision often leads to the diagnosis of **(cataract, amblyopia, glaucoma),** or lazy eye.

2. Stella's vision became progressively worse as she aged. Her physician told her that she had a common condition called **(presbyopia, detached retina, anisocoria),** which many elderly patients develop.

3. Matthew rubbed his itchy eyes constantly and thus spread his "pink eye" or **(conjunctivitis, blepharitis, myringitis)** from one eye to the other. Dr. Chang prescribed antibiotics for this common condition.

4. As David's **(mastoiditis, otitis media, tinnitus)** became progressively worse, his doctor worried that this ringing in his ears might be caused by a benign brain tumor, a(an) **(cholesteatoma, acoustic neuroma, glaucoma).**

5. Baby Sally had so many episodes of **(vertigo, otosclerosis, suppurative otitis media)** that Dr. Sills recommended the placement of PE tubes.

VI. Answers to Exercises

A

1. E	5. F	9. A
2. G	6. I	10. D
3. H	7. B	
4. J	8. C	

B

1. optic disc (disk)	5. refraction	9. anterior chamber
2. accommodation	6. optic chiasm	10. fundus
3. macula	7. cones	
4. fovea centralis	8. rods	

C

1. cranial nerve that carries impulses from the retina to the brain
2. having two sides that are rounded, elevated, and curved evenly
3. condition of pupils of unequal (anis/o) size
4. pertaining to paralysis of the ciliary muscles
5. pertaining to the eyelid
6. condition of enlargement of the pupil
7. condition of narrowing of the pupil
8. swelling in the region of the optic disc
9. condition of sensitivity to ("fear of") light
10. blind spot; area of darkened (diminished) vision surrounded by clear vision

D

1. blepharitis
2. conjunctivitis
3. dacryoadenitis
4. iritis
5. keratitis
6. scleritis
7. retinitis
8. blepharoptosis
9. lacrimal
10. intraocular

E

1. corneal ulcer
2. uveitis
3. xerophthalmia
4. hemianopsia
5. exotropia
6. ophthalmologist
7. optometrist
8. optician
9. aphakia
10. esotropia

F

1. dimness of vision; lazy eye (resulting from strabismus and diplopia)
2. farsightedness
3. decreased vision resulting from old age
4. nearsightedness
5. night blindness; decreased vision at night
6. double vision
7. defective curvature of the lens and cornea leading to blurred vision

G

1. retina; long; strong; front; concave
2. short; weak; back; convex
3. constricts
4. dilates

H

1. diabetic retinopathy
2. retinal detachment
3. strabismus
4. cataract
5. macular degeneration
6. hordeolum (style)
7. chalazion
8. glaucoma
9. retinitis pigmentosa

I

3 stroke (hemianopsia)—loss of half of the visual field caused by a stroke occurring in the left visual cortex.

Glaucoma would cause loss of peripheral vision (darkness around the edges of the picture). A cataract would cause blurred vision. Macular degeneration would produce loss of central vision.

J

1. tears
2. tears
3. cornea
4. cornea
5. eyelid
6. eyelid
7. pupil
8. pupil
9. lens
10. lens
11. eye
12. eye
13. eye
14. darkness

K

1. phacoemulsification
2. visual acuity test
3. tonometry
4. laser photocoagulation
5. LASIK
6. fluorescein angiography
7. scleral buckle
8. visual field examination
9. vitrectomy
10. ophthalmoscopy
11. slit lamp ocular examination
12. keratoplasty

L

1. each eye
2. visual acuity
3. right eye
4. left eye
5. visual field
6. intraocular lens
7. intraocular pressure
8. pupils equal, round, reactive to light and accommodation

Continued on following page

M

1. pinna (auricle)
2. external auditory canal
3. tympanic membrane
4. malleus

5. incus
6. stapes
7. oval window
8. cochlea

9. auditory liquids and receptors
10. auditory nerve fibers
11. cerebral cortex

N

1. cochlea and organs of equilibrium (semicircular canals and vestibule)
2. organ of equilibrium in the inner ear
3. passageway between the middle ear and the throat
4. third ossicle (little bone) of the middle ear

5. region in the cochlea that contains auditory receptors
6. auditory fluids circulating within the inner ear
7. wax in the external auditory meatus
8. central cavity of the inner ear that

connects the semicircular canals and the cochlea
9. delicate membrane between the middle and the inner ears
10. eardrum

O

1. otoscope
2. stapedectomy
3. salpingopharyngeal
4. otopyorrhea

5. audiometer
6. myringotomy (tympanotomy)
7. tympanoplasty (myringoplasty)
8. presbycusis

9. microtia
10. otitis media

P

1. sensation of irregular or whirling motion either of oneself or of external objects
2. disorder of the labyrinth marked by elevation of ear fluids and pressure within the cochlea (tinnitus, vertigo, and nausea result)
3. hardening of the bony tissue of the labyrinth of the inner ear

4. noise (ringing, buzzing) in the ears
5. inflammation of the labyrinth of the inner ear
6. collection of skin cells and cholesterol in a sac within the middle ear
7. inflammation of the middle ear with bacterial infection and pus collection

8. benign tumor arising from the acoustic nerve in the brain
9. inflammation of the mastoid process (behind the ear)
10. inflammation of the eardrum

Q

1. both ears
2. left ear
3. right ear

4. eyes, ears, nose, and throat
5. ears, nose, and throat
6. ventilating tube placed in the eardrum

R

1. amblyopia
2. presbyopia
3. conjunctivitis

4. tinnitus; acoustic neuroma
5. suppurative otitis media

Answers to Practical Applications

1. I
2. B
3. C

4. D
5. G
6. A

7. H
8. E
9. F

VII. Pronunciation of Terms

Pronunciation Guide

ā as in āpe   ă as in ăpple
ē as in ēven   ĕ as in ĕvery
ī as in īce   ĭ as in ĭnterest
ō as in ōpen   ŏ as in pŏt
ū as in ūnit   ŭ as in ŭnder

To test your understanding of the terminology in this chapter, write the meaning of each term in the space provided. In addition, you may wish to cover the terms and write them by looking at your definitions. Make sure your spelling is correct. The page number after each term indicates where it is defined or used in the text so you can easily check your responses.

Vocabulary and Terminology

Eye

Term	Pronunciation	Meaning
accommodation (642)	ă-kŏm-ō-DĀ-shŭn	_____
amblyopia (647)	ăm-blē-Ō-pē-ă	_____
anisocoria (644)	ăn-ī-sō-KŌ-rē-ă	_____
anterior chamber (642)	ăn-TĒ-rē-ŏr CHĀM-bĕr	_____
aphakia (646)	ă-FĀ-kē-ă	_____
aqueous humor (643)	ĂK-wē-ŭs or Ā-kwē-ŭs HŪ-mĕr	_____
astigmatism (648)	ă-STĬG-mă-tĭsm	_____
biconvex (643)	bī-KŎN-vĕks	_____
blepharitis (644)	blĕf-ă-RĪ-tĭs	_____
blepharoptosis (644)	blĕf-ă-rŏp-TŌ-sĭs	_____
cataract (650)	KĂT-ă-răkt	_____
chalazion (650)	kă-LĀ-zē-ŏn	_____
choroid layer (643)	KŎR-oyd LĀ-ĕr	_____
ciliary body (643)	SĬL-ē-ăr-ē BŎD-ē	_____
cones (643)	kōnz	_____
conjunctiva (643)	kŏn-jŭnk-TĪ-vă	_____
conjunctivitis (644)	kŏn-jŭnk-tĭ-VĪ-tĭs	_____

cornea (643)	KŎR-nē-ă	_____
corneal ulcer (644)	KŎR-nē-ăl ŬL-sĕr	_____
corneoscleral (646)	kŏr-nē-ō-SKLĔ-răl	_____
cycloplegic (644)	sī-klō-PLĒ-jĭk	_____
dacryoadenitis (645)	dăk-rē-ō-ăd-ĕ-NĪ-tĭs	_____
diabetic retinopathy (650)	dī-ă-BĔT-ĭk rĕ-tĭn-NŎP-ă-thē	_____
diplopia (647)	dĭp-LŌ-pē-ă	_____
enucleation (654)	ē-nū-klē-Ā-shun	_____
esotropia (648)	ĕs-ō-TRŌP-pē-ă	_____
exotropia (648)	ĕk-sō-TRŌ-pē-ă	_____
fluorescein angiography (653)	flōō-ō-RĔS-ē-ĭn ăn-jē-ŎG-ră-fē	_____
fovea centralis (643)	FŌ-vē-ă sĕn-TRĂ-lĭs	_____
fundus (643)	FŬN-dŭs	_____
glaucoma (650)	glăw-KŌ-mă	_____
hemianopsia (648)	hĕ-mē-ă-NŎP-sē-ă	_____
hordeolum (650)	hŏr-DĒ-ō-lŭm	_____
hyperopia (648)	hī-pĕr-Ō-pē-ă	_____
hypertensive retinopathy (646)	hī-pĕr-TĔN-sĭv rĕ-tĭ-NŎP-ă-thē	_____
intraocular (645)	ĭn-tră-ŎK-ū-lăr	_____
iridectomy (645)	ĭr-ĭ-DĔK-tō-mē	_____
iridic (645)	ĭ-RĬD-ĭk	_____
iris (643)	Ī-rĭs	_____
iritis (645)	ī-RĪ-tĭs	_____
keratitis (645)	kĕr-ă-TĪ-tĭs	_____
keratoplasty (654)	kĕr-ă-tō-PLĂS-tē	_____

keratotomy (645)	kĕ-ră-TŎT-ō-mē	
lacrimal (645)	LĂK-rĭ-măl	
lacrimation (645)	lă-krĭ-MĀ-shŭn	
laser photocoagulation (654)	LĀ-zĕr fō-tō-kō-ăg-ū-LĀ-shŭn	
lens (643)	lĕnz	
macula (643)	MĂK-ū-lă	
macular degeneration (653)	MĂK-ū-lăr dē-jĕn-ĕ-RĀ-shŭn	
miosis (647)	mī-Ō-sĭs	
miotic (647)	mī-ŎT-ĭk	
mydriasis (647)	mĭ-DRĪ-ă-sĭs	
myopia (648)	mī-Ō-pē-ă	
nyctalopia (647)	nĭk-tă-LŌ-pē-ă	
ophthalmic (645)	ŏf-THĂL-mĭk	
ophthalmologist (645)	ŏf-thăl-MŎL-ō-jĭst	
ophthalmoplegia (645)	ŏf-thăl-mō-PLĒ-jă	
ophthalmoscopy (653)	ŏf-thăl-MŎS-kō-pē	
optic chiasm (643)	ŎP-tĭk KĪ-azm	
optic disc (643)	ŎP-tĭk dĭsk	
optician (646)	ŏp-TĬSH-ăn	
optic nerve (643)	ŎP-tĭk nĕrv	
optometrist (646)	ŏp-TŎM-ĕ-trĭst	
palpebral (646)	PĂL-pĕ-brăl	
papilledema (646)	păp-ĕ-lĕ-DĒ-mă	
phacoemulsification (646)	făk-ō-ĕ-mŭl-sĭ-fĭ-KĀ-shŭn	
photophobia (647)	fō-tō-FŌ-bē-ă	
presbyopia (649)	prĕz-bē-Ō-pē-ă	
pupil (643)	PŪ-pĭl	

pupillary (646)	PŪ-pĭ-lăr-ē	_____
refraction (643)	rē-FRĂK-shŭn	_____
retina (644)	RĚT-ĭ-nă	_____
retinal detachment (653)	RĚ-tĭ-năl dē-TĂCH-měnt	_____
retinitis pigmentosa (646)	rět-ĭ-NĪ-tĭs pĭg-měn-TŌ-să	_____
sclera (644)	SKLĚ-ră	_____
scleral buckle (656)	SKLĚ-răl BŬK'l	_____
scleritis (646)	sklě-RĪ-tĭs	_____
scotoma (647)	skō-TŌ-mă	_____
slit lamp ocular examination (654)	slĭt lămp ŏk-ū-lăr ěk-zăm-ĭ-NĀ-shŭn	_____
strabismus (653)	stră-BĬZ-mŭs	_____
tonometry (654)	tō-NŎM-ě-trē	_____
uveitis (646)	ū-vē-Ī-tĭs	_____
visual acuity (654)	VĬZ-ū-ăl ă-KŪ-ĭ-tē	_____
visual field examination (654)	VĬZ-ū-ăl fēld ěk-zăm-ĭ-NĀ-shŭn	_____
vitrectomy (656)	vĭ-TRĚK-tō-mē	_____
vitreous humor (644)	VĬT-rē-ŭs Ū-měr	_____
xerophthalmia (647)	zěr-ŏf-THĂL-mē-ă	_____

Ear

Term	Pronunciation	Meaning
acoustic (660)	ă-KOOS-tĭk	_____
acoustic neuroma (663)	ă-KOOS-tĭk nū-RŌ-mă	_____
audiogram (660)	ĂW-dē-ō-grăm	_____
audiometer (660)	ăw-dē-ŎM-ě-těr	_____
audiometry (664)	ăw-dē-ŎM-ě-trē	_____
auditory canal (659)	ăw-dĭ-TŌ-rē kă-NĂL	_____

auditory meatus (659)	ăw-dĭ-TŌ-rē mē-Ā-tŭs	_____
auditory tube (659)	ăw-dĭ-TŌ-rē to͞ob	_____
aural (660)	ĂW-răl	_____
auricle (659)	ĂW-rĭ-k'l	_____
cerumen (659)	sĕ-RO͞O-mĕn	_____
cholesteatoma (663)	kō-lē-stē-ă-TŌ-mă	_____
cochlea (659)	KŎK-lē-ă	_____
cochlear (660)	KŎK-lē-ăr	_____
deafness (663)	DĔF-nĕs	_____
endolymph (659)	ĔN-dō-lŭmí	_____
eustachian tube (659)	ū-STĀ-shŭn or ū-STĀ-kē-ăn	_____
hyperacusis (662)	hī-pĕr-ă-kū-sis	_____
incus (659)	ĬNG-kŭs	_____
labyrinth (659)	LĂB-ĭ-rĭnth	_____
macrotia (662)	măk-RŌ-shē-ă	_____
malleus (659)	MĂL-ē-ŭs	_____
mastoiditis (660)	măs-toy-DĪ-tĭs	_____
Ménière disease (663)	mĕn-ē-ĀRZ dĭ-ZĒZ	_____
microtia (662)	mī-KRŌ-shē-ă	_____
myringitis (661)	mĭr-ĭn-JĪ-tĭs	_____
myringotomy (661)	mĭr-ĭn-GŎT-ō-mē	_____
ossicle (659)	ŎS-ĭ-k'l	_____
ossiculoplasty (661)	ŏs-ĭ-kū-lō-PLĂS-tē	_____
otic (661)	Ō-tĭk	_____
otolaryngologist (661)	ō-tō-lă-rĭn-GŎL-ō-jĭst	_____
otomycosis (661)	ō-tō-mī-KŌ-sĭs	_____
otopyorrhea (661)	ō-tō-pī-ō-RĒ-ă	_____

otosclerosis (663)   ō-tō-sklĕ-RŌ-sĭs   _____

otoscopy (664)   ō-TŎS-kō-pē   _____

oval window (659)   Ō-văl WĬN-dō   _____

perilymph (660)   PĔR-ĭ-lĭmf   _____

pinna (660)   PĬN-ă   _____

pneumatic otoscopy (664)   nū-MĂ-tĭk ō-TŎS-kō-pē   _____

postauricular (660)   pōst-ăw-RĬK-ū-lăr   _____

presbycusis (662)   prĕz-bē-KŪ-sĭs   _____

salpingopharyngeal (661)   săl-pĭng-gō-fă-RĬN-gē-ăl _____

semicircular canals (660)   sĕ-mē-SĔR-kū-lăr kă-NĂLZ _____

serous otitis media (663)   SĔR-ŭs ō-TĪ-tĭs MĒ-dē-ă   _____

stapedectomy (661)   stā-pĕ-DĔK-tō-mē   _____

stapes (660)   STĀ-pēz   _____

suppurative otitis   SŪ-pĕr-ă-tĭv ō-TĪ-tĭs   _____
  media (663)   MĒ-dē-ă

tinnitus (663)   tĭ-NĪ-tĭs   _____

tuning fork tests (664)   TOO-nĕng fort tests   _____

tympanic membrane (660)   tĭm-PĂN-ĭk MĔM-brān   _____

tympanoplasty (662)   tĭm-pă-nō-PLĂS-tē   _____

vertigo (664)   VĔR-tĭ-gō   _____

vestibule (660)   VĔS-tĭ-būl   _____

vestibulocochlear (662)   vĕs-tĭb-ū-lō-KŌK-lē-ăr   _____

VIII. Review Sheet

Write the meaning of the word parts in the spaces provided and test yourself. Check your answers with the information in the chapter or in the glossary (Medical Terms—English) at the end of the book.

COMBINING FORMS

Combining Form	Meaning	Combining Form	Meaning
acous/o		kerat/o	
ambly/o		lacrim/o	
anis/o		mastoid/o	
aque/o		mi/o	
audi/o		myc/o	
audit/o		mydr/o	
aur/o		myring/o	
auricul/o		nyct/o	
blephar/o		ocul/o	
conjunctiv/o		ophthalm/o	
cor/o		opt/o	
corne/o		optic/o	
cycl/o		ossicul/o	
dacry/o		ot/o	
dipl/o		palpebr/o	
glauc/o		papill/o	
ir/o		phac/o	
irid/o		phak/o	

Continued on following page

phot/o	_____	staped/o	_____
presby/o	_____	tympan/o	_____
pupill/o	_____	uve/o	_____
retin/o	_____	vestibul/o	_____
salping/o	_____	vitre/o	_____
scler/o	_____	xer/o	_____
scot/o	_____		

SUFFIXES

Suffix	Meaning	Suffix	Meaning
-acusis	_____	-otia	_____
-cusis	_____	-phobia	_____
-opia	_____	-plegic	_____
-opsia	_____	-tropia	_____

CHAPTER

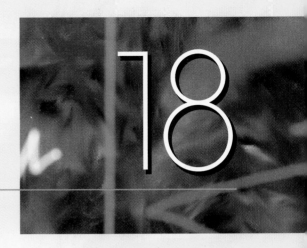

18

Endocrine System

This chapter is divided into the following sections

In this chapter you will

- Identify the endocrine glands and their hormones;
- Gain an understanding of the functions of these hormones in the body;
- Analyze medical terms related to the endocrine glands and their hormones;
- Describe the abnormal conditions resulting from excessive and deficient secretions of the endocrine glands;
- Identify laboratory tests, clinical procedures, and abbreviations related to endocrinology; and
- Apply your new knowledge to understanding medical terms in their proper contexts, such as medical reports and records.

I. Introduction

The endocrine system is an information signaling system much like the nervous system. However, the nervous system uses nerves to conduct information, whereas the endocrine system uses blood vessels as information channels. **Glands** located in many regions of the body release into the bloodstream specific chemical messengers called **hormones** (from the Greek work *hormōn,* meaning urging on), which regulate the many and varied functions of an organism. For example, one hormone stimulates the growth of bones, another causes the maturation of sex organs and reproductive cells, and another controls the metabolic rate (metabolism) within all the individual cells of the body. In addition, one powerful endocrine gland near the brain secretes a wide variety of different hormones that travel through the bloodstream and regulate the activities of other endocrine glands.

Hormones produce their effects by binding to **receptors,** which are recognition sites in the various **target** tissues on which the hormones act. The receptors initiate specific biological effects when the hormones bind to them. Each hormone has its own receptor, and binding of a receptor by a hormone is much like the interaction of a key and a lock.

All the **endocrine glands,** no matter which hormones they produce, secrete their hormones directly into the bloodstream rather than into ducts leading to the exterior of the body. Those glands that send their chemical substances into ducts and out of the body are called **exocrine glands.** Examples of exocrine glands are sweat, mammary, mucous, salivary, and lacrimal (tear) glands.

The ductless, internally secreting **endocrine glands** are listed below. Locate these glands on Figure 18–1.

[1] thyroid gland

[2] parathyroid glands (four glands)

[3] adrenal glands (one pair)

[4] pancreas (islets of Langerhans)

[5] pituitary gland

[6] ovaries in female (one pair)

[7] testes in male (one pair)

[8] pineal gland

[9] thymus gland

The last two glands on this list, the pineal and the thymus glands, are included as endocrine glands because they are ductless, although little is known about their endocrine function in the human body. The **pineal gland,** located in the central portion of the brain, is believed to secrete a substance called **melatonin.** Melatonin contributes to the process of skin pigmentation in lower animals, such as frogs and fishes. In mammals, melatonin is believed to affect the brain and influence the rate of gonad (ovary and testis) maturation. Calcification of the pineal gland can occur and can be an important radiological landmark when x-rays of the brain are examined.

The **thymus gland,** located behind the sternum in the mediastinum, resembles a lymph gland in structure. It contains lymphatic tissue and T cell lymphocytes. The gland produces a hormone, **thymosin,** and is important in the development of immune responses in newborns (it is large in childhood but shrinks in adulthood). Its endocrine function is not well understood. Removal of the thymus gland is helpful in treating a muscular-neurological disorder called myasthenia gravis.

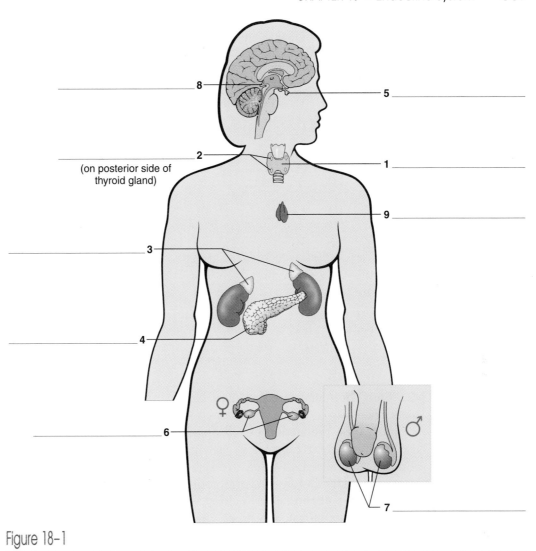

Figure 18-1

The endocrine system.

Table 18-1. **ENDOCRINE TISSUE (APART FROM MAJOR GLANDS): LOCATION, SECRETION, AND ACTION**

Location	Secretion	Action
Body cells	Prostaglandins	Contract uterus Lower blood pressure Clump platelets Lower acid secretion in stomach
Gastrointestinal tract	Cholecystokinin Gastrin Secretin	Contracts gallbladder Stimulates gastric secretion Stimulates pancreatic enzymes
Kidney	Erythropoietin	Stimulates erythrocyte production
Pineal gland	Melatonin	Affects brain and releases hormones (gonadotropins)
Placenta	hCG	Sustains pregnancy
Skin	Vitamin D	Affects absorption of calcium
Thymus gland	Thymosin	Affects immune response

Some hormones are produced by organs other than the endocrine glands already mentioned. For example, the kidney secretes a hormone called **erythropoietin,** which stimulates the production of red blood cells by the bone marrow. The gastrointestinal tract secretes three hormones, **gastrin, secretin,** and **cholecystokinin.** These hormones stimulate the secretion of gastric acid and enzymes (gastrin), the secretion of pancreatic enzymes (secretin), and the contraction of the gallbladder (cholecystokinin). The skin produces **vitamin D,** which is also considered a hormone. Vitamin D stimulates the absorption of calcium from the gastrointestinal tract and is necessary for the maintenance of proper amounts of calcium in the bones and in the bloodstream. During pregnancy, the placenta secretes **hCG (HCG; human chorionic gonadotropin),** which helps to sustain the fetus in the womb.

Prostaglandins are hormone-like substances that affect the body in many ways. First found in semen (produced by the prostate gland) but now recognized in cells throughout the body, prostaglandins stimulate the contraction of the uterus; regulate body temperature, platelet aggregation, and acid secretion in the stomach; and have the ability to lower blood pressure.

Endocrine tissue (apart from the major glands) is reviewed in Table 18–1. Use it as a reference.

II. Thyroid Gland

A. Location and Structure

Label Figure 18–2.

The **thyroid gland** [1] is composed of a right and a left lobe on either side of the **trachea** [2], just below a large piece of cartilage called the **thyroid cartilage** [3]. The thyroid cartilage covers the larynx and produces the prominence on the neck known as the Adam's apple. The **isthmus** [4] of the thyroid gland is a narrow strip of glandular tissue that connects the two lobes on the ventral (anterior) surface of the trachea.

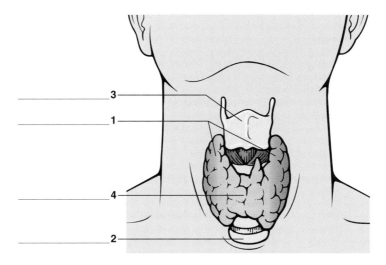

Figure 18-2

The thyroid gland, anterior view.

B. Function

Two of the hormones secreted by the thyroid gland are **thyroxine** or **tetraiodothyronine (T_4)** and **triiodothyronine (T_3).** These hormones are synthesized in the thyroid gland from **iodine,** which is picked up from the blood circulating through the gland, and from an amino acid called tyrosine. T_4 (containing four atoms of iodine) is much more concentrated in the blood, whereas T_3 (containing three atoms of iodine) is far more potent in affecting the metabolism of cells. Most thyroid hormone is bound to protein molecules as it travels in the bloodstream.

T_4 and T_3 are necessary in the body to maintain a normal level of metabolism in all body cells. Cells need oxygen to carry on metabolic processes, one aspect of which is the burning of food to release the energy stored within the food. Thyroid hormone aids cells in their uptake of oxygen and thus supports the metabolic rate in the body. Injections of thyroid hormone raise the metabolic rate, whereas removal of the thyroid gland, diminishing thyroid hormone content in the body, results in a lower metabolic rate, heat loss, and poor physical and mental development.

A more recently discovered hormone produced by the thyroid gland is called **calcitonin (thyrocalcitonin).** Calcitonin is secreted when calcium levels in the blood are high. It stimulates calcium to leave the blood and enter the bones, thus lowering blood calcium back to normal. Figure 18–3 summarizes the hormones secreted by the thyroid glands.

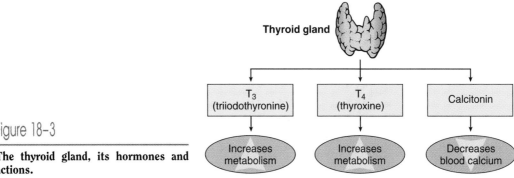

Figure 18-3

The thyroid gland, its hormones and actions.

III. Parathyroid Glands

A. Location and Structure

Label Figure 18–4.

The **parathyroid glands** [1] are four small oval bodies located on the dorsal aspect of the **thyroid gland** [2].

B. Function

Parathyroid hormone (PTH) is secreted by the parathyroid glands. This hormone (also known as **parathormone**) mobilizes **calcium** (a mineral substance) from bones into the bloodstream, where calcium is necessary for the proper functioning of body tissues, especially muscles. Normally, calcium in the food we eat is absorbed from the intestine and carried, by the blood, to the bones, where it is stored. The adjustment of the level of calcium in the blood is a good example of the way hormones in general control the **homeostasis** (equilibrium or constancy in the internal environment) of the body. If there is a decrease in blood calcium (as in pregnancy or rickets, a vitamin D–deficiency disease), parathyroid hormone is secreted in larger amounts to cause calcium to leave the bones and enter the bloodstream. Thus, blood calcium levels are brought back to normal (Fig. 18–5). Conversely, any situation of increase in calcium in the bloodstream, such as excess quantity of calcium or vitamin D in the diet, will lead to decreased parathyroid hormone secretion (calcium then leaves the blood to enter bones), decreasing blood calcium, so that homeostasis is again achieved.

IV. Adrenal Glands

A. Location and Structure

Label Figure 18–6.

The **adrenal glands,** also called the **suprarenal glands,** are two small glands; one is situated on top of each **kidney** [1]. Each gland consists of two parts, an outer portion called the **adrenal cortex** [2] and an inner portion called the **adrenal medulla** [3]. The cortex and medulla are two glands in one, each secreting its own different endocrine hormones. The cortex secretes hormones called **corticosteroids** (complex chemicals derived from cholesterol), and the medulla secretes hormones called **catecholamines** (chemicals derived from amino acids).

B. Function

The **adrenal cortex** secretes three types of steroid hormones called **corticosteroids.**

1. **Glucocorticoids**—These steroid hormones have an important influence on the metabolism of sugars, fats, and proteins within all body cells and have a powerful anti-inflammatory effect.

    Cortisol (also called **hydrocortisone**) is the most important glucocorticoid hormone. Cortisol increases the ability of cells to make new sugars out of fats and proteins (gluconeogenesis) and regulates the quantity of sugars, fats, and proteins in the blood and cells.

    Cortisone is a hormone very similar to cortisol and can be prepared synthetically. Cortisone is useful in treating inflammatory conditions such as rheumatoid arthritis.

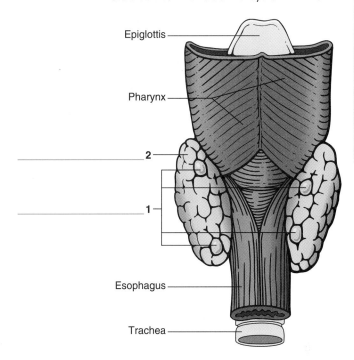

Epiglottis

Pharynx

2

1

Esophagus

Trachea

Figure 18-4

The parathyroid glands, posterior view.

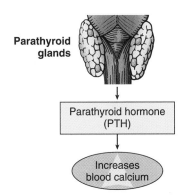

Parathyroid glands

Parathyroid hormone (PTH)

Increases blood calcium

Figure 18-5

The parathyroid glands, their hormone and actions.

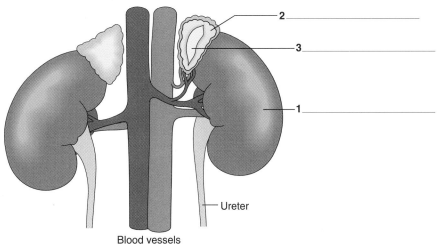

2

3

1

Ureter

Blood vessels

Figure 18-6

The adrenal (suprarenal) glands.

2. **Mineralocorticoids**—These hormones are essential to life because they regulate the amounts of mineral salts (also called **electrolytes**) that are retained in the body. A proper balance of water and salts in the blood and tissues is essential to the normal functioning of the body.

    Aldosterone is a mineralocorticoid hormone. The secretion of aldosterone by the adrenal cortex increases the reabsorption into the bloodstream of **sodium** (a mineral electrolyte commonly found in salts) by the kidney tubules. At the same time, aldosterone stimulates the excretion of another electrolyte called **potassium.**

    The secretion of aldosterone increases manyfold in the face of a severely sodium-restricted diet, thereby enabling the body to hold needed salt in the bloodstream.

3. **Sex hormones: Androgens, Estrogens, and Progestins**—These are male and female hormones that maintain the secondary sex characteristics, such as beard and breast development, and are necessary for reproduction. These hormones are also produced in the ovaries and testes. Excess adrenal androgen secretion in females leads to **virilism** (development of male characteristics), and excess adrenal estrogen and progesten secretion in males produces feminization (development of feminine characteristics).

The **adrenal medulla** secretes two types of **catecholamine** hormones:

1. **Epinephrine (adrenaline)**—This hormone increases cardiac rate, dilates bronchial tubes, and stimulates the production of glucose from a storage substance called glycogen when glucose is needed by the body.
2. **Norepinephrine (noradrenaline)**—This hormone constricts vessels and raises blood pressure.

Both epinephrine and norepinephrine are called **sympathomimetic** agents because they mimic, or copy, the actions of the sympathetic nervous system. During times of stress, these hormones are secreted by the adrenal medulla in response to nervous stimulation. They help the body respond to crisis situations by raising blood pressure, increasing heartbeat and respiration, and bringing sugar out of storage in the cells.

    Figure 18–7 summarizes the hormones that are secreted by the adrenal glands and notes their actions.

V. Pancreas

A. Location and Structure

Label Figure 18–8.

The **pancreas** [1] is located near and partially behind the **stomach** [2] in the region of the first and second lumbar vertebrae. The endocrine tissue of the pancreas consists of specialized hormone-producing cells called the **islets of Langerhans** [3]. More than 98 per cent of the pancreas consists of exocrine cells (glands and ducts). These cells secrete digestive enzymes into the gastrointestinal tract.

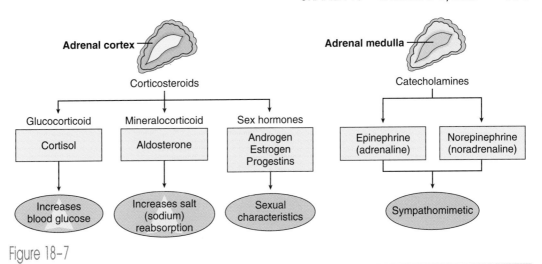

Figure 18–7

The adrenal cortex and adrenal medulla, their hormones and actions.

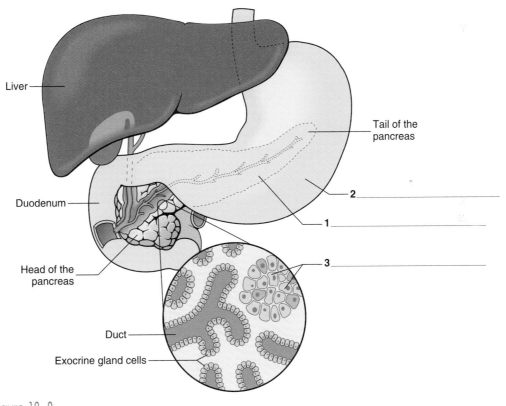

Figure 18–8

The pancreas and surrounding organs.

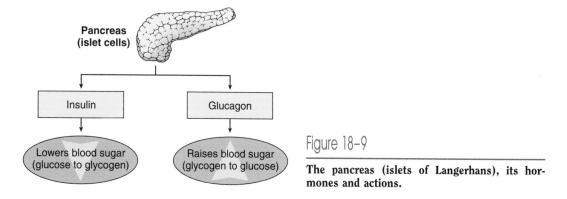

Figure 18-9

The pancreas (islets of Langerhans), its hormones and actions.

B. Function

The islets of Langerhans produce two hormones, **insulin** (produced by beta cells) and **glucagon** (produced by alpha cells). Both of these hormones play a role in the proper metabolism of sugars and starches in the body. Insulin is necessary in the bloodstream so that sugars can pass from the blood into the cells of the body where they are burned to release energy. When blood sugar **(glucose)** is above normal level, insulin is released by the beta islet cells of the pancreas. Insulin causes glucose to enter body cells to be used for energy and stimulates the conversion of **glucose** to **glycogen** (a starch-storage form of sugar) in the liver. Thus, sugar can leave the blood to be stored (as glycogen) or used to release energy. Glucagon, the opposite "twin" of insulin, is released into the blood when sugar levels are below normal. It causes the breakdown of stored liver **glycogen** to **glucose,** so that there is a rise in the sugar content of blood leaving the liver.

Figure 18–9 reviews the secretions of the islet cells and their actions.

VI. Pituitary Gland

A. Location and Structure

Label Figure 18–10.

The **pituitary gland,** also called the **hypophysis,** is a small, pea-sized gland located at the base of the brain in a small, pocket-like depression of the skull called the **sella turcica.** It is a well-protected gland with the entire mass of the brain above it and the nasal cavity below. The ancient Greeks imagined that its function was to produce *pituita* or nasal secretion.

The pituitary consists of two distinct parts: an **anterior lobe** called the **adenohypophysis** [1], which is formed by an upgrowth from the pharynx and is glandular in nature; and a **posterior lobe** called the **neurohypophysis** [2], which is derived from a downgrowth from the base of the brain and is composed of nervous tissue. The **hypothalamus** [3] is a region of the brain that is in close proximity to the pituitary gland. Signals transmitted from the hypothalamus control the secretions by the pituitary gland. Neurons in the hypothalamus send releasing and inhibiting factors (hormones) via capillaries to the anterior pituitary gland. These factors stimulate or inhibit secretion of hormones from the anterior pituitary (Fig. 18–11A). The hypothalamus also produces and secretes hormones directly to the posterior pituitary gland, where the hormones are stored and then released (Fig. 18–11B).

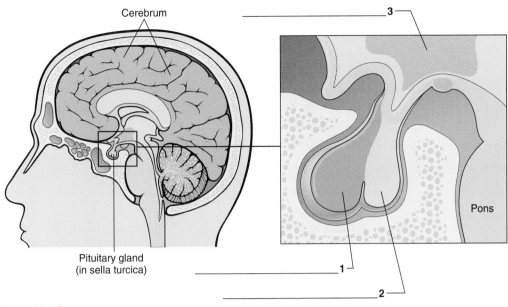

Cerebrum

Pituitary gland
(in sella turcica)

Pons

3

1

2

Figure 18–10

The pituitary gland.

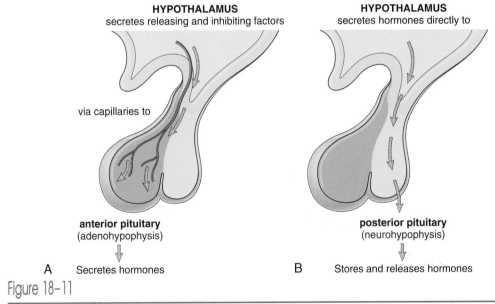

HYPOTHALAMUS
secretes releasing and inhibiting factors

via capillaries to

anterior pituitary
(adenohypophysis)

A   Secretes hormones

HYPOTHALAMUS
secretes hormones directly to

posterior pituitary
(neurohypophysis)

B   Stores and releases hormones

Figure 18–11

(A) The relationship of the **hypothalamus** to the **anterior pituitary gland** and **(B)** its relationship to the **posterior pituitary gland.**

B. Function

The hormones of the **anterior pituitary gland** are

1. **Growth hormone (GH;** also called **somatotropin)**—This hormone promotes protein synthesis that results in the growth of bone and other tissues. Growth hormone also stimulates the liver to make insulin-like growth factor (IGF1) or somatomedin C, which stimulates the growth of bones.
2. **Thyroid-stimulating hormone (TSH;** also called **thyrotropin)**—This hormone stimulates the growth of the thyroid gland and its secretion of thyroxine.
3. **Adrenocorticotropic hormone (ACTH)**—This hormone stimulates the growth of the adrenal cortex and increases its secretion of steroid hormones (primarily cortisol).
4. **Gonadotropic hormones**—There are several gonadotropic hormones that influence the growth and hormone secetion of the ovaries in females and the testes in males. In the female, **follicle-stimulating hormone (FSH)** and **luteinizing hormone (LH)** stimulate the growth of eggs in the ovaries, the production of hormones, and ovulation.

    In the male, FSH influences the production of sperm and LH (as interstitial cell–stimulating hormone) stimulates the testes to produce testosterone.
5. **Prolactin (PRL)**—This hormone stimulates and sustains milk production after birth.
6. **Melanocyte-stimulating hormone (MSH)**—This hormone influences the formation of melanin and causes increased pigmentation of the skin. This effect is observed only when hypersecretion of the hormone occurs.

The **posterior pituitary gland** secretes two important hormones. These hormones are formed in the hypothalamus but secreted through the posterior pituitary gland:

1. **Antidiuretic hormone (ADH)**—This hormone, also known as **vasopressin,** stimulates the reabsorption of water by the kidney tubules. In addition, ADH can also increase blood pressure by constricting arterioles.
2. **Oxytocin**—This hormone stimulates the uterus to contract during childbirth and maintains labor during childbirth. Oxytocin is also secreted during suckling and causes the production of milk from the mammary glands.

Figure 18–12 reviews the hormones secreted by the pituitary gland and their functions.

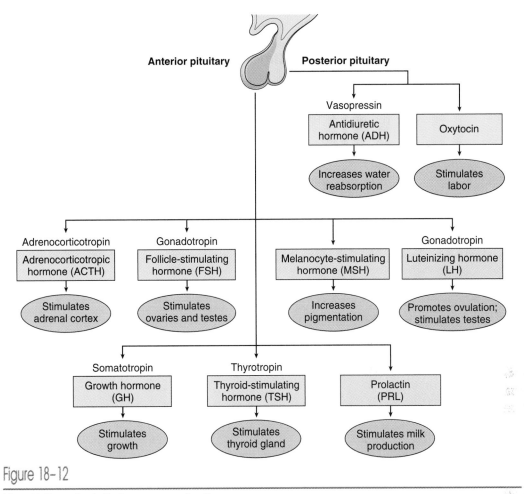

Anterior pituitary   Posterior pituitary

Vasopressin

Antidiuretic hormone (ADH)

Oxytocin

Increases water reabsorption

Stimulates labor

Adrenocorticotropin

Adrenocorticotropic hormone (ACTH)

Stimulates adrenal cortex

Gonadotropin

Follicle-stimulating hormone (FSH)

Stimulates ovaries and testes

Melanocyte-stimulating hormone (MSH)

Increases pigmentation

Gonadotropin

Luteinizing hormone (LH)

Promotes ovulation; stimulates testes

Somatotropin

Growth hormone (GH)

Stimulates growth

Thyrotropin

Thyroid-stimulating hormone (TSH)

Stimulates thyroid gland

Prolactin (PRL)

Stimulates milk production

Figure 18-12

The pituitary gland, its hormones and actions.

VII. Ovaries

A. Location and Structure

The **ovaries** are two small glands located in the lower abdominal region of the female. The ovaries produce the female gamete, the ovum, as well as hormones that are responsible for female sex characteristics and regulation of the menstrual cycle.

B. Function

The ovarian hormones are **estradiol** (an estrogen) and **progesterone.** Estradiol is responsible for the development and maintenance of secondary sex characteristics, such as hair and breast development. Progesterone is responsible for the preparation and maintenance of the uterus in pregnancy.

VIII. Testes

A. Location and Structure

The **testes** are two small, ovoid glands suspended from the inguinal region of the male by the spermatic cord and surrounded by the scrotal sac. The testes produce the male gametes, spermatozoa, as well as the male hormone called **testosterone.**

B. Function

Testosterone is an **androgen** (male steroid hormone) that stimulates and promotes the growth of secondary sex characteristics in the male (development of beard and pubic hair, deepening of voice, and distribution of fat).

Figure 18–13 reviews the hormones secreted by the ovaries and testes.

Table 18–2 lists the major endocrine glands, their hormones, and the actions they produce.

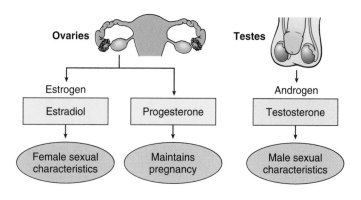

Figure 18-13

The ovaries and testes, their hormones and actions.

Table 18-2. MAJOR ENDOCRINE GLANDS, THE HORMONES THEY PRODUCE, AND THEIR ACTIONS

Endocrine Gland	Hormone	Action
Thyroid	Thyroxine; triiodothyronine	Increases metabolism in body cells
	Calcitonin	Lowers blood calcium
Parathyroids	Parathyroid hormone	Increases blood calcium
Adrenals		
Cortex	Cortisol (glucocorticoid)	Increases blood sugar
	Aldosterone (mineralocorticoid)	Increases reabsorption of sodium
	Sex hormones: androgens, estrogens, and progestins	Maintain secondary sex characteristics
Medulla	Epinephrine (adrenaline)	Sympathomimetic
	Norepinephrine (noradrenaline)	Sympathomimetic
Pancreas		
Islet cells	Insulin	Decreases blood sugar (glucose to glycogen)
	Glucagon	Increases blood sugar (glycogen to glucose)
Pituitary		
Anterior lobe	Growth hormone (GH; somatotropin)	Increases bone and tissue growth
	Thyroid-stimulating hormone (TSH)	Stimulates production of thyroxine and growth of the thyroid gland
	Adrenocorticotropic hormone (ACTH)	Stimulates secretion of hormones from the adrenal cortex, especially cortisol
	Gonadotropins	
	Follicle-stimulating hormone (FSH)	Oogenesis and spermatogenesis
	Luteinizing hormone (LH); or ICSH in a male	Promotes ovulation; testosterone secretion
	Prolactin (PRL)	Promotes growth of breast tissue and milk secretion
	Melanocyte-stimulating hormone (MSH)	Increases pigmentation of the skin
Posterior lobe	Antidiuretic hormone (ADH; vasopressin)	Stimulates reabsorption of water by kidney tubules
	Oxytocin	Stimulates contraction of the uterus during labor and childbirth
Ovaries	Estradiol	Develops and maintains secondary sex characteristics in the female
	Progesterone	Prepares and maintains the uterus in pregnancy
Testes	Testosterone	Promotes growth and maintenance of secondary sex characteristics in the male

IX. Vocabulary

This list will help you review many of the new terms introduced in the text. Short definitions will reinforce your understanding of the terms. See Section XVIII of this chapter for help in pronouncing the more difficult terms.

Major Glands

adrenal cortex	The outer section of each adrenal gland.
adrenal medulla	The inner section of each adrenal gland.
ovaries	Two endocrine glands in a female's lower abdomen; responsible for egg production and estrogen and progesterone secretion.
pancreas	Endocrine gland behind the stomach. Islet cells (islets of Langerhans) secrete hormones from the pancreas.
parathyroid glands	Four small endocrine glands on the posterior side of the thyroid gland.
pituitary gland (hypophysis)	Endocrine gland at the base of the brain; composed of an anterior lobe **(adenohypophysis)** and a posterior lobe **(neurohypophysis).**
testes	Two endocrine glands enclosed in the scrotal sac of a male; responsible for sperm production and testosterone secretion.
thyroid gland	Endocrine gland in the neck.

Hormones

adrenaline	Produced by the adrenal medulla; also called **epinephrine.** Adrenaline increases heart rate and blood pressure.
adrenocorticotropic hormone (ACTH)	Produced by the anterior lobe of the pituitary gland (adenohypophysis); also called **adrenocorticotropin.** ACTH stimulates the adrenal cortex.
aldosterone	Produced by the adrenal cortex; increases salt (sodium) reabsorption.
androgen	Male hormone produced by the testes and to a lesser extent by the adrenal cortex; testosterone is an example.
antidiuretic hormone (ADH)	Secreted by the posterior lobe of the pituitary gland (neurohypophysis). ADH increases reabsorption of water by the kidney and is also known as **vasopressin.**
calcitonin	Produced by the thyroid gland. Calcitonin lowers blood calcium. Also called **thyrocalcitonin.**
cortisol	Produced by the adrenal cortex; increases blood sugar.

epinephrine	Produced by the adrenal medulla; also called **adrenaline.** Epinephrine (a sympathomimetic) increases heart rate and blood pressure and dilates airways.
estradiol	An estrogen (female hormone) produced by the ovaries.
estrogen	Female hormone produced by the ovaries and to a lesser extent by the adrenal cortex.
follicle-stimulating hormone (FSH)	Hormone produced by the anterior lobe of the pituitary gland (adenohypophysis). FSH stimulates hormone secretion and egg production by the ovaries and sperm production by the testes.
glucagon	Hormone produced by the islet cells of the pancreas; increases blood sugar by conversion of glycogen (starch) to glucose.
growth hormone (GH)	Produced by the anterior lobe of the pituitary gland (adenohypophysis); also called **somatotropin.** GH stimulates the growth of bones and tissues.
insulin	Produced by the islet cells (**insula** means island) of the pancreas. Insulin lowers blood sugar by transport and conversion of glucose to glycogen (starch).
luteinizing hormone (LH)	Produced by the anterior lobe of the pituitary gland (adenohypophysis). LH stimulates ovulation in females and (as ICSH) stimulates testosterone secretion in males.
melanocyte-stimulating hormone (MSH)	Produced by the anterior lobe of the pituitary gland (adenohypophysis). High levels of MSH increase the pigmentation of the skin.
norepinephrine	Produced by the adrenal medulla; also called **noradrenaline.** Norepinephrine (a sympathomimetic) increases heart rate and blood pressure. Nor- in chemistry means a parent compound from which another is derived.
oxytocin	Secreted by the posterior lobe of the pituitary gland (neurohypophysis). Oxytocin stimulates contraction of the uterus during labor and childbirth.
parathormone (PTH)	Produced by the parathyroid gland; also called **parathyroid hormone.** PTH increases blood calcium.
progesterone	Produced by the ovaries. Progesterone prepares the uterus for pregnancy.
prolactin (PRL)	Produced by the anterior lobe of the pituitary gland (adenohypophysis). PRL promotes milk secretion.
somatotropin	Produced by the anterior lobe of the pituitary gland (adenohypophysis); also called **growth hormone.**

testosterone	Male hormone produced by the testes.
thyroid-stimulating hormone (TSH)	Produced by the anterior lobe of the pituitary gland (adenohypophysis). TSH acts on the thyroid gland to promote its functioning; also called **thyrotropin.**
thyroxine (T$_4$)	Produced by the thyroid gland; also called **tetraiodothyronine.** T$_4$ increases metabolism in cells.
triiodothyronine (T$_3$)	Produced by the thyroid gland; T$_3$ increases metabolism in cells.
vasopressin	Secreted by the posterior lobe of the pituitary gland (neurohypophysis); also called **antidiuretic hormone.**

Related Terms

catecholamines	Hormones derived from an amino acid and secreted by the adrenal medulla. Epinephrine is a catecholamine.
corticosteroids	Hormones (steroid) produced by the adrenal cortex. Glucocorticoids and mineralocorticoids are examples.
electrolyte	A mineral salt found in the blood and tissues and necessary for proper functioning of cells; potassium, sodium, and calcium are examples.
glucocorticoid	Hormone secreted by the adrenal cortex; necessary for use of sugars, fats, and proteins by the body and for the body's normal response to stress. Cortisol is an example.
homeostasis	The tendency of an organism to maintain a constant internal environment.
hormone	A substance that is produced by an endocrine gland and that travels through the blood to a distant organ or gland where it acts to modify the structure or function of that organ or gland.
hypothalamus	A region of the brain that lies below the thalamus and above the pituitary gland. It produces releasing factors that stimulate the pituitary gland to release hormones.
mineralocorticoid	Steroid hormone produced by the adrenal cortex to regulate the mineral salts (electrolytes) and water balance in the body. Aldosterone is an example.
sella turcica	The cavity in the skull that contains the pituitary gland.
steroid	Complex substance related to fats (derived from a sterol, such as cholesterol) and of which many hormones are made. Examples of steroids are estrogens, androgens, glucocorticoids and mineralocorticoids. **Ster/o** means solid, **-ol** means oil.

sympathomimetic   Pertaining to mimicking or copying the effect of the sympathetic nervous system. Adrenaline is a sympathomimetic hormone (raises blood pressure and heart rate and dilates airways).

X. Combining Forms, Suffixes, Prefixes, and Terminology: Glands and Related Terms

Write the meanings of the medical terms in the spaces provided.

Glands

Combining Forms			
Combining Form	Meaning	Terminology	Meaning
aden/o	gland	adenectomy _____	
adren/o	adrenal glands	adrenopathy _____	
adrenal/o	adrenal glands	adrenalectomy _____	
gonad/o	sex glands (ovaries and testes)	gonadotropin _____	
		-tropin means to act upon, to turn. A gonadotropin acts on (stimulates) the gonads. Examples are FSH and LH.	
		hypogonadism _____	
		Deficiency of gonadotropins can produce hypogonadism.	
pancreat/o	pancreas	pancreatectomy _____	
parathyroid/o	parathyroid gland	parathyroidectomy _____	
pituitar/o	pituitary gland, hypophysis	hypopituitarism _____	
		Pituitary dwarfism (see page 712, Section XI, Abnormal Conditions) is caused by hypopituitarism.	
thyr/o	thyroid gland	thyrotropin hormone _____	
		Thyroid-stimulating hormone (TSH).	
thyroid/o	thyroid gland	thyroiditis _____	

Related Terms

Combining Forms			
Combining Form	Meaning	Terminology	Meaning
andr/o	male	androgen _____	
		Androgens are produced by the testes in males and by the adrenal cortex in males and females.	
calc/o	calcium	hypercalcemia _____	
		hypocalcemia _____	
cortic/o	cortex, outer region	corticosteroid _____	
		Cortisol is an example of a corticosteroid.	
crin/o	secrete	endocrinologist _____	
dips/o	thirst	polydipsia _____	
		Symptom associated with both diabetes mellitus and diabetes insipidus (see page 712, Section XI, Abnormal Conditions).	
estr/o	female	estrogenic _____	
gluc/o	sugar	glucagon _____	
		-agon means to assemble or gather together. Glucagon raises blood sugar by stimulating its release from glycogen into the bloodstream.	
glyc/o	sugar	hyperglycemia _____	
		glycemic _____	
		A patient with diabetes mellitus requires glycemic control.	
		glycogen _____	
		Glycogen is animal starch that can be broken down into glucose by the hormone glucagon.	
home/o	sameness	homeostasis _____	
		-stasis means to control.	

hormon/o	hormone	<u>hormon</u>al _____
insulin/o	insulin	hypo<u>insulin</u>ism _____
kal/i	potassium (an electrolyte)	hypo<u>kal</u>emia _____

This condition can occur in dehydration and with excessive vomiting and diarrhea. The heart is particularly sensitive to potassium loss.

lact/o	milk	pro<u>lact</u>in _____

-in means a substance.

myx/o	mucus	<u>myx</u>edema _____

Mucus-like material accumulates under the skin. See page 708, Section XI, Abnormal Conditions, under hypothyroidism.

natr/o	sodium (an electrolyte)	hypo<u>natr</u>emia _____

Occurs with hyposecretion of the adrenal cortex as salts and water leave the body.

phys/o	growing	hypo<u>phys</u>ectomy _____

The hypophysis is the pituitary gland, which is so named because it grows from the undersurface (hypo-) of the brain.

somat/o	body	<u>somat</u>otropin _____

Also called growth hormone.

ster/o	solid structure	<u>ster</u>oid _____

This complex, solid, ring-shaped molecule resembles a sterol (such as cholesterol); many hormones (androgens, estrogens, glucocorticoids, and mineralocorticoids) are steroids.

toc/o	childbirth	oxy<u>toc</u>in _____

oxy- means swift, rapid.

toxic/o	poison	thyro<u>toxic</u>osis _____

This condition is caused by excessive thyroid gland activity and oversecretion of thyroid hormone. Symptoms are sweating, weight loss, tachycardia, and nervousness.

ur/o	urine	antidi<u>ur</u>etic hormone _____

This posterior pituitary hormone affects the kidneys and reduces water loss.

Suffixes

Suffix	Meaning	Terminology	Meaning
-agon	assemble, gather together	glucagon _____	
-in, ine	a substance	epinephrine _____	
-tropin	stimulating the function of (to turn or act upon)	adrenocorticotropin _____	
		-tropic is the adjective form (adrenocorticotropic hormone).	
-uria	urine condition	glycosuria _____	
		A symptom of diabetes mellitus.	

Prefixes

Prefix	Meaning	Terminology	Meaning
eu-	good, normal	euthyroid _____	
oxy-	rapid, sharp, acid	oxytocin _____	
pan-	all	panhypopituitarism _____	
tetra-	four	tetraiodothyronine _____	
		iod/o means iodine.	
tri-	three	triiodothyronine _____	

XI. Abnormal Conditions

Thyroid Gland

Enlargement of the thyroid gland is known as **goiter** (Fig. 18–14A). Goiter may be a symptom of many different conditions. **Endemic (en-** means in; **dem/o** means people) **goiter** occurs in certain regions and peoples as a result of deficiency of **iodine** in the diet. A glue-like or gelatinous material called **colloid** collects in the thyroid, and the gland enlarges as it works harder to compensate for the scarcity of iodine. Treatment of this type of goiter is to increase the supply of iodine in the diet.

Another type of goiter is **nodular** or **adenomatous goiter,** in which hyperplasia occurs as well as nodules and adenomas. Some patients develop hyperthyroidism with symptoms such as rapid pulse, tremors, nervousness, and excessive sweating. Treatment consists of use of thyroid hormone to suppress the normal thyroid functioning (by reducing TSH production).

Hypersecretion

hyperthyroidism   **Overactivity of the thyroid gland.**

The most common form of this condition is known as **thyrotoxicosis** or **Graves disease.** Hyperplasia of the thyroid parenchyma (glandular cells) occurs, so that excessive hormone is produced. The metabolic rate in cells is increased, leading to thyrotoxic symptoms as in nodular or adenomatous goiter. The term **thyroid storm** is used to indicate the abrupt onset of severe hyperthyroidism. In addition, **exophthalmos** (protrusion of the eyeballs) occurs as a result of the swelling of tissue behind the eyeball. The cause is unclear, although it is currently thought to be an immunological disorder. Treatment may include thyroidectomy, management with antithyroid drugs that reduce the amount of thyroid hormone produced by the gland, or administration of radioactive iodine, which destroys the overactive glandular tissue. Figure 18–14B shows a patient with exophthalmos and Graves disease.

Figure 18–14

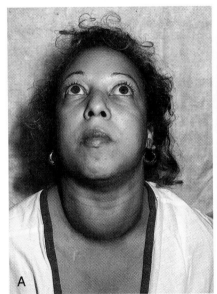
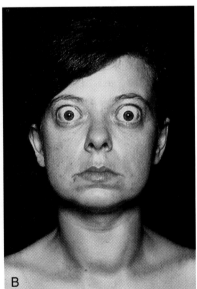

(A) Goiter. Notice the wide neck, indicating enlargement of the thyroid gland. **(B) Exophthalmos** in Graves disease. Note the staring or startled expression. (A from Jarvis C: Physical Examination and Health Assessment, 2nd ed. Philadelphia, WB Saunders, 1996, page 296; B from Seidel H et al: Mosby's Guide to Physical Examination, 4th ed. St. Louis, Mosby, 1998, page 264.)

Hyposecretion

hypothyroidism

Underactivity of the thyroid gland.

Any one of several conditions can produce hypothyroidism (thyroidectomy, endemic goiter, destruction of the gland by irradiation), but all have similar physiological effects. These include fatigue, muscular and mental sluggishness, and constipation. Two examples of hypothyroidism are

Myxedema—This is advanced hypothyroidism in adulthood. Atrophy of the thyroid gland occurs, and practically no hormone is produced. The skin becomes dry and puffy (edema) because of the collection of mucus-like (**myx/o** means mucus) material under the skin. Many patients also develop atherosclerosis because lack of thyroid hormone increases the quantity of blood lipids (fats). Recovery may be complete if thyroid hormone is given soon after symptoms appear. Figure 18–15A shows a patient with myxedema.

Cretinism—Extreme hypothyroidism during infancy and childhood leads to a lack of normal physical and mental growth. Skeletal growth is more inhibited than soft tissue growth, so the **cretin** has the appearance of an obese, short, and stocky child. Treatment consists of the administration of thyroid hormone, which may be able to reverse some of the hypothyroid effects.

Neoplasms

thyroid carcinoma

Cancer of the thyroid gland.

Some tumors are very slow growing, and others may metastasize widely. Adenomas (benign growths) can be distinguished from carcinomas (malignant growths) by radioactive iodine tracer scans. "Hot" tumor areas (those collecting more radioactivity than surrounding tissues) usually indicate hyperthyroidism and benign growth; "cold," nonfunctional nodules can be either benign or malignant. Ultimately, fine-needle aspiration, surgical biopsy, or excision is often required to make the diagnosis.

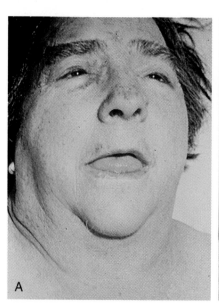
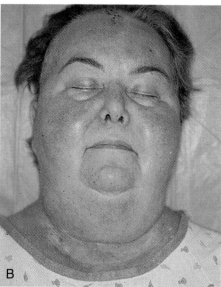

Figure 18–15

(A) Myxedema. Note the dull, puffy, yellowed skin; coarse, sparse hair; periorbital (around the orbits of the eyes) edema; prominent tongue. **(B) Cushing syndrome.** Facial features include a rounded, or moon-shaped, face with thin, erythematous skin. Hirsutism may also be present. (A courtesy of Paul W. Ladenson, M.D., The Johns Hopkins University and Hospital, Baltimore, MD; B from Seidel HM et al: Mosby's Guide to Physical Examination, 4th ed. St. Louis, Mosby, 1998, page 263.)

Parathyroid Glands
Hypersecretion

hyperparathyroidism   **Excessive production of parathormone.**

Hypercalcemia occurs as calcium leaves the bones and enters the bloodstream. Bones become decalcified and susceptible to fractures and cysts, as in **osteitis fibrosa cystica.** Kidney stones can occur as a result of hypercalcemia. The cause is often a parathyroid tumor, which is resected as treatment of the condition.

Hyposecretion

hypoparathyroidism   **Deficient production of parathyroid hormone.**

Hypocalcemia results as calcium remains in bones and is unable to enter the bloodstream. This leads to muscle and nerve weakness with spasms of muscles, a condition called **tetany** (constant muscle contraction). Administration of calcium plus large quantities of vitamin D (to promote absorption of calcium) can control the calcium level in the bloodstream.

Adrenal Cortex
Hypersecretion

adrenal virilism   **Excessive output of adrenal androgens.**

Adrenal hyperplasia or tumor can cause this condition in adult women. Symptoms include amenorrhea, and virilism, including **hirsutism** (excessive hair on the face and body), acne, and deepening of the voice. Drug therapy to suppress androgen production and adrenalectomy are possible treatments.

Cushing syndrome   **A group of symptoms produced by excess of cortisol from the adrenal cortex.**

Obesity, moon-like fullness of the face, excess deposition of fat in the thoracic region of the back (so-called buffalo hump), hyperglycemia, hypernatremia, hypokalemia, osteoporosis, and hypertension occur with hypercortisolism. The cause may be excess ACTH secretion (called Cushing syndrome) or tumor of the adrenal cortex. Tumors and disseminated cancers can be associated with ectopic secretion of hormone, such as ectopic ACTH produced by nonendocrine neoplasms (lung and thyroid tumors). Figure 18–15B shows a woman with Cushing syndrome.

In clinical practice, most cases of Cushing syndrome are caused by the administration of exogenous (from outside the body) glucocorticoids in the treatment of immune disorders, such as rheumatoid arthritis, lupus erythematosus, asthma, and renal and skin conditions.

Hyposecretion

Addison disease   **Hypofunctioning of the adrenal cortex.**

Mineralocorticoids and glucocorticoids are produced in deficient amounts. Hypoglycemia (from deficient glucocorticoids), hyponatremia (excretion of large amounts of water and salts from deficient mineralocorticoids), fatigue, weakness, weight loss, low blood pressure, syncope and darker pigmentation of the skin (because of increased blood levels of MSH) are symptoms of the condition. Most cases are caused by an autoimmune adrenalitis. Treatment consists of daily cortisone administration and intake of salts or administration of a synthetic form of aldosterone.

Adrenal Medulla

Hypersecretion

pheochromocytoma

Benign tumor of the adrenal medulla (tumor cells stain a dark or dusky [phe/o] color [chrom/o]).

The tumor cells produce excess secretion of epinephrine and norepinephrine. Symptoms are hypertension, palpitations, severe headaches, sweating, flushing of the face, and muscle spasms. Surgery to remove the tumor and administration of antihypertensive drugs are possible treatments.

Pancreas

Hypersecretion

hyperinsulinism

Excess secretion of insulin causing hypoglycemia.

The cause may be a tumor of the pancreas (benign adenoma or carcinoma) or an overdose of insulin. Hypoglycemia occurs as insulin draws sugar out of the bloodstream. Fainting spells, convulsions, and loss of consciousness are common because a minimal level of blood sugar is necessary for proper mental functioning.

Hyposecretion

diabetes mellitus

Lack of insulin secretion or resistance of insulin in promoting sugar, starch, and fat metabolism in cells.

In diabetes mellitus (mellitus means sweet or sugary), insulin insufficiency or ineffectiveness prevents sugar from leaving the blood and entering the body cells, where it is normally used to produce energy. There are two major types of diabetes mellitus.

Type 1 diabetes, with onset usually in childhood, involves destruction of the beta islet cells of the pancreas and complete deficiency of insulin in the body. Patients are usually thin and require frequent injections of insulin to maintain a normal level of glucose in the blood.

Type 2 diabetes is a separate disease from type 1 and has a different inheritance pattern. Patients are usually older, and obesity is very common. The islet cells are not destroyed, and there is a relative deficiency of insulin secretion with a resistance by target tissues to the action of insulin. Treatment is with diet, weight reduction, exercise and, if necessary, insulin or oral hypoglycemic agents. The oral hypoglycemic agents can stimulate the release of insulin from the pancreas and improve the body's sensitivity to insulin.

Table 18–3 compares the features, symptoms, and treatments of type 1 and type 2 diabetes.

Both type 1 and type 2 diabetes are associated with primary and secondary complications. **Primary complications** of type 1 include **ketoacidosis** (fats are improperly burned, leading to an accumulation of ketones in the body) and **coma** when blood sugar concentration gets too high or the patient receives an insufficient amount of insulin. **Hypoglycemia** occurs when too much insulin is taken by the patient.

Secondary (long-term) **complications** appear many years after the patient develops diabetes. These include eye disorders such as glaucoma and cataract and destruction of the blood vessels of the retina **(diabetic retinopathy),** causing visual loss and blindness; destruction of the kidneys **(diabetic nephropathy),** causing renal insufficiency and often requiring hemodialysis or renal transplantation; destruction of blood vessels, with **atherosclerosis** leading to

Table 18-3. COMPARISON OF TYPE 1 AND TYPE 2 DIABETES MELLITUS

	Type 1	Type 2
FEATURES	Usually occurs **before age 30** **Abrupt, rapid onset** **Little or no insulin** production **Thin** or **normal** body weight at onset **Ketoacidosis** often occurs	Usually occurs **after age 30** **Gradual onset; asymptomatic** **Insulin usually present** 85% are **obese** **Ketoacidosis** seldom occurs
SYMPTOMS	**Polyuria** (kidneys fail to reabsorb water) **Polydipsia** (dehydration causes thirst) **Polyphagia** (tissue breakdown causes hunger)	**Polyuria** sometimes seen **Polydipsia** sometimes seen **Polyphagia** sometimes seen
TREATMENT	Insulin	**Diet; oral hypoglycemics** or **insulin**

stroke, heart disease, and peripherovascular ischemia (gangrene, infection, and loss of limbs); and destruction of nerves **(diabetic neuropathy)** involving pain or loss of sensation, most commonly in the extremities. Figure 18–16 reviews the secondary complications of diabetes mellitus.

As a result of hormonal changes, **gestational diabetes** can occur in pregnant women during the 2nd or 3rd trimester of pregnancy. After delivery, blood glucose usually returns to normal. Type 2 diabetes may develop in these women within 5 to 15 years postpartum.

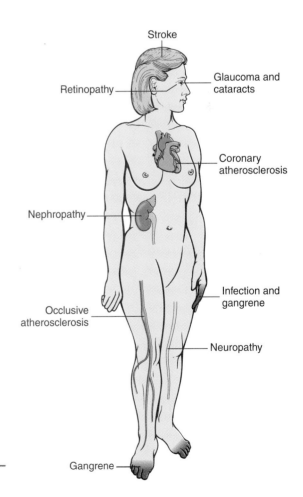

Figure 18-16

Secondary complications of diabetes mellitus.

Pituitary Gland (Anterior Lobe)

Hypersecretion

acromegaly

Enlargement of the extremities (acr/o means extremities) caused by hypersecretion of the anterior pituitary *after* puberty.

An excess of growth hormone (GH) is produced by adenomas of the pituitary gland that occur during adulthood. This excess GH stimulates the liver to secrete a hormone (somatomedin C, or IGF) that causes the clinical manifestations of acromegaly. Bones in the hands, feet, face, and jaw grow abnormally large, producing a characteristic Frankenstein-type facial appearance. The pituitary adenoma can be irradiated or surgically removed. Figure 18–17 shows a woman with acromegaly. Measurement of blood levels of somatomedin C as GH fluctuates is a test for acromegaly.

gigantism

Hyperfunctioning of the pituitary gland *before* puberty, leading to abnormal overgrowth of the body.

Benign adenomas of the pituitary gland that occur before a child reaches puberty produce an excess of growth hormone. Gigantism can be corrected by early diagnosis in childhood, followed by resection of the tumor or irradiation of the pituitary.

Hyposecretion

dwarfism

Congenital hyposecretion of growth hormone; hypopituitary dwarfism.

The children affected are normal mentally, but their bones remain small and underdeveloped. Treatment consists of administration of growth hormone. Achondroplastic dwarfs differ from hypopituitary dwarfs in that they suffer from a genetic defect in cartilage formation that adversely affects the growth of bones.

panhypopituitarism

All pituitary hormones are deficient.

Tumors of the sella turcica as well as arterial aneurysms may be etiological factors. Functions of target glands (adrenals, thyroid, ovaries, and testes) are also adversely affected.

Pituitary Gland (Posterior Lobe)

Hypersecretion

syndrome of inappropriate ADH (SIADH)

Excessive secretion of antidiuretic hormone (ADH).

Hypersecretion of ADH produces excess water retention in the body. Treatment consists of dietary water restriction. Tumor, drug reactions, and head injury are some of the possible causes.

Hyposecretion

diabetes insipidus

Insufficient secretion of antidiuretic hormone (vasopressin).

Deficient antidiuretic hormone causes the kidney tubules to fail to hold back (reabsorb) needed water and salts. Clinical symptoms include polyuria and polydipsia. Synthetic preparations of ADH are administered with nasal sprays or intramuscularly as treatment. **Insipidus** means tasteless, reflecting the condition of dilute urine.

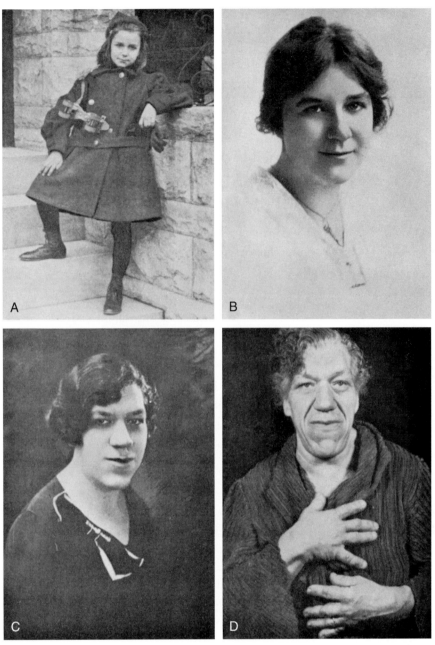

Figure 18-17

Progression of acromegaly: (A) patient at age 9; **(B)** age 16, with possible early features of acromegaly; **(C)** age 33, well-established acromegaly; **(D)** age 52, end-stage acromegaly. (A–D from Clinical Pathological Conference. Am J Med 1956; 20:133.)

Table 18-4. ABNORMAL CONDITIONS OF ENDOCRINE GLANDS

Endocrine Gland	Hypersecretion	Hyposecretion
Adrenal cortex	Adrenal virilism Cushing syndrome	Addison disease
Adrenal medulla	Pheochromocytoma	
Pancreas	Hyperinsulinism	Diabetes mellitus
Parathyroid glands	Hyperparathyroidism (osteitis fibrosa cystica)	Hypoparathyroidism (tetany, hypocalcemia)
Pituitary (anterior lobe)	Acromegaly Gigantism	Dwarfism Panhypopituitarism
Pituitary (posterior lobe)	Syndrome of inappropriate antidiuretic hormone	Diabetes insipidus
Thyroid gland	Exophthalmic goiter (Graves disease, thyrotoxicosis) Nodular (adenomatous) goiter	Cretinism (children) Endemic goiter Myxedema (adults)

Table 18–4 reviews the abnormal conditions associated with hypersecretions and hyposecretions of the endocrine glands.

XII. Laboratory Tests

serum and urine tests
These tests measure hormones and other substances (electrolytes and glucose) in blood and urine as indicators of endocrine function.

fasting blood sugar (FBS)
This test measures the glucose levels in a blood sample taken from a fasting patient **(fasting blood sugar)** and in specimens taken 30 minutes, 1 hour, 2 hours, and 3 hours after ingestion of 75 gm of glucose. Delayed return of blood glucose to normal levels indicates diabetes mellitus.

An **oral glucose tolerance test** (not fasting) is used in the diagnosis of gestational diabetes. The **glycosylated hemoglobin test** measures long-term control of blood glucose. A urinary microalbumin test measures small quantities of albumin in the urine as a marker or harbinger of diabetic neuropathy.

radioimmunoassay (RIA)
This test measures hormone levels in plasma. The test is based on the ability of antibodies to bind specifically to radioactively labeled hormone molecules and to nonradioactively labeled molecules.

thyroid function tests
These tests measure the levels of T_4, T_3, and TSH in the bloodstream.

XIII. Clinical Procedures

exophthalmometry

This test measures the extent of eyeball protrusion (exophthalmos) as evidenced in Graves disease.

computed tomography (CT) scans

These transverse x-ray views of the pituitary gland and other endocrine organs are useful in the diagnosis of pathological conditions.

magnetic resonance imaging (MRI) of the head

Magnetic and radiofrequency pulses are used to produce images of the hypothalamus and pituitary gland and locate abnormalities in that region.

thyroid scan

A radioactive compound is administered and localizes in the thyroid gland. The gland is then visualized with a scanner device to detect tumors or nodules.

radioactive iodine uptake

Radioactive iodine is administered orally, and its uptake into the thyroid gland is measured as evidence of thyroid function.

XIV. ABBREVIATIONS

ACTH	adrenocorticotropic hormone	**LH**	luteinizing hormone
ADH	antidiuretic hormone (vasopressin)	**MSH**	melanocyte-stimulating hormone
BMR	basal metabolic rate (an indicator of thyroid function, but not in current use)	**Na**	sodium
		NIDDM	non–insulin-dependent diabetes mellitus; type 2 diabetes
DI	diabetes insipidus		
DM	diabetes mellitus	**17-OH**	17-hydroxycorticosteroids
FBG	fasting blood glucose	**PRL**	prolactin
FBS	fasting blood sugar	**PTH**	parathyroid hormone (parathormone)
FSH	follicle-stimulating hormone	**RIA**	radioimmunoassay; measures hormone levels in plasma
GH	growth hormone		
ICSH	interstitial cell-stimulating hormone	**SIADH**	syndrome of inappropriate ADH
IDDM	insulin-dependent diabetes mellitus; type 1 diabetes	T_3	triiodothyronine
		T_4	thyroxine
IGF	insulin-like growth factors; also called somatomedins (produced in the liver, they stimulate the growth of bones)	**TFT**	thyroid function test
		TSH	thyroid-stimulating hormone
K	potassium		

XV. Practical Applications

Answers to the questions in each case report are on page 725 after Answers to Exercises.

Case Report 1

A 24-year-old college student, known diabetic, was admitted for treatment of ketoacidosis. He had a several-year history of diabetes and had been taking insulin in the morning and in the evening. After the history was pieced together from the patient and his friends, it appeared that he had been getting progressively ill over several days following a flu-like episode and may well not have taken his insulin on the day of admission. He was found, slightly drowsy and confused, by class-mates. His respirations were rapid, his pulse was 126, and he offered no sensible answers to questions. Blood sugar level was elevated at 728 mg/dL [100 mg/dL is normal], and blood ketones were positive. The patient was treated with insulin intravenously, and over the course of the next 24 hours the ketoacidosis cleared.

Questions

1. Ketoacidosis is a complication of
   (A) diabetes insipidus
   (B) diabetes mellitus
   (C) both A and B

2. A symptom of ketoacidosis is
   (A) tachypnea
   (B) bradycardia
   (C) hypoglycemia

3. Ketoacidosis occurs when
   (A) insulin blood levels are high
   (B) sugar is not transported to cells and fats are burned improperly
   (C) insulin is given intravenously

Case Report 2

A 42-year-old woman presented with a 6-month history of progressive weakness. She had facial and central obesity with muscle wasting in the extremities. As an initial screening test, a 24-hour urine collection for cortisol determination revealed high levels. Her ACTH level was low. On CT scan a 3-cm mass was found in the left adrenal. When the mass was resected, it proved to be a 3-cm, smooth, yellow adrenocortical adenoma that secreted cortisol. The patient's condition (Cushing syndrome) normalized after surgery.

Questions

1. Symptoms of Cushing syndrome are
   (A) hirsutism and hypergonadism
   (B) palpitations
   (C) moon-like fullness of the face and deposition of fat
2. What factors pointed to a diagnosis of Cushing syndrome?
   (A) pituitary gland tumor on CT scan
   (B) hypersecretion of ACTH
   (C) hypersecretion of cortisol and adrenal mass on CT scan
3. Surgery performed to correct this condition was
   (A) adrenocortical adenoma resection
   (B) hypophysectomy
   (C) both A and B

Case Report 3

Graves disease, as characterized by exophthalmos and stare, was diagnosed in a 51-year-old man. Examination revealed a history of nervousness, palpitation, weight loss, diarrhea, dyspnea on exertion, insomnia, heat intolerance, and fatigue. An ECG showed atrial fibrillation with a ventricular rate of about 180 beats per minute, which was treated with digoxin and propranolol. A chest x-ray film disclosed cardiomegaly. Thyroid function tests showed T_4 and T_3 levels to be elevated, and a thyroid scan showed diffuse enlargement of the gland. The patient was treated with radioactive iodine and is now euthyroid. The exophthalmos has not resolved, however.

Questions

1. Symptoms of Graves disease are
   (A) bulging eyeballs
   (B) difficult breathing on exertion
   (C) A and B
2. Atrial fibrillation means that
   (A) the heart is enlarged
   (B) the heart rate is less than 180 beats per minute
   (C) the heart rate is rapid and irregular
3. Blood tests revealed that
   (A) the thyroid gland was hypersecreting
   (B) the thyroid gland was hyposecreting
   (C) goiter was present
4. The patient was treated and
   (A) exophthalmia has regressed
   (B) is still having palpitations
   (C) his thyroid gland is functioning normally

XVI. Exercises

Remember to check your answers carefully with those given in Section XVII, Answers to Exercises.

A. Name the endocrine organs (including appropriate lobe or region) that produce the following hormones.

1. follicle-stimulating hormone _____

2. vasopressin _____

3. aldosterone _____

4. insulin _____

5. thyroxine _____

6. cortisol _____

7. gonadotropic hormones _____

8. epinephrine _____

9. oxytocin _____

10. prolactin _____

11. growth hormone _____

12. glucagon _____

13. adrenocorticotropic hormone _____

14. estradiol _____

15. progesterone _____

16. testosterone _____

17. melanocyte-stimulating hormone _____

B. Give the meanings of the following abbreviations for hormones.

1. ADH _____

2. ACTH _____

3. LH _____

4. FSH _____

5. TSH _____

6. PTH _____

7. GH _____

8. PRL _____

9. T_4 _____

10. T_3 _____

C. Match the following hormones with their actions.

insulin   aldosterone   estradiol
parathyroid hormone   epinephrine   ACTH
testosterone   thyroxine   cortisol
ADH

1. sympathomimetic; raises heart rate and blood pressure _____

2. promotes growth and maintenance of male sex characteristics _____

3. stimulates water reabsorption by kidney tubules; decreases urine output _____

4. increases metabolism in body cells _____

5. raises blood calcium _____

6. increases reabsorption of sodium by kidney tubules _____

7. stimulates secretion of hormones from the adrenal cortex _____

8. increases blood sugar _____

9. helps transport glucose to cells and decreases blood sugar _____

10. develops and maintains female sex characteristics _____

D. Indicate whether the following conditions are related to hypersecretion or hyposecretion. Also, select from the following the endocrine gland and hormone involved in each disease.

Glands

thyroid	neurohypophysis
adrenal cortex	adenohypophysis
pancreas	parathyroid gland
testes	ovaries
adrenal medulla	

Hormones

GH	ADH
parathyroid hormone	insulin
cortisol	aldosterone
thyroxine	epinephrine

Disease	*Hypo or Hyper*	*Gland and Hormone*
1. Cushing syndrome	_____	_____
2. tetany	_____	_____
3. Graves disease	_____	_____
4. diabetes insipidus	_____	_____
5. acromegaly	_____	_____
6. myxedema	_____	_____
7. osteitis fibrosa cystica	_____	_____
8. diabetes mellitus	_____	_____
9. Addison disease	_____	_____
10. gigantism	_____	_____
11. endemic goiter	_____	_____
12. cretinism	_____	_____
13. pheochromocytoma	_____	_____

E. Build medical terms based on the definitions and word parts given.

1. abnormal condition (poison) of the thyroid gland: thyro _____

2. removal of the pancreas: _____ ectomy

3. condition of deficiency or underdevelopment of the sex organs: hypo _____

4. pertaining to producing female (characteristics): _____ genic

5. removal of the pituitary gland: _____ ectomy

6. deficiency of calcium in the blood: hypo _____

7. excessive sugar in the blood: _____ emia

8. inflammation of the thyroid gland: _____ itis

9. specialist in the study of hormone disorders: _____ ist

10. disease condition of the adrenal glands: adren _____

F. Give the meanings of the following conditions.

1. hyponatremia _____

2. polydipsia _____

3. hyperkalemia _____

4. hypercalcemia _____

5. hypoglycemia _____

6. glycosuria _____

7. euthyroid _____

8. hyperthyroidism _____

9. tetany _____

10. ketoacidosis _____

G. The following hormones are all produced by the anterior lobe of the pituitary gland (note that they all have the same suffix, -tropin). Name the target tissue they act on or stimulate in the body.

1. gonadotropins _____

2. somatotropin _____

3. thyrotropin _____

4. adrenocorticotropin _____

H. Give the meanings of the following medical terms.

1. steroids _____

2. catecholamines _____

3. adenohypophysis _____

4. tetany _____

5. exophthalmos _____

6. mineralocorticoids _____

7. homeostasis _____

8. sympathomimetic _____

9. glucocorticoids _____

10. epinephrine _____

11. glycogen _____

12. androgen _____

13. corticosteroid _____

14. oxytocin _____

15. tetraiodothyronine _____

16. adrenal virilism _____

17. thyroid carcinoma _____

18. hirsutism _____

19. acromegaly _____

20. estradiol _____

I. Give the meanings of the following terms related to diabetes mellitus.

1. Type 1 _____

2. diabetic neuropathy _____

3. ketoacidosis _____

4. hypoglycemia _____

5. Type 2 _____

6. diabetic retinopathy _____

7. diabetic coma _____

8. diabetic nephropathy _____

9. atherosclerosis _____

10. hyperglycemia _____

J. Explain the following laboratory tests or clinical procedures related to the endocrine system.

1. thyroid scan _____

2. fasting blood sugar _____

3. RIA _____

4. exophthalmometry _____

K. Circle the term that best fits the meaning of the sentence.

1. Phyllis was diagnosed with Graves disease when her husband noticed her (**panhypopituitarism, hirsutism, exophthalmos**). Her eyes seemed to be bulging out of their sockets.

2. Helen had a primary brain tumor called a (**pituitary, thyroid, adrenal**) adenoma. Her entire endocrine system was disrupted and her physician recommended surgery and radiation to help relieve her symptoms.

3. Bessie's facial features gradually became "rough" in her late 30s and 40s. By the time she was 50, her children noticed her very large hands and recommended that she see an endocrinologist, who diagnosed her chronically progressive condition as (**hyperinsulism, gigantism, acromegaly**).

4. Bobby was brought into the emergency room because he was found passed out in the kitchen. He had forgotten his insulin and had developed (**Cushing disease, hyperparathyroidism, diabetic ketoacidosis**).

5. Because her 1-hour test of blood sugar was slightly abnormal, Selma's obstetrician ordered a (**glucose tolerance test, thyroid function test, Pap smear**) to rule out gestational (**hyperthyroidism, chlamydial infection, diabetes**).

XVII. Answers to Exercises

A

1. anterior lobe of the pituitary gland (adenohypophysis)
2. posterior lobe of the pituitary gland (neurohypophysis)
3. adrenal cortex
4. islet cells of the pancreas
5. thyroid gland
6. adrenal cortex
7. anterior lobe of the pituitary gland; these hormones are FSH and LH
8. adrenal medulla
9. posterior lobe of the pituitary gland
10. anterior lobe of the pituitary gland
11. anterior lobe of the pituitary gland
12. islet cells of the pancreas
13. anterior lobe of the pituitary gland
14. ovaries
15. ovaries
16. testes
17. anterior lobe of the pituitary gland

B

1. antidiuretic hormone
2. adrenocorticotropic hormone
3. luteinizing hormone
4. follicle-stimulating hormone
5. thyroid-stimulating hormone
6. parathyroid hormone
7. growth hormone
8. prolactin
9. thyroxine
10. triiodothyronine

C

1. epinephrine
2. testosterone
3. ADH
4. thyroxine
5. parathyroid hormone
6. aldosterone
7. ACTH
8. cortisol
9. insulin
10. estradiol

D

1. hypersecretion; adrenal cortex; cortisol
2. hyposecretion; parathyroid gland; parathyroid hormone
3. hypersecretion; thyroid gland; thyroxine
4. hyposecretion; neurohypophysis; ADH
5. hypersecretion; adenohypophysis; GH
6. hyposecretion; thyroid gland; thyroxine
7. hypersecretion; parathyroid gland; parathyroid hormone
8. hyposecretion; pancreas; insulin
9. hyposecretion; adrenal cortex; aldosterone and cortisol
10. hypersecretion; adenohypophysis; GH
11. hyposecretion; thyroid gland; thyroxine
12. hyposecretion; thyroid gland; thyroxine
13. hypersecretion; adrenal medulla; epinephrine

E

1. thyrotoxicosis
2. pancreatectomy
3. hypogonadism
4. estrogenic
5. hypophysectomy
6. hypocalcemia
7. hyperglycemia
8. thyroiditis
9. endocrinologist
10. adrenopathy

F

1. deficient sodium in the blood
2. condition of excessive thirst
3. excessive potassium in the blood
4. excessive calcium in the blood
5. deficient sugar in the blood
6. condition of sugar in the urine
7. normal thyroid function
8. condition of increased secretion from the thyroid gland
9. constant muscle contraction (result of hypoparathyroidism)
10. condition of excessive ketones (acids) in the blood as a result of diabetes mellitus

G

1. the male and female sex organs (ovaries and testes); examples of gonadotropins are FSH and LH
2. bones; another name for somatotropin is growth hormone
3. thyroid gland; another name for thyrotropin is thyroid-stimulating hormone
4. adrenal cortex; another name for adrenocorticotropin is adrenocorticotropic hormone (ACTH)

H

1. Complex substances derived from cholesterol; hormones from the adrenal cortex and sex hormones are steroids.
2. Complex substances derived from an amino acid; epinephrine (adrenaline) and norepinephrine (noradrenaline) are examples.
3. Anterior lobe of the pituitary gland.
4. Continuous contractions of muscles associated with low levels of parathyroid hormone.
5. Eyeballs that bulge outward; associated with hyperthyroidism.
6. Steroid hormones from the adrenal cortex (outer region of the adrenal gland) that influence salt (minerals such as sodium and potassium) metabolism.

7. A state of equilibrium in the body with respect to function, fluids, and times.
8. A substance that mimics the action of the sympathetic nerves; epinephrine (adrenaline) is an example.
9. Steroid hormones from the adrenal cortex that influence sugar metabolism in the body.
10. Catecholamine hormone from the adrenal medulla; adrenaline.
11. Animal starch; storage form of glucose.
12. Male hormone; testosterone is an example.
13. Hormone secreted by the adrenal cortex; cortisol is an example.

14. Hormone from the posterior lobe of the pituitary that stimulates contraction of the uterus during labor.
15. Major hormone from the thyroid gland; thyroxine (contains four iodine atoms).
16. Abnormal secretion of androgens from the adrenal cortex produces masculine characteristics in a female.
17. Cancerous tumor of the thyroid gland.
18. Excessive hair on the body (result of excessive secretion of androgens).
19. Enlargement of extremities (excessive secretion of growth hormone after puberty).
20. Female hormone; an estrogen.

I

1. Destruction of the beta islets of Langerhans; insulin is not produced (insulin-dependent diabetes mellitus, IDDM)
2. Destruction of nerves as a secondary complication of diabetes mellitus.
3. Abnormal condition of high levels of ketones (acids) in the blood as a result of improper burning of fats. Fats are burned because the cells do not have sugar available as a result of lack of insulin or inability of insulin to act.

4. Too little sugar in the blood. This can occur if too much insulin is taken by a diabetic patient.
5. Insulin deficiency and resistance by target tissue to the action of insulin; (non–insulin-dependent diabetes mellitus, NIDDM)
6. Destruction of blood vessels in the retina as a secondary complication of diabetes mellitus.
7. Unconsciousness due to high levels of sugar in the blood. Water leaves cells

to balance the large amounts of sugar in the blood, leading to cellular dehydration.
8. Destruction of the kidneys as a secondary complication of diabetes mellitus.
9. Collection of fatty plaque in arteries.
10. High level of sugar in the blood; insulin is unavailable or unable to transport sugar from the blood into cells.

J

1. A radioactive compound is given, and the thyroid gland is pictured using a scanning device.
2. Measurement of blood sugar levels in a fasting patient and after intervals of 30

minutes and 1, 2, and 3 hours following ingestion of glucose.
3. Radioimmunoassay; hormone concentrations are measured by using antibodies, nonradioactively labeled

hormone, and radioactively labeled hormone.
4. Measurement of eyeball protrusion (symptom of Graves disease).

K

1. exophthalmos
2. pituitary
3. acromegaly

4. diabetic ketoacidosis
5. glucose tolerance test; diabetes

Answers to Practical Applications

Case Report 1—1. B, 2. A, 3. B
Case Report 2—1. C, 2. C, 3. A
Case Report 3—1. C, 2. C, 3. A, 4. C

XVIII. Pronunciation of Terms

Pronunciation Guide

ā as in āpe   ă as in ăpple
ē as in ēven   ĕ as in ĕvery
ī as in īce   ĭ as in ĭnterest
ō as in ōpen   ŏ as in pŏt
ū as in ūnit   ŭ as in ŭnder

To test your understanding of the terminology in this chapter, write the meaning of each term in the space provided. In addition, you may wish to cover the terms and write them by looking at your definitions. Make sure your spelling is correct. The page number after each term indicates where it is defined or used in the text so you can easily check your responses.

Vocabulary and Terminology

Term	Pronunciation	Meaning
adenectomy (703)	ăd-ĕ-NĔK-tō-mē	_____
adenohypophysis (700)	ăd-ĕ-nō-hī-PŎF-ĭ-sĭs	_____
adrenal cortex (700)	ă-DRĒ-năl KŎR-tĕks	_____
adrenalectomy (703)	ă-drē-năl-ĔK-tō-mē	_____
adrenaline (700)	ă-DRĔN-ă-lĭn	_____
adrenal medulla (700)	ă-DRĒ-năl mĕ-DŪ-lă	_____
adrenocorticotropic hormone (700)	ă-drē-nō-kŏr-tĭ-kō-TRŌP-ĭk HŎR-mōn	_____
adrenocorticotropin (706)	ă-drē-nō-kŏr-tĭ-kō-TRŌ-pĭn	_____
adrenopathy (703)	ă-drē-NŎP-ă-thē	_____
aldosterone (700)	ăl-DŎS-tĕ-rōn or ăl-dō-STĔR-ŏn	_____
androgen (700)	ĂN-drō-jĕn	_____
antidiuretic hormone (700)	ăn-tĭ-dī-ū-RĔT-ĭk HŎR-mōn	_____
calcitonin (700)	kăl-sĭ-TŌ-nĭn	_____
catecholamines (702)	kăt-ĕ-KŌL-ă-mēnz	_____
corticosteroid (702)	kŏr-tĭ-kō-STĔ-royd	_____
cortisol (700)	KŎR-tĭ-sōl	_____
electrolyte (702)	ĕ-LĔK-trō-līt	_____
endocrinologist (704)	ĕn-dō-krĭ-NŎL-ō-jĭst	_____

epinephrine (701)	ĕp-ĭ-NĔF-rĭn	_____
estradiol (701)	ĕs-tră-DĪ-ŏl	_____
estrogen (701)	ĔS-trō-jĕn	_____
estrogenic (704)	ĕs-trō-JĔN-ĭk	_____
euthyroid (706)	ū-THĪ-royd	_____
follicle-stimulating hormone (701)	FŎL-ĭ-k'l STĬM-ū-lā-ting HŎR-mōn	_____
glucagon (701)	GLOO-kă-gŏn	_____
glucocorticoid (702)	gloo-kō-KŎR-tĭ-koyd	_____
glycemic (704)	glī-SĒ-mĭk	_____
glycogen (704)	GLĪ-kō-jĕn	_____
glycosuria (706)	glī-kōs-Ū-rē-ă	_____
gonadotropin (703)	gō-năd-ō-TRŌ-pĭn	_____
growth hormone (701)	GRŌ-TH HŎR-mōn	_____
homeostasis (702)	hō-mē-ō-STĀ-sĭs	_____
hormonal (705)	hŏr-MŎ-năl	_____
hormone (702)	HŎR-mōn	_____
hypercalcemia (704)	hī-pĕr-kăl-SĒ-mē-ă	_____
hyperglycemia (704)	hī-pĕr-glī-SĒ-mē-ă	_____
hypocalcemia (704)	hī-pō-kăl-SĒ-mē-ă	_____
hypogonadism (703)	hī-pō-GŌ-năd-ĭzm	_____
hypoinsulinism (705)	hī-pō-ĬN-sū-lĭn-ĭzm	_____
hypokalemia (705)	hī-pō-kā-LĒ-mē-ă	_____
hyponatremia (705)	hī-pō-nā-TRĒ-mē-ă	_____
hypophysectomy (705)	hī-pō-fĭ-SĔK-tō-mē	_____
hypophysis (700)	hī-PŎF-ĭ-sĭs	_____
hypopituitarism (703)	hī-pō-pĭ-TOO-ĭ-tă-rĭzm	_____
hypothalamus (702)	hī-pō-THĂL-ă-mŭs	_____

insulin (701)   ĬN-sū-lĭn _____

luteinizing hormone (701)   LŪ-tē-ĭn-īz-ĭng HŎR-mōn _____

mineralocorticoid (702)   mĭn-ĕr-ăl-ō-KŎR-tĭ-koyd _____

neurohypophysis (700)   nū-rō-hī-PŎF-ĭ-sĭs _____

norepinephrine (701)   nŏr-ĕp-ĭ-NĔF-rĭn _____

oxytocin (701)   ŏk-sĕ-TŌ-sĭn _____

pancreas (700)   PĂN-krē-ăs _____

pancreatectomy (703)   păn-krē-ă-TĔK-tō-mē _____

parathormone (701)   păr-ă-THŎR-mōn _____

parathyroidectomy (703)   păr-ă-thī-roy-DĔK-tō-mē _____

parathyroid glands (700)   păr-ă-THĪ-royd glănz _____

pineal gland (686)   pī-NĒ-ăl glănd _____

pituitary gland (700)   pĭ-TOO-ĭ-tĕr-ē glănd _____

polydipsia (704)   pŏl-ē-DĬP-sē-ă _____

progesterone (701)   prō-JĔS-tĕ-rōn _____

prolactin (701)   prō-LĂK-tĭn _____

sella turcica (702)   SĔL-ă TŬR-sĭ-kă _____

somatotropin (701)   sō-mă-tō-TRŌ-pĭn _____

steroid (702)   STĔR-oyd _____

sympathomimetic (703)   sĭm-pă-thō-mĭ-MĔT-ĭk _____

testosterone (702)   tĕs-TŎS-tĕ-rōn _____

tetraiodothyronine (706)   tĕ-tră-ī-ō-dō-THĪ-rō-nēn _____

thyroid gland (700)   THĪ-royd glănd _____

thyroiditis (703)   thī-royd-Ī-tĭs _____

thyrotropin (702)   thī-rō-TRŌ-pĭn _____

thyroxine (702)   thī-RŎK-sĭn _____

triiodothyronine (706)   trī-ī-ō-dō-THĪ-rō-nĕn _____

vasopressin (702)   văz-ō-PRĔS-ĭn _____

Abnormal Conditions, Laboratory Tests, and Clinical Procedures

Term	Pronunciation	Meaning
acromegaly (712)	ăk-rō-MĔG-ă-lē	_____
Addison disease (709)	ĂD-ĭ-sŏn dĭ-ZĒZ	_____
adrenal virilism (709)	ă-DRĒ-năl VĬR-ĭ-lĭzm	_____
cretinism (708)	KRĒ-tĭn-ĭzm	_____
Cushing syndrome (709)	KŬSH-ĭng SĬN-drōm	_____
diabetes insipidus (712)	dī-ă-BĒ-tēz ĭn-SĬP-ĭ-dŭs	_____
diabetes mellitus (710)	dī-ă-BĒ-tēz MĔL-ĭ-tŭs or mĕ-LĪ-tŭs	_____
dwarfism (712)	DWARF-izm	_____
endemic goiter (707)	ĕn-DĔM-ĭk GOY-tĕr	_____
exophthalmos (707)	ĕk-sŏf-THĂL-mōs	_____
exophthalmometry (715)	ĕk-sŏf-thăl-MŎM-ĕ-trē	_____
fasting blood sugar (714)	FĂS-tĭng blŭd SŬG-ăr	_____
gigantism (712)	JĪ-găn-tĭzm	_____
glucose tolerance test (714)	GLŪ-kōs TŎL-ĕr-ăns test	_____
goiter (707)	GOY-tĕr	_____
Graves disease (707)	GRĀVZ dĭ-ZĒZ	_____
hirsutism (709)	HĔR-soot-ĭzm	_____
hyperinsulinism (710)	hī-pĕr-ĬN-sū-lĭn-ĭzm	_____
hyperparathyroidism (709)	hī-pĕr-pă-ră-THĪ-royd-ĭzm	_____
hyperthyroidism (707)	hī-pĕr-THĪ-royd-ĭsm	_____
hypoparathyroidism (709)	hī-pō-pă-ră-THĪ-royd-ĭzm	_____
hypothyroidism (708)	hī-pō-THĪ-royd-ĭzm	_____
ketoacidosis (710)	kē-tō-ă-sĭ-DŌ-sĭs	_____
myxedema (708)	mĭk-sĕ-DĒ-mă	_____

nodular goiter (707)	NŎD-ū-lăr GOY-tĕr	_____
osteitis fibrosa cystica (709)	ŏs-tē-Ī-tĭs fĭ-BRŌ-să sĭs-tĭ-kă	_____
panhypopituitarism (712)	păn-hī-pō-pĭ-TŪ-ĭ-tăr-ĭzm	_____
pheochromocytoma (710)	fē-ō-krō-mō-sī-TŌ-mă	_____
radioactive iodine uptake (715)	rā-dē-ō-ĂK-tĭv Ī-ō-dīn ŬP-tāk	_____
radioimmunoassay (714)	rā-dē-ō-ĭm-ū-nō-ĂS-ā	_____
syndrome of inappropriate ADH (712)	SĬN-drōm of ĭn-ă-PRŌ-prē-ĭt ADH	_____
tetany (709)	TĔT-ă-nē	_____
thyroid carcinoma (708)	THĪ-royd kăr-sĭ-NŌ-mă	_____
thyroid function tests (714)	THĪ-royd FŬNK-shŭn tests	_____
thyroid scan (715)	THĪ-royd skăn	_____
thyrotoxicosis (707)	thī-rō-tŏk-sĭ-KŌ-sis	_____

XIX. Review Sheet

Write the meanings of the word parts in the spaces provided and test yourself. Check your answers with the information in the chapter or in the glossary (Medical Terms—English) at the end of the book.

COMBINING FORMS

Combining Form	Meaning	Combining Form	Meaning
aden/o		lact/o	
adren/o		myx/o	
adrenal/o		natr/o	
andr/o		pancreat/o	
calc/o		parathyroid/o	
cortic/o		phys/o	
crin/o		pituitar/o	
dips/o		somat/o	
estr/o		ster/o	
gluc/o		thyr/o	
glyc/o		thyroid/o	
gonad/o		toc/o	
home/o		toxic/o	
kal/i		ur/o	

Continued on following page

SUFFIXES

Suffix	Meaning	Suffix	Meaning
-agon	_____	-osis	_____
-ectomy	_____	-physis	_____
-emia	_____	-stasis	_____
-genic	_____	-tocin	_____
-in, -ine	_____	-tropin	_____
-megaly	_____	-uria	_____
-oid	_____		

PREFIXES

Prefix	Meaning	Prefix	Meaning
eu-	_____	pan-	_____
hyper-	_____	poly-	_____
hypo-	_____	tetra-	_____
oxy-	_____	tri-	_____

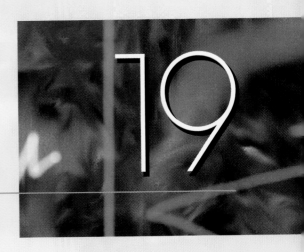

CHAPTER 19

Cancer Medicine (Oncology)

This chapter is divided into the following sections

In this chapter you will

- Learn medical terms that describe the growth and spread of tumors;
- Become familiar with terms related to the causes, diagnosis, and treatment of cancer;
- Recognize how tumors are classified and described by pathologists;
- Understand the x-rays, laboratory tests, and procedures used by physicians for determining the presence and extent of spread (staging) of tumors;
- Recognize procedures, tests, and abbreviations that pertain to the care of cancer patients; and
- Apply your new knowledge to understanding medical terms in their proper contexts, such as medical reports and records.

733

I. Introduction

Cancer is a disease characterized by unrestrained and excessive growth of cells in the body. It may occur in any tissue and at any time of life, although cancer increases in likelihood of occurrence with age. Cancer cells accumulate as growths called **malignant tumors,** which compress, invade, and ultimately destroy the surrounding normal tissue. In addition to their local growth, cancerous cells are able to spread throughout the body by way of the bloodstream or lymphatic vessels. In most patients, the spread of cancers from their site of primary origin to distant organs occurs early in the course of tissue growth and ultimately is responsible for causing death.

Although more than half of all patients who develop cancer are cured of their disease, it is currently the cause of about one fifth of all deaths in the United States. Lung cancer, followed by breast and colorectal cancers, are the most common causes of cancer death for women, whereas lung, colorectal, and prostate cancers are the leading causes of death due to cancer in men. This chapter explores the terminology related to this common and potentially fatal disease process.

II. Characteristics of Tumors

Tumors (also called **neoplasms**) are masses, or growths, that arise from normal tissue. They may be either **malignant** (capable of invasion and spread to other sites) or **benign** (noninvasive and not spreading to other sites). There are several differences between benign and malignant tumors. Some of these differences are:

1. Benign tumors **grow slowly,** and malignant tumor cells **multiply rapidly.**
2. Benign tumors are often **encapsulated** (contained within a fibrous capsule or cover), so that the tumor cells do not invade the surrounding tissue. Malignant tumor growth is characteristically **invasive** and **infiltrative,** extending beyond the tissue of origin into adjacent organs.
3. Benign tumors are composed of organized and specialized **(differentiated)** cells that closely resemble the normal, mature tissue from which they are derived. For example, benign tumors derived from cells that line the gastrointestinal tract or glands

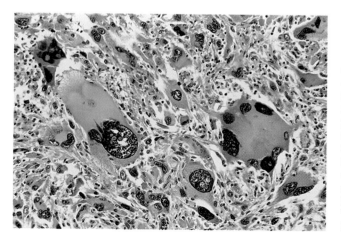

Figure 19-1

Anaplastic tumor cells of the skeletal muscle (rhabdomyosarcoma). Note the marked cellular and nuclear pleomorphism, which is variation in size and shape: (pleo = many, morph/o = shape), hyperchromatic nuclei, and tumor giant cells (which possess either one enormous nucleus or several nuclei). (Courtesy of Dr. Trace Worrell, Department of Pathology, University of Texas Southwestern Medical School, Dallas, TX.)

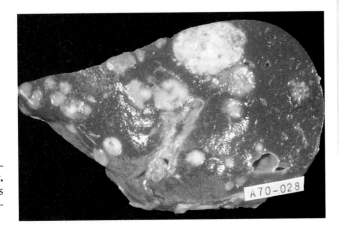

Figure 19-2

A liver studded with **metastatic cancer.** (From Kumar V, Cotran RS and Robbins SL: Basic Pathology, 6th ed. Philadelphia, WB Saunders, 1997, page 139.)

look very much like gastrointestinal cells, their normal counterparts. Malignant tumors are composed of cancerous cells that resemble primitive, or embryonic, cells that lack the capacity to perform mature cellular functions. This characteristic of malignant tumors is called **anaplasia.** Anaplasia (ana- means backward and -plasia means growth) indicates that the cancerous cells are **dedifferentiated,** or **undifferentiated** (reverting to a less developed state), in contrast to the normal, differentiated tissue of their origin. Anaplastic cells lack an orderly arrangement. Thus, tumor cells vary in size and shape and are piled one on top of the other in a disorganized fashion. The nuclei in these cells are hyperchromatic (stain excessively with increased genetic material) and large. Figure 19–1 shows anaplasia in skeletal muscle tumor cells.

4. Cells from benign tumors do not spread or **metastasize** to form secondary tumor masses in distant places in the body. Malignant tumors, however, can detach themselves from the primary tumor site, penetrate a blood vessel or lymphatic vessel, travel through the bloodstream or lymphatic system, and establish a new tumor site at a distant tissue, such as the lung, liver, or bone marrow. The secondary growth is called a **metastasis.** Figure 19–2 shows a liver infiltrated by metastatic cancer.

Figure 19–3 reviews the differences between benign and malignant tumors.

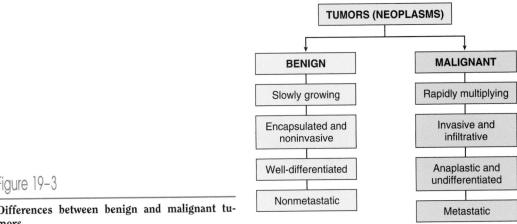

Figure 19-3

Differences between benign and malignant tumors.

III. Carcinogenesis

What Causes Cancer?

The process of transformation from a normal cell to a cancerous one (carcinogenesis) is only partially understood at the present time. What is clear is that malignant transformation results from damage to the genetic material, or **DNA (deoxyribonucleic acid),** of the cell. Strands of DNA in the cell nucleus form **chromosomes,** which become readily visible under a microscope when a cell is preparing to divide into two (daughter) cells. In order to understand what causes cancer, it is necessary to learn more about DNA and its functions in a normal cell.

DNA has two main functions in a normal cell. First, DNA controls the production of new cells (cell division). When a cell divides, the DNA material in each chromosome copies itself, so that exactly the same DNA is passed to the two new daughter cells that are formed. This process of cell division is called **mitosis** (Fig. 19–4A).

Second, between cycles of mitosis, DNA controls the production of new proteins **(protein synthesis)** in the cell. DNA contains about 100,000 separate and distinct codes or programs called **genes** that direct the process of protein synthesis. DNA (as coded genes) sends a molecular message outside the nucleus to the cytoplasm of the cell, directing the synthesis of specific proteins (such as hormones and enzymes) essential for normal cell function and growth. This message is transmitted in the following way. In the nucleus, the coded message with instructions for making a specific protein is copied from DNA onto another molecule called **RNA (ribonucleic acid).** Then RNA travels from the nucleus to the cytoplasm of the cell, carrying the coded message to direct the formation of specific proteins (Fig. 19–4B).

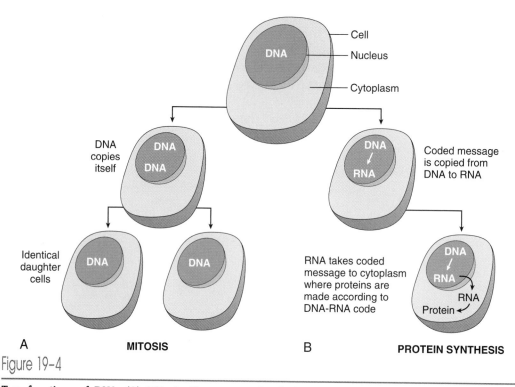

Figure 19-4

Two functions of DNA. (A) Mitosis (the process of cell division). **(B) Protein synthesis** (creating new proteins for cellular growth).

When a cell becomes malignant, however, the processes of mitosis and protein synthesis are disturbed. Cancer cells reproduce almost continuously, and abnormal proteins are made. Malignant cells are anaplastic; that is, their DNA stops making codes that allow the cells to carry on their normal function. Instead, altered DNA and altered cellular programs make new signals that lead to movement of cells, invasion of adjacent tissue, and metastasis.

The damage to DNA that results in malignancy may be caused by environmental factors, such as toxic chemicals, sunlight, tobacco smoke, and viruses. Once these changes are established in a cell, they are passed on to daughter cells. Such an inheritable change in DNA is called a **mutation.** Mutations, particularly those that affect cell growth or DNA repair, lead to malignant growths.

Although most DNA changes, or mutations, lead to higher-than-normal rates of growth, some mutations found in cancer cells actually prevent the cells from dying. In recent years, scientists have recognized that some types of cancers have lost the normal blueprints that direct aging or damaged cells to die. Normal cells undergo spontaneous disintegration by a process known as **apoptosis,** or programmed cell death. Some cancer cells have lost elements of this program and thus can live indefinitely.

Environmental Agents

Agents from the environment, such as chemicals, drugs, tobacco smoke, radiation, and viruses, can cause damage to DNA and thus produce cancer. These environmental agents are called **carcinogens.**

Chemical carcinogens are found in a variety of products and drugs including **hydrocarbons** (in cigarette, cigar, and pipe smoke and automobile exhaust), insecticides, dyes, industrial chemicals, insulation, and hormones. For example, the hormone diethylstilbestrol (DES) causes a malignant tumor, carcinoma of the vagina, in daughters of women treated with DES during pregnancy. Drugs such as estrogens can cause cancer by stimulating the proliferation of cells in target organs such as the lining of the uterus.

Radiation, whatever its source—sunlight, x-rays, radioactive substances, nuclear fission—is a wave of energy. When this energy interacts with DNA, it causes DNA damage and mutations that lead to cancer. Thus, leukemia (a cancerous condition of white blood cells) may be an occupational hazard of radiologists, who are routinely exposed to x-rays. There is a high incidence of leukemia and other cancers among survivors of atomic bomb explosions, as at Hiroshima and Nagasaki. Ultraviolet radiation given off by the sun can cause skin cancer, especially in persons with lightly pigmented, or fair, skin.

Some **viruses** are carcinogenic. For example, the human T-cell leukemia virus (HTLV) causes a form of leukemia in adults. A related virus, HIV (human immunodeficiency virus), causes a tumor (Kaposi sarcoma) associated with AIDS. Other viruses are known to cause cervical cancer (papilloma virus) and a tumor of lymph nodes called Burkitt lymphoma (Epstein-Barr virus). These tumor-producing viruses, called **oncogenic viruses,** fall into two categories: **RNA viruses** (composed of RNA and known as retroviruses) and **DNA viruses** (composed of DNA).

In addition to transmission of cancer by whole viruses, pieces of DNA called **oncogenes** can cause normal cells to become malignant if they are activated by mutations. An oncogene (cancer-causing gene) is a piece of DNA whose activation is associated with the conversion of a normal cell into a cancerous cell. Some examples of

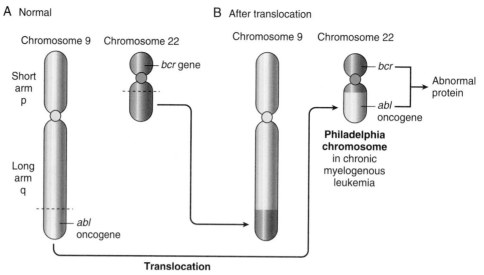

Figure 19–5

Chromosomal (oncogene) translocation leading to the Philadelphia chromosome and chronic myelogenous leukemia (CML). **(A)** Normal chromosomes 9 and 22. **(B)** Translocation of the *abl* oncogene from the long arm (q) of chromosome 9 to the long arm of chromosome 22 (next to the *bcr* gene). This forms a combination oncogene *bcr-abl* that produces an abnormal protein (tyrosine kinase), which leads to malignant transformation (CML).

oncogenes are **ras** (colon cancer), **myc** (lymphoma), and **bcr-abl** (chronic myelogenous leukemia).

In chronic myelogenous leukemia the oncogene *bcr-abl* is activated when pieces from two different chromosomes switch locations. This genetic change (mutation) is called a **translocation.** The oncogene *abl* on chromosome 9 moves to a new location on the base of chromosome 22, close to a gene called *bcr*. When these two genes are located near each other, they cause the production of an abnormal protein that makes the leukocyte divide and causes a malignancy (chronic myelogenous leukemia). The new chromosome formed from the translocation is called the **Philadelphia chromosome** (it was discovered in 1960 in Philadelphia) (Fig. 19–5).

Heredity

Cancer may be caused not only by environmental factors, but also by inherited factors. Susceptibility to some forms of cancer is transmitted from parents to offspring through defects in the DNA of the egg and sperm cells. Examples of known inherited cancers are retinoblastoma (tumor of the retina of the eye), polyposis coli syndrome (polyps that grow in the colon and rectum), and certain other forms of colon, breast, and kidney cancer.

Each of these diseases is caused by specific breaks or rearrangements of the DNA code. Detection of these changes in the DNA code is possible by analysis of genes on a chromosome. This is accomplished through DNA sequencing, a step-by-step analysis of the components of the affected gene, or by small DNA probes that test the overall fit of a person's gene to a normal gene sequence. If the DNA damage affects a large segment of a chromosome, it can be visualized by examining a microscopic picture of an appropriately stained chromosome preparation called a **karyotype.**

Table 19-1. GENES IMPLICATED IN HEREDITARY CANCERS

Cancer	Gene	Chromosomal Location
Breast; ovarian	*BRCA1*	17q21
Breast	*BRCA2*	13q12-13
Polyposis coli syndrome	*APC*	5q21
Li-Fraumeni (multiple cancers)	*p53*	17p13
Retinoblastoma	*Rb1*	13q14
Wilms tumor	*WT1*	11p13

Note: The first number is the chromosome; p is the short arm of the chromosome, and q is the long arm of the chromosome; the second number is the region (band) of the chromosome.

In many cases, it is believed that these tumors arise because of inherited or acquired abnormalities in certain genes called **suppressor genes.** In normal individuals, these suppressor genes regulate growth, promote differentiation, and suppress oncogenes from causing cancer. Loss of a normal suppressor gene takes the brake off the process of cell division and leads to cancer. Examples of suppressor genes are the **retinoblastoma gene (Rb-1)** and the **p53** gene (named after the molecular weight of the protein that it codes for). A loss or mutation of the p53 gene (located on chromosome 17) can lead to numerous human cancers, such as colon and breast cancer.

Because inherited changes can be detected in all tissues of the body, not simply cancerous cells, family members can be tested to determine whether they have inherited the cancer-causing gene. This is known as **genetic screening.** Affected individuals may be watched carefully to detect tumors at an early stage. Table 19–1 lists several hereditary cancers and the name of the responsible gene. Figure 19–6 reviews the role of environmental agents and heredity in carcinogenesis.

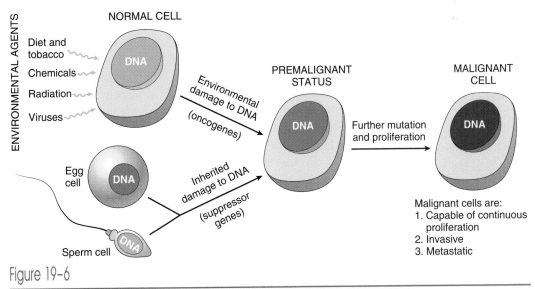

Figure 19-6

The role of environmental agents and heredity in carcinogenesis (transformation of a normal to malignant cell).

IV. Classification of Cancerous Tumors

Almost half of all cancer deaths are caused by malignancies that originate in lung, breast, or colon. However, in all there are more than 100 distinct types of cancer, each having a unique set of symptoms and requiring a specific type of therapy. It is possible to divide these types of cancer into three broad groups on the basis of **histogenesis**— that is, by identifying the particular type of tissue **(hist/o)** from which the tumor cells arise **(-genesis)**. These major groups are **carcinomas, sarcomas,** and **mixed tissue tumors.**

Carcinomas

Carcinomas, the largest group, are solid tumors that are derived from epithelial tissue that lines external and internal body surfaces, including skin, glands, and digestive, urinary, and reproductive organs. Approximately 90 per cent of all malignancies are carcinomas.

Table 19–2 gives examples of specific carcinomas and the epithelial tissue from which they derive. Benign tumors of epithelial origin are usually designated by the term **adenoma,** which indicates that the tumor is of epithelial or glandular **(aden/o)** origin. For example, a gastric adenoma is a benign tumor of the glandular epithelial cells lining the stomach. Malignant tumors of epithelial origin are named by using the term **carcinoma** and adding the type of tissue in which the tumor occurs. Thus, a **gastric adenocarcinoma** is a cancerous tumor arising from glandular cells lining the stomach.

Sarcomas

Sarcomas are less common (less than 5 per cent of all malignant tumors) than carcinomas and are derived from connective tissues in the body, such as bone, fat, muscle, cartilage, and bone marrow and from cells of the lymphatic system. Often, the term **mesenchymal tissue** is used to describe embryonic connective tissue from which sarcomas are derived. The middle, or mesodermal, layer of the embryo gives rise to the connective tissues of the body as well as to blood and lymphatic vessels.

Table 19–3 gives examples of specific types of sarcomas and the connective tissues from which they derive. Benign tumors of connective tissue origin are named by adding the suffix **-oma** to the type of tissue in which the tumor occurs. For example, a benign tumor of bone is called an **osteoma.** Malignant tumors of connective tissue origin are frequently named by using the term **sarcoma (sarc/o** means **flesh).** For example, an **osteosarcoma** is a malignant tumor of bone.

In addition to the solid tumors of connective tissue origin, sarcomas include tumors arising from blood-forming tissue. **Leukemias** are tumors derived from bone marrow, whereas **lymphomas** are derived from immune cells of the lymphatic system. Connective tissue within the brain (neuroglial cells) and embryonic tissue of the nervous system give rise to **gliomas** (such as astrocytomas of the brain) and **neuroblastomas.**

Table 19-2. **CARCINOMAS AND THE EPITHELIAL**
TISSUES FROM WHICH THEY DERIVE

Type of Epithelial Tissue	Malignant Tumor
GASTROINTESTINAL TRACT	
Stomach	Gastric adenocarcinoma
Esophagus	Esophageal carcinoma
Colon	Adenocarcinoma of the colon
Liver	Hepatocellular carcinoma, also called hepatoma
GLANDULAR TISSUE	
Thyroid	Carcinoma of the thyroid
Adrenal glands	Carcinoma of the adrenals
Pancreas	Carcinoma of the pancreas (pancreatic adenocarcinoma)
Breast	Carcinoma of the breast
Prostate	Carcinoma of the prostate
SKIN	
Squamous cell layer	Squamous cell carcinoma
Basal cell layer	Basal cell carcinoma
Melanocyte	Malignant melanoma
LUNG	
	Adenocarcinoma of the lung
	Small cell carcinoma
	Epidermoid carcinoma
KIDNEY AND BLADDER	
	Renal cell carcinoma (hypernephroma)
	Transitional cell carcinoma of the bladder
REPRODUCTIVE ORGANS	
	Cystadenocarcinoma of the ovaries
	Adenocarcinoma of the uterus
	Squamous cell (epidermoid) carcinoma of the vagina or cervix
	Carcinoma of the penis
	Seminoma and embryonal cell carcinoma (testes)
	Choriocarcinoma of the uterus or testes

Table 19-3. SARCOMAS AND THE CONNECTIVE TISSUES FROM WHICH THEY DERIVE

Type of Connective Tissue	Malignant Tumor
BONE	
	Osteosarcoma (osteogenic sarcoma)
	Ewing sarcoma
MUSCLE	
Smooth (visceral) muscle	Leiomyosarcoma
Striated (skeletal) muscle	Rhabdomyosarcoma
CARTILAGE	
	Chondrosarcoma
FAT	
	Liposarcoma
FIBROUS TISSUE	
	Fibrosarcoma
BLOOD VESSEL TISSUE	
	Angiosarcoma
BLOOD-FORMING TISSUE	
All leukocytes	Leukemias
Lymphocytes	Hodgkin disease
	Non-Hodgkin lymphomas
	Burkitt lymphoma
Plasma cells	Multiple myeloma
NERVE TISSUE	
Embryonic nerve tissue	Neuroblastoma
Neuroglial tissue	Astrocytoma (tumor of neuroglial cells called astrocytes)

Mixed-tissue Tumors

Mixed-tissue tumors are derived from tissue that is capable of differentiating into both epithelial and connective tissue. These uncommon tumors are thus composed of several different types of cells. Examples of mixed-tissue tumors (Table 19–4) can be found in the kidney, ovaries, and testes.

Table 19-4. MIXED-TISSUE TUMORS

Type of Tissue	Malignant Tumor
Kidney	Wilms tumor (embryonal adenosarcoma)
Ovaries and testes	Teratoma (tumor composed of bone, muscle, skin, gland cells, cartilage, etc.)

V. Pathological Descriptions

The following terms are used to describe the appearance of a malignant tumor, on either gross (visual) or on microscopic examination.

Gross Descriptions

cystic
Forming large open spaces filled with fluid. **Mucinous** tumors are filled with mucus (thick, sticky fluid), and **serous** tumors are filled with a thin, watery fluid resembling serum. The most common site of cystic tumors is in ovaries.

fungating
Mushrooming pattern of growth in which tumor cells pile one on top of another and project from a tissue surface. Tumors found in the colon are often of this type.

inflammatory
Having the features of inflammation; that is, redness, swelling, and heat. Inflammatory changes result from tumor blockage of the lymphatic drainage of the skin, as in breast cancer.

medullary
Pertaining to large, soft, fleshy tumors. Thyroid and breast tumors may be medullary.

necrotic
Containing dead tissue. Any type of tumor can outgrow its blood supply and undergo necrosis.

polypoid
Growths that are like projections extending outward from a base. **Sessile** polypoid tumors extend from a broad base, and **pedunculated** polypoid tumors extend from a stem or stalk. Both benign and malignant tumors of the colon may grow as polyps.

ulcerating
Characterized by an open, exposed surface resulting from the death of overlying tissue. Ulcerating tumors are often found in the stomach, breast, colon, and skin.

verrucous
Resembling a wart-like growth. Tumors of the gingiva (cheek) are frequently verrucous.

Microscopic Descriptions

alveolar   Tumor cells form patterns resembling small, microscopic sacs; commonly found in tumors of muscle, bone, fat, and cartilage.

carcinoma *in situ*   Referring to localized tumor cells that have not invaded adjacent structures. Cancer of the cervix may begin as carcinoma *in situ*.

diffuse   Spreading evenly throughout the affected tissue. Malignant lymphomas may display diffuse involvement of lymph nodes.

dysplastic   Pertaining to abnormal formation of cells. These tumors display a highly abnormal but not clearly cancerous appearance. Dysplastic nevi (moles on skin) are an example.

epidermoid   Resembling squamous epithelial cells (thin, plate-like), often occurring in the respiratory tract.

follicular   Forming small, microscopic, gland-type sacs. Thyroid gland cancer is an example.

nodular   Forming multiple areas of tightly packed clusters of cells with lightly populated areas in between. Malignant lymphomas may display a nodular pattern of lymph node involvement.

papillary   Forming small, finger-like or nipple-like projections of cells. Bladder cancer may be described as papillary.

pleomorphic   Composed of a variety of types of cells. Mixed-cell tumors are examples.

scirrhous   Densely packed (scirrhous means hard) tumors, overgrown with fibrous tissue; commonly found in breast or stomach cancers.

undifferentiated   Lacking microscopic structures typical of normal mature cells.

VI. Grading and Staging Systems

Tumors are classified on the basis of their location, microscopic appearance, and extent of spread. Of particular importance are the tumor's **grade** (its degree of maturity or differentiation under the microscope) and its **stage** (its extent of spread within the body). These two properties influence the prognosis (the chances of successful treatment and survival) and determine the specific treatment to be used.

When grading a tumor, the pathologist is concerned with the microscopic appearance of the tumor cells, specifically with their degree of maturation or differentiation. Often, three or four grades are used. **Grade I** tumors are very well differentiated, so that they closely resemble the normal parent tissue of their origin. **Grade IV** tumors are so undifferentiated or anaplastic that even recognition of the tumor's tissue of origin may be difficult. **Grades II** and **III** are intermediate in appearance, moderately or poorly differentiated, as opposed to well differentiated (grade I) and undifferentiated (grade IV).

Grading is often of value in determining the prognosis of certain types of cancers, such as cancer of the urinary bladder, prostate gland, ovary, and brain tumors (astrocytomas). Patients with grade I tumors have a high survival rate, and patients with grades II, III, and IV tumors have a poorer survival rate. Grading is also used in evaluating cells obtained from body fluids in preventive screening tests, such as **Papanicolaou (Pap) smears** of the uterine cervix, tracheal secretions, or stomach secretions.

The staging of cancerous tumors is based on the extent of spread of the tumor rather than on its microscopic appearance. An example of a staging system is the **TNM staging system.** It has been applied to malignancies such as lung cancer, as well as to many other tumors. **T** refers to the size and degree of local extension of the **tumor; N** refers to the number of regional lymph **nodes** that have been invaded by tumor; and **M** refers to the presence or absence of **metastases** (spreads to distant sites) of the tumor cells. Subscripts are used to denote size and degree of involvement: For example, 0 indicates undetectable, and 1, 2, 3, and 4 a progressive increase in size or involvement. A tumor may be described as $T_1N_2M_0$ (a small tumor with spread to regional nodes, but no distant metastases). Table 19–5 presents the notations in the TNM staging system.

Other staging systems use letters such as A, B, C, and D or I, II, III, and IV to indicate the extent of spread of tumor in the body. For example, in the Duke staging system for colon cancer, A = disease confined to the colon; B = penetration of the muscle lining in the wall of the colon; C = involvement of lymph nodes; D = metastasis.

Table 19-5. A TNM STAGING SYSTEM

TUMOR

T_0	No evidence of primary tumor
T_{IS}	Carcinoma *in situ*
$T_1\ T_2\ T_3\ T_4$	Progressive increase in tumor size and in local invasion
T_x	Tumor cannot be assessed

NODES

N_0	Regional lymph nodes not demonstrably abnormal
$N_1\ N_2\ N_3\ N_4$	Increasing numbers or increasingly distant location of spread to regional lymph nodes
N_x	Regional lymph nodes cannot be assessed clinically

METASTASIS

M_0	No evidence of distant metastasis
M_1	Distant metastasis

VII. Cancer Treatment

Four major approaches to cancer treatment are **surgery, radiation therapy, chemotherapy,** and **biological therapy.** Each method **(modality)** may be used alone, but often they are used together in combined-modality programs to improve the overall treatment result.

Surgery

In many patients with cancer, the tumor is discovered before it has spread, and it may be cured by surgical excision. Some common cancers in which surgery may be curative are those of the stomach, breast, and uterus (endometrium). Often, surgical removal of the primary tumor is indicated to prevent local spread or complications, even in the presence of distant disease.

The following is a list of terms that describe surgical procedures used in treating cancer.

cryosurgery	Malignant tissue is frozen and thus destroyed. This procedure is occasionally used to treat bladder and prostate tumors.
electrocauterization	Malignant tissue is destroyed by burning. Electrocauterization is often used in treating tumors of the rectum and colon, when surgical removal is not possible.
en bloc resection	Tumor is removed along with a large area of surrounding tissue containing lymph nodes. Modified radical mastectomy, colectomy, and gastrectomy are examples.
excisional biopsy	Removal of tumor and a margin of normal tissue. This procedure provides a specimen for diagnosis and may be curative for small tumors.
exenteration	A wide resection involving removal of the tumor, its organ of origin, and all surrounding tissue in the body space. Pelvic exenteration may be performed to treat large primary tumors of the uterus.
fulguration	Destruction of tissue by electric sparks generated by a high-frequency current.
incisional biopsy	A piece of tumor is removed for examination to establish a diagnosis. A more extensive surgical procedure or other forms of treatment, such as chemotherapy or x-ray, may then be used to treat the bulk of the tumor.

Radiation

The goal of radiation therapy is to deliver a maximal dose of ionizing radiation (irradiation) to the tumor tissue and a minimal dose to the surrounding normal tissue. In reality, this goal is difficult to achieve, and usually one accepts a degree of residual normal cell damage **(morbidity)** as a side effect of the destruction of the tumor. High-dose radiation produces damage to DNA. Newer techniques of radiation utilize high-energy beams of **protons** (atomic particles) to improve the focus of the beam and limit damage to normal tissues. Radiation damage to normal tissue leads to **fibrosis** (an increase in connective tissue), loss of epithelial (surface lining) cells, and damage to blood vessels.

Terms used in the field of radiation therapy for cancer are as follows:

brachytherapy	Implantation of seeds of radioactive material directly into the tumor; used in prostatic cancer and brain tumors.
electron beams	Low-energy beams for treatment of skin or surface tumors.
fields	Defined areas that will be bombarded by radiation.
fractionation	A method of dividing radiation into small, repeated doses rather than providing fewer large doses. Fractionation allows larger total doses to be given while causing less damage to normal tissue.
linear accelerator	A large electronic device that produces high-energy x-ray beams for the treatment of deep-seated tumors.
proton therapy	Highly focused, high-energy irradiation. This treatment requires large machinery such as a cyclotron to generate particles.
radiocurable tumor	Tumor that can be completely eradicated by radiation therapy. Usually, this is a localized tumor with no evidence of metastasis. Lymphomas and Hodgkin disease are examples.
radioresistant tumor	Tumor that requires large doses of radiation to produce death of the cells. Connective tissue tumors are the most radioresistant.
radiosensitive tumor	Tumor in which irradiation can cause the death of cells without serious damage to surrounding tissue. Tumors of hematopoietic (blood-forming) and lymphatic origins are radiosensitive.
radiosensitizers	Drugs that increase the sensitivity of tumors to x-rays. Many cancer chemotherapy drugs, especially 5-fluorouracil and cisplatin, sensitize tumors and normal tissue to radiation and improve the outcome of treatment.

Chemotherapy and Biological Therapy

Chemotherapy

Cancer chemotherapy is the treatment of cancer using chemicals (drugs). It is the standard treatment for many types of cancer, and it produces cures in most patients who have choriocarcinoma, testicular cancer, acute lymphocytic leukemia, and Hodgkin disease. Chemotherapy may be used alone or in combination with surgery and radiation to improve cure rates.

The field of **pharmacokinetics** (-kinetic means pertaining to movement) is concerned with measuring the amount of drug that is present over time in various body compartments (such as blood, urine, and spinal fluid). These measurements require specialized equipment.

The ideal is to develop drugs that kill large numbers of tumor cells without harming normal cells. Because normal cells, such as bone marrow and gastrointestinal lining cells, have a rapidly dividing cell population, they suffer considerable damage from antitumor drugs. Scientists working in the field of pharmacokinetics use information from research to design better routes (oral, intravenous) and schedules of administration to achieve the greatest tumor kill with the least toxicity (harm) to normal cells.

Combination chemotherapy is the use of two or more antitumor drugs together to kill a specific type of malignant growth. In chemotherapy, drugs are given according to a written **protocol,** or plan, that details exactly how the drugs will be given. Usually, drug therapy is continued until the patient achieves a complete **remission,** which is the absence of all signs of disease. At times, chemotherapy is given as an **adjuvant** (an aid) to surgery. This means that drugs are used to kill possible hidden disease in patients who, after surgery, are otherwise free of any evidence of malignancy.

Drugs cause tumor cells to die by damaging their DNA. Tumor cells with damaged DNA undergo **apoptosis,** or self-destruction. Tumors have impaired capacity to repair their DNA and, in general, appear to be less able to survive DNA damage due to drugs and radiation.

The following are categories of cancer chemotherapeutic agents. Table 19–6 lists the specific drugs in each of these categories and the particular cancers they are used to treat.

1. **Alkylating agents.** These are synthetic compounds containing two or more chemical groups called alkyl groups. They interfere with the process of DNA synthesis by attaching to DNA molecules. Toxic side effects include nausea and vomiting, diarrhea, bone marrow depression (myelosuppression), and alopecia (hair loss). These are common side effects because cells in the gastrointestinal tract, bone marrow, and scalp are rapidly dividing cells, which along with tumor cells, are susceptible to the lethal effects of chemotherapeutic drugs. Most side effects disappear after treatment is suspended.
2. **Antibiotics.** These drugs are produced by bacteria or fungi. They act by binding to DNA in the cell, thus promoting DNA strand breaks and preventing normal replication. Toxic side effects include alopecia, stomatitis (inflammation of the mouth), myelosuppression, and gastrointestinal disturbances.
3. **Antimetabolites.** These drugs inhibit the synthesis of substances that are the necessary components of DNA, or they may directly block the replication of DNA. Toxic side effects are myelosuppression with leukopenia, thrombocytopenia, and bleeding; and oral and digestive tract toxicity, including stomatitis, nausea, and vomiting.
4. **Antimitotics (natural products and marine extracts).** These chemicals are derived

Table 19-6. SELECTED CANCER CHEMOTHERAPEUTIC AGENTS AND THE CANCERS THEY TREAT

Chemotherapeutic Agent	Type of Cancer
ALKYLATING AGENTS	
Carmustine (BCNU)	Brain
Carboplatin (Paraplatin)	Ovarian
Chlorambucil (Leukeran)	Chronic lymphocytic leukemia (CLL)
Cisplatin (Platinol)	Testicular; ovarian
Cyclophosphamide (Cytoxan)	Lymphoma
Dacarbazine (DTIC-Dome)	Hodgkin lymphoma
Mechlorethamine, nitrogen mustard (Mustargen)	Lymphoma
Melphalan (Alkeran)	Multiple myeloma
ANTIBIOTICS	
Bleomycin (Blenoxane)	Testicular
Daunorubicin (Cerubidine)	Acute myelogenous leukemia (AML)
Doxorubicin (Adriamycin, Doxil)	Breast
Idarubicin (Idamycin)	Acute myelogenous leukemia (AML)
Mitomycin-C (Mutamycin)	Lung
ANTIMETABOLITES	
Cladribine (Leustatin)	Hairy cell leukemia
Cytarabine (ara-C, Cytosar-U)	Acute myelogenous leukemia (AML)
Fludarabine (Fludara)	Chronic lymphocytic leukemia (CLL)
5-Fluorouracil, 5-FU (various)	Colon
Methotrexate, MTX (Folex, Mexate)	Acute lymphocytic leukemia (ALL)
Pentostatin, DCF (Nipent)	Hairy cell leukemia
ANTIMITOTICS (NATURAL PRODUCTS)	
Docetaxel (Taxotere)	Breast
Paclitaxel (Taxol)	Breast
Vinca alkaloids	Lymphoma
Vinblastine (Velban)	
Vincristine (Oncovin)	
Vinorelbine (Navelbine)	Breast
HORMONES	
Dexamethasone (Decadron)	Lymphoma
Flutamide (Eulexin)	Prostate
Leuprolide (Lupron)	Prostate
Prednisone (various)	Acute lymphocytic leukemia (ALL)
Tamoxifen (Nolvadex)	Breast

Note: Brand names are in parenthesis.

from plants and animals found on coral reefs or in the ocean. **Taxol,** and the vinca alkaloids, are isolated from plants and block the function of the cell structural protein, the microtubule, which is essential for mitosis. They are used frequently in combination with other chemotherapeutic agents. Side effects include myelosuppression, alopecia, and nerve damage.

5. **Hormonal agents.** Hormones are a class of chemicals made by endocrine glands in the body. Examples are estrogens and androgens. They act by attaching to receptor proteins in target tissues. Hormones are key factors in promoting the growth of human tumors. Some steroid (cholesterol-derived) hormones, such as prednisone, estrogens, and androgens, have growth-inhibiting effects on leukemias and breast

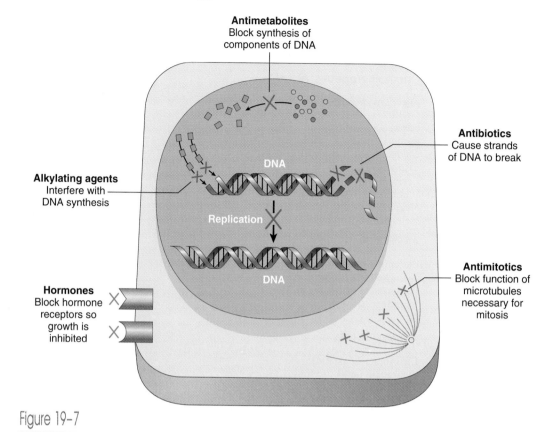

Figure 19-7

Mechanisms of action of cancer chemotherapeutic agents.

Table 19-7. CANCERS AND CHEMOTHERAPEUTIC REGIMENS

Type of Cancer	Combination Regimen	
Breast	CMF	**C**yclophosphamide
		Methotrexate
		5-**F**luorouracil
Bladder	CMV	**C**isplatin
		Methotrexate
		Vinblastine
Hodgkin disease	ABVD	Doxorubicin (**A**driamycin)
		Bleomycin
		Vinblastine
		Dacarbazine
Ovarian	Carbo-Tax	**Carbo**platin
		Pacli**tax**el (Taxol)

Note: Brand names are in parenthesis.

cancer. Other compounds, designed to block the growth-promoting effects of estrogens or androgens, are used in breast cancer and prostate cancer, respectively. Some breast cancers have **estrogen receptors.** These tumors respond to the removal of estrogen by oophorectomy or the use of antiestrogen drugs such as **tamoxifen,** which block estrogenic effects. Others such as **flutamide** block androgen action and cause regression of prostate cancer.

Figure 19–7 illustrates the mechanisms of action of cancer chemotherapeutic agents. Often, drugs are administered in combination, according to carefully planned regimens. Table 19–7 gives examples of drug combination regimens (protocols).

Tumor cells grow by establishing a new blood supply via **angiogenesis** (growth of new blood vessels). **Antiangiogenic drugs** interfere with angiogenesis. Examples of these drugs are **endostatin** and **angiostatin,** which prevent tumor growth (in mice) by inhibiting the growth of new blood vessels. Trials are under way to test these drugs in humans.

Biological Therapy

A more recent approach to cancer treatment is the use of the body's own defenses to fight tumor cells. Investigators are exploring how the elements of the immune system can be restored, enhanced, mimicked, and manipulated to destroy cancer cells. Substances produced by normal cells that directly block tumor growth or that stimulate the immune system and other body defenses are called **biological response modifiers.** Examples of these substances are **interferons** (made by lymphocytes), **monoclonal antibodies** (made by mouse cells and capable of binding to human tumors), **colony-stimulating factors (CSFs)** that stimulate blood-forming cells to combat the myelosuppressive side effects of chemotherapy, and **interleukins** that stimulate the immune system to destroy tumors. Table 19–8 lists various biological agents and their modes of action.

Table 19-8. BIOLOGICAL AGENTS AND THEIR MODES OF ACTION

Biological Agent	Mode of Action
Filgrastin (Neupogen)	Colony-stimulating factor; promotes the growth of white blood cells (leukocytes)
Interferons (Roferon, Intron)	Promote broad immune response
Interleukin 2, IL-2 (Interleukin-2)	Promotes immune response of T lymphocytes
Rituximab (Rituxan)	Monoclonal antibody binding to cell surface receptor; induces apoptosis
Trastuzumab (Herceptin)	Monoclonal antibody binding to cell surface; blocks growth-signaling pathways in a cell; induces apoptosis

Note: Brand names are in parenthesis.

VIII. Vocabulary

This list will help you review many of the new terms introduced in the text. Short definitions will reinforce your understanding of the terms. See Section XVI of this chapter for help in pronouncing the more difficult terms.

adjuvant therapy	Assisting primary treatment. Drugs are given early in the course of treatment, along with surgery or radiation to attack cancer cells that may be too small to be detected by diagnostic techniques.
alkylating agents	Synthetic chemicals containing alkyl groups that interfere with DNA synthesis.
anaplasia	Loss of differentiation of cells; reversion to a more primitive cell type.
antibiotics	Chemical substances, produced by bacteria, that inhibit the growth of cells; used in cancer chemotherapy.
antimetabolites	Chemicals that prevent cell division by inhibiting the formation of substances necessary to make DNA; used in cancer chemotherapy.
apoptosis	Programmed cell death. Apo- means off, away, and -ptosis means to fall. Normal cells undergo apoptosis when they are damaged or aging. Some cancer cells have lost the ability to undergo apoptosis and live forever.
benign tumor	Noncancerous.
biological response modifiers	Substances produced by normal cells that either directly block tumor growth or stimulate the immune system.
biological therapy	Use of the body's own defense mechanisms to fight tumor cells.
carcinogens	Agents that cause cancer; chemicals and drugs, radiation, and viruses.
carcinoma	Cancerous tumor made up of cells of epithelial origin.
cellular oncogenes	Pieces of DNA that, when broken or dislocated, can cause a normal cell to become malignant.
chemotherapy	Treatment with drugs.
combination chemotherapy	Use of several chemotherapeutic agents together for the treatment of tumors.
dedifferentiation	Loss of differentiation of cells; reversion to a more primitive, embryonic cell type; anaplasia or undifferentiation.
deoxyribonucleic acid (DNA)	Genetic material within the nucleus of a cell; controls cell division and protein synthesis.

differentiation	Specialization of cells.
electron beams	Low-energy beams of radiation for treatment of skin or surface tumors.
encapsulated	Surrounded by a capsule; benign tumors are encapsulated.
fractionation	Giving radiation in small, repeated doses.
genetic screening	Family members are tested to determine whether they have inherited a cancer-causing gene.
grading of tumors	Evaluating the degree of maturity of tumor cells.
gross description of tumors	Visual appearance of tumors: cystic, fungating, inflammatory, medullary, necrotic, polypoid, ulcerating, and verrucous.
infiltrative	Extending beyond normal tissue boundaries.
invasive	Having the ability to enter and destroy surrounding tissue.
linear accelerator	Device that produces high-energy x-ray beams for treatment of deep-seated tumors.
malignant tumor	Tending to become worse and result in death; having the characteristics of invasiveness, anaplasia, and metastasis.
mesenchymal	Embryonic connective tissue; mes = middle, enchym/o = to pour.
metastasis	Spread of a malignant tumor to a secondary site; literally, beyond (meta-) control (-stasis).
microscopic description (of tumors)	The appearance of tumors when viewed under a microscope: alveolar, carcinoma *in situ,* diffuse, dysplastic, epidermoid, follicular, nodular, papillary, pleomorphic, scirrhous, undifferentiated.
mitosis	Replication of cells; a stage in a cell's life cycle involving the production of two identical cells from a parent cell.
mixed-tissue tumors	Tumors composed of different types of tissue (epithelial as well as connective tissue).
modality	Method of treatment, such as surgery, chemotherapy, or radiation.
morbidity	The condition of being diseased.
mucinous	Containing mucus.
mutation	Change in the genetic material (DNA) of a cell; may be caused by chemicals, radiation, or viruses or may occur spontaneously.

neoplasm   New growth; benign or malignant tumors.

oncogene   A region of DNA (genetic material) found in tumor cells (cellular oncogene) or in viruses that cause cancer (viral oncogene). Oncogenes are designated by a three-letter word, such as *abl, erb, jun, myc, ras,* and *src.*

pedunculated   Possessing a stem or stalk (peduncle); characteristic of some polypoid tumors.

pharmacokinetics   Study of the distribution in and removal of drugs from the body over a period of time.

protocol   An explicit, detailed plan for treatment.

radiation   Energy carried by a stream of particles. Various forms of radiation can cause cancer.

radiocurable tumor   Cells that are eradicated by radiation therapy.

radioresistant tumor   Cells that require large doses of radiation to be destroyed.

radiosensitive tumor   A tumor in which radiation can cause the death of cells.

radiosensitizers   Drugs that increase the sensitivity of tumors to x-rays.

radiotherapy   Treatment using radiation.

relapse   Return of symptoms of disease.

remission   Absence of symptoms of disease.

ribonucleic acid (RNA)   Cellular substance (located within and outside the nucleus) that, along with DNA, plays an important role in the synthesis of proteins in a cell.

sarcoma   Cancerous tumor derived from connective tissue.

serous   Pertaining to a thin, watery fluid (serum).

sessile   Having no stem; characteristic of some polypoid tumors.

solid tumor   Tumor composed of a mass of cells.

staging of tumors   System of evaluating the extent of spread of tumors. An example is the TNM system (tumor, nodes, and metastasis).

steroids   Complex, naturally occurring chemicals, such as hormones, that are used as chemotherapeutic agents.

surgical procedures to treat cancer	Methods of removing cancerous tissue: cryosurgery, electrocauterization, en bloc resection, excisional biopsy, exenteration, fulguration, incisional biopsy.
ultraviolet radiation	Rays given off by the sun.
viral oncogenes	Pieces of DNA from viruses that infect a normal cell and cause it to become malignant.
virus	An infectious agent that reproduces by entering a host cell and using the host's genetic material to make copies of itself.

IX. Combining Forms, Suffixes, Prefixes, and Terminology

Write the meanings of the medical terms in the spaces provided.

Combining Forms

Combining Form	Meaning	Terminology	Meaning
alveol/o	small sac	alveolar _____ *Microscopic description of tumor cell arrangement (found in connective tissue tumors).*	
cac/o	bad	cachexia _____ *General ill health and malnutrition associated with chronic disease (-hexia means habit).*	
carcin/o	cancer, cancerous	carcinoma *in situ* _____ *Localized cancer; confined to the site of origin.*	
cauter/o	burn, heat	electrocauterization _____	
chem/o	chemical, drug	chemotherapy _____	
cry/o	cold	cryosurgery _____	
cyst/o	sac of fluid	cystic tumor _____	
fibr/o	fibers	fibrosarcoma _____	

follicul/o	small glandular sacs	follicular _____
		A microscopic description of cellular arrangement in glandular tumors.
fung/o	fungus, mushroom	fungating tumor _____
medull/o	soft, inner part	medullary tumor _____
mut/a	genetic change	mutation _____
		-ation means process.
mutagen/o	causing genetic change	mutagenic _____
onc/o	tumor	oncology _____
papill/o	nipple-like	papillary _____
		A microscopic description of tumor cell growth.
pharmac/o	chemical, drug	pharmacokinetics _____
		-kinetic means pertaining to movement.
plas/o	formation	dysplastic _____
		Microscopic description of cells that are highly abnormal but not clearly cancerous.
ple/o	many, more	pleomorphic _____
		Microscopic description of tumors that are composed of a variety of cells.
polyp/o	polyp	polypoid tumor _____
		-oid means resembling.
radi/o	rays, x-rays	radiotherapy _____
sarc/o	flesh, connective tissue	osteosarcoma _____
scirrh/o	hard	scirrhous _____
		Microscopic description of densely packed, fibrous tumor cell composition.

XIII. Practical Applications

This section contains an actual medical report using terms that you have studied in this and previous chapters. Answers to the questions are on page 769 after Answers to Exercises.

Case Report

A 52-year-old married woman presented to her physician with a painless mass in her left breast. During breast examination a 2-cm, firm, nontender mass was palpated in the upper outer quadrant located at the 2 o'clock position, 3 cm from the areola. The mass was not fixed to the skin, and there was no cutaneous erythema or edema. No axillary or supraclavicular lymphadenopathy was noted.

An excisional biopsy of the mass was performed. The pathology report described a gross specimen of fatty breast tissue. Microscopic evaluation of the nodule revealed a scirrhous carcinoma. The margins of the excision were free of tumor. Axillary dissection of lymph nodes was performed, and all 12 lymph nodes were free of tumor.

A portion of the specimen was sent for estrogen receptor assay and proved positive. The patient was informed of the diagnosis and underwent additional studies, including chest x-ray, liver chemistries, CBC, and bone scan—all of which were negative.

The patient was staged as having a $T_1N_0M_0$, stage 1 carcinoma of the left breast. She was referred to a radiation therapist for primary radiation therapy. After completion of radiotherapy, she was treated with tamoxifen. Prognosis is excellent for cure.

Questions on the Case Report

1. Where was the breast lesion located?
   (A) under the pigmented area of the breast
   (B) about an inch and a half to the upper left of the nipple and pigmented area
   (C) near the axilla and under the shoulder blade

2. Other associated findings were
   (A) redness and swelling
   (B) enlarged lymph nodes under the armpit
   (C) none of the above

3. The tumor was composed of
   (A) dense connective tissue, giving it a hard structure
   (B) soft, glandular tissue
   (C) cells that had extended beyond the borders of the mass

4. What procedure gave evidence that the tumor had not yet metastasized?
   (A) estrogen receptor assay
   (B) excisional biopsy of the mass
   (C) removal of lymph nodes under the arm

Continued on following page

5. What additional therapy was undertaken?
   (A) bone scan, liver chemistries, CBC, and chest x-ray
   (B) radiation to the breast
   (C) radiation to the breast and hormonal treatment

6. Tamoxifen was prescribed because
   (A) the tumor was found to be nonresponsive to estrogen
   (B) the tumor was found to be responsive to estrogen, and tamoxifen is an antiestrogen
   (C) the tumor was a stage 1 carcinoma

XIV. Exercises

Remember to check your answers carefully with those given in Section XV, Answers to Exercises.

A. Identify the following characteristics of malignant tumors based on their definitions as given below. Word parts are given as clues.

1. loss of differentiation of cells and reversion to a more primitive cell type: ana _____

2. extending beyond the normal tissue boundaries: in _____

3. having the ability to enter and destroy surrounding tissue: in _____

4. spreading to a secondary site: meta _____

B. Match the following terms or abbreviations with their meanings below.

mutation	chemical carcinogen	virus
RNA	oncogene	radiation
ultraviolet radiation	DNA	ionizing
mitosis		

1. replication of cells; two identical cells are produced from a parent cell _____

2. change in the genetic material of a cell _____

3. genetic material within the nucleus that controls replication and protein synthesis _____

4. cellular substance (ribonucleic acid) that is important in protein synthesis _____

5. rays given off by the sun; can be carcinogenic _____

6. energy carried by a stream of particles; can be carcinogenic _____

7. infectious agent that reproduces by entering a host cell and using the host's genetic material to make copies of itself _____

8. a region of genetic material found in tumor cells and in viruses that cause cancer _____

9. an agent (hydrocarbon, insecticide, hormone) that causes cancer _____

C. Give the meanings of the following terms.

1. solid tumor _____

2. adenoma _____

3. adenocarcinoma _____

4. osteoma _____

5. osteosarcoma _____

6. mixed-tissue tumor _____

7. neoplasm _____

8. pharmacokinetics _____

9. benign _____

10. differentiation _____

D. Name the terms that describe microscopic tumor growth. Definitions and word parts are given.

1. small nipple-like projections: pap _____

2. abnormal formation of cells: dys _____

3. localized growth of cells: carcin _____

4. densely packed; containing fibrous tissue: _____ ous

5. patterns resembling small, microscopic sacs: alv _____

6. small, gland-type sacs: foll _____

7. variety of cell types: pleo _____

8. lacking structures typical of mature cells: un _____

9. spreading evenly throughout the tissue: di _____

10. many areas of tightly packed clusters of cells: nod _____

11. resembling epithelial cells: epiderm _____

E. Match the following gross descriptions of tumors with their meanings as given below.

polypoid   medullary   inflammatory
ulcerating   necrotic   verrucous
cystic   fungating

1. containing dead tissue _____

2. mushrooming pattern of growth: tumor cells pile on top of each other _____

3. characterized by large, open, exposed surfaces _____

4. characterized by redness, swelling, and heat _____

5. growths are projections from a base; sessile and pedunculated tumors are examples _____

6. tumors from large, open spaces filled with fluid; serous and mucinous tumors are examples

_____

7. tumors resemble wart-like growths _____

8. tumors are large, soft, and fleshy _____

F. Select or supply the appropriate medical terms.

1. A (carcinoma/sarcoma) is a cancerous tumor composed of cells of epithelial tissue. An example of such a cancerous tumor is a (an) _____ .

2. A (carcinoma/sarcoma) is a cancerous tumor composed of connective tissue. An example of such a cancerous tumor is a (an) _____ .

3. Retinoblastoma and polyposis coli syndrome are examples of (chemical carcinogens/inherited cancers).

4. The assessment of a tumor's degree of maturity or microscopic differentiation is (grading/staging) of the tumor.

5. The assessment of a tumor's extent of spread within the body is known as (grading/staging).

6. In the TNM staging system, T stands for (tissue/tumor), N stands for (node/necrotic), and M stands for (mitotic/metastasis).

7. The transformation of adult, differentiated tissue to differentiated tissue of another type is called (metaplasia/anaplasia).

8. The formation of new blood vessels is known as (apoptosis/angiogenesis).

G. Match the surgical procedure in column I with its meaning in column II. Write the letter of the meaning in the space provided.

Column I

1. fulguration _____

2. en bloc resection _____

3. incisional biopsy _____

4. excisional biopsy _____

5. cryosurgery _____

6. electrocauterization _____

7. exenteration _____

Column II

A. removal of tumor and a margin of normal tissue for diagnosis and possible cure of small tumors
B. burning a lesion to destroy tumor cells
C. wide resection involving removal of tumor, its organ of origin, and surrounding tissue in the body space
D. destruction of tissue by electric sparks generated by a high-frequency current
E. removal of entire tumor and regional lymph nodes
F. freezing a lesion to kill tumor cells
G. cutting into tumor and removing a piece to establish a diagnosis

H. Give medical terms for the following.

1. The method of treating cancer by use of high-energy radiation waves is called

_____ .

2. If tumor tissue requires large doses of radiation to kill cells, it is called a (an)

_____ tumor.

3. If radiation can cause loss of tumor cells without much damage to surrounding regions, the

tumor is called _____ .

4. A tumor that can be completely eradicated by irradiation is known as a (an)

_____ tumor.

5. The method of giving radiation in small, repeated doses is called _____ .

6. Drugs that increase the sensitivity of tumors to x-rays are called _____ .

7. Treatment of cancerous tumors with drugs is called _____ .

8. The study of the distribution and disappearance of drugs in the body is called _____ .

9. The use of two or more drugs to kill tumor cells is called _____ .

10. A large electronic device that produces high-energy x-ray beams for treatment of deep-seated tumors is called a (an) _____ .

11. Alkylating agents, antimetabolites, hormones, antibiotics, and antimitotics are all types of

_____ agents.

12. Implantation of seeds of radioactive material directly into a tumor is called _____ .

I. Give the meanings of the following medical terms.

1. modality _____

2. adjuvant therapy _____

3. protocol _____

4. remission _____

5. relapse _____

6. morbidity _____

7. biological therapy _____

8. biological response modifiers _____

9. interferon _____

10. monoclonal antibodies _____

J. Match the test or procedure with its description below.

laparoscopy   beta-HCG test   bone marrow biopsy
exfoliative cytology   staging laparotomy   needle biopsy
lymphangiography   estrogen receptor assay   PSA test
CEA test   bone marrow transplant

1. test for the presence of a portion of human chorionic gonadotropin hormone (a marker for testicular cancer) _____

2. incision of the abdomen to determine extent of disease _____

3. contrast injected into lymph vessels and x-rays taken _____

4. visual examination of the abdominal cavity; peritoneoscopy _____

5. test for the presence of a hormone receptor on breast cancer cells _____

6. removal and microscopic examination of bone marrow tissue _____

7. aspiration of tissue for microscopic examination _____

8. blood test for the presence of an antigen related to prostate cancer _____

9. blood test for carcinogenic antigen (marker for GI cancer) _____

10. cells are scraped off tissue and microscopically examined _____

11. blood-forming cells are infused intravenously _____

K. Select the correct term to complete each sentence.

1. Pauline was diagnosed with a meningioma, which is usually a (an) **(benign, anaplastic, necrotic)** tumor. The doctor told her that it was not malignant, but that it should be removed because of the pressure it was causing on the surrounding tissues.

2. Marlene underwent surgical resection of her breast mass. Dr. Smith recommended **(dedifferentiated, modality, adjuvant)** therapy because her tumor was large and she had one positive lymph node.

3. Unfortunately, at the time of diagnosis, the tumor had spread to distant sites because it was **(pleomorphic, metastatic, mutagenic).** The oncologist recommended beginning chemotherapy as soon as possible.

4. The polyp in Lisa's colon was *not* pedunculated, and Dr. Sidney described it as flat and **(fungating, scirrhous, sessile).**

5. Mr. Elder had difficulty urinating and had an elevated PSA test. Dr. Jones examined him and found a hard prostate gland. **(Staging laparotomy, electrocauterization, biopsy)** demonstrated adenocarcinoma.

XV. Answers to Exercises

A

1. anaplasia
2. infiltrative
3. invasive
4. metastasis

B

1. mitosis
2. mutation
3. DNA (deoxyribonucleic acid)
4. RNA (ribonucleic acid)
5. ultraviolet radiation
6. ionizing radiation
7. virus
8. oncogene
9. chemical carcinogen

C

1. tumor composed of a mass of cells
2. tumor of glandular tissue (benign)
3. cancerous tumor of glandular tissue (malignant)
4. tumor of bone (benign)
5. flesh (connective tissue) tumor of bone (malignant)
6. tumor composed of different types of tissue (both epithelial and connective tissues)
7. new formation (tumor)
8. study of the distribution and removal of drugs in the body over a period of time
9. noncancerous
10. specialization of cells

D

1. papillary
2. dysplastic
3. carcinoma *in situ*
4. scirrhous
5. alveolar
6. follicular
7. pleomorphic
8. undifferentiated
9. diffuse
10. nodular
11. epidermoid

E

1. necrotic
2. fungating
3. ulcerating
4. inflammatory
5. polypoid
6. cystic
7. verrucous
8. medullary

F

1. carcinoma; thyroid adenocarcinoma, squamous cell carcinoma
2. sarcoma; liposarcoma, chondrosarcoma, osteogenic sarcoma
3. inherited cancers
4. grading
5. staging
6. tumor; node; metastasis
7. metaplasia
8. angiogenesis

G

1. D
2. E
3. G
4. A
5. F
6. B
7. C

H

1. radiation therapy
2. radioresistant
3. radiosensitive
4. radiocurable
5. fractionation
6. radiosensitizers
7. chemotherapy
8. pharmacokinetics
9. combination chemotherapy
10. linear accelerator
11. chemotherapeutic agents
12. brachytherapy

I

1. method of treatment
2. assisting treatment
3. report or plan of steps taken in an experiment or disease case
4. absence of all signs of disease
5. symptoms of disease return
6. conditions of damage to normal tissue; disease
7. treatment that uses the body's own defense mechanisms to fight tumor cells
8. substances produced by normal cells that directly block tumor growth or that stimulate the immune system
9. a biological response modifier that is made by lymphocytes
10. biological response modifiers that are made by mouse cells and are able to bind to tumor cells

J

1. beta-HCG test
2. staging laparotomy
3. lymphangiography
4. laparoscopy
5. estrogen receptor assay
6. bone marrow biopsy
7. needle biopsy
8. PSA test
9. CEA test
10. exfoliative cytology
11. bone marrow transplant

K

1. benign
2. adjuvant
3. metastatic
4. sessile
5. biopsy

Answers to Practical Applications Case Report

1. B
2. C

3. A
4. C

5. C
6. B

XVI. Pronunciation of Terms

Pronunciation Guide	
ā as in āpe	ă as in ăpple
ē as in ēven	ĕ as in ĕvery
ī as in īce	ĭ as in ĭnterest
ō as in ōpen	ŏ as in pŏt
ū as in ūnit	ŭ as in ŭnder

To test your understanding of the terminology in this chapter, write the meaning of each term in the space provided. In addition, you may wish to cover the terms and write them by looking at your definitions. Make sure your spelling is correct. The page number after each term indicates where it is defined or used in the text so you can easily check your responses.

Vocabulary and Terminology

Term	Pronunciation	Meaning
adenocarcinoma (757)	ăd-ĕ-nŏ-kăr-sĭ-NŌ-mă	_____
adjuvant therapy (752)	ĂD-jū-vănt THĔR-ă-pē	_____
alkylating agents (752)	ĂL-kĭ-lā-tĭng Ā-jents	_____
alveolar (755)	ăl-vē-Ō-lăr or ăl-VĒ-ō-lăr	_____
anaplasia (752)	ăn-ă-PLĀ-zē-ă	_____
angiogenesis (757)	ăn-jē-ō-GĔN-ĕ-sĭs	_____
antibiotics (752)	ăn-tĭ-bī-ŎT-ĭks	_____
antimetabolites (752)	ăn-tĭ-mĕ-TĂB-ō-līts	_____
antimitotics (748)	ăn-tĭ-mī-TŎT-ĭks	_____
apoptosis (752)	ăp-ō-TŌ-sĭs or ā-pŏp-TŌ-sĭs	_____
benign (752)	bē-NĪN	_____
biological response modifier (752)	bī-ō-LŎJ-ĭ-kăl rĕ-SPŎNS MŎD-ĭ-fī-ĕr	_____

biological therapy (752)	bī-ō-LŎJ-ĭ-kăl THĔR-ă-pē	
bone marrow biopsy (758)	bōn MĂ-rō BĪ-ŏp-sē	
bone marrow transplantation (758)	bōn MĂ-rō TRĂNZ-plăn-tā-shŭn	
cachexia (755)	kă-KĔK-sē-ă	
carcinogen (752)	kăr-SĬN-ō-jĕn	
carcinoma *in situ* (755)	kăr-sĭ-NŌ-ma ĭn SĪ-too	
cellular oncogenes (752)	SĔL-ū-lăr ŎNGK-ō-jēnz	
chemotherapy (752)	kē-mō-THĔR-ă-pē	
colonoscopy (758)	kō-lŏn-ŎS-kō-pē	
cryosurgery (755)	krī-ō-SŬR-jĕr-ē	
cystic tumor (755)	SĬS-tĭk TOO-mŏr	
differentiation (753)	dĭf-ĕr-ĕn-shē-Ā-shŭn	
dysplastic (744)	dĭs-PLĂS-tĭk	
electrocauterization (755)	ē-lĕk-trō-kăw-tĕr-ĭ-ZĀ-shŭn	
en bloc resection (746)	ĕn blŏk rē-SĔK-shŭn	
encapsulated (753)	ĕn-KĂP-sū-lāt-ĕd	
epidermoid (744)	ĕp-ĭ-DĔR-moyd	
excisional biopsy (746)	ek-SIZH-unal BĪ-ŏp-sē	
exenteration (746)	ĕks-ĕn-tĕ-RĀ-shŭn	
exfoliative cytology (759)	ĕks-FŌ-lē-ā-tĭv sī-TŎL-ō-jē	
fibrosarcoma (755)	fī-brō-săr-KŌ-ma	
follicular (756)	fō-LĬK-ū-lăr	
fractionation (753)	frăk-shă-NĀ-shŭn	
fulguration (746)	fŭl-gū-RĀ-shŭn	
fungating tumor (756)	fŭng-GĀ-tĭng or FŬNG-gā-tĭng TOO-mŏr	
genetic screening (753)	gĕ-NĔT-ik SCRĒ-ning	
grading of tumors (753)	GRĀ-ding of TOO-mŏrz	

hyperplasia (757)	hī-pĕr-PLĀ-zē-ă	_____
incisional biopsy (746)	ĭn-SĪZH-ŭn-ăl BĪ-ŏp-sē	_____
infiltrative (753)	ĬN-fĭl-trā-tĭv	_____
invasive (753)	ĭn-VĀ-sĭv	_____
laparoscopy (759)	lă-păr-ŎS-kō-pē	_____
lymphangiography (759)	lĭm-făn-jē-ŎG-ră-fē	_____
malignant (753)	mă-LĬG-nănt	_____
mammography (759)	mă-MŎG-ră-fē	_____
medullary tumor (743)	MĔD-ū-lār-ē TOO-mŏr	_____
metaplasia (757)	mĕ-tă-PLĀ-zē-ă	_____
metastasis (753)	mĕ-TĂS-tă-sĭs	_____
mitosis (753)	mī-TŌ-sĭs	_____
modality (753)	mō-DĂL-ĭ-tē	_____
morbidity (753)	mŏr-BĬD-ĭ-tē	_____
mucinous (753)	MŪ-sĭ-nŭs	_____
mutagenic (756)	mū-tă-JĔN-ĭk	_____
mutation (753)	mū-TĀ-shŭn	_____
necrotic tumor (743)	nĕ-KRŎT-ĭk TOO-mŏr	_____
neoplasm (754)	NĒ-ō-plăzm	_____
neuroblastoma (757)	nŭ-rō-blăs-TŌ-mă	_____
nodular (744)	NŎD-ū-lăr	_____
oncogene (754)	ŎNGK-ō-jēn	_____
oncology (756)	ŏn-KŎL-ō-jē	_____
osteosarcoma (756)	ŏs-tē-ō-săr-KŌ-mă	_____
papillary (744)	PĂP-ĭ-lăr-ē	_____
pedunculated (754)	pĕ-DŬNG-kū-lāt-ĕd	_____
pharmacokinetics (754)	făr-mă-kō-kī-NĔT-ĭks	_____
pleomorphic (744)	plē-ō-MŎR-fĭk	_____

polypoid tumor (743)	PŎL-ĭ-poyd TOO-mŏr	_____
protocol (754)	PRŌ-tō-kŏl	_____
radiation (754)	rā-dē-Ā-shŭn	_____
radiocurable tumor (754)	rā-dē-ō-KŪR-ă-b'l TOO-mŏr	_____
radionuclide scans (760)	rā-dē-ō-NŪ-klīd skănz	_____
radioresistant tumor (754)	rā-dē-ō-rĕ-ZĬS-tănt TOO-mŏr	_____
radiosensitive tumor (754)	rā-dē-ō-SĔN-sĭ-tĭv TOO-mŏr	_____
radiosensitizer (754)	rā-dē-ō-SĔN-sĭ-tī-zer	_____
radiotherapy (754)	rā-dē-ō-THĔR-ă-pē	_____
relapse (754)	rē-LĂPS	_____
remission (754)	rē-MĬSH-ŭn	_____
retinoblastoma (757)	rĕt-ĭ-nō-blăs-TŌ-mă	_____
ribonucleic acid (754)	rī-bō-nū-KLĒ-ik ĂS-ĭd	_____
sarcoma (754)	săr-KŌ-mă	_____
scirrhous (744)	SKĬR-ŭs	_____
serous (754)	SĒ-rŭs	_____
sessile (754)	SĔS-ĭl	_____
solid tumor (754)	SŎL-ĭd TOO-mŏr	_____
staging laparotomy (760)	STĀ-jing lă-pă-RŎT-ō-mē	_____
staging of tumors (754)	STĀ-jĭng of TOO-mŏrz	_____
steroids (754)	STĒ-roydz	_____
ulcerating tumor (743)	ŬL-sĕ-rā-tĭng TOO-mŏr	_____
ultraviolet radiation (755)	ŭl-tră-VĪ-ō-lĕt rā-dē-Ā-shun	_____
verrucous tumor (743)	vĕ-ROO-kŭs or VĔR-oo-kŭs TOO-mŏr	_____
viral oncogenes (755)	VĪ-răl ŎNGK-ō-jĕnz	_____
virus (755)	VĪ-rŭs	_____

XVII. Review Sheet

Write the meanings of the combining forms in the spaces provided and test yourself. Check your answers with the information in the chapter or in the glossary (Medical Terms—English) at the back of the book.

COMBINING FORMS

Combining Form	Meaning	Combining Form	Meaning
aden/o	_____	mut/a	_____
alveol/o	_____	mutagen/o	_____
cac/o	_____	onc/o	_____
carcin/o	_____	papill/o	_____
cauter/o	_____	pharmac/o	_____
chem/o	_____	plas/o	_____
cry/o	_____	ple/o	_____
cyst/o	_____	polyp/o	_____
fibr/o	_____	radi/o	_____
follicul/o	_____	sarc/o	_____
fung/o	_____	scirrh/o	_____
medull/o	_____		

SUFFIXES

Suffix	Meaning	Suffix	Meaning
-ary	_____	-plasia	_____
-blast	_____	-plasm	_____
-oid	_____	-ptosis	_____
-oma	_____	-stasis	_____

Continued on following page

PREFIXES

Prefix	Meaning	Prefix	Meaning
ana-	_____	epi-	_____
anti-	_____	hyper-	_____
apo-	_____	meta-	_____
dys-	_____		

Radiology, Nuclear Medicine, and Radiation Therapy

This chapter is divided into the following sections

In this chapter you will
- Learn the physical properties of x-rays;
- Become familiar with diagnostic and therapeutic techniques used by radiologists and radiotherapists;
- Identify the x-ray views and patient positions used in x-ray examinations;
- Learn about the role of radioactivity in the diagnosis and treatment of disease;
- Become familiar with medical terms used in the specialties of radiology, nuclear medicine, and radiation therapy; and
- Apply your new knowledge to understanding medical terms in their proper contexts, such as medical reports and records.

I. Introduction

Radiology (also called **roentgenology** after its discoverer, Wilhelm Conrad Roentgen) is the medical specialty concerned with the study of x-rays. **X-rays** are invisible waves of energy that are produced by an energy source (x-ray machine, cathode ray tube) and are useful in the diagnosis and treatment of disease.

Nuclear medicine is the medical specialty that studies the characteristics and uses of **radioactive substances** in the diagnosis of disease. Radioactive substances are materials that emit high-speed particles and energy-containing rays from the interior of their matter. The emitted particles and rays are called **radioactivity** and can be of three types: **alpha particles, beta particles,** and **gamma rays. Gamma rays** are similar to x-rays in that they have no mass and are used effectively as a diagnostic label to trace the path and uptake of chemical substances in the body.

Radiation therapy (radiation oncology) is the treatment of disease using either an external source of high-energy rays (photons, electrons, protons, gamma rays) or internally implanted radioactive substances. These rays and substances are effective in damaging the DNA of cancer cells and halting their growth.

The personnel involved in these medical fields are varied. A **radiologist** is a physician who specializes in the practice of diagnostic radiology. A **nuclear physician** is a radiologist who specializes in the practice of administering diagnostic nuclear medicine procedures. A **radiation oncologist,** also a physician, specializes in the practice of radiotherapy (treatment of disease using radiation).

Allied health care professionals who work with physicians in the fields of radiology, nuclear medicine, and radiotherapy are called **radiologic technologists.** Radiologic technologists can be divided into three categories: **radiographers** (aid physicians in administering diagnostic x-ray procedures), **nuclear medicine technologists** (attend to patients undergoing nuclear medicine procedures and operate devices under the direction of a nuclear physician), and **radiation therapy technologists** (deliver courses of radiation therapy prescribed by a radiation oncologist).

II. Radiology

A. Characteristics of X-Rays

Several characteristics of x-rays are useful to physicians in the diagnosis and treatment of disease. Some of these characteristics are

1. **Ability to cause exposure of a photographic plate.** If a photographic plate is placed in front of a beam of x-rays, the x-rays, traveling unimpeded through the air, will expose the silver coating of the plate and cause it to blacken.

2. **Ability to penetrate different substances to varying degrees.** X-rays pass through the different types of substances in the human body (air in the lungs, water in blood vessels and lymph, fat around muscles, and metal such as calcium in bones) with varying ease. Air is the least dense substance and exhibits the greatest transmission. Fat is denser, water is next, followed by metal, which is the densest and transmits least. If the x-rays are absorbed (stopped) by the denser body substance (e.g., calcium in bones), they do not reach the photographic plate held behind the patient, and white areas are left in the x-ray film (plate). Figure 20–1 is an example of an x-ray photograph.

    A substance is said to be **radiolucent** if it permits passage of most of the x-rays. Lung tissue (containing air) is an example of a radiolucent substance, and it appears

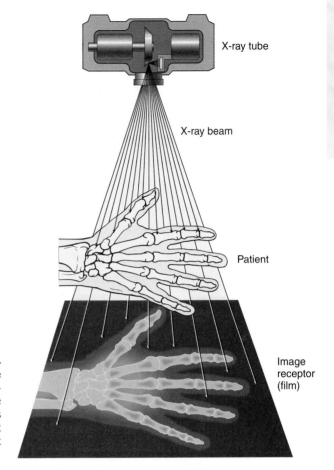

X-ray tube

X-ray beam

Patient

Image receptor (film)

Figure 20-1

X-ray photograph (radiograph) of the hand. Relative position of x-ray tube, patient (hand), and film necessary to make the x-ray photograph is shown. Bones tend to stop diagnostic x-rays, but soft tissue does not. This results in the light and dark regions that form the image.

black on an x-ray image. **Radiopaque** substances (bones) are those that absorb most of the x-rays they are exposed to, allowing only a small fraction of the x-rays to reach the x-ray plate. Thus, normally radiopaque, calcium-containing bone appears white on an x-ray image.

3. **Invisibility.** X-rays cannot be detected by sight, sound, or touch. Workers exposed to x-rays must wear a **film badge** to detect and record the amount of radiation to which they have been exposed. The film badge contains a special film that is exposed by x-rays. The amount of blackness on the film is an indication of the amount of x-rays or gamma rays received by the wearer.

4. **Travel in straight lines.** This property allows the formation of precise shadow images on the x-ray plate and also permits x-ray beams to be directed accurately at a tissue site during radiotherapy.

5. **Scattering of radiation.** Scattering occurs when x-rays come in contact with any material. Greater scatter occurs with dense objects and less scatter with those substances that are radiolucent. Scatter can be a serious occupational hazard to those in the vicinity of a source of x-rays, such as an x-ray machine. In addition, because scatter can blur images and expose areas of film that otherwise would be in shadow, a grid (containing thin lead strips arranged parallel to the x-ray beams) is placed in front of the film to absorb scattered radiation before it strikes the x-ray film.

6. **Ionization.** X-rays have the ability to ionize substances through which they pass. Ionization is a chemical process in which the energy of an x-ray beam causes rearrangement and disruption within a substance, so that previously neutral parti-

cles are changed to charged particles called **ions.** This strongly ionizing ability of x-rays is a double-edged sword. In x-ray therapy, the ionizing effect of x-rays can help kill cancerous cells and stop tumor growth; however, ionizing x-rays in small doses can affect normal body cells, leading to tissue damage and malignant changes. Thus, persons exposed to high doses of x-rays are at risk of developing leukemia, thyroid tumors, breast cancer, or other malignancies.

B. Diagnostic Techniques

X-Rays

X-rays are used in a variety of ways to detect pathological conditions. The most common use of the diagnostic x-ray is dental, to locate cavities (caries) in teeth. Other areas examined include the digestive, nervous, reproductive, and endocrine systems and the chest bones. Some special diagnostic x-ray techniques are the following:

Computed Tomography or Computerized Axial Tomography (CT, CAT). Machines called **CT scanners** (also called **CAT scanners**) beam ionizing x-rays through a patient at multiple angles around a specific section of the body (Fig. 20–2). The absorption of the x-rays at these angles as they pass through the body is detected and relayed to a computer that is programmed with a knowledge of the absorption capacities of the various body tissues. The computer then synthesizes all the information it receives from the many different x-ray views and projects a single composite picture of a specific "slice" of the abdomen, chest, or head on a screen. The ability of CT scanners to detect abnormalities is enhanced by the use of iodine-containing contrast agents, which outline blood vessels.

The CT scanners are highly sensitive in detecting disease in bony structures and can actually provide images of internal organs that are impossible to visualize with ordinary x-ray technique. CT scans also involve the use of contrast dyes and can detect brain tumors, hematomas, spinal cord lesions, and masses in the chest, liver, kidneys, and pancreas. Figure 20–3 shows a series of CT scans through various regions of the body.

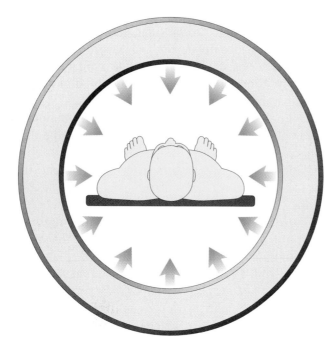

Figure 20–2

Representation of a patient inside a CT scanner. Arrows indicate the x-ray tubes that are positioned around the patient.

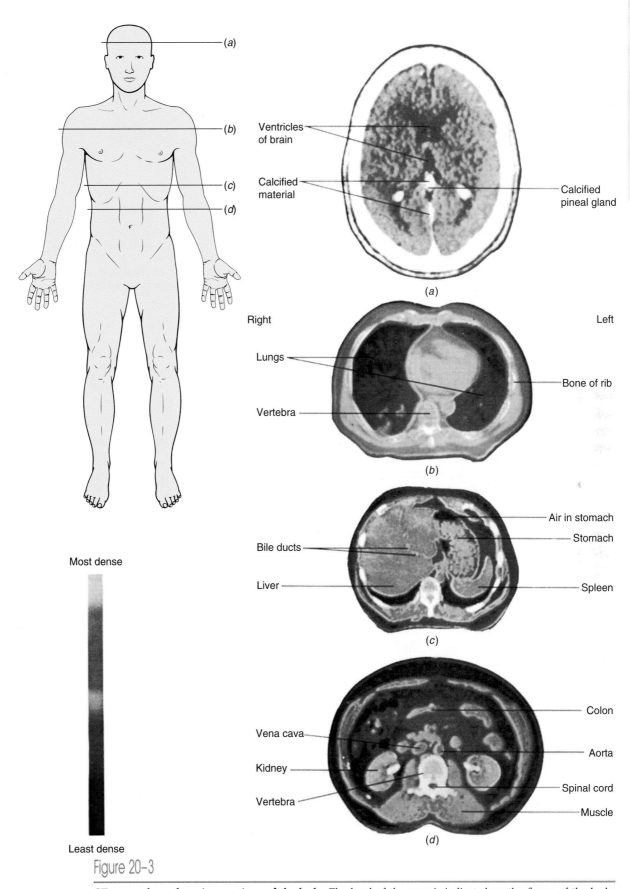

Most dense

Least dense

Figure 20-3

CT scans through various regions of the body. The level of the scan is indicated on the figure of the body. The bar below the figure indicates the gradient of structure density as represented by black (least dense, such as air) and white (most dense, such as bone). (CT scan courtesy of Professor Jan H. Ehringer.)

779

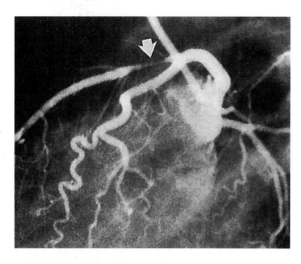

Figure 20-4

Coronary angiography shows stenosis (see arrow) of the left anterior descending coronary artery. (From Braunwald E: Heart Disease: A Textbook of Cardiovascular Medicine, 4th ed. Philadelphia, WB Saunders, 1992.)

Contrast Studies. In x-ray film, the natural differences in the density of body tissues (e.g., air in lung, calcium in bone) produce contrasting shadow images on the x-ray film. However, when x-rays pass through two adjacent body parts composed of substances of the same density, for example, the digestive organs in the abdomen, their images cannot be distinguished on the film or on the screen. It is necessary, then, to inject a **contrast medium** into the structure or fluid to be visualized so that the specific part, organ, tube, or liquid can be visualized as a negative imprint on the dense contrast agent.

The following are artificial contrast materials used in diagnostic radiological studies:

Barium Sulfate. Barium sulfate is a metallic powder that is mixed in water and used for examination of the upper and lower GI (gastrointestinal) tract. A **barium swallow (upper GI series)** involves oral ingestion of barium sulfate so that the esophagus, stomach, and duodenum can be visualized. A **small bowel follow-through** traces the passage of barium in a sequential manner as it passes through the small intestine. A **barium enema (lower GI series)** opacifies the lumen (passageway) of the large intestine using an enema containing barium sulfate.

A **double-contrast study** uses both a radiopaque and a radiolucent contrast medium. For example, the walls of the stomach or intestine are coated with barium and the lumen is filled with air. The radiographs show the pattern of mucosal ridges (see Fig. 6–1A).

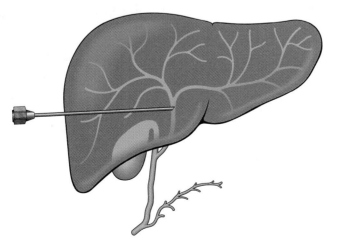

Figure 20-5

Percutaneous transhepatic cholangiography. Under fluoroscopic visualization, the aspirating needle is passed through the skin and liver tissue until the tip penetrates the hepatic duct. Contrast medium is then introduced, and x-rays are taken to visualize the biliary tree.

Iodine Compounds. Radiopaque fluids containing up to 50 per cent iodine are used in the following tests:

angiography	An x-ray image (angiogram) of blood vessels and heart chambers is obtained after injecting a water-soluble dye through a catheter (tube) into the appropriate blood vessel or heart chamber. In clinical practice, the terms angiogram and arteriogram are used interchangeably. Figure 20–4 shows coronary angiography which determines the degree of obstruction of the arteries that supply blood to the heart.
arthrography	Dye or air, or both, is injected into a joint, and x-rays are taken of the joint.
bronchography	An x-ray image of the bronchial tubes after injecting an iodized oil suspension into the bronchi through the trachea.
cholangiography	X-ray images are taken after injecting contrast into the bile ducts intravenously or after surgery of the gallbladder and biliary tract (directly into the tube left in the tract since surgery). An alternative route for injection of contrast is via a needle through the skin and into the liver. This is called **percutaneous transhepatic cholangiography** (Fig. 20–5).
digital subtraction angiography (DSA)	An x-ray image of contrast-injected blood vessels is produced by taking two x-rays (the first without contrast) and using a computer to subtract obscuring shadows from the image.
hysterosalpingography	An x-ray record of the fallopian tubes is obtained after injecting dye into the uterus via the vagina. This procedure determines the patency of the fallopian tubes.
myelography	An x-ray of the spinal cord (myel/o) after injecting radiopaque contrast (Pantopaque) into the subarachnoid space surrounding the spinal cord. Myelography identifies protrusion of an intervertebral disc (disk), bone, or tumor pressing on the spinal cord or nerve roots. This procedure is performed less frequently now because of the availability of MRI (magetic resonance imaging).
pyelography	X-ray images are made of the renal pelvis and urinary tract after contrast is injected into a vein **(intravenous pyelogram)** or after dye is injected directly into the urethra, bladder, and ureters **(retrograde pyelogram).**

    Urography is another term used to describe the process of recording x-ray images of the urinary tract after the introduction of contrast.

Some individuals experience side effects caused by the iodine-containing contrast substances. These effects can range from mild reactions such as flushing, nausea, warmth, or tingling sensations to severe, life-threatening reactions characterized by airway spasm, hives, laryngeal edema (swelling of the larynx), vasodilation, and tachycardia. Treatment involves immediate establishment of an airway and ventilation followed by injections of epinephrine (adrenaline), corticosteroids, or antihistamines.

Fluoroscopy. This x-ray procedure uses a fluorescent screen instead of a photographic plate to derive a visual image from the x-rays that pass through the patient. The fact that ionizing radiation such as x-rays can produce **fluorescence** (rays of light energy emitted as a result of exposure to and absorption of radiation from another source) is the basis for fluoroscopy. The fluorescent screen glows when it is struck by the x-rays. Opaque tissue such as bone appears as a dark shadow image on the fluorescent screen.

A major advantage of fluoroscopy over normal radiography is that internal organs, such as the heart and digestive tract organs, can be observed in motion. In addition, the patient's position can be changed constantly to provide the right view at the right time so that the most useful diagnostic information can be obtained.

Digital computerized imaging techniques can be used to enhance conventional and fluoroscopic x-ray images. A lower dose of x-ray is used to achieve higher quality images, and computerized digital images can be sent via networks to other locations and computer monitors so that many people can share information and assist in diagnoses.

Interventional Radiology. These therapeutic procedures are performed by a radiologist while the patient is undergoing fluoroscopy (or ultrasound). Interventional radiology may be used for placement of drainage catheters, drainage of abscesses, occlusion of bleeding vessels, and installation of antibiotics or chemotherapy through catheters.

Image-intensifier systems for fluoroscopy can brighten fluoroscopic images and can be combined with television and movie cameras and videotape recorders to obtain a permanent record of either a fluoroscopic or an x-ray examination. This procedure is called **cineradiography** (cine- means motion).

Ultrasound

This technique employs high-frequency, inaudible sound waves that bounce off body tissues and are then recorded to give information about the anatomy of an internal organ. An instrument is placed near or on the skin, which is covered with a thin coating of mineral oil to assure good transmission of sound waves. This instrument emits sound waves in short, repetitive pulses. The ultrasound waves move with different speeds through body tissues and detect interfaces between tissues of different densities. An echo reflection of the sound waves is formed as the waves hit the various body tissues and pass back to the ultrasound monitor.

These ultrasonic echoes are then recorded as a composite picture of the area of the body over which the instrument has passed. The record produced by ultrasound is called a **sonogram** or **echogram.**

Ultrasound is used as a diagnostic tool not only by radiologists but also by neurosurgeons and ophthalmologists to detect intracranial and ophthalmic lesions, by cardiologists to detect heart valve and blood vessel disorders **(echocardiography),** by gastroenterologists to locate abdominal masses outside the digestive organs, and by obstetricians and gynecologists to differentiate single and multiple pregnancies as well as to help in performing amniocentesis and in locating tumors or cysts. Fetal size and age can also be measured using ultrasound. The measurements are made of the

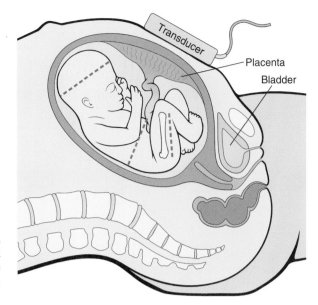

Figure 20-6

Fetal measurements taken with ultrasound imaging. Dashed lines indicate the image planes for measurements of the fetal head, abdomen, and femur.

head, abdomen, and femur based on ultrasound images taken in various fetal planes (Fig. 20–6).

Ultrasound has several advantages in that the sound waves are nonionizing and noninjurious to tissues at the energy ranges utilized for diagnostic purposes. Because water is an excellent conductor of the ultrasonic beams, patients are requested to drink large quantities of water prior to examination so that the urinary bladder will be distended and enable better viewing of pelvic and abdominal organs.

Two ultrasound techniques, Doppler ultrasound and color-flow imaging, make it possible to record blood velocity (in diagnosing vascular disease) and to image major blood vessels in patients at risk for stroke. Figure 20–7 shows color-flow imaging in a patient with aortic regurgitation (blood flowing backward from the aorta into the left ventricle).

Ultrasound, like fluoroscopy, has also been used in interventional radiology to guide needle biopsies for the puncture of cysts and for the placement of needles for amniocentesis.

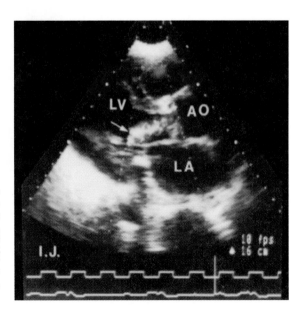

Figure 20-7

Color-flow imaging in a patient with aortic regurgitation. The brightly colored, high-velocity jet *(arrow)* can be seen passing from the aorta (AO) to the left ventricle (LV). The center of the jet is white, and the edges are shades of blue. (From Braunwald E: Heart Disease: A Textbook of Cardiovascular Medicine, 5th ed. Philadelphia, WB Saunders, 1997.)

Magnetic Imaging or Magnetic Resonance Imaging (MRI)

This is a type of diagnostic radiography that uses electromagnetic energy. The technique produces sagittal, coronal (frontal), and axial (cross-sectional) images, the latter being similar to CT scanning. MRI, however, uses no x-rays and does not require a contrast medium. It is based on the fact that the nuclei of some atoms behave like little magnets when a larger magnetic field is applied. The nuclei spin and emit radio waves that create an image as the nuclei move back to an equilibrium position. Hydrogen nuclei, present in water and abundant in living tissue, are the nuclei used to create the image. MRI is useful for providing soft-tissue images, detecting edema in the brain, projecting a direct image of the spinal cord, detecting tumors in the chest and abdomen, and visualizing the cardiovascular system. Figure 20–8 shows three different MRI images (frontal, transverse, and sagittal).

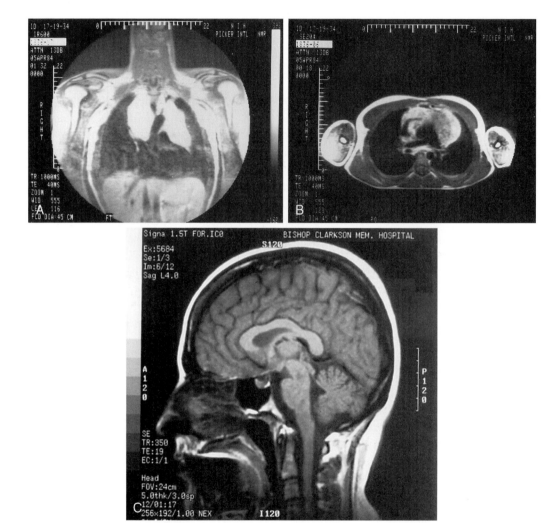

Figure 20–8

Magnetic resonance images. (A) Frontal (coronal) view of the upper body. White masses in the chest are Hodgkin disease lesions. **(B)** Transverse view of the same patient with chest mass. **(C)** Sagittal section of the head (normal magnetic resonance image) showing cerebrum, ventricles, cerebellum, and medulla oblongata. (C from Black JM, Matassarin-Jacobs E: Medical-Surgical Nursing, 5th ed. Philadelphia, WB Saunders, 1997.)

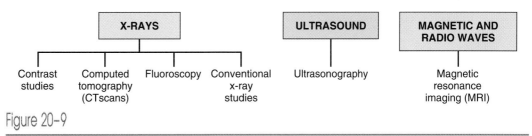

Figure 20-9

Review of radiological diagnostic techniques.

MRI is not used for patients with pacemakers or metallic implants because the powerful MRI magnet can interfere with the position and functioning of such devices. The sounds (loud tapping) heard during the test are caused by the pulsing of the magnetic field as it scans the body.

Figure 20–9 reviews the radiological diagnostic techniques discussed.

C. X-Ray Positioning

In order to take the best view of the part of the body being radiographed, the patient, film, and x-ray tube must be positioned in the most favorable alignment possible. There are special terms used by radiologists to designate the position or direction of the x-ray beam, the patient's position, and the motion and position of the part of the body to be examined. Some of the x-ray terms describing the position of the x-ray beam are as follows:

1. **AP view** (**a**nteroposterior). In this view, the patient is usually supine (lying on the back), and the x-ray tube is aimed from above at the anterior of the body, with the beam passing from anterior to posterior. The film lies underneath the patient. The AP view may also be taken with the patient in the upright position.
2. **PA view** (**p**osteroanterior). In this view, the patient is upright—back to the x-ray machine and the film to the chest. The x-ray machine is aimed horizontally from a distance of about 6 feet from the film.
3. **Lateral view.** In this view, the x-ray beam passes from one side of the body to the opposite side. In taking a right lateral view, the right side of the body is held closely against the x-ray film and the x-ray beam passes from the left to the right through the body.
4. **Oblique view.** In this view, the x-ray tube is positioned at an angle from the perpendicular plane. Oblique views are used to show regions that would be hidden and superimposed in routine AP and PA views.

The following terms are used to describe the position of the patient or part of the body in the x-ray examination:

abduction	Moving the part of the body away from the midline of the body or away from the body.
adduction	Moving the part of the body toward the midline of the body or toward the body.
eversion	Turning outward.
extension	Lengthening or straightening a flexed limb.
flexion	Bending a part of the body.
inversion	Turning inward.
lateral decubitus	Lying down on the side with the x-ray beam horizontally positioned; sometimes called **cross-table lateral.**
prone	Lying on the belly (face down).
recumbent	Lying down (may be prone or supine).
supine	Lying on the back (face up).

III. Nuclear Medicine

A. Radioactivity and Radionuclides

The emission of energy in the form of particles or rays coming from the interior of a substance is called **radioactivity.** A **radionuclide** (or **radioisotope**) is a substance that gives off high-energy particles or rays as it disintegrates. Radionuclides are produced in either a nuclear reactor or a charged-particle accelerator (cyclotron) or by irradiating stable substances, causing disruption and instability. **Half-life** is the time required for a radioactive substance (radionuclide) to lose half of its radioactivity by disintegration. Knowledge of a radionuclide's half-life is important in determining how long the radioactive substance will emit radioactivity when in the body. The half-life must be long enough to allow for diagnostic imaging but as short as possible to minimize patient exposure to radiation. Technetium-99m (^{99m}Tc), with a half-life of 6 hours, is an ideal radionuclide and is used most frequently in diagnostic imaging.

Radionuclides emit three types of radioactivity: **alpha particles, beta particles,** and **gamma rays.** Gamma rays, which have greater penetrating ability than alpha and beta particles, and more ionizing power, are especially useful to physicians in both the diagnosis and the treatment of disease.

B. Nuclear Medicine Tests: *In Vitro* and *In Vivo* Procedures

Nuclear medicine physicians use two types of tests in the diagnosis of disease: ***in vitro*** (in the test tube) procedures and ***in vivo*** (in the body) procedures. ***In vitro*** procedures involve analysis of blood and urine specimens using radioactive chemicals. For example, a **radioimmunoassay (RIA)** is an *in vitro* procedure that combines the use of radioactive chemicals and antibodies to detect hormones and drugs in a patient's blood. The test allows the detection of minute amounts of drug. RIA is used to monitor the amount of digitalis, a drug used to treat heart disease, in a patient's bloodstream and can detect hypothyroidism in newborn infants.

In vivo tests trace the amounts of radioactive substances within the body. They are given directly to a patient to evaluate the function of an organ or to image it. For example, in **tracer studies** a specific radionuclide is incorporated into a chemical substance and administered to a patient. The combination of the radionuclide and a drug or chemical is called a **radiopharmaceutical** (or **labeled compound**). Each radiopharmaceutical is designed to concentrate in a certain organ. The organ can then be imaged with the radiation given off by the radionuclide.

A sensitive, external detection instrument called a **scintiscanner** (or **gamma camera**) is used to determine the distribution and localization of the radiopharmaceutical in various organs, tissues, and fluids. The amount of radiopharmaceutical at a given location is proportional to the rate at which the gamma rays are emitted. Nuclear medicine studies depict the physiological behavior (how the organ works) rather than the specific anatomy of an organ.

The procedure of making an image to follow the distribution of radioactive substance in the body is called **scintigraphy (radionuclide scanning),** and the image produced is called a **scintiscan. Uptake** refers to the rate of absorption of the radiopharmaceutical into an organ or tissue.

Radiopharmaceuticals may be administered by many different routes to obtain a scan of a specific organ in the body. For example, in the case of a **lung scan,** the radiopharmaceutical can be given intravenously (**perfusion studies,** which rely on passage of the radioactive compound through the capillaries of the lungs) or by inhalation of xenon-133 (^{133}Xe) gas (**ventilation studies),** which fills the air sacs (alveoli). The combination of these tests permits sensitive and specific diagnosis of clots in the lung (pulmonary emboli).

Other examples of diagnostic procedures that utilize radionuclides are as follows:

1. **Bone scan.** ^{99m}Tc (technetium) is used to label phosphate substances and is injected intravenously. The phosphate compound is taken up preferentially by bone, and the skeleton can be imaged in 2 or 3 hours by use of a scintiscanner. Waiting 2–3 hours allows much of the radiopharmaceutical to be excreted in urine and allows for better visualization of the skeleton. The scan is useful in demonstrating malignant metastases to the skeleton, which appear as areas of high uptake ("hot spots") on the scan.
2. **Gallium scan.** The radioisotope gallium-67 is injected intravenously and has an affinity for tumors and non-neoplastic lesions such as abscesses. Because gallium has an affinity for areas of inflammation such as that which occurs in pneumonitis, it is used to differentiate between a pulmonary embolism and pneumonitis.
3. **Liver and spleen scans.** To visualize the liver and spleen, a radiopharmaceutical (^{99m}Tc and sulfur colloid) is injected intravenously, and images are taken with a scintiscanner (gamma camera). Areas of tumor or abscess are shown as blank spots (regions of reduced uptake). Abnormalities such as cirrhosis, abscesses, tumor, hepatomegaly, and hepatitis can be detected by liver scanning, and splenomegaly due to tumor, cyst, abscess, or rupture can be diagnosed with spleen scanning.
4. **MUGA scan.** This test (**mu**ltiple **g**ated **a**cquisitions scan) studies the motion of the left ventricular wall and the ventricle's ability to eject blood (ejection fraction).

Technetium-99m (^{99m}Tc) is injected intravenously, the patient is put on a heart monitor, and images are observed. If a coronary artery is narrowed, causing ischemia, the portion of the heart muscle that it supplies shows diminished wall motion, or contractility.

5. **Positron emission tomography (PET scan).** This radionuclide technique produces a cross-sectional (transverse) image of the distribution of radioactivity (through emission of positrons) in a region of the body. It is similar to the CT scan, but radioisotopes are used instead of contrast and x-rays. The radionuclides are incorporated (by intravenous injection) into the tissues to be scanned, and an image is made showing where the radionuclide (such as carbon-11 [^{11}C] glucose, oxygen-15 [^{15}O] oxygen) is or is not being metabolized. For example, PET scanning has determined that schizophrenics do not metabolize glucose equally in all parts of the brain and that drug treatment can bring improvement to these regions. Thus, areas of metabolic deficiency can be pinpointed by PET, making it helpful in diagnosing and treating other neurological disorders such as stroke, epilepsy, Alzheimer disease, and brain tumors, as well as cardiac, pulmonary, and abdominal disorders.

6. **Single-photon emission computed tomography (SPECT).** This technique involves an intravenous injection of radioactive tracer and the computer reconstruction of a three-dimensional image based on a composite of many views. Clinical applications include detecting liver tumors, detecting cardiac ischemia, and evaluating bone disease of the spine.

7. **Thallium (Tl) scan.** Thallium 201 is injected intravenously to allow for myocardial perfusion. A high concentration of thallium 201 is present in well-perfused heart muscle cells, but infarcted or scarred myocardium does not extract any Tl, showing up as "cold spots." If the defective area is ischemic, the cold spots fill in (become "warm") on delayed images. Thallium is a widely used isotope for myocardial perfusion because of its short (73 hours) half-life and low total body radiation dose. The study may be performed before or after an exercise ECG study or as a resting study only.

8. **Thyroid scan.** Radionuclide is administered intravenously. The scan produced can help determine the size and shape of the thyroid gland. Hyperfunctioning thyroid nodules (adenomas) accumulate higher amounts of ^{131}I radioactivity and are termed "hot." Thyroid carcinoma does not concentrate radioiodine well and, therefore, is seen as a "cold" spot on the scan. Figure 20–10 shows thyroid scans.

Figure 20–11 reviews *in vitro* and *in vivo* nuclear medicine diagnostic tests.

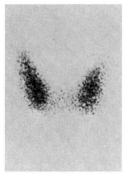
Normal

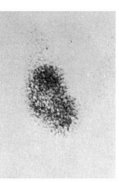
"Hot nodule"

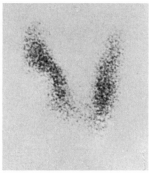
"Cold nodule"

Figure 20-10

Thyroid scans. The scan of a "hot nodule" shows a darkened area of increased uptake, which indicates a diseased thyroid gland. The scan of a "cold nodule" shows an area of decreased uptake, which indicates a nonfunctioning region, a common occurrence when normal tissue is replaced by malignancy. (From Beare PG, Myers JL: Adult Health Nursing, 3rd ed. St. Louis, Mosby, 1998.)

NUCLEAR MEDICINE TESTS

IN VITRO	Radioimmunoassay

IN VIVO	Tracer Studies:
	Bone scan
	Gallium scan
	Liver/spleen scan
	Lung scan (ventilation/perfusion)
	Positron emission tomography (PET)
	Single-photon emission computed tomography (SPECT)
	Thyroid scan

Figure 20-11

In vitro and *in vivo* **nuclear medicine diagnostic tests.**

IV. Radiation Therapy (Radiation Oncology)

Not only are x-rays and radionuclides helpful in detecting disease, but they can be used as therapy as well. Large doses of ionizing radiation to body tissues can be **lethal** (killing) to the cells that are **irradiated.** Radiation oncology has been particularly helpful as a method for the treatment of cancers, as discussed in Chapter 19.

The machines used for radiation oncology are different from those used for diagnosis. Therapy machines deliver rays that are many times higher in intensity. **Orthovoltage** machines deliver low-energy radiation, which in modern treatment centers is used in the treatment of superficial skin cancers. **Megavoltage** machines generate high-energy radiation and are used to treat deeper tissues in curative radiotherapy for cancer. Two examples of such machines are the **betatron** and the **linear accelerator;** they deliver a sharply defined radiation beam to a specific area of the body while sparing overlying superficial tissue.

Radiation may be applied to a tumor from some distance **(external beam radiation)** or implanted within the tumor itself **(brachytherapy).** External beam machines (such as the linear accelerator) direct a beam of photons toward the tumor. The higher the energy of the photons, the greater the penetration of the beam. Photons can also be produced from a radioactive source (cobalt-60 [^{60}Co]); both sources of high-energy photons (linear accelerator and cobalt) are well suited for the treatment of deep-seated tumors.

Brachytherapy includes **interstitial therapy** and **intracavitary therapy.** In order to deliver interstitial therapy, a radioactive element (such as radium, gold-198 [^{198}Au], iodine-125 [^{125}I], or iridium-192 [^{192}Ir]) is surgically inserted into the tumor. This results in a very localized form of treatment, sparing normal tissues in the vicinity. The radionuclide is implanted in strands, in small sealed containers called **seeds,** or in removable needles. Intracavitary therapy is delivered by placing radioactive sources (radium, cesium-137 [^{137}Ce], or phosphorus-32 [^{32}P]) within a body cavity and adjacent to a tumor. This form of therapy is particularly suited for gynecological malignancies (uterus, cervix, or vagina).

Another form of radiotherapy is the administration of radioactive materials into the bloodstream. ^{131}I is used to treat hyperthyroidism and thyroid carcinoma. In hyperthyroidism, the ^{131}I, given orally, passes into the blood and accumulates in the thyroid gland, irradiating the tissue there and reducing the activity of the gland. ^{131}I is also taken up by thyroid tumors. In treating thyroid carcinoma, ^{131}I is used after partial or total thyroidectomy to inactivate any residual thyroid tissue and to treat metastases.

Radiation delivered to tissues is measured in a unit called a **gray (Gy).** A gray is equal to 100 **rad** (radiation absorbed dose). Tumors and body tissues are classified as **radiosensitive** or **radioresistant,** according to the number of grays necessary to kill or injure cells. Examples of radiosensitive organs are the ovaries and testes. Radioresistant organs (such as the pituitary and adrenal glands) are less susceptible to the effects of radiation. Lymphomas are generally radiosensitive, whereas sarcomas are generally very radioresistant.

Radiotherapy, although it may be either a palliative or a curative agent, can produce undesirable side effects on normal body tissues that are incidentally irradiated. Some of these complications are reversible with time, and recovery takes place soon after the period of radiotherapy is completed. These acute reversible effects may include

1. Ulceration of mucous membranes **(mucositis);** for example, in the mouth, pharynx, vagina, bladder, or large and small intestine. **Xerostomia** (dryness of mouth) occurs after radiation to the mouth or pharynx.
2. **Nausea and vomiting** as a reaction to radiotherapy to the brain or gastrointestinal organs.
3. Bone marrow suppression **(myelosuppression),** with leukopenia and thrombocytopenia.
4. **Alopecia** (baldness).

With higher doses of radiotherapy, these complications can be associated with permanent organ damage. In addition, radiotherapy delivered in therapeutic doses may produce chronic (long-lasting) injury to any body organ that happens to be in or near the path of the radiation beam. Chronic side effects depend on the site of treatment delivery and can include pericarditis, pneumonitis, vasculitis (inflammation of blood vessels), and fibrosis of the skin and lungs.

V. Vocabulary

This list will help you review many of the new terms introduced in the text. Short definitions will reinforce your understanding of the terms. See Section XI of this chapter for help in pronouncing the more difficult terms.

betatron	A machine used in radiotherapy to deliver a dose of radiation to a patient.
brachytherapy	Radiation therapy using an implanted radioisotope radiation source (brachy- means short).
cineradiography	Use of motion picture techniques to record a series of x-ray images during fluoroscopy.
cobalt-60	A radioactive substance used in radiotherapy.

computed tomography (CT)	Diagnostic x-ray procedure whereby a cross-section image of a specific body segment is produced; also known as computed axial tomography (CAT).
contrast studies	Materials (contrast media) are injected to obtain contrast with surrounding tissue when shown on the x-ray film.
external beam radiation	Radiation applied using a distant source.
fluorescence	The emission of glowing light that results from exposure to and absorption of radiation from x-rays.
fluoroscopy	The process of using x-rays to produce a fluorescent image on a screen.
gamma rays	High-energy rays emitted by radioactive substances.
gray (Gy)	Unit of absorbed radiation dose (equal to 100 rad).
half-life	Time required for a radioactive substance to lose half its radioactivity by disintegration.
interstitial therapy	Radioisotopes surgically inserted into a tumor (-stitial means to set).
interventional radiology	Therapeutic procedures that are performed by a radiologist.
intracavitary therapy	Radioisotopes are placed within a body cavity adjacent to a tumor.
in vitro	A process, test, or procedure in which something is measured or observed outside a living organism.
in vivo	A process, test, or procedure in which something is measured or observed in a living organism.
ionization	The separation of stable substances into charged particles called ions.
irradiation	Administering radiation treatment to a patient (ir- stands for in-, meaning into).
lethal	Pertaining to that which is deadly or fatal.
linear accelerator	Machine that delivers radiation therapy.
magnetic resonance imaging (MRI)	A magnetic field and radio waves are used to form sagittal, coronal, and axial images of the body.
megavoltage	High-energy radiation generated by a machine and used in curative x-ray therapy for cancer.

nuclear medicine

Medical specialty that studies the uses of radioactive substances (radionuclides) in diagnosis and treatment of disease.

orthovoltage

Low-energy radiation used in palliative radiation therapy and superficial skin cancers.

palliative

Relieving symptoms, but not curing.

positron emission tomography (PET)

Radioactive substances are given intravenously and then emit positrons, which create a cross-sectional image of the metabolism of the body, representing local concentration of the radioactive substance.

rad

Radiation absorbed dose; a unit of absorbed radiation in the body.

radiation oncology

Treatment of tumors using high-energy radiation. Also called radiotherapy or radiation therapy.

radioimmunoassay

Test that combines the use of radioactive chemicals and antibodies to detect minute quantities of substances in a patient's blood.

radioisotope

A radioactive form of a substance; radionuclide.

radiology

Medical specialty concerned with the study of x-rays and their use in the diagnosis of disease; includes other forms of energy, such as ultrasound and magnetic waves.

radiolucent

Permitting the passage of most x-rays. Radiolucent structures appear black on x-ray film.

radionuclide

A radioactive chemical element that gives off energy in the form of radiation; radioisotope.

radiopaque

Obstructing the passage of x-rays. Radiopaque structures appear white on the x-ray film.

radiopharmaceutical

A radioactive drug (radionuclide plus chemical) that is administered safely for diagnostic and therapeutic purposes.

roentgenology

Study of x-rays; radiology.

scan

A general term for images of organs, parts, or transverse sections of the body produced in various ways. Most frequently used to describe images obtained from ultrasound, radioactive tracer studies, or computed tomography.

scintiscanner

Machine used to detect radiopharmaceuticals in the body for diagnostic imaging. Scinti/i means spark. Also called **gamma camera.**

scintigraphy	The production of two-dimensional images of the distribution of radioactivity in tissues after the administration of a radiopharmaceutical imaging agent.
single-photon emission computed tomography (SPECT)	A radioactive tracer substance is injected intravenously and a computer is used to create a three-dimensional image.
tagging	Attaching a radionuclide to a chemical and following its course in the body.
tracer studies	Radionuclides are used as tags, or labels, attached to chemicals and followed as they migrate through the body.
ultrasound (US, U/S)	Diagnostic technique that projects and retrieves high-frequency sound waves as they echo off of parts of the body.
uptake	The rate of absorption of a radionuclide into an organ or tissue.
ventilation/perfusion studies	Radiopharmaceutical is inhaled (ventilation) and injected (perfusion) and its passage through the respiratory tract is imaged.

VI. Combining Forms, Suffixes, Prefixes, and Terminology

Write the meanings of the medical terms in the spaces provided.

Combining Forms			
Combining Form	**Meaning**	**Terminology**	**Meaning**
fluor/o	luminous, fluorescence	fluoroscopy _____	
		In this term, -scopy does not refer to visual examination with an endoscope. In fluoroscopy, x-rays can be viewed directly, without taking and developing x-ray photographs. Light is emitted from the fluorescent screen when it is exposed to x-rays.	
is/o	same	radioisotope _____	
		top/o means place; radioisotopes of an element have similar structures but different weights and electric charges. A radioisotope (radionuclide) is an unstable form of an element that emits radioactivity.	
leth/o	death	lethal _____	

mucos/o	mucous membrane, mucosa	mucositis _____ _This may be a side effect of radiotherapy._	
pharmaceut/o	drug	radiopharmaceutical _____ _In this term, radi/o stands for radioisotope (radionuclide)._	
radi/o	x-rays	radioresistant _____ _Radioresistant tumors are not easily treated with radiotherapy._ radiosensitive _____ _Radiosensitive tumors respond to radiotherapy and can be treated by x-rays or other radiation._	
roentgen/o	x-rays	roentgenology _____	
scint/i	spark	scintigraphy _____	
son/o	sound	sonogram _____	
therapeut/o	treatment	therapeutic _____	
tom/o	to cut	tomography _____ _A series of x-ray images (taken as if to make slices or cuts) are made of the body to show an organ in depth. Changing the depth of focus allows each tomogram to focus on the one slice that is to be viewed._	
vitr/o	glass	_in vitro_ _____	
viv/o	life	_in vivo_ _____	
xer/o	dry	xerostomia _____ _Radiation to the mouth and pharynx can affect the salivary glands and produce this condition. Stom- comes from stomat/o meaning mouth._	

Suffixes			
Suffix	**Meaning**	**Terminology**	**Meaning**
-gram	record	angiogram _____	
		hysterosalpingogram _____	
		pyelogram _____	

-graphy	process of recording	computed tomo<u>graphy</u> _____

-lucent	to shine	radio<u>lucent</u> _____

Radiolucent (indicating that x-rays pass through easily) areas on x-ray film appear dark on the exposed film.

-opaque	obscure	radio<u>paque</u> _____

Radiopaque (indicating that x-rays do not penetrate) areas on x-ray film appear white or light on exposed film.

-suppression	to stop	myelo<u>suppression</u> _____

Myelosuppression may be a side effect of treatment with radiation. Myel/o means bone marrow in this term.

-therapy	treatment	radio<u>therapy</u> _____

Prefixes

Prefix	Meaning	Terminology	Meaning
brachy-	short, short distance	<u>brachy</u>therapy _____	
cine-	movement	<u>cine</u>radiography _____	
echo-	a repeated sound	<u>echo</u>cardiography _____	
inter-	between	<u>inter</u>stitial therapy _____	

stit/o means to stand, put, place, or set.

intra-	within	<u>intra</u>cavitary therapy _____	

cavit/o means a space.

ultra-	beyond	<u>ultra</u>sonography _____	

Sound waves are beyond the normal range of those that a human can hear.

VII. ABBREVIATIONS

Angio	angiography	**LAT**	lateral
AP	anteroposterior	**LS Films**	lumbosacral spine films
Ba	barium	**mCi**	millicurie (measure of radiation)
CAT	computerized axial tomography	**μCi**	microcurie (measure of radiation)
cGy	centigray (a rad—one hundredth of a gray)	**MRI**	magnetic resonance imaging
C-spine	cervical spine films	**MUGA**	multiple-gated acquisitions scan (radioactive test to show heart function)
CT	computed tomography	**PA**	posteroanterior
CXR	chest x-ray	**PET**	positron emission tomography
Decub	decubitus (lying down)	**rad**	radiation absorbed dose
DI	diagnostic imaging	**SPECT**	single-photon emission computed tomography; radioactive substances and a computer are used to create three-dimensional images
DSA	digital subtraction angiography		
^{67}Ga	radioactive gallium (used in whole-body scans)	**^{99m}Tc**	radioactive technetium (used in brain, skull, thyroid, liver, spleen, bone, and lung scans)
Gy	gray (unit of radiation and equal to 100 rads)	**^{201}Tl**	radioisotope (thallium) used in scanning heart muscle
^{131}I	radioactive iodine (used in thyroid, liver, and kidney scans and treatment of malignant and nonmalignant conditions of the thyroid)	**UGI**	upper gastrointestinal series
		US, U/S	ultrasound
IVP	intravenous pyelogram	**VQ scan**	ventilation-perfusion scan of the lungs
KUB	kidneys, ureters, bladder (x-ray without contrast medium)	**XRT**	radiation therapy

VIII. Practical Applications

This section contains actual medical reports using terms that you have studied in this and previous chapters. Answers to the questions are on page 805 after Answers to Exercises.

CT Upper Abdomen Using IV Contrast

Comparison was also made with prior examination. The extensive retroperitoneal and mesenteric lymphadenopathy has shown marked reduction in size. The celiac lymph nodes are also reduced, and the outlines of the lymph nodes are in the top limits of normal at this point. In images 8 and 9 the celiac lymph nodes are no longer visible. Previously described right pleural effusion is also not present. The obstructed right kidney shows atrophy and now measures approximately 7–8 cm in size. The left kidney remains much the same as before. The adrenal glands are symmetrical with normal aorta and inferior vena cava as well as abdominal wall.

Chart Note

DX. Stage T3 N0 M0 colon carcinoma.

TX. 5-FU plus XRT.

Mr. Dean Smith returns today for general follow-up and is currently ready to begin his 5-FU and concurrent XRT in his right lower quadrant. He is without symptoms and denies any abdominal pain, diarrhea, nausea, vomiting, melena, or hematochezia. Vital signs stable, afebrile. HEENT [head, ears, eyes, nose, and throat] entirely benign. Axillary, cervical, and inguinal lymph nodes benign. Chest: lungs clear to auscultation and percussion. Abdomen: notable only for a well-healing midline abdominal scar with moderate smooth hepatomegaly.

Laboratory. This time notable for SGOT 26 [normal: 8–20]; LDH 541 [normal 48–115]. HCT 32.2 [normal 40–54]; platelet 400,000 [normal 200,000–400,000]; WBC 10.1 [normal 4,500–11,000] with normal differential.

Impression and Plan. Mr. Smith should begin his XRT and chemotherapy some time early next week.

Chart Rounds: Center for Radiation Oncology

(A) Patient has metastatic carcinoma and is being treated to the costovertebral junction with 3000 cGy palliatively.

(B) Patient is being treated for cervical esophageal carcinoma. Previously treated with a hockey field technique [RT given covering the area in the shape of a hockey stick] for breast cancer and recurrent field is only being taken to 3000 cGy.

(C) Patient is being treated for a pathological stage II-B Hodgkin disease on the mantle [upper chest and neck]-only protocol.

(D) The patient is being treated for a parietal GBM [glioblastoma multiforme]. The plan needs to be signed. The films look fine.

Questions on the Case Studies

1. Which patient is being treated for a brain tumor?   _____

2. Which patient is being treated for lesions in the ribs?   _____

3. Which patient has disease in cervical and thoracic lymph nodes?   _____

4. Which patient is being treated for gastrointestinal cancer?   _____

General Hospital—Nuclear Medicine Dept.—Radionuclides Available

Radionuclide	Radiopharmaceutical	Admission Route	Target Organ
^{133}Xe	xenon gas	inhaled	lungs
^{99m}Tc	albumin microspheres	IV	lungs
^{87m}Sr (strontium)	solution	IV	bone
^{99m}Tc	diphosphonate	IV	bone
^{99m}Tc	pertechnetate	IV	brain
^{99m}Tc	sulfur colloid	IV	liver/spleen
^{198}Au	colloid	IV	liver
^{199}Au	colloid	IV	spleen
^{131}I	rose bengal	IV	colon
^{99m}Tc	DTPA* or HIDA†	IV	kidney
^{197}Hg (mercury)	chlormerodrin	IV	kidney
^{131}I	iodide	IV	thyroid
^{42}K (potassium)	solution	IV	heart
^{201}Tl (thallium)	thallium chloride	IV	heart
^{99m}Tc	pyrophosphate	IV	heart
^{67}Ga (gallium)	citrate	IV	tumors and abscesses

*DTPA = diethylenetriaminepentaacetic acid
†HIDA = N-(2.6-dimethyl)iminodiacetic acid

IX. Exercises

Remember to check your answers carefully with those given in Section X, Answers to Exercises.

A. Complete the medical terms based on the definitions and word parts given.

1. obstructing the passage of x-rays: radio _____

2. permitting the passage of x-rays: radio _____

3. administering radiation to a patient: irr _____

4. separation of stable substances into charged particles: _____ ization

5. deadly or fatal: _____ al

6. treatment of disease (usually cancer) by means of high-energy rays: _____

   oncology or radio _____

7. a physician who specializes in diagnostic radiology: radi _____

8. study of the uses of radioactive substances in the diagnosis of disease: _____

   _____ medicine

B. Match the special diagnostic techniques below with their definitions.

fluoroscopy   interventional radiology   cineradiography
ultrasonography   magnetic resonance imaging   contrast studies
computed tomography   tomography

1. radiopaque substances are given and conventional x-rays taken _____

2. use of motion picture techniques to record x-ray images _____

3. series of x-rays are taken at different depths of an organ _____

4. use of echoes of high-frequency sound waves to diagnose disease _____

5. x-ray beams are focused from the body onto a screen that glows as a result of the ionizing effect of

   x-rays _____

6. a magnetic field and radio waves are used to form images of the body _____

7. x-ray pictures are taken circularly around an area of the body, and a computer synthesizes the

   information into a composite cross-section picture _____

8. therapeutic procedures are performed by a radiologist under the guidance of fluoroscopy or

   ultrasound _____

C. Match the diagnostic x-ray test in column I with the part of the body that is imaged in column II.

Column I

1. myelography   _____

2. intravenous pyelography   _____

3. angiography   _____

4. arthrography   _____

5. barium swallow   _____

6. bronchography   _____

7. cholangiography   _____

8. barium enema   _____

9. hysterosalpingography   _____

Column II

A. joints
B. spinal cord
C. uterus and fallopian tubes
D. tubes within the lungs
E. blood vessels
F. upper gastrointestinal tract
G. lower gastrointestinal tract
H. renal pelvis of kidney and urinary tract
I. bile vessels (ducts)

D. Match the following x-ray views or positions in column I with their meanings in column II. Write the letter of the answer in the space provided.

Column I

1. PA _____

2. supine _____

3. prone _____

4. AP _____

5. lateral _____

6. oblique _____

7. lateral decubitus _____

8. adduction _____

9. inversion _____

10. abduction _____

11. recumbent _____

12. eversion _____

13. flexion _____

14. extension _____

Column II

A. on the side
B. turned inward
C. movement away from the midline
D. lying on the belly
E. x-ray tube positioned on an angle
F. bending a part
G. straightening a limb
H. lying on the back
 I. lying down on the side; cross-table lateral position
 J. lying down; prone or supine
K. anterior to posterior view
L. turning outward
M. posterior to anterior view
N. movement toward the midline

E. Give the meanings of the following medical terms.

1. *in vitro* _____

2. *in vivo* _____

3. radiopharmaceutical _____

4. tracer studies _____

5. uptake _____

6. perfusion lung scan _____

7. ventilation lung scan _____

8. bone scan _____

9. gallium scan _____

10. thyroid scan _____

11. thallium scan _____

F. Match the following terms with their meanings below.

palliative   scintiscanner   external beam radiation
positron emission tomography (PET)   orthovoltage   brachytherapy
lethal   megavoltage   radionuclide
linear accelerator

1. Low-energy radiation used in treating superficial skin cancers is called _____ .

2. High-energy radiation used to treat deeper tissues is called _____ .

3. Radiation therapy delivered from a shielded, distant unit is called _____ .

4. Radiation therapy using an implanted radioactive substance is called _____ .

5. A machine that delivers radiation therapy is called a (an) _____ .

6. A machine used to detect rays emitted by radioactive substances is a (an) _____ .

7. Pertaining to that which is deadly or fatal _____ .

8. Relieving symptoms but not curative _____ .

9. A radioactive form of a substance is called a (an) _____ .

10. In this test, radioactive substances are given and metabolized by body cells; a cross-sectional image

    is then produced as radioactivity (positrons) is emitted from the body _____ .

G. Give the meanings of the following terms.

1. radiosensitive _____

2. radioresistant _____

3. radioisotope _____

4. myelosuppression _____

5. interstitial therapy _____

6. echocardiography _____

7. intracavitary therapy _____

H. Give the meanings of the following terms that describe side effects produced by radiotherapy.

1. alopecia _____

2. dysphagia _____

3. hyperemesis _____

4. leukopenia _____

5. mucositis _____

6. pericarditis _____

7. xerostomia _____

8. pneumonitis _____

I. Give the meanings of the following combining forms and prefixes.

1. xer/o _____   6. viv/o _____

2. leth/o _____   7. pharmaceut/o _____

3. fluor/o _____   8. son/o _____

4. tom/o _____   9. brachy- _____

5. vitr/o _____   10. inter- _____

J. Give the meanings of the following abbreviations and then select from the sentences that follow the best association for each.

Column I

1. MRI _____ ____

2. SPECT _____ ____

3. MUGA _____ ____

4. Gy _____ ____

5. CXR _____ ____

6. DSA _____ ____

7. XRT _____ ____

8. LAT _____ ____

9. U/S _____ ____

10. ^{131}I _____ ____

Column II

A. This treatment procedure may involve both brachytherapy and machines such as linear accelerators.

B. This diagnostic procedure is frequently used to assess fetal size and development.

C. This unit of radiation is equal to 100 rads.

D. This is an x-ray of blood vessels made by taking two images (with and without contrast) and subtracting one from the other.

E. A radioisotope used in nuclear medicine (tracer studies) and radiotherapy.

F. Radioactive substances and a computer are used to create three-dimensional images.

G. This diagnostic procedure produces images of all three planes of the body and visualizes soft tissue in the nervous and musculoskeletal systems.

H. Radioactive substances are injected intravenously to assess heart function.

I. This is an x-ray position (side view).

J. This diagnostic procedure (x-rays are used) is necessary to investigate thoracic disease.

K. Select the correct term to complete each sentence.

1. Mr. Jones was scheduled for ultrasound-guided removal of his pleural effusion. He was sent to the **(interventional radiology, radiation oncology, nuclear medicine)** department for the procedure.

2. In order to better visualize Mr. Smith's colon, Dr. Wong ordered a **(perfusion study, hysterosalpingography, barium enema).** She hoped to determine why he was having blood in his stools.

3. After the head-on collision, Sam was taken to the emergency room in an unconscious state. The paramedics suspected head trauma, and the doctors ordered an emergency **(PET scan, U/S, CT scan)** of his head.

4. After her mastectomy, Lucy was referred to the department of **(radiology, radiation oncology, nuclear medicine)** for adjuvant treatment to her chest wall and lymph nodes.

5. In light of Sue's symptoms of fever, cough, and malaise, the doctors thought that the consolidated, hazy **(radioisotope, radiolucent, radiopaque)** area on the chest x-ray represented a pneumonia.

X. Answers to Exercises

A

1. radiopaque
2. radiolucent
3. irradiation
4. ionization
5. lethal
6. radiation oncology or radiotherapy
7. radiologist
8. nuclear medicine

B

1. contrast studies
2. cineradiography; a type of fluoroscopy
3. tomography
4. ultrasonography
5. fluoroscopy
6. magnetic resonance imaging
7. computed tomography
8. interventional radiology

C

1. B
2. H
3. E
4. A
5. F
6. D
7. I
8. G
9. C

D

1. M
2. H
3. D
4. K
5. A
6. E
7. I
8. N
9. B
10. C
11. J
12. L
13. F
14. G

E

1. Process, test, or procedure in which something is measured or observed outside a living organism.
2. Process, test, or procedure in which something is measured or observed in a living organism.
3. Radioactive drug (radionuclide plus chemical) that is given for diagnostic or therapeutic purposes.
4. Tests in which radioactive substance (radioisotopes) are used with chemicals and followed as they travel throughout the body.
5. The rate of absorption of a radionuclide into an organ or tissue.
6. A radiopharmaceutical is injected intravenously and traced within the blood vessels of the lung.
7. A radiopharmaceutical is inhaled, and its passage through the respiratory tract is imaged.
8. A radiopharmaceutical is given intravenously and taken up by bone tissue. An image allows the radioactive substance to be traced in the bone.
9. The radioisotope gallium 67 is injected intravenously, and the body is scanned.
10. Radioactive substance is given intravenously, and a scan (image) is made of its uptake in the thyroid gland.
11. Thallium 201 is given intravenously, and myocardial perfusion is assessed.

F

1. orthovoltage
2. megavoltage
3. external beam radiation
4. brachytherapy
5. linear accelerator
6. scintiscanner
7. lethal
8. palliative
9. radionuclide
10. positron emission tomography

G

1. tissue that is sensitive to radiation therapy
2. tissue that is resistant to the effects of radiation therapy
3. a radioactive form (radionuclide) of a substance; gives off radiation
4. bone marrow stops functioning (may be a side effect of radiation therapy)
5. radioisotopes placed in a tumor; a form of brachytherapy
6. ultrasound used to create an image of the heart
7. radioisotopes placed in a body cavity near a tumor; a form of brachytherapy

H

1. baldness
2. difficulty swallowing
3. excessive vomiting
4. deficiency of white blood cells
5. inflammation of mucous membranes
6. inflammation of the membrane surrounding the heart
7. dry mouth
8. inflammation of the lungs

I

1. dry
2. death
3. luminous, fluorescence
4. to cut
5. glass
6. life
7. drug
8. sound
9. short, short distance
10. between

J

1. Magnetic resonance imaging. G
2. Single-photon emission computed tomography. F
3. Multiple-gated acquisitions scan. H
4. Gray. C
5. Chest x-ray. J
6. Digital subtraction angiography. D
7. Radiation therapy. A
8. Lateral. I
9. Ultrasound. B
10. Radioactive iodine. E

K

1. interventional radiology
2. barium enema
3. CT scan
4. radiation oncology
5. radiopaque

Answers to Practical Applications

1. D
2. A
3. C
4. B

XI. Pronunciation of Terms

Pronunciation Guide

ā as in āpe
ē as in ēven
ī as in īce
ō as in ōpen
ū as in ūnit

ă as in ăpple
ĕ as in ĕvery
ĭ as in ĭnterest
ŏ as in pŏt
ŭ as in ŭnder

To test your understanding of the terminology in this chapter, write the meaning of each term in the space provided. In addition, you may wish to cover the terms and write them by looking at your definitions. Make sure your spelling is correct. The page number after each term indicates where it is defined or used in the text so you can easily check your responses.

Term	Pronunciation	Meaning
abduction (786)	ăb-DŬK-shŭn	
adduction (786)	ă-DŬK-shŭn	
angiogram (794)	ĂN-jē-ō-grăm	
anteroposterior (785)	ăn-tĕr-ō-pōs-TĔ-rē-ŏr	
arthrography (781)	ăr-THRŎG-ră-fē	
betatron (790)	BĀ-tă-trŏn	
brachytherapy (790)	brā-kē-THĔR-ă-pē or brăk-ē-THĔR-ă-pē	
cholangiography (781)	kō-lăn-jē-ŎG-ră-fē	
cineradiography (790)	sĭn-ē-rā-dē-ŎG-ră-fē	
computed tomography (791)	kŏm-PŪ-tĕd tō-MŎG-ră-fē	

echocardiography (782)	ĕk-ō-kăr-dē-ŎG-ră-fē	_____
eversion (786)	ē-VĔR-zhŭn	_____
extension (786)	ĕk-STĔN-shŭn	_____
external beam radiation (791)	ĕks-TĔR-năl bēm ră-dē-Ā-shŭn	_____
flexion (786)	FLĔK-shŭn	_____
fluorescence (791)	flū-RĔS-ĕns	_____
fluoroscopy (791)	flū-RŎS-kō-pē	_____
gallium scan (787)	GĂ-lē-ŭm skăn	_____
hysterosalpingogram (794)	hĭs-tĕr-ō-săl-PĬNG-gō-grăm	_____
interstitial therapy (791)	ĭn-tĕr-STĬSH-ăl THĔR-ă-pē	_____
interventional radiology (791)	ĭn-tĕr-VĔN-shŭn-ăl rā-dē-ŎL-ō-je	_____
intracavitary therapy (791)	ĭn-tră-KAV-ĭ-tār-ē THĔR-ă-pē	_____
inversion (786)	ĭn-VĔR-zhŭn	_____
in vitro (791)	in VĒ-trō	_____
in vivo (791)	in VĒ-vō	_____
ionization (791)	ī-ŏn-ĭ-ZĀ-shŭn	_____
irradiation (791)	ĭ-rā-dē-Ā-shŭn	_____
lateral decubitus (786)	LĂ-tĕr-ăl de-KŪ-bĭ-tus	_____
lethal (791)	LĒ-thăl	_____
magnetic resonance imaging (791)	măg-NĔT-ik RĔZ-ō-nans IM-a-jĭng	_____
megavoltage (791)	MĔG-ă-vōl-tăj	_____
mucositis (794)	mū-kō-SĪ-tĭs	_____
myelography (781)	mī-ĕ-LŎG-ră-fē	_____
myelosuppression (795)	mī-ĕ-lō-sŭ-PRĔSH-ŭn	_____
nuclear medicine (792)	NU-klē-ar MĔD-ĭ-sĭn	_____
oblique (785)	ŏ-BLĒK	_____

orthovoltage (792)   ŎR-thō-vŏl-tăj   _____

palliative (792)   PĂL-ē-ă-tĭv   _____

positron emission tomography (792)   pŏs-ĭ-trŏn ē-MĬSH-ŭn tō-MŎG-ră-fē   _____

posteroanterior (785)   pōs-tĕr-ō-ăn-TĒ-rē-ŏr   _____

prone (786)   prōn   _____

pyelogram (794)   PĪ-ē-lō-grăm   _____

radioimmunoassay (792)   rā-dē-ō-ĭ-mū-nō-ĂS-ā   _____

radioisotope (792)   rā-dē-ō-Ī-sō-tōp   _____

radiolucent (792)   rā-dē-ō-LŪ-sĕnt   _____

radionuclide (792)   rā-dē-ō-NŪ-klīd   _____

radiopaque (792)   rā-dē-ō-PĀK   _____

radiopharmaceutical (792)   rā-dē-ō-făr-mă-SŪ-tĭ-kăl   _____

radiotherapy (795)   rā-dē-ō-THĔR-ă-pē   _____

recumbent (786)   rē-KŬM-bĕnt   _____

roentgenology (792)   rĕnt-gĕ-NŎL-ō-jĕ   _____

scintigraphy (793)   sin-TĬG-ră-fē   _____

scintiscanner (792)   sĭn-tĭ-SKĂN-ĕr   _____

sonogram (782)   SŎN-ō-grăm   _____

supine (786)   SŪ-pīn   _____

therapeutic (794)   thĕr-ă-PŪ-tik   _____

tomography (794)   tō-MŎG-ră-fē   _____

tracer studies (793)   TRĀ-sĕr STŬ-dēz   _____

ultrasound (793)   ŭl-tră-SOWND   _____

uptake (793)   ŬP-tāk   _____

urography (781)   ūr-ŎG-ră-fē   _____

ventilation/perfusion studies (793)   vĕn-tĭ-LĀ-shŭn/pĕr-FŪ-shŭn STŬ-dēz   _____

xerostomia (794)   zĕ-rō-STŌ-mē-ă   _____

XII. Review Sheet

Write the meanings of the combining forms in the spaces provided and test yourself. Check your answers with the information in the text or in the glossary (Medical Terms—English) at the back of the book.

COMBINING FORMS

Combining Form	Meaning	Combining Form	Meaning
fluor/o		roentgen/o	
ion/o		scint/i	
is/o		son/o	
leth/o		therapeut/o	
mucos/o		tom/o	
myel/o		vitr/o	
pharmaceut/o		viv/o	
radi/o		xer/o	

SUFFIXES

Suffix	Meaning	Suffix	Meaning
-gram		-opaque	
-graphy		-suppression	
-lucent		-therapy	

PREFIXES

Prefix	Meaning	Prefix	Meaning
brachy-		inter-	
cine-		intra-	
echo-		ultra-	

CHAPTER 21

Pharmacology

This chapter is divided into the following sections

In this chapter you will

- Learn of the various subspecialty areas of pharmacology;
- Identify the various routes of drug administration;
- Differentiate among the various classes of drugs and learn their actions and side effects;
- Define medical terms using combining forms, prefixes, and suffixes that relate to pharmacology; and
- Apply your new knowledge to understanding medical terms in their proper contexts, such as medical reports and records.

I. Introduction

Drugs are chemical or biological substances used in the prevention or treatment of disease or to alter bodily functions, such as mood, behavior, or performance, in a beneficial way. Drugs can come from many different sources. Some drugs are obtained from parts of **plants,** such as the roots, leaves, and fruit. Examples of such drugs are digitalis (from the foxglove plant) and antibiotics such as penicillin and erythromycin (from lower plants called molds). Drugs can also be obtained from **animals;** for example, certain hormones are secretions from the glands of animals. Drugs can be made as chemical substances that are **synthesized** in the laboratory. Anticancer drugs, such as methotrexate and prednisone, are examples of laboratory-synthesized drugs. Some drugs are isolated from plant or animal sources and are contained in food substances; these drugs are called **vitamins.**

Drugs are prepared and dispensed by a **pharmacist** through a drugstore or **pharmacy** on written order from a physician or dentist. A pharmacist must complete a B.S. (bachelor of science) degree in pharmacy (5 years) and many hospital pharmacists complete a Pharm.D. (doctor of pharmacy) after 6 or 7 years of study. As a health care professional, a pharmacist cooperates with, consults with, and sometimes advises licensed practitioners concerning drugs. In addition, the pharmacist answers patients' questions concerning their prescription needs.

The field of medicine that studies drugs—their nature, origin, and effect on the body—is called **pharmacology.** Pharmacology is a broad medical specialty and contains many subdivisions of study, including **medicinal chemistry, pharmacodynamics, pharmacokinetics, molecular pharmacology, chemotherapy,** and **toxicology.**

Medicinal chemistry is the study of new drug synthesis and the relationship between chemical structure and biological effects. **Pharmacodynamics** involves the study of drug effects in the body. Scientists may also study the processes of drug **absorption** (how drugs pass into the bloodstream), **metabolism** (changes drugs undergo within the body), and **excretion** (removal of the drug from the body). The mathematical description of drug disposition (appearance and disappearance) in the body over time is called **pharmacokinetics.**

Molecular pharmacology concerns the study of the interaction of drugs and subcellular entities, such as DNA, RNA, and enzymes. These studies provide important information about the mechanism of action of drugs.

Chemotherapy is the study of drugs that destroy microorganisms, parasites, or malignant cells within the body. Chemotherapy includes treatment of infectious diseases and cancer.

Toxicology is the study of the harmful effects of drugs and chemicals on the body. Toxicological studies in animals are required by law before new drugs can be tested in humans. A toxicologist is also interested in finding proper **antidotes** to any harmful effects of drugs. Antidotes are substances given to neutralize unwanted effects of drugs.

Figure 21–1 reviews the subspecialty areas of pharmacology.

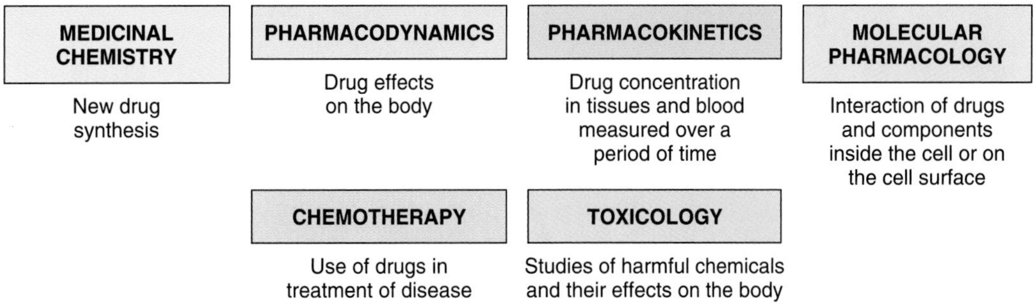

MEDICINAL CHEMISTRY	PHARMACODYNAMICS	PHARMACOKINETICS	MOLECULAR PHARMACOLOGY
New drug synthesis	Drug effects on the body	Drug concentration in tissues and blood measured over a period of time	Interaction of drugs and components inside the cell or on the cell surface

	CHEMOTHERAPY	TOXICOLOGY	
	Use of drugs in treatment of disease	Studies of harmful chemicals and their effects on the body	

Figure 21-1

Subspecialty areas of pharmacology.

II. Drug Names, Standards, and References

Names

A drug can have three different names. The **chemical name** is the chemical formula for the drug. This name, often long and complicated, is useful for the chemist because it shows the structure of the drug.

The **generic,** or **official, name** is a shorter, less complicated name that is recognized as identifying the drug for legal and scientific purposes. The generic name becomes public property after 17 years of use by the original manufacturer, and any drug manufacturer may use it thereafter. There is only one generic name for each drug.

The **brand (trade or proprietary) name** is the private property of the individual drug manufacturer, and no competitor may use it. A brand name often has the superscript ® after or before the name, indicating that it is a registered trade name. Drugs may have several brand names because each manufacturer producing a drug gives it a different name. When a specific brand name is ordered on a prescription by a physician, it must be dispensed by the pharmacist; no other brand name may be substituted. It is usual practice to capitalize the first letter of a brand name.

The following list shows the chemical, generic, and brand names of the antibiotic drug ampicillin; note that the drug can have several names but only one generic, or official, name:

Chemical Name	Generic Name	Brand Name
derivative of 6-aminopenicillanic acid	ampicillin	Omnipen Polycillin Principen Totacillin

Standards

The U.S. **Food and Drug Administration (FDA)** has the legal responsibility for deciding whether a drug may be distributed and sold. It sets rigorous standards for efficacy (effectiveness) and purity and requires extensive experimental testing in animals and people before it approves a new drug for sale in the United States. An independent committee of physicians, pharmacologists, pharmacists, and manufacturers, called the **United States Pharmacopeia (U.S.P.)** reviews the available commercial drugs and continually reappraises their effectiveness. Two important standards of the U.S.P. are that the drug be clinically useful (useful for patients) and available in pure form (made by good manufacturing methods). If a drug has U.S.P. after its name, it has met with the standards of the Pharmacopeia.

References

Libraries and hospitals have two large reference listings of drugs. The most complete and up-to-date is the **Hospital Formulary,** which gives information about the characteristics of drugs and their clinical usage (application to patient care) as approved by that particular hospital.

The **Physicians' Desk Reference (PDR)** is published by a private firm, and drug manufacturers pay to have their products listed. The PDR is a useful reference with several different indices to identify drugs, along with precautions, warnings about side effects, and information about the recommended dosage and administration of each drug.

III. Administration of Drugs

The route of administration of a drug (how it is introduced into the body) is very important in determining the rate and completeness of its absorption into the bloodstream and the speed and duration of the drug's action in the body.

The various methods of administering drugs are described here:

Oral Administration. Drugs are given by mouth and are slowly absorbed into the bloodstream through the stomach or intestinal wall. This method, although convenient for the patient, has several disadvantages. If the drug is destroyed in the digestive tract by digestive juices, or if the drug is unable to pass through the intestinal mucosa, it will be ineffective. Oral administration is also disadvantageous if time is a factor in therapy.

Sublingual Administration. Drugs are not swallowed but are placed under the tongue and allowed to dissolve in the saliva. For some agents, absorption may be rapid. Nitroglycerin tablets are taken in this way to treat attacks of angina pectoris.

Rectal Administration. Suppositories (cone-shaped objects containing drugs) and aqueous solutions are inserted into the rectum. At times, drugs are given by rectum when oral administration presents difficulties, such as when the patient is nauseated and vomiting.

Parenteral Administration. This type of administration is accomplished by injection of the drug from a **syringe** (tube) through a hollow needle placed under the skin, into a muscle, into a vein, or into a body cavity. There are several types of parenteral injections:

1. **Subcutaneous injection (SC).** This is also called a **hypodermic injection,** and it is given just under the skin. The outer surface of the thigh is a usual location for this injection.
2. **Intradermal injection.** This shallow injection is made into the upper layers of the skin and is used chiefly in skin testing for allergic reactions.
3. **Intramuscular injection (IM).** The buttock or upper arm is usually the site for this injection into muscle. When drugs are irritating to the skin or when a large volume of a long-acting drug is needed, IM injections are advisable.
4. **Intravenous injection (IV).** This injection is given directly into a vein. It is used when an immediate effect from the drug is desired or when the drug cannot be safely introduced into other tissues. Good technical skill is needed to administer this injection because leakage of a drug into surrounding tissues may result in irritation and inflammation.
5. **Intrathecal injection.** This injection is made into the space underlying the membranes (meninges) that surround the spinal cord and brain. Methotrexate (a cancer chemotherapeutic drug) is injected intrathecally for treatment of leukemia.
6. **Intracavitary injection.** This injection is made into a body cavity, such as the peritoneal or pleural cavity. For example, nitrogen mustard is injected into the pleural cavity in people who have pleural effusions due to malignant disease. The drug causes the pleural surfaces to adhere, thus obliterating the pleural space and preventing the accumulation of fluid.

Inhalation. Vapors, or gases, are taken into the nose or mouth and are absorbed into the bloodstream through the thin walls of the air sacs in the lungs. **Aerosols** (particles of drug suspended in air) are administered by inhalation, as are many anesthetics. Examples of aerosols are pentamidine, used to treat a form of pneumonia associated with acquired immunodeficiency syndrome (AIDS), and various aerosolized medicines used to treat asthma (spasm of the lung airways).

Topical Application. Drugs are locally applied on the skin or mucous membranes of the body. **Antiseptics** (against infection) and **antipruritics** (against itching) are commonly used as ointments, creams, and lotions. **Transdermal patches** are used to deliver drugs (such as estrogen, pain medications, and nicotine) continuously through the skin.

Table 21–1 summarizes the various routes of drug administration.

Table 21-1. ROUTES OF DRUG ADMINISTRATION

Oral	Sublingual	Rectal	Parenteral	Inhalation	Topical
Tablets	Tablets	Suppositories	Injections Subcutaneous Intradermal Intramuscular Intravenous Intrathecal Intracavitary	Aerosols	Lotions Creams Ointments Transdermal patches

IV. Terminology of Drug Action

When a drug enters the body, the target substance with which the drug interacts to produce its effects is called a **receptor.** A drug may cross the cell membrane to reach its intracellular receptor or may react with a receptor on the cell's surface.

The following terms describe the action and interaction of drugs in the body after they have been absorbed into the bloodstream:

Additive Action. The combination of two similar drugs is equal to the **sum** of the effects of each. For example, if drug A gives 10 per cent tumor kill as a chemotherapeutic agent and drug B gives 20 per cent tumor kill, using A and B together would give 30 per cent tumor kill.

Idiosyncrasy. This is any **unexpected effect** that may appear in the patient following administration of a drug. Idiosyncratic reactions (due to genetic deficiencies in enzymes) are produced in very few patients but may be life-threatening in those few instances. For example, in some individuals penicillin is known to cause an idiosyncratic reaction such as **anaphylaxis** (acute type of hypersensitivity, including asthma and shock).

Synergism (Potentiation). A combination of two drugs can sometimes cause an effect that is **greater** than the sum of the individual effects of each drug given alone. For example, penicillin and streptomycin, two antibiotic drugs, are given together in the treatment of bacterial endocarditis because of their synergistic effect.

Tolerance. The effects of a given dose diminish as treatment goes on, and increasing amounts are needed to produce the same effect. Tolerance is a feature of addiction to drugs such as morphine and meperidine hydrochloride (Demerol). **Addiction** is the physical and psychological dependence on and craving for a drug and the presence of clear effects when that drug or other agent is withdrawn.

V. Drug Toxicity

Drug toxicity is the poisonous and potentially dangerous effects of some drugs. Idiosyncrasy is an example of an unpredictable type of drug toxicity.

Other types of drug toxicity are more predictable and are based on the dosage of the drug given. Physicians are trained to be aware of the potential toxic effects of all drugs that they prescribe. **Iatrogenic** (produced by treatment) disorders can occur, however, as a result of mistakes in drug use or of individual sensitivity to a given agent.

Side effects are toxic effects that routinely result from the use of a drug. They often occur with the usual therapeutic dosage of a drug and are generally tolerable. For example, nausea, vomiting, and alopecia are common side effects of the chemotherapeutic drugs used to treat cancer.

Contraindications are factors in a patient's condition that make the use of a drug dangerous and ill advised. For example, in the presence of renal failure, it is unwise to administer a drug that is normally eliminated by the kidneys because excess drug will accumulate in the body and cause side effects.

VI. Classes of Drugs

The following are major classes of drugs and explanations of their uses in the body. The names of specific drugs are included in tables for your reference (trade or brand names are capitalized; generic names begin with a small letter).

Analgesics

An analgesic (alges/o means sensitivity to pain) is a drug that relieves pain. Mild analgesics are used for mild to moderate pain, such as that caused by myalgias, headaches, and toothaches. More potent analgesics are **narcotics** or **opioids,** so called because they contain or are derived from opium. They induce stupor (a condition of near unconsciousness and reduced mental and physical activity). They are used only to relieve severe pain because they may produce dependence (habit formation) and tolerance. Morphine is an example of a narcotic analgesic.

Some non-narcotic analgesics reduce fever, pain, and inflammation and are used in rheumatic (joint) disorders. These agents are not steroid hormones (such as cortisone) and are known as **nonsteroidal anti-inflammatory drugs (NSAIDs).** NSAIDs act on tissues to inhibit prostaglandins (hormone-like substances that sensitize peripheral pain receptors).

Examples of analgesics are listed in Table 21–2.

Anesthetics

An anesthetic is an agent that reduces or eliminates sensation. This can affect the whole body **(general anesthetic)** or a particular region **(local anesthetic).** General anesthetics are used for surgical procedures; they depress the activity of the central nervous system, producing loss of consciousness. Local anesthetics inhibit the conduction of impulses in sensory nerves in the region in which they are injected or applied.

Table 21–2 gives examples of specific anesthetics.

Table 21-2. ANALGESICS AND ANESTHETICS

Analgesics	Anesthetics
MILD acetaminophen (Tylenol) aspirin	**GENERAL** ether halothane (Fluothane) nitrous oxide thiopental (Pentothal)
NARCOTIC (opioid) codeine hydromorphone (Dilaudid) meperidine (Demerol) morphine oxycodone (Percodan) propoxyphene (Darvon)	**LOCAL** hydrocortisone acetate (Orabase) lidocaine (Xylocaine) procaine (Novocaine)
NONSTEROIDAL ANTI-INFLAMMATORY DRUG (NSAID) diclofenac (Voltaren) ibuprofen (Motrin, Advil) indomethacin (Indocin) naproxen (Naprosyn, Aleve)	

Note: Brand names are in parentheses.

Antibiotics and Antivirals

An antibiotic is a chemical substance produced by a microorganism (bacterium, yeast, or mold) that inhibits **(bacteriostatic)** or kills **(bactericidal)** bacteria, fungi, and parasites. The use of antibiotics (penicillin was first in general use in 1945) has largely controlled many diseases such as pneumonia, rheumatic fever, and mastoiditis. Caution about the use of antibiotics is warranted because they are powerful agents. With indiscriminate use, pathogenic organisms can develop resistance to the antibiotic and thus destroy the antibiotic's disease-fighting capability.

Antiviral drugs are used against viruses, such as the herpesvirus, Epstein-Barr virus, cytomegalovirus (CMV), and human immunodeficiency virus (HIV).

Table 21–3 lists types of antibiotics and antiviral drugs and gives specific examples of each.

Anticoagulants and Antiplatelet Drugs

Anticoagulants prevent the clotting (coagulation) of blood. They prevent the formation of clots or break up clots in blood vessels in conditions such as thrombosis and embolism. They are also used to prevent coagulation in preserved blood used for transfusions. **Heparin** is a natural anticoagulant produced by liver cells and some white blood cells. Other anticoagulants, including **warfarin (Coumadin),** are manufactured. **Tissue-type plasminogen activator (tPA)** dissolves clots and is used to open vessels after myocardial infarction.

Antiplatelet drugs reduce the tendency of platelets to stick together. Aspirin is an example of an antiplatelet drug; it is recommended for patients with coronary artery disease and for those who have had heart attacks.

Table 21–4 lists anticoagulants and antiplatelet drugs.

Anticonvulsants

An anticonvulsant prevents or reduces the frequency of convulsions in various types of epilepsy. Ideally, anticonvulsants depress abnormal spontaneous activity of the brain arising from areas of scar or tumor, without affecting normal brain function. Table 21–4 lists examples of anticonvulsants.

Antidepressants

These drugs treat symptoms of depression. They can elevate mood, increase physical activity and mental alertness, and improve appetite and sleep patterns. Many antidepressants are also mild sedatives and treat mild forms of depression associated with anxiety.

The largest class of antidepressants increases the action of neurotransmitters by blocking their removal (reuptake) from the synapses (spaces between nerve cells). These drugs include **tricyclics (TCAs)** and **selective serotonin reuptake inhibitors (SSRIs).** Other antidepressants are **monoamine oxidase inhibitors (MAOIs),** which increase the length of time neurotransmitters work by blocking monoamine oxidase, an enzyme that normally inactivates neurotransmitters.

Lithium is a drug that is used to stabilize the mood swings and unpredictable behavior of people with bipolar depressive illness (manic-depressive illness).

Table 21–4 gives examples of antidepressants.

Table 21-3. ANTIBIOTICS AND ANTIVIRALS

ANTIFUNGALS

amphotericin B (Fungizone)
fluconazole (Diflucan)
miconazole (Monistat)
nystatin (Nilstat)

ANTITUBERCULARS

isoniazid or INH (Nydrazid)
rifampin (Rifadin)

ANTIVIRALS

acylovir (Zovirax)
* indinavir (Crixivan)
† lamivudine (Epivir)
† zidovudine or AZT (Retrovir)

CEPHALOSPORINS: BACTERICIDAL AND SIMILAR TO PENICILLINS

cefprozil (Cefzil)
cefuroxime axetil (Ceftin)

ERYTHROMYCINS: BACTERIOSTATIC

azithromycin (Zithromax)
clarithromycin (Biaxin)

PENICILLINS: BACTERICIDAL

amoxicillin (Amoxil, Trimox)
amoxicillin with clavulanate (Augmentin)

QUINOLONES: BACTERICIDAL AND WIDE-SPECTRUM

ciprofloxacin (Cipro)
ofloxacin (Floxin)

SULFONAMIDES OR SULFA DRUGS: BACTERICIDAL

sulfamethoxazole with trimethoprim
    (Bactrim, Sulfatrim)
sulfisoxazole (Gantrisin)

TETRACYCLINES: BACTERIOSTATIC

doxycycline
tetracycline

* Anti-HIV (protease inhibitor)
† Anti-HIV (reverse transcriptase inhibitor)
Note: Brand names are in parentheses.

Table 21-4. ANTICOAGULANTS, ANTICONVULSANTS, ANTIDEPRESSANTS, ANTIDIABETICS, AND ANTIHISTAMINES

ANTICOAGULANTS AND ANTIPLATELET DRUGS

aspirin
dicumarol
heparin
tissue plasminogen activator (tPA)
warfarin (Coumadin)

ANTICONVULSANTS

carbamazepine (Tegretol)
phenobarbital
phenytoin (Dilantin)

ANTIDEPRESSANTS

* amitriptyline (Elavil)
† fluoxetine (Prozac)
lithium carbonate (Eskalith)
* nortriptyline (Pamelor)
# phenelzine (Nardil)
† sertraline (Zoloft)

ANTIDIABETICS

Insulins
    rDNA human insulin N (Humulin N)
    rDNA human insulin lispro (Humalog)
Oral drugs
    acarbose (Precose): alphaglucosidase inhibitor
    glipizide (Glucotrol XL): sulfonylurea
    glyburide: sulfonylurea
    metformin (Glucophage): biguanide
    repaglinide (Prandin)-meglitinide
    troglitazone (Rezulin)—thiazolidinedione

ANTIHISTAMINES

    cetirizine (Zyrtec)
    chlorpheniramine maleate (Chlor-Trimeton)
    dimenhydrinate (Dramamine)
    diphenhydramine (Benadryl)
    fexofenadine (Allegra)

* tricyclic drug
† selective serotonin reuptake inhibitor (SSRI)
# monoamine oxidase inhibitor (MAOI)
Note: Brand names are in parentheses.

Antidiabetics

These drugs are used to treat diabetes mellitus (a condition in which the hormone insulin is either not produced by the pancreas or is not effective in the body). Patients with type 1 (insulin-dependent) diabetes must receive daily injections of **insulin.** In the past, most insulin was obtained from animals (pork or beef insulin). Now, much purer human insulin is produced by recombinant DNA research (biosynthesis), and it has replaced animal-derived insulin in the management of diabetes.

Patients with type 2 (non–insulin-dependent) diabetes are given **oral antidiabetic drugs.** These include **sulfonylureas** (lower the levels of glucose in the blood by stimulating the production of insulin), **biguanides** (increase the body's sensitivity to insulin and reduce the production of glucose by the liver), **alpha-glucosidase inhibitors** (temporarily block enzymes that digest sugars), **thiazolidinediones** (enhance glucose uptake into tissues), and **meglitinides** (stimulate the beta cells in the pancreas to produce insulin).

An **insulin pump** is a device strapped to the patient's waist that periodically delivers (via needle) the desired amount of insulin.

Table 21–4 lists antidiabetic drugs.

Antihistamines

These drugs block the action of histamine, which is normally released in the body in allergic reactions. Histamine causes allergic symptoms such as hives, bronchial asthma, hay fever, and in severe cases **anaphylactic shock** (dyspnea, hypotension, and loss of consciousness). Antihistamines cannot cure the allergic reaction, but they can relieve its symptoms. Many antihistamines have strong **antiemetic** (prevention of nausea) activity and are used to prevent motion sickness. The most common side effects of antihistamines are drowsiness, blurred vision, tremors, digestive upset, and lack of motor coordination.

Table 21–4 lists common antihistamines.

Cardiovascular Drugs

Cardiovascular drugs act on the heart or the blood vessels to treat hypertension, angina (pain due to decreased oxygen delivery to heart muscle), heart attack, congestive heart failure, and arrhythmias. Often, before other drugs are used, daily aspirin therapy (to prevent clots in blood vessels) and sublingual nitroglycerin (to dilate coronary blood vessels) are prescribed. **Digoxin (Lanoxin),** comes from a plant of the foxglove family. It slows the heart rate (to control arrhythmias) and helps the heart to pump more forcefully (to treat congestive heart failure). Other cardiovascular drugs are:

Angiotensin-Converting Enzyme (ACE) Inhibitors. These drugs keep blood vessels dilated to lower blood pressure, improve the performance of the heart, and reduce its workload. They prevent the conversion of angiotensin I into angiotensin II, which is a powerful vasopressor (vasoconstrictor). ACE inhibitors are used in treating hypertension, congestive heart failure, and heart attack (myocardial infarction), especially if patients show evidence of a weakened heart.

Beta-Blockers. These drugs decrease the muscular tone in blood vessels (vasodilation), decrease the output of heart, and reduce blood pressure by blocking the action of epinephrine at receptor sites in the heart muscle and in blood vessels. They are used to treat angina, hypertension, and arrhythmias and to treat patients after heart attacks.

Table 21-5. CARDIOVASCULAR DRUGS

ANGIOTENSIN-CONVERTING ENZYME (ACE) INHIBITORS
enalapril (Vasotec)
lisinopril (Zestril)

BETA-BLOCKERS
atenolol (Tenormin)
metoprolol (Lopressor)
propranolol (Inderal)

CALCIUM ANTAGONISTS
amlodipine (Norvasc)
diltiazem (Cardizem)
nifedipine (Cardizem)

CHOLESTEROL-LOWERING
atorvastatin (Lipitor)
cholestyramine (Questran)
lovastatin (Mevacor)
pravastatin (Pravachol)
simvastatin (Zocor)

DIURETICS
furosemide (Lasix)
spironolactone (Aldactone)

Note: Brand names are in parentheses.

Calcium Antagonists or **Calcium Channel Blockers.** As with beta-blockers, they dilate blood vessels and lower blood pressure; they are used to treat angina and arrhythmias. They inhibit the entry of calcium (necessary for blood vessel contraction) into the muscles of the heart and blood vessels.

Cholesterol-Lowering Drugs. They reduce hypercholesterolemia (high levels of cholesterol in the blood), which is a major factor in the development of heart disease. **Cholestyramine (Questran)** lowers cholesterol by promoting its excretion in feces. Other drugs, called **statins** or **HMG-CoA reductase inhibitors,** lower cholesterol by reducing its production in the liver.

Diuretics. These are drugs that reduce the volume of blood in the body by promoting the kidney to remove water and salt through urine. They are used to treat hypertension (high blood pressure) and congestive heart failure.

Table 21–5 reviews and gives examples of cardiovascular drugs.

Endocrine Drugs

These drugs act in much the same manner as the naturally occurring (endogenous) hormones discussed in Chapter 19. **Androgens** are hormones made by the testes and adrenal glands. They are used for male hormone replacement and to treat endometriosis and breast cancer in women. An androgen antagonist (antiandrogen) is **flutamide,** which is used to treat prostate cancer. **Estrogens** are female hormones, normally produced by the ovaries, that are used for symptoms associated with menopause (estrogen replacement therapy) and to prevent postmenopausal osteoporosis. They are also used as chemotherapy for some types of cancer (for example, prostate cancer). An important **antiestrogen** drug is **tamoxifen (Nolvadex),** which is used to prevent recurrence of breast cancer and to treat metastatic breast cancer.

A **SERM (selective estrogen receptor modulator)** is a drug that has estrogen-like effects on bone (increase in bone mineral density) and on lipid (decrease in cholesterol levels) metabolism. However, it seems to lack estrogenic effects on uterus and breast tissue. **Progestins** are prescribed for abnormal uterine bleeding due to hormonal imbalance and, together with estrogen, in hormone replacement therapy and oral contraceptives. **Levonorgestrel (Norplant)** is a contraceptive drug that is imbedded under the skin.

Thyroid hormone is administered when there is a low output of hormone from the thyroid gland. **Glucocorticoids** (adrenal corticosteroids) are prescribed for reduction of inflammation and a wide range of other disorders, including arthritis, severe skin and allergic conditions, respiratory and blood disorders, gastrointestinal ailments, and malignant conditions.

Table 21–6 gives examples of endocrine drugs.

Gastrointestinal Drugs

These drugs are often used to relieve uncomfortable and potentially dangerous symptoms, rather than as cures for specific diseases. **Antacids** neutralize the hydrochloric acid in the stomach to relieve symptoms of peptic ulcer, esophagitis, and epigastric discomfort. **Antiulcer** drugs block secretion of acid by cells in the lining of the stomach and are prescribed for patients with gastric and duodenal ulcers and gastroesophageal reflux disease (GERD). Histamine H_2 receptor antagonists such as **ranitidine (Zantac)** and **cimetidine (Tagamet)** turn off the system (histamine) that produces stomach acid. Another drug, **omeprazole (Prilosec)** works by stopping acid production by a different method (proton-pump inhibition).

Antidiarrheal drugs relieve diarrhea and decrease the rapid movement of the walls of the colon. **Cathartics** relieve constipation and promote defecation for diagnostic and operative procedures and are used in the treatment of disorders of the gastrointestinal tract. Some cathartics increase the intestinal salt content to cause fluid to fill the intestines; others increase the bulk of the feces to promote peristalsis (movement of the intestinal wall). Another type of cathartic lubricates the intestinal tract to produce soft stools. **Laxatives** are mild cathartics, and **purgatives** are strong cathartics.

Antinauseants (antiemetics) relieve nausea and vomiting and also overcome vertigo, dizziness, motion sickness, and labyrinthitis (inflammation of the inner ear).

Table 21–7 lists the various types of gastrointestinal drugs and examples of each.

Respiratory Drugs

These drugs are prescribed for the treatment of emphysema, asthma, and respiratory infections, such as pneumonia and bronchitis. **Bronchodilators** are used to open the air passages (bronchial tubes) and can be administered by injection or aerosol inhalers. Table 21–8 lists common bronchodilators and **steroid drugs** that are used as inhalants or intranasal products to reduce inflammation in nasal passages.

Table 21-6. ENDOCRINE DRUGS

ANDROGEN
fluoxymesterone (Halotestin)
methyltestosterone (Virilon)

ANTIANDROGEN
flutamide (Eulexin)

ESTROGEN
estrogens (Premarin, Estradiol)

ANTIESTROGEN
tamoxifen (Novadex)

GLUCOCORTICOID
dexamethasone (Decadron)
prednisone (Deltasone)

PROGESTIN
medroxyprogesterone (Provera)
megestrol (Megace)

SERM
raloxifene (Evista)

THYROID HORMONE
levothyroxine (Synthroid)
liothyronine (Cytomel)
liotrix (Euthroid)

Note: Brand names are in parentheses.

Table 21-7. GASTROINTESTINAL DRUGS

ANTACID
aluminum and magnesium antacid (Gaviscon)
magnesium antacid (milk of magnesia)
aluminum antacid (Rolaids)

ANTIDIARRHEAL
diphenoxylate and atropine (Lomotil)
loperamide (Imodium)
paregoric

ANTINAUSEANT (ANTIEMETIC)
meclizine (Antivert)
metoclopramide (Reglan)
ondansetron (Zofran)
prochlorperazine maleate (Compazine)

ANTIULCER
cimetidine (Tagamet)
omeprazole (Prilosec)
ranitidine (Zantac)

CATHARTIC
casanthranol and docusate sodium (Peri-Colace)

Note: Brand names are in parentheses.

Table 21-8. RESPIRATORY DRUGS

BRONCHODILATORS
albuterol (Proventil)
epinephrine
salmeterol (Serevent)
theophylline (Theo-Dur)

STEROIDS
beclomethasone (Vanceril)
flunisolide (AeroBid)
triamcinolone (Azmacort)

Note: Brand names are in parentheses.

Sedatives and Hypnotics

Sedatives and hypnotics are medications that depress the central nervous system and promote drowsiness and sleep. They are prescribed for insomnia and sleep disorders. These products have a very high abuse potential and should be used only for short periods of time and under close supervision.

Low doses of **benzodiazepines** (that influence the part of the brain responsible for emotions) may act as sedatives and, in higher doses, as hypnotics (that promote sleep). Table 21–9 gives examples of sedatives/hypnotics.

Stimulants

These drugs act on the brain and are used to speed up vital processes (heart and respiration) in cases of shock and collapse. They also increase alertness and inhibit hyperactive behavior in children. High doses can produce restlessness, insomnia, and hypertension. Examples of stimulants are **amphetamines**—used to prevent narcolepsy (seizures of sleep), to suppress appetite, and to calm hyperkinetic children. **Caffeine** is also a cerebral stimulant. It is used in drugs to relieve certain types of headache by constricting cerebral blood vessels. Table 21–9 lists examples of stimulants.

Tranquilizers

These drugs are useful for controlling anxiety. Minor tranquilizers **(benzodiazepines)** control minor symptoms of anxiety. Major tranquilizers **(phenothiazines)** control more severe disturbances of behavior. Table 21–9 lists examples of minor and major tranquilizers.

Table 21–9. SEDATIVES/HYPNOTICS, STIMULANTS, TRANQUILIZERS

SEDATIVES/HYPNOTICS	TRANQUILIZERS
butabarbital (Butisol)	**Minor**
phenobarbital	* alprazolam (Xanax)
* temazepam (Restoril)	buspirone (BuSpar)
* triazolam (Halcion)	* diazepam (Valium)
zolpidem (Ambien)	* lorazepam (Ativan)
STIMULANTS	**Major**
caffeine	† chlorpromazine (Thorazine)
dextroamphetamine sulfate (Dexedrine)	lithium
methylphenidate (Ritalin)	† thioridazine (Mellaril)
	† trifluoperazine (Stelazine)

* benzodiazepine
† phenothiazine
Note: Brand names are in parentheses.

VII. Vocabulary

This list will help you review many of the new terms introduced in the text. Short definitions will reinforce your understanding of the terms. See Section XIII of this chapter for help in pronouncing the more difficult terms.

General Terms

addiction	Physical and psychological dependence on and craving for a drug.
additive action	Drug action in which the combination of two similar drugs is equal to the sum of the effects of each.
aerosol	Particles of drug suspended in air.
anaphylaxis	An exaggerated hypersensitivity reaction of the body to a drug or foreign organism.
antidote	Agent given to counteract an unwanted effect of a drug.
brand name	Commercial name for a drug; trade name.
chemical name	Chemical formula for a drug.
contraindications	Factors in the patient's condition that prevent the use of a particular drug or treatment.
Food and Drug Administration (FDA)	Governmental agency having the legal responsibility for enforcing proper drug manufacture and clinical use.
generic name	The legal noncommercial name for a drug.
iatrogenic	An effect that is produced as a result of mistakes in drug use or of individual sensitivity to a drug.
idiosyncrasy	An unexpected effect produced in a particularly sensitive individual but not seen in most patients.
inhalation	Administration of drugs in gaseous or vapor form through the nose or mouth.
medicinal chemistry	Study of new drug synthesis; relationship between chemical structure and biological effects.

molecular pharmacology	Study of interaction of drugs and subcellular entities such as DNA, RNA, and enzymes.
oral administration	Drugs are given by mouth.
parenteral administration	Drugs are given by injection into the skin, muscles, or veins (any route other than through the digestive tract).
pharmacodynamics	Study of the effects of a drug within the body.
pharmacokinetics	The calculation of drug concentration in tissues and blood over a period of time.
Physicians' Desk Reference (PDR)	Reference book that lists drug products.
receptor	Target substance with which a drug interacts in the body.
rectal administration	Drugs are inserted through the anus into the rectum.
side effect	A toxic effect that routinely results from the use of a drug.
sublingual administration	Drugs are given by placement under the tongue.
synergism	Drug action in which the combination of two drugs causes an effect that is greater than the sum of the individual effects of each drug alone; potentiation.
syringe	Instrument (tube) for introducing or withdrawing fluids from the body.
tolerance	Drug action in which larger and larger doses must be given to achieve the desired effect. The patient becomes resistant to the action of a drug as treatment progresses.
topical application	Drugs are applied locally on the skin or mucous membranes of the body; ointments, creams, and lotions are applied topically.
toxicity	Harmful effects of a drug.
toxicology	A branch of pharmacology that studies harmful chemicals and their effects on the body.
transport	Movement of a drug across a cell membrane into body cells.
United States Pharmacopeia (U.S.P.)	An authoritative list of drugs, formulas, and preparations that sets a standard for drug manufacturing and dispensing.
vitamin	Substance found in foods and essential in small quantities for growth and good health.

Classes of Drugs and Related Terms

ACE inhibitor
Lowers blood pressure. Angiotensin-converting enzyme (ACE) inhibitors block the conversion of angiotensin I to angiotensin II (a powerful vasoconstrictor).

amphetamine
Central nervous system stimulant.

analgesic
Drug that relieves pain.

anesthetic
Drug that reduces or eliminates sensation.

antacid
Gastrointestinal drug that neutralizes acid in the stomach.

antibiotic
Chemical substance, produced by a plant or microorganism, that has the ability to inhibit or kill foreign organisms in the body. Examples are antifungals, cephalosporins, erythromycin, tetracycline, antituberculars, penicillins, quinolones, and sulfonamides.

anticoagulant
Drug that prevents blood clotting.

anticonvulsant
Drug that prevents convulsions (abnormal brain activity).

antidepressant
Drug used to relieve symptoms of depression.

antidiabetic
Drug used to prevent diabetes mellitus.

antidiarrheal
Drug used to prevent diarrhea.

antiemetic
Agent that prevents nausea and vomiting.

antihistamine
Drug that blocks the action of histamine and helps prevent symptoms of allergy.

antinauseant
Agent that relieves nausea and vomiting; antiemetic.

antiplatelet
Drug that reduces the tendency of platelets to stick together.

antiulcer
Drug that inhibits the secretion of acid by cells of the lining of the stomach.

antiviral
Drug that acts against viruses such as the herpesvirus and HIV.

bactericidal
Drug that kills bacteria (-cidal means to kill).

bacteriostatic
Drug that inhibits bacterial growth (-static means to stop or control).

beta-blocker
Drug that blocks the action of epinephrine at sites on receptors of heart muscle cells, the muscle lining of blood vessels, and bronchial tubes; antiarrhythmic, antianginal, and antihypertensive.

caffeine	Central nervous system stimulant.
calcium antagonist	Drug that blocks the entrance of calcium into heart muscle and muscle lining of blood vessels; used as an antiarrhythmic, antianginal, and antihypertensive; **calcium channel blocker.**
cardiovascular	Drug that acts on the heart and blood vessels. This category of drug includes ACE inhibitors, beta-blockers, calcium antagonists, cholesterol-lowering drugs, and diuretics.
cathartic	Drug that relieves constipation.
diuretic	Drug that increases the production of urine and thus reduces the volume of fluid in the body; antihypertensive.
emetic	Drug that promotes vomiting.
endocrine	A hormone or hormone-like drug. Examples are androgens, estrogens, progestins, SERMs, thyroid hormone, and glucocorticoids.
gastrointestinal	Drug that relieves symptoms of diseases in the gastrointestinal tract. Examples are antacids, antiulcer drugs, antidiarrheal drugs, cathartics, laxatives, purgatives, and antinauseants (antiemetics).
glucocorticoid	Hormone from the adrenal cortex that raises blood sugar and reduces inflammation.
hypnotic	Agent that produces sleep.
laxative	Weak cathartic.
narcotic	Habit-forming drug (potent analgesic) that relieves pain by producing stupor or insensibility.
purgative	Strong cathartic.
respiratory	Drug prescribed for the treatment of asthma, emphysema, and infections of the respiratory system. Bronchodilators are examples.
sedative	A mildly hypnotic drug that relaxes without necessarily producing sleep. Benzodiazepines are examples.
stimulant	Agent that excites and promotes activity. Caffeine and amphetamines are examples.
tranquilizer	Drug used to control anxiety and severe disturbances of behavior.

VIII. Combining Forms, Prefixes, and Terminology

Write the meaning of the medical term in the space provided.

Combining Forms

Combining Form	Meaning	Terminology	Meaning
aer/o	air	aerosol _____
		-sol means solution.
alges/o	sensitivity to pain	analgesic _____
bronch/o	bronchial tube	bronchodilator _____
		Theophylline is a smooth-muscle relaxant used to treat asthma, emphysema, and chronic bronchitis.
chem/o	drug	chemotherapy _____
cras/o	mixture	idiosyncrasy _____
		idi/o means individual, peculiar; syn- means together. An idiosyncrasy is an abnormal, unexpected effect of a drug that is peculiar to an individual.
cutane/o	skin	subcutaneous _____
derm/o	skin	hypodermic _____
erg/o	work	synergism _____
esthes/o	feeling, sensation	anesthesia _____
hist/o	tissue	antihistamine _____
		-amine indicates a nitrogen-containing compound. Histamine is a substance found in all body tissues (it causes capillary dilation and gastric acid secretion and constricts bronchial tube smooth muscle); an excess of histamine is released when the body comes in contact with substances to which it is sensitive.
hypn/o	sleep	hypnotic _____
iatr/o	treatment	iatrogenic _____
lingu/o	tongue	sublingual _____

myc/o	mold, fungus	erythro<u>myc</u>in _____	
narc/o	stupor	<u>narc</u>otic _____	
pharmac/o	drug	<u>pharmac</u>ology _____	
prurit/o	itching	anti<u>prurit</u>ic _____	
pyret/o	fever	anti<u>pyret</u>ic _____	
thec/o	sheath (of brain and spinal cord)	intra<u>thec</u>al _____	
tox/o	poison	<u>tox</u>ic _____	
toxic/o	poison	<u>toxic</u>ology _____	
vas/o	vessel	<u>vas</u>odilator _____	
ven/o	vein	intra<u>ven</u>ous _____	
vit/o	life	<u>vit</u>amin _____	

The first vitamins discovered were nitrogen-containing substances called amines. Table 21–10 lists vitamins, their medical names, and foods that are a major source of each.

Prefixes			
Prefix	Meaning	Terminology	Meaning
ana-	upward, excessive, again	<u>ana</u>phylaxis _____ *-phylaxis means protection.*	
anti-	against	<u>anti</u>dote _____ *-dote comes from the Greek, meaning what is given.* <u>anti</u>biotic _____	
contra-	against, opposite	<u>contra</u>indication _____	
par-	other than, apart from	<u>par</u>enteral _____ *enter/o means intestine.*	
syn-	together, with	<u>syn</u>ergistic _____	

Table 21-10. VITAMINS

Vitamin	Name	Food Source
Vitamin A	Retinol; dehydroretinol	Green leafy and yellow vegetables; liver, eggs, cod liver oil
Vitamin B_1	Thiamine	Yeast, ham, liver, peanuts, milk
Vitamin B_2	Riboflavin	Milk, liver, green vegetables
Niacin	Nicotinic acid	Yeast, liver, peanuts, fish, poultry
Vitamin B_6	Pyridoxine	Liver, fish, yeast
Vitamin B_{12}	Cyanocobalamin	Milk, eggs, liver
Vitamin C	Ascorbic acid	Citrus fruits, vegetables
Vitamin D	Calciferol	Cod liver oil, milk, egg yolk
Vitamin E	α-Tocopherol	Wheat germ oil, cereals, egg yolk
Vitamin K	Phytonadione; menaquinone; menadione	Alfalfa, spinach, cabbage

IX. ABBREVIATIONS

ac	before meals (*ante cibum*)	**pc**	after meals (*post cibum*)
ACE	angiotensin-converting enzyme	**PCA**	patient-controlled administration
ad lib	freely as desired (*ad libitum*)	**PDR**	Physicians' Desk Reference
APAP	acetaminophen (Tylenol)	**po**	by mouth (*per os*)
bid	two times a day (*bis in die*)	**prn**	when requested; *pro re nata* (required)
c̄	with	**Q(q)**	every (*quaque*)
caps	capsule	**qd**	every day (*quaque die*)
cc	cubic centimeter	**qh**	every hour (*quaque hora*)
FDA	Food and Drug Administration	**qhs**	at bedtime (*quaque hora somni*)
gm	gram	**qid**	four times a day (*quater in die*)
gt, gtt	drops (*gutta*)	**qns**	quantity not sufficient
h	hour (*hora*)	**qs**	sufficient quantity (*quantum satis*)
H_2 blocker	histamine H_2 receptor antagonist	**s̄**	without (*sine*)
HRT	hormone replacement therapy	**SERM**	selective estrogen receptor modulator
IM	intramuscular	**sig.**	let it be labeled (*signetur*)
INH	isoniazid (antitubercular agent)	**sos**	if necessary (*si opus sit*)
IV	intravenous	**SSRI**	selective serotonin reuptake inhibitor; antidepressant
MAOI	monoamine oxidase inhibitor; antidepressant	**subcu, subq**	subcutaneous injection
mg	milligram	**tab**	tablet
NPO	nothing by mouth (*nil per os*)	**TCA**	tricyclic antidepressant
NSAID	nonsteroidal anti-inflammatory drug	**tid**	three times a day (*ter in die*)
os	mouth		
oz.	ounce		

X. Practical Applications

The following are the top 25 prescription drugs dispensed in U.S. community pharmacies, new and refill prescriptions, in 1998 (from American Druggist, February 1999, pp. 42–43).

Top 25 Prescription Drugs—1998

Drug (Trade Name)	Generic Name	Type/Use
1. Premarin	estrogen	Hormone (HRT)
2. Synthroid	levothyroxine	Hormone (thyroid gland)
3. Trimox	amoxicillin	Antibiotic (penicillin-type)
4. Hydrocodone w/APAP	hydrocodone w/APAP	Analgesic (narcotic)
5. Prozac	fluoxetine	Antidepressant (SSRI)
6. Prilosec	omeprazole	Gastric acid pump inhibitor
7. Zithromax	azithromycin	Antibiotic (erythromycin-type)
8. Lipitor	atorvastatin	Cholesterol-lowering agent
9. Norvasc	amlodipine	Antihypertensive (calcium channel blocker)
10. Claritin	lovatadine	Antihistamine-decongestant
11. Lanoxin	digoxin	Congestive heart failure
12. Zoloft	sertraline	Antidepressant (SSRI)
13. Albuterol aerosol	albuterol	Bronchodilator
14. Paxil	paroxetine	Antidepressant (SSRI)
15. Amoxicillin	amoxicillin	Antibiotic (penicillin-type)
16. Prempro	conjugated estrogen-medroxyprogesterone	Hormone (HRT)
17. Zestril	lisinopril	Antihypertensive (ACE inhibitor)
18. Vasotec	enalapril	Antihypertensive (ACE inhibitor)
19. Augmentin	amoxicillin/clavulanate	Antibiotic (penicillin-type)
20. Cephalexin	cephalexin	Antibiotic (cephalosporin-type)
21. Zocor	simvastatin	Cholesterol-lowering agent

22. Glucophage	metformin	Antidiabetic (biguanide antihyperglycemic)
23. Coumadin	warfarin	Anticoagulant
24. Acetaminophen/ Codeine	acetaminophen/codeine	Analgesic (narcotic)
25. Ibuprofen	ibuprofen	Nonsteroidal anti-inflammatory drug (NSAID)

Prescriptions

The usual order of drug prescription is name of the drug, dosage, route of administration, time of administration. At times the physician will include a qualifying phrase to indicate why the prescription is being written. Not all information is listed with every prescription. Consider the following:

1. Fluoxetine (Prozac) 20 mg po bid
2. Dimenhydrinate (Dramamine) 10 mg 2 tab q 4–6h
3. Ondansetron (Zofran) 4 mg 1 tab/cap tid prn for nausea
4. Ranitidine (Zantac) 300 mg 1 tab pc qd
5. Pseudoephedrine (Sudafed) 60 mg 1 cap qid for 15 days
6. Acetaminophen (300 mg) & codeine (30 mg) 1 tab qid prn for pain

XI. Exercises

Remember to check your answers carefully with those given in Section XII, Answers to Exercises.

A. *Match the pharmacological specialty with its description below.*

1. use of drugs in the treatment of disease _____

2. study of new drug synthesis _____

3. study of how drugs interact with subcellular parts _____

4. study of the harmful effects of drugs _____

5. study of drug effects in the body _____

6. measurement of drug concentrations in tissues and in blood over a period of time

B. Select from the following terms to complete the sentences below.

antidote   trade (brand) name   toxicologist
generic name   Food and Drug Administration   chemical name
Physicians' Desk Reference   pharmacologist   pharmacist
United States Pharmacopeia

1. A person specializing in the study of the harmful effects of drugs on the body is known as a (an)

   _____.

2. An agent given to counteract harmful effects of a drug is a (an) _____.

3. The governmental agency that has legal responsibility for enforcing proper drug manufacture and

   clinical use is known as the _____.

4. The _____ is the commercial name for a drug.

5. The _____ is the complicated chemical formula for a drug.

6. The _____ is the legal noncommercial name for a drug.

7. A person who dispenses drugs from a store is known as a (an) _____.

8. A person (often a medical doctor) who specializes in the study of the actions of drugs is known as

   a (an) _____.

9. A reference book that lists drug products is known as the _____.

10. An authoritative list of drugs, formulas, and preparations that sets a standard for drug manufac-

    turing and dispensing is known as the _____.

C. Name the route of drug administration based on its description as given below.

1. Drug is administered via suppository or fluid into the anus. _____

2. Drug is administered via vapor or gas into the nose or mouth. _____

3. Drug is administered under the tongue. _____

4. Drug is applied locally on skin or mucous membrane. _____

5. Drug is injected via syringe under the skin or into a vein, muscle, or body cavity.

   _____

6. Drug is given by mouth and absorbed through the stomach or intestinal wall. _____

D. Give the meanings of the following terms.

1. intravenous _____

2. intrathecal _____

3. antiseptic _____

4. antipruritic _____

5. aerosol _____

6. intramuscular _____

7. subcutaneous _____

8. intracavitary _____

9. addiction _____

E. Match the routes of drug administration in column I with the medications or procedures in column II. Write the letter of the answer in the space provided.

Column I

1. intravenous _____

2. rectal _____

3. oral _____

4. topical _____

5. inhalation _____

6. intrathecal _____

7. intramuscular _____

8. intradermal _____

Column II

A. lotions, creams, ointments
B. tablets and capsules
C. skin testing for allergy
D. lumbar puncture
E. deep injection, usually in buttock
F. suppositories
G. blood transfusions
H. aerosol medications

F. The following are descriptions of drug actions. Supply the word that fits the description.

1. the combination of two drugs that is greater than the total effects of each drug operating by itself _____

2. the combination of two drugs that is equal to the sum of the effects of each _____

3. the effects of a given drug dose become less as treatment continues, and larger and larger doses must be given to achieve the desired effect _____

4. any unexpected effect that may appear in a patient following administration of a drug

_____

G. Give the meanings of the following terms that describe classes of drugs.

1. antibiotic _____

2. antidepressant _____

3. antihistamine _____

4. analgesic _____

5. anticoagulant _____

6. anesthetic _____

7. antidiabetic _____

8. sedative _____

9. stimulant _____

10. tranquilizer _____

H. Match the term in column I with the associated term in column II. Write the letter of the answer in the space provided.

Column I

1. antihistamine _____

2. analgesic _____

3. antidiabetic _____

4. anticoagulant _____

5. antibiotic _____

6. stimulant _____

7. sedative/hypnotic _____

8. tranquilizer _____

Column II

A. caffeine or amphetamines
B. penicillin or erythromycin
C. insulin
D. benzodiazepine
E. heparin
F. nonsteroidal anti-inflammatory drug
G. phenothiazine
H. anaphylactic shock

I. Give the meanings of the following terms.

1. beta-blocker _____

2. androgen _____

3. glucocorticoid _____

4. calcium antagonist _____

5. estrogen _____

6. antacid _____

7. cathartic _____

8. antiemetic _____

9. bronchodilator _____

10. hypnotic _____

11. diuretic _____

12. cholesterol-lowering drug _____

J. Match the type of drug in column I with the condition it treats in column II. Write the letter of the answer in the space provided.

Column I

1. anticonvulsant _____

2. anticoagulant _____

3. antacid _____

4. progestins _____

5. antibiotic _____

6. ACE inhibitor _____

7. bronchodilator _____

8. antihistamine _____

9. tranquilizer _____

10. analgesic _____

Column II

A. abnormal uterine bleeding due to hormonal imbalance
B. severe behavior disturbances and anxiety
C. epilepsy
D. congestive heart failure and hypertension
E. epigastric discomfort
F. myalgia and neuralgia
G. anaphylactic shock
H. thrombosis and embolism
I. bacterial pneumonia
J. asthma

K. Complete the following terms based on definitions given.

1. an agent that reduces fever: anti _____

2. an agent that reduces itching: anti _____

3. a habit-forming analgesic: _____ tic

4. two drugs cause an effect greater than the sum of each alone: syn _____

5. an antibiotic derived from a red mold: _____ mycin

6. the legal nonproprietary name of a drug: _____ name

7. a factor in a patient's condition that prevents the use of a particular drug: contra _____

8. drug that produces an absence of sensation or feeling: an _____

L. Using the terms listed below, complete the following sentences.

anesthetic	anticonvulsant	diuretic
NSAID	antiestrogen	antidepressant
antiviral	oral antidiabetic	ACE inhibitor
bactericidal	antihistamine	SERM

1. Cephalosporins (such as cefuroxime and cefprozil) and penicillins are examples of a (an)

   _____ drug.

2. Advil (ibuprofen) is an example of a (an) _____.

3. Tegretol (carbamazepine) and phenytoin (Dilantin) are examples of a (an) _____
   drug.

4. Zovirax (acyclovir) and Crixivan (indinavir) are both types of a (an) _____
   drug.

5. Novadex (tamoxifen), used to treat estrogen receptor positive breast cancer in women, is an

   example of a (an) _____ drug.

6. Patients with high blood pressure may need Vasotec (enalapril) or Zestril (lisinopril). Both of these

   are examples of a (an) _____.

7. Glucophage (metformin) and Rezulin (troglitazone) are two types of _____
   drugs.

8. Evista (raloxifene), used to treat osteoporosis in postmenopausal women, is an example of an estrogen-like drug, known as a (an) _____.

9. Elavil (amitriptyline) and fluoxetine (Prozac) are two types of _____ drug.

10. If you have an allergy, your doctor may prescribe Allegra (fexofenadine), which is a (an) _____ drug.

11. Two agents that reduce the amount of fluid in the blood and thus lower blood pressure are Lasix (furosemide) and Aldactone (spironolactone). These are _____ drugs.

12. Xylocaine (lidocaine) and Pentothal (thiopental) are examples of a (an) _____ drug.

M. Give the meanings of the following abbreviations.

1. NSAID _____   8. s̄ _____

2. prn _____   9. NPO _____

3. qid _____   10. pc _____

4. ad lib _____   11. bid _____

5. tid _____   12. qh _____

6. mg _____   13. po _____

7. c̄ _____   14. q _____

N. Circle the term that best completes the meaning of the sentence.

1. After his heart attack, Bernie was supposed to take many drugs including diuretics and a(an) **(progestin, laxative, anticoagulant)** to prevent blood clots.

2. Estelle was always anxious and had a hard time sleeping. Dr. Max felt that a mild **(antacid, anticonvulsant, tranquilizer)** would help her relax and concentrate on her work.

3. During chemotherapy Helen was very nauseated. Dr. Cohen prescribed an **(antihypertensive, antiemetic, antianginal)** to relieve her symptoms of queasy stomach.

4. The two antibiotics worked together and were therefore **(idiosyncratic, generic, synergistic)** in killing the bacteria in Susan's bloodstream.

5. The label warned that the drug might impair fine motor skills. It listed the **(side effects, antidote, pharmacodynamics)** of taking the sedative.

XII. Answers to Exercises

A

1. chemotherapy
2. medicinal chemistry
3. molecular pharmacology
4. toxicology
5. pharmacodynamics
6. pharmacokinetics

B

1. toxicologist
2. antidote
3. Food and Drug Administration
4. trade (brand) name
5. chemical name
6. generic name
7. pharmacist
8. pharmacologist
9. Physicians' Desk Reference
10. United States Pharmacopeia

C

1. rectal
2. inhalation
3. sublingual
4. topical
5. parenteral
6. oral

D

1. within a vein
2. within a sheath (membranes around the spinal cord or brain)
3. an agent that works against infection
4. an agent that works against itching
5. a solution of particles (drug) in air (vapor or gas)
6. within a muscle
7. under the skin
8. within a cavity
9. physical and psychological dependence on a drug

E

1. G
2. F
3. B
4. A
5. H
6. D
7. E
8. C

F

1. synergism (potentiation)
2. additive action
3. tolerance
4. idiosyncrasy

G

1. an agent that inhibits or kills germ life (microorganisms)
2. an agent that relieves the symptoms of depression
3. an agent that blocks the action of histamine and relieves allergic symptoms
4. an agent that relieves pain
5. an agent that prevents blood clotting
6. an agent that reduces or eliminates sensation
7. an agent used to prevent diabetes mellitus
8. an agent (mildly hypnotic) that relaxes and calms nervousness
9. an agent that excites and promotes activity
10. a drug used to control anxiety and severe disturbances of behavior

H

1. H
2. F
3. C
4. E
5. B
6. A
7. D
8. G

I

1. drug that blocks the action of epinephrine at sites of receptors of heart muscles, blood vessels, and bronchial tubes (antihypertensive, antianginal, and antiarrhythmic)
2. a drug that produces male sexual characteristics
3. a hormone from the adrenal glands that reduces inflammation and raises blood sugar
4. a drug that blocks the entrance of calcium into heart muscle and blood vessel walls (antianginal, antiarrhythmic, and antihypertensive)
5. a hormone that produces female sexual characteristics
6. a drug that neutralizes acid in the stomach
7. a drug that relieves constipation
8. a drug that prevents nausea and vomiting
9. a drug that opens air passages
10. an agent that produces sleep
11. a drug that reduces the volume of blood and lowers blood pressure
12. a drug that reduces hypercholesterolemia

J

1. C
2. H
3. E
4. A
5. I
6. D
7. J
8. G
9. B
10. F

838

K

1. antipyretic
2. antipruritic
3. narcotic
4. synergism
5. erythromycin
6. generic
7. contraindication
8. anesthetic

L

1. bactericidal
2. NSAID
3. anticonvulsant
4. antiviral
5. antiestrogen
6. ACE inhibitor
7. oral antidiabetic
8. SERM (selective estrogen receptor modulator)
9. antidepressant
10. antihistamine
11. diuretic
12. anesthetic

M

1. nonsteroidal anti-inflammatory drug
2. when requested
3. four times a day
4. freely as desired
5. three times a day
6. milligram
7. with
8. without
9. nothing by mouth
10. after meals
11. twice a day
12. every hour
13. by mouth
14. every

N

1. anticoagulant
2. tranquilizer
3. antiemetic
4. synergistic
5. side effects

XIII. Pronunciation of Terms

Pronunciation Guide

ā as in āpe   ă as in ăpple
ē as in ēven   ĕ as in ĕvery
ī as in īce   ĭ as in ĭnterest
ō as in ōpen   ŏ as in pŏt
ū as in ūnit   ŭ as in ŭnder

To test your understanding of the terminology in this chapter, write the meaning of each term in the space provided. In addition, you may wish to cover the terms and write them by looking at your definitions. Make sure your spelling is correct. The page number after each term indicates where it is defined or used in the text so you can easily check your responses.

Term	Pronunciation	Meaning
addiction (823)	ă-DIK-shun	_____
additive action (823)	AD-ĭ-tĭv ĂK-shŭn	_____
aerosol (823)	Ā-ĕr-ō-sōl	_____
amphetamine (825)	ăm-FĔT-ă-mēn	_____
analgesic (825)	ăn-ăl-JĒ-zĭk	_____
anaphylaxis (823)	ăn-ă-fĭ-LĂK-sĭs	_____
androgen (819)	ĂN-drō-jĭn	_____
anesthesia (827)	ăn-ĕs-THĒ-zē-ă	_____
anesthetic (825)	ăn-ĕs-THĔ-tĭk	_____

antacid (825)	ănt-ĂS-ĭd	
antibiotic (825)	ăn-tĭ-bī-ŎT-ĭk	
anticoagulant (825)	ăn-tĭ-kō-ĂG-ū-lănt	
anticonvulsant (825)	ăn-tĭ-kŏ-VŬL-sănt	
antidepressant (825)	ăn-tĭ-dĕ-PRĔS-ănt	
antidiabetic (825)	ăn-tĭ-dī-ă-BĔ-tĭk	
antidiarrheal (825)	ăn-tĭ-dī-ă-RĒ-ăl	
antidote (823)	ĂN-tĭ-dōt	
antiemetic (825)	ăn-tĭ-ĕ-MĔ-tĭk	
antihistamine (825)	ăn-tĭ-HĬS-tă-mēn	
antinauseant (825)	ăn-tĭ-NAW-zē-ănt	
antiplatelet (825)	ăn-tĭ-PLĀT-lĕt	
antipyretic (828)	ăn-tĭ-pĭ-RĔT-ĭk	
antiulcer (825)	ăn-tĭ-ŬL-ser	
bactericidal (825)	băk-tē-rĭ-SĪ-dăl	
bacteriostatic (825)	băk-te-rē-ō-STĂ-tĭk	
beta-blocker (825)	BĀ-tă-BLŎK-er	
bronchodilator (827)	brŏng-kō-DĪ-lā-tĕr	
benzodiazepine (822)	bĕn-zō-dī-ĂZ-ĕ-pēn	
caffeine (826)	kăf-ĒN	
calcium antagonist (826)	KĂL-sē-ŭm ăn-TĂ-gōn-ĭst	
cathartic (826)	kă-THĂR-tĭk	
chemotherapy (827)	kē-mō-THĔR-ă-pē	
contraindication (823)	kōn-tră-ĭn-dĭ-KĀ-shŭn	
diuretic (826)	dī-ū-RĔT-ĭk	
emetic (826)	ĕ-MĔT-ĭk	
erythromycin (828)	ĕ-rīth-rō-MĪ-sĭn	
estrogen (819)	ĔS-trō-jŭn	
generic name (823)	jĕ-NĔR-ĭk năm	

glucocorticoid (826)   gloo͞-kō-KOR-tĭ-koyd   _____

hypnotic (826)   hĭp-NOT-ĭk   _____

hypodermic (827)   hī-pō-DĔR-mĭk   _____

iatrogenic (827)   ī-ăt-rō-JĔN-ĭk   _____

idiosyncrasy (827)   ĭd-ē-ō-SĬN-kră-sē   _____

inhalation (823)   ĭn-hă-LĀ-shŭn   _____

intrathecal (828)   ĭn-tră-THĒ-kăl   _____

laxative (826)   LĂK-să-tĭv   _____

medicinal chemistry (823)   mĕ-DĬ-sĭ-năl KĔM-ĭs-trē   _____

molecular pharmacology (824)   mō-LĔK-ū-lăr făr-mă-KOL-ō-jē   _____

narcotic (826)   năr-KOT-ĭk   _____

parenteral (828)   pă-RĔN-tĕr-ăl   _____

pharmacodynamics (824)   făr-mă-kō-dī-NĂM-ĭks   _____

pharmacokinetics (824)   făr-mă-kō-kĭ-NĔT-ĭks   _____

progestin (819)   prō-GĔS-tĭn   _____

purgative (826)   PŬR-gă-tĭv   _____

sedative (826)   SĔD-ă-tĭv   _____

stimulant (826)   STĬM-ū-lănt   _____

sublingual (827)   sŭb-LĬNG-wăl   _____

synergism (824)   SĬN-ĕr-jĭzm   _____

synergistic (828)   sĭn-ĕr-JĬS-tĭk   _____

syringe (824)   sĭ-RĬNJ   _____

tolerance (824)   TOL-ĕr-ănz   _____

toxicity (824)   tŏk-SĬS-ĭ-tē   _____

toxicology (824)   tŏk-sĭ-KOL-ō-jē   _____

tranquilizer (826)   TRĂN-kwĭ-lī-zĕr   _____

vasodilation (818)   văz-ō-dī-LĀ-shŭn   _____

vitamin (824)   VĪ-tă-mĭn   _____

XIV. Review Sheet

Write the meanings of the word parts in the spaces provided and test yourself. Check your answers with the information in the chapter or in the glossary (Medical Terms—English) at the back of the book.

COMBINING FORMS

Combining Form	Meaning	Combining Form	Meaning
aer/o	_____	lingu/o	_____
alges/o	_____	myc/o	_____
bronchi/o	_____	narc/o	_____
chem/o	_____	pharmac/o	_____
cras/o	_____	prurit/o	_____
cutane/o	_____	pyret/o	_____
derm/o	_____	thec/o	_____
enter/o	_____	tox/o	_____
erg/o	_____	toxic/o	_____
esthes/o	_____	vas/o	_____
hist/o	_____	ven/o	_____
hypn/o	_____	vit/o	_____
iatr/o	_____		

SUFFIXES

Suffix	Meaning	Suffix	Meaning
-amine	_____	-in	_____
-dote	_____	-phylaxis	_____
-genic	_____	-sol	_____

PREFIXES

Prefix	Meaning	Prefix	Meaning
ana-	_____	par-	_____
anti-	_____	syn-	_____
contra-	_____		

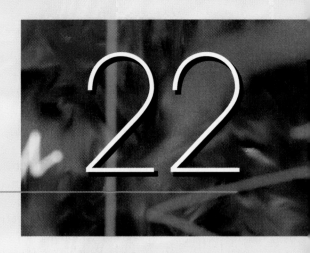

CHAPTER 22

Psychiatry

This chapter is divided into the following sections

In this chapter you will

- Differentiate among a psychiatrist, a psychologist, and other mental health specialists;
- Learn of tests used by clinical psychologists to evaluate a patient's mental health and intelligence;
- Define terms that describe major psychiatric disorders;
- Identify terms that describe psychiatric symptoms;
- Compare different types of therapy for psychiatric disorders;
- Learn the categories and names of common psychiatric drugs;
- Define combining forms, suffixes, prefixes, and abbreviations related to psychiatry; and
- Apply your new knowledge to understanding medical terms in their proper contexts, such as medical reports and records.

I. Introduction

You will find this chapter different from others in the book. Most psychiatric disorders are not readily explainable in terms of abnormalities in the structure or chemistry of an organ or tissue, as are other illnesses. In addition, the causes of mental disorders are complex and include significant psychological and social as well as chemical and structural elements. Our purpose here will be to provide a simple outline and definitions of major psychiatric terms. For more extensive and detailed information, you may wish to consult the **Diagnostic and Statistical Manual of Mental Disorders: DSM-IV** (American Psychiatric Association, Washington, DC, 1994), as well as other textbooks of psychiatry.

Psychiatry (psych/o means mind, **iatr/o** means treatment) is the branch of medicine that deals with the diagnosis, treatment, and prevention of mental illness. It is a specialty of clinical medicine comparable to surgery, internal medicine, pediatrics, and obstetrics.

Psychiatrists complete the same medical training (4 years of medical school) as other physicians and receive an M.D. degree. Then they spend a varying number of years training in the methods and practice of **psychotherapy** (psychological techniques of treating mental disorders) and drug therapy. Psychiatrists can also take additional years of training to specialize in various aspects of psychiatry. **Child psychiatrists** specialize in the treatment of children; **forensic psychiatrists** specialize in the legal aspects of psychiatry, such as the determination of mental competence in criminal cases. **Psychoanalysts** complete 3–5 years of training in a special psychotherapeutic technique called **psychoanalysis** in which the patient freely relates her or his thoughts to the analyst, who does not interfere in the flow of thoughts.

A **psychologist** is a nonmedical person who is trained in methods of psychotherapy, analysis, and research and completes a master's or doctor of philosophy (Ph.D.) degree in a specific field of interest, such as **clinical** (patient-oriented) **psychology, experimental psychology,** or **social psychology** (focusing on social interaction and the ways the actions of others influence the behavior of the individual). A clinical psychologist, like a psychiatrist, can use various methods of psychotherapy to treat patients but, unlike the psychiatrist, cannot prescribe drugs or electroconvulsive therapy. Other nonphysicians trained in the treatment of mental illness are licensed clinical social workers and psychiatric nurses.

Clinical psychologists are trained in the use of tests to evaluate various aspects of a patient's mental health and intelligence. Examples are intelligence (I.Q.) tests such as the **Wechsler Adult Intelligence Scale (WAIS)** and the **Stanford-Binet Intelligence Scale.** Projective (personality) tests are the **Rorschach technique** (inkblots, as shown in Fig. 22–1, are used to bring out associations) and the **Thematic Apperception Test (TAT),** in which pictures are used as stimuli for making up a story (Fig. 22–2). Both tests are especially revealing of personality structure. Graphomotor projection tests are the **Draw a Person Test,** in which the patient is asked to draw a body, and the **Bender-Gestalt Test,** in which the patient is asked to draw certain geometric designs. The Bender-Gestalt Test picks up deficits in mental processing and memory caused by brain damage. The **Minnesota Multiphasic Personality Inventory (MMPI)** contains true-false questions that reveal aspects of personality, such as sense of duty or responsibility, ability to relate to others, and dominance. This test is widely used as an objective measure of psychological disorders in adolescents and adults. A patient's responses to questions are compared with responses made by patients with diagnoses of schizophrenia, depression, and so on.

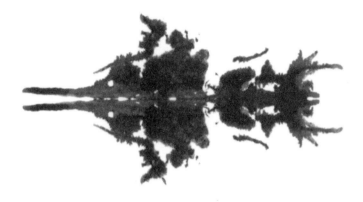

Figure 22-1

Inkblots like this one are presented on 10 cards in the Rorschach test. The patient describes images seen in the blot.

II. Psychiatric Clinical Symptoms

These terms describe abnormalities in behavior that are evident to an examining mental health professional. They will help you to understand Section III, Psychiatric Disorders.

amnesia	Loss of memory.
anxiety	Varying degrees of uneasiness, apprehension, or dread often accompanied by palpitations, tightness in the chest, breathlessness, and choking sensations.
apathy	Absence of emotions; lack of interest or emotional involvement.
autism	Severe lack of responsiveness to others, preoccupation with inner thoughts; withdrawal and retarded language development. Auto- means self.

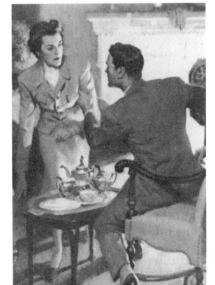

Figure 22-2

A sample picture from the **Thematic Apperception Test.** The patient is asked to tell the story that the picture illustrates. (From Gleitman H: Psychology. New York, WW Norton, 1991.)

compulsion	Uncontrollable urge to perform an act repeatedly.
conversion	Anxiety becomes a bodily symptom, such as blindness, deafness, or paralysis, that does not have an organic basis.
delusion	A fixed, false belief that cannot be changed by logical reasoning or evidence.
dissociation	Uncomfortable feelings are separated from their real object. In order to avoid mental distress, the feelings are redirected toward a second object or behavior pattern.
dysphoria	Sadness, hopelessness; depressive mood.
euphoria	Exaggerated feeling of well-being ("high").
hallucination	False or unreal sensory perception as, for example, hearing voices when none is present; an **illusion** is a false perception of an actual sensory stimulus.
labile	Unstable; undergoing rapid emotional change.
mania	State of excessive excitability; hyperactivity and agitation.
mutism	Nonreactive state; stupor.
obsession	An involuntary, persistent idea, emotion, or urge.
paranoia	Delusions of persecution or grandeur or combinations of the two.

III. Psychiatric Disorders

Sigmund Freud's ideas of personality structure play an important role in the understanding of many types of psychiatric disorders. Freud believed that personality is made up of three major parts: the **id**, the **ego**, and the **superego.** The **id** represents the unconscious instincts and psychic energy present at birth and thereafter. From the id arises basic drives that, operating according to the pleasure principle, seek immediate gratification regardless of the reality of the situation. The id is believed to predominate in the thinking of infants and to be manifest in the uncontrolled actions of certain mentally ill patients.

The **ego** is the central coordinating branch of the personality. It is the mediator between the id and the outside world. It is the part of the personality that evaluates and assesses the reality of a situation **(reality testing)** and, if necessary, postpones the gratification of a need or drive (id) until a satisfactory object or situation arises. The ego is perceived as being "self" by the individual.

The **superego** is the internalized conscience and moral part of the personality. It encompasses the sense of discipline derived from parental authority and society. Guilt feelings, for example, arise from behavior and thoughts that do not conform to the standards of the superego.

Freud believed that certain psychological disorders occur when conflicts arise between two or more of these aspects of the personality. **Defense mechanisms,** such as denial, are the techniques people employ to ward off the anxiety produced by these conflicts. For example, a person afflicted with a serious illness may avoid confronting his or her present or future problems by denial. Thus, he or she may refuse to believe the diagnosis, may miss appointments, may neglect medication, or may ignore symptoms. Whereas all persons utilize defense mechanisms to cope with difficult problems, the use of these mechanisms may be regarded as abnormal or normal according to whether that use makes a constructive or destructive contribution to the individual's personality.

The term **psychosis** is frequently used to describe mental illness. A **psychosis** involves significant impairment of reality testing, with symptoms such as **delusions** (false beliefs), **hallucinations** (false sensory perceptions), and bizarre behavior. Schizophrenic disorders are examples of psychoses. Patients exhibit a disturbed sense of self, inappropriate affect (emotional reactions), and withdrawal from the external world.

Psychiatric disorders that will be discussed in this section are **anxiety disorders, delirium** and **dementia, dissociative disorders, eating disorders, mood disorders, personality disorders, schizophrenia, sexual** and **gender identity disorders, somatoform disorders,** and **substance-related disorders.**

Anxiety Disorders

These disorders are characterized by anxiety—the experience of unpleasant tension, distress, troubled feelings, and avoidance behavior. A **panic attack (disorder),** marked by intense fear or discomfort and symptoms such as palpitations, sweating, trembling, and dizziness, can occur on its own with no symbolic meaning for the patient (that is, it occurs "out of the blue"), or it can occur in the context of the following anxiety disorders: **phobic disorders, obsessive-compulsive disorder,** and **post-traumatic stress disorder.**

Phobic disorders are characterized by irrational or debilitating fears associated with a specific object or situation. The patient with a phobic disorder goes to extreme lengths to avoid the object of her or his fear. The object that is feared is often symbolic of an unconscious conflict that is the cause of the phobia and thus diverts the patient's attention from the conflict, keeping it unconscious.

Agoraphobia (**agora** means marketplace) is the fear of being alone or in open, crowded, public places from which escape would be difficult or in which help might not be available. Persons with agoraphobia limit their normal activities to avoid situations that trigger their anxiety. Thus, they may feel comfortable only by remaining at home or in the company of a friend or relative. Panic attacks (periods of intense apprehension and fear) can occur in anticipation of the phobic situation.

A **social phobia (social anxiety disorder)** is the fear of situations in which the individual is open to public scrutiny which could result in possible embarrassment and humiliation. Fear of speaking in public, using public lavatories, or eating in public are examples of social phobias.

Other specific phobias are **claustrophobia** (fear of closed-in places; **claustr/o** means barrier), **acrophobia** (fear of heights; **acr/o** means extremity), and **zoophobia** (fear of animals; **zo/o** means animals).

Obsessive-compulsive disorder (OCD) involves recurrent thoughts **(obsessions)** and repetitive acts **(compulsions)** that dominate the patient's behavior. The patient experiences anxiety if he or she is prevented from performing special rituals, which are used to shield against overwhelming anxiety or fear. Often the OCD consumes time and significantly interferes with the individual's social or occupational functioning. Several antidepressant drugs, including clomipramine, have been used for the treatment of OCD with considerable success, particularly when combined with cognitive-behavioral therapy.

Post-traumatic stress disorder is the development of symptoms (intense fear, helplessness, insomnia, nightmares, and diminished responsiveness to the external world) following exposure to a traumatic event.

Delirium and Dementia

Delirium and **dementia** are both disorders of abnormal **cognition** (mental processes of thinking, perception, reasoning, judgment).

Delirium is acute, temporary disturbance of consciousness and mental confusion. It is characterized by rambling, irrelevant, or incoherent speech, sensory misperceptions, and disorientation as to time, place, or person and by memory impairment. Delirium is caused by a variety of conditions, including drug intoxication or withdrawal, seizures or head trauma, and metabolic disturbances such as hypoxia, hypoglycemia, electrolyte imbalances, or hepatic or renal failure. **Delirium tremens** is brought on by withdrawal after prolonged periods of heavy alcohol ingestion.

Dementia is a general loss of intellectual abilities that involves impairment of judgment, memory, and abstract thinking as well as changes in personality. Dementia may be caused by conditions, some reversible and some progressive, involving damage to the brain. The most common cause is Alzheimer disease, but others are cerebrovascular disease, central nervous system (CNS) infection, brain trauma, tumors, and Parkinson and Huntington disease.

Dissociative Disorders

Dissociative disorders are chronic or sudden disturbances of memory, identity, consciousness, or perception of the environment that are not caused by the direct effects of brain damage or drug abuse. Symptoms hide the pain and anxiety of unconscious conflicts. Examples of dissociative disorders are **dissociative identity disorder,** which is the existence within the individual of two or more distinct personalities that take hold of the individual's behavior (illustrated in literature by Dr. Jekyll and Mr. Hyde); **dissociative amnesia** (inability to remember important personal information that is too extensive to be explained by ordinary forgetfulness); and **dissociative fugue** (sudden, unexpected travel away from home or customary work locale). The fugue (fugue means flight) disorder includes the assumption of a new identity and an inability to recall one's previous identity.

Eating Disorders

Eating disorders are severe disturbances in eating behavior. Examples are **anorexia nervosa** and **bulimia nervosa.** Anorexia nervosa is a refusal to maintain a minimally normal body weight. An individual is intensely afraid of gaining weight and has a disturbance in the perception of the shape or size of his or her body. (The term anorexia, meaning lack of appetite, is a misnomer because lack of appetite is rare). The condition predominantly affects adolescent females, and its principal symptom is a conscious, relentless attempt to diet along with excessive, compulsive overactivity, such as exercise, running, or gymnastics. Most postmenarcheal females with this disorder are amenorrheic.

Bulimia nervosa (bulimia means abnormal increase in hunger) is characterized by binge eating (uncontrolled indulgence in food) followed by purging (eliminating food from the body). Bulimic individuals maintain normal or nearly normal weight because after binging they engage in inappropriate purging. Examples are self-induced vomiting and the misuse of laxatives or enemas.

Mood Disorders

A mood disorder is prolonged emotion such as depression or mania (elation) that dominates a patient's entire mental life. Examples of mood disorders are **bipolar disorders** and **depressive disorders.**

Bipolar disorders (**bi-** means two; **pol/o** means extreme) are characterized by one or more **manic** episodes alternating with depressive episodes. A manic episode is a period during which the predominant mood is excessively elevated (euphoria), expansive, or irritable. Associated symptoms include inflated self-esteem, or grandiosity, decreased need for sleep, a nearly continuous flow of rapid speech with quick changes of topic, distractibility, an increase in goal-directed activity, and excessive involvement in pleasurable activities that have a high potential for painful consequences. Often there is increased sociability and participation in multiple activities marked by intrusive, domineering, and demanding behavior. **Hypomania** (hypo- means decrease) describes a mood resembling mania, but of lesser intensity. **Bipolar I** is one or more manic episodes, often with a major depressive episode. **Bipolar II** is recurrent major depressive episodes with hypomanic episodes.

Cyclothymic disorder (**cycl/o** means cycle, **thym/o** means mind) is a mild form of bipolar disorder characterized by at least 2 years of hypomania and numerous depressive episodes that do not meet the criteria that define a major depressive episode.

Depressive disorders are marked by one or more major depressive episodes without a history of mania or hypomania. **Major depression** involves episodes of severe **dysphoria** (sadness, hopelessness, worry, discouragement). Other symptoms are appetite disturbances and changes in weight, sleep disorders such as insomnia or hypersomnia, fatigue or low energy, feelings of worthlessness, hopelessness, or excessive or inappropriate guilt, difficulty thinking or concentrating, and recurrent thoughts of death or suicide. **Dysthymia** (or **dysthymic disorder**) is a depressive disorder involving depressed mood (feeling sad or "down in the dumps") that persists over a 2-year period but is not as severe as major depression. Also, there are no psychotic features (delusions, hallucinations, incoherent thinking) as are sometimes found in major depression. Dysthymic disorder can be very impairing but commonly responds well to medication.

Physicians have noted a relationship between the onset of an episode of depressive disorder and a particular 60-day period of the year. A regular appearance of depression may occur between the beginning of October and the end of November every year. This is referred to as **seasonal affective** (mood) **disorder (SAD).** A change from depression to mania or hypomania also may occur within a 60-day period from mid-February to mid-April.

Personality Disorders

Personality traits are established patterns of thinking and ways of relating to and perceiving the environment and one's self. However, when these traits become inflexible and rigid, causing impairment of functioning, distress, and conflict with others, they constitute personality disorders. Examples of personality disorders are

antisocial	No loyalty to or concern for others, and without moral standards; acts only in response to desires and impulses; cannot tolerate frustration and blames others when she or he is at fault.
borderline	Instability in interpersonal relationships and sense of self; characterized by alternating involvement with and rejection of people. Frantic efforts are made to avoid real or imagined abandonment.
histrionic	Emotional, attention-seeking, immature, and dependent; irrational outbursts and tantrums; flamboyant and theatrical; having general dissatisfaction with one's self and angry feelings about the world.
narcissistic	Grandiose sense of self-importance or uniqueness and preoccupation with fantasies of success and power. **Narcissism** is a pervasive interest in one's self with a lack of empathy for others.
paranoid	Continually suspicious and mistrustful of other people but not to a psychotic or delusional degree; jealous and overly concerned with hidden motives of others; quick to take offense.
schizoid	Emotionally cold and aloof; indifferent to praise or criticism or to the feelings of others; few friendships and rarely appears to experience strong emotions, such as anger or joy.

Schizophrenia

This disorder is characterized by withdrawal from reality into an inner world of disorganized thinking and conflict. There is mental deterioration from a previous level of function in areas such as work, social relations, and self-care. Some characteristic symptoms of schizophrenia are:

Delusions such as thought broadcasting (the belief that one's thoughts, as they occur, are broadcast from one's head to the external world so that others can hear them).

Hallucinations, which may involve many voices the person perceives as coming from outside her or his head.

Disorganized thinking such as loosening of associations (ideas shift from one subject to another, completely unrelated or only obliquely connected). This may result in incoherent, incomprehensible speech.

Flat affect (external expression of emotion) marked by monotonous voice, immobile face, and no signs of expression. Affect may also be inappropriate (giggling and laughing when talking about torture and illness).

Impaired interpersonal functioning and relationship to the external world such as emotional detachment and social withdrawal. **Autism** (preoccupation with self-centered, illogical ideas and fantasies that exclude the external world) is often a feature of schizophrenia.

Physicians describe several types of schizophrenia, such as **catatonic type** (characterized by catatonic stupor in which the patient is mute and does not move or react to the outside environment); **disorganized type** (disorganized speech and behavior and flat or inappropriate affect); and **paranoid type** (presence of prominent delusions of grandeur or persecution and auditory hallucinations).

Sexual and Gender Identity Disorders

Sexual disorders are divided into two types: **paraphilias** and **sexual dysfunctions. Paraphilias (para** means abnormal, **philia** means attraction to or love) are characterized by recurrent intense sexual urges, fantasies, or behaviors that involve unusual objects, activities, or situations. Sexual dysfunctions are disturbances in sexual desire or psychosexual changes in sexual response, such as premature ejaculation and dyspareunia (painful sexual intercourse) that are not the result of a general medical condition.

Examples of paraphilias are

exhibitionism	Compulsive need to expose one's body, particularly the genitals, to an unsuspecting stranger.
fetishism	The use of nonliving objects (articles of clothing) as substitutes for a human sexual love object.
pedophilia	Sexual urges and fantasies involving sexual activity with a prepubescent child (age 13 or younger).
sexual masochism	Sexual gratification is gained by being humiliated, beaten, bound, or otherwise made to suffer by another person.
sexual sadism	Sexual gratification is gained by inflicting physical or psychological pain or humiliation on others.
transvestic fetishism	Cross-dressing; wearing clothing of the opposite sex. This disorder has been described only in heterosexual males who have intense sexually arousing fantasies, urges, or behaviors involving cross-dressing.
voyeurism	Sexual excitement is achieved by observing unsuspecting people who are naked, undressing, or engaging in sexual activity.

A **gender identity disorder** is a strong and persistent cross-gender identification with the opposite sex. This identification is manifested in preference for cross-dressing and cross-sex roles in make-believe play or in persistent fantasies of being the other sex.

Somatoform Disorders

These are a group of disorders in which the patient's mental conflicts are expressed as physical symptoms. The physical symptoms, such as abdominal or chest pain, nausea, vomiting, diarrhea, palpitations, deafness, blindness, and paralysis, are not adequately explained by a physical or other mental disorder or by injury and are not side effects of medication, drugs, or alcohol. There is no diagnosable medical condition such as depression that fully accounts for a physical symptom.

Examples of somatoform (**somat/o** means body) disorders are **conversion disorder** and **hypochondriasis.**

Conversion disorder is a loss of physical functioning that suggests a physical disorder but that instead is an expression of a psychological conflict or need. The patient usually has a feared or unconscious conflict that threatens to escape from **repression** (a defense mechanism in which a person removes unacceptable ideas or impulses from consciousness), but the energies associated with this conflict are experienced as a physical symptom. The conversion symptom (examples are paralysis, blindness, seizures, paresthesias, and dyskinesia) enables the individual to avoid the conflict and get support from the surrounding environment. For example, a person with repressed anger and desire to physically harm a family member may suddenly develop paralysis of the arm (conversion symptom). Another example of conversion disorder is shell shock or combat fatigue, in which a soldier becomes paralyzed and cannot participate in battle.

Hypochondriasis is a preoccupation with bodily aches, pains, and discomforts in the absence of real illness. Appropriate physical evaluation does not support the diagnosis of any physical disorder that can account for the symptoms or the person's unwarranted interpretation of them.

Substance-Related Disorders

These disorders are characterized by symptoms and behavioral changes associated with regular use of substances that affect the central nervous system. Continued or periodic use of certain drugs produces a state of dependence. **Psychological dependence** is a compulsion to continue taking a drug despite adverse consequences, and **physical dependence** is characterized by the onset of withdrawal symptoms when the drug is discontinued abruptly. A significant feature of dependence is **tolerance.** Tolerance is the declining effect of the drug, so that the dose must be increased to give the same effect.

Examples of substances that are associated with drug abuse (use of a drug for purposes other than those for which it is prescribed) and dependence are:

Alcohol. Alcohol dependence is often associated with the use and abuse of other psychoactive drugs (cannabis, cocaine, heroin, amphetamines). Signs of alcohol dependence and intoxication include slurred speech, incoordination, unsteady gait, nystagmus (rapid, rhythmic movement of the eyeball), impairment in attention or memory, stupor or coma. It is also associated with depression, as either a cause or a consequence of the drinking.

Amphetamines. These central nervous system stimulants are taken orally or intravenously. Examples are **amphetamine (Benzedrine), dextroamphetamine (Dexedrine), and methamphetamine (Desoxyn,** or speed). Appetite suppressants (diet pills) are amphetamine-like drugs. Psychological and behavioral changes associated with amphetamine dependence include anger, tension or anxiety, impaired judgment, inability to enjoy what was previously pleasurable, and social isolation. Physical symptoms include tachycardia or bradycardia, pupillary dilation, nausea, elevated or low blood pressure, and muscular weakness.

Cannabis. This class of drugs includes all substances with psychoactive properties derived from the cannabis plant plus chemically similar synthetic substances. Examples are **marijuana,** hashish, and purified delta-9-tetrahydrocannabinol (THC), the major psychoactive ingredient in these substances. Psychological and physical symptoms following the smoking of cannabis include euphoria, impaired motor coordination, anxiety, sensation of slowed time, social withdrawal, and impaired memory and judgment. Other signs of cannabis intoxication are increased appetite, dry mouth, and tachycardia.

Cocaine. Cocaine is a stimulant drug that produces euphoria as well as vasoconstriction, tachycardia, and hypertension. It comes from the leaves of the coca tree, which grows in Central and South America. The form of cocaine most commonly used in the United States is cocaine hydrochloride powder, which is inhaled through the nostrils and then absorbed into the bloodstream through mucous membranes. It can also be injected intravenously and mixed with heroin (speedball). This mixture is particularly dangerous because cocaine and heroin act synergistically in depressing respiratory function. If the cocaine is separated from its powdered salt form (with ether, ammonia, or baking soda), the resulting cocaine alkaloid is commonly called freebase. This form can be smoked and is known as crack or rock. Often, the user of cocaine is also dependent on alcohol or sedatives, which are taken in an attempt to alleviate the unpleasant aftereffects (anxiety, depression, and fatigue) of cocaine intoxication.

Hallucinogens. These drugs produce a state of central nervous system excitement, hyperactivity, hallucinations, delusions, hypertension, and mood changes. Examples of hallucinogens are **lysergic acid diethylamide (LSD), mescaline (peyote),** and **phencyclidine (PCP).** The use of hallucinogens is generally episodic because their psychoactive effects are so potent; frequent use may lead to marked tolerance.

Opioids. This group of drugs includes **heroin** and **morphine** and synthetic drugs with morphine-like action, such as **codeine** and meperidine (Demerol). These compounds are prescribed as analgesics, anesthetics, or cough-suppressants. Typical symptoms of opioid intoxication are pupillary constriction, euphoria, slowness in movement, drowsiness, and slurred speech. Effects of overdose are slow and shallow breathing, convulsions, coma, and possible death. Symptoms of opioid withdrawal are watery eyes, rhinorrhea, pupillary dilation, abdominal cramps and diarrhea, and muscle and joint pain.

Sedatives, hypnotics, or anxiolytics. These drugs have a soothing, relaxing, euphoric effect and can also produce sleep (hypnotics). Sleeping pills include **barbiturates** such as phenobarbital and secobarbital. Other drugs that produce a barbiturate-like effect are **benzodiazepines,** including temazepam (Restoril), alprazolam (Xanax), and diazepam (Valium). Intoxication is characterized by slurred speech and disorientation. Effects of overdose are shallow respiration, cold and clammy skin, dilated pupils, weak and rapid pulse, coma, and possibly death. Sudden cessation of these drugs results in seizures.

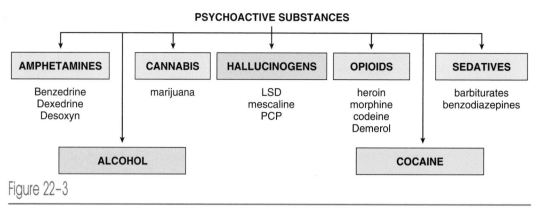

Figure 22-3

Psychoactive substances that lead to drug dependence.

Table 22-1. PSYCHIATRIC DISORDERS

Disorder	Examples
Anxiety disorders	Panic disorder Phobic disorders Obsessive-compulsive disorder Post-traumatic stress disorder
Delirium and dementia	Delirium tremens
Dissociative disorders	Dissociative identity disorder Dissociative amnesia Dissociative fugue
Eating disorders	Anorexia nervosa Bulimia nervosa
Mood disorders	Bipolar I Bipolar II Cyclothymic disorder Depressive disorders Seasonal affective disorder
Personality disorders	Antisocial, borderline, histrionic, narcissistic, paranoid, schizoid
Schizophrenia	Catatonic, disorganized, and paranoid types
Sexual and gender identity disorders	Paraphilias Sexual dysfunction Gender identity disorder
Somatoform disorders	Conversion disorder Hypochondriasis
Substance-related disorders	Alcohol, amphetamines, cannabis, cocaine, hallucinogens, opioids, sedatives

Figure 22–3 reviews the types of psychoactive substances that lead to drug dependence and abuse.

Table 22–1 reviews psychiatric disorders and gives examples of each type.

IV. Therapeutic Terminology

Some major therapeutic techniques that are used to treat psychiatric disorders are **psychotherapy, electroconvulsive therapy,** and **drug therapy (psychopharmacology).**

Psychotherapy

This is the treatment of emotional problems by using psychological techniques. The following are psychotherapeutic techniques used by psychiatrists, psychologists, and other mental health professionals.

Behavior Therapy. Conditioning (changing behavior patterns and responses by training and repetition) is used to relieve anxiety and treat phobias.

Family Therapy. Treatment of an entire family to resolve and understand their conflicts and problems.

Group Therapy. A group of patients with similar problems gain insight into their own personalities through discussions and interaction with each other. In **psychodrama,** patients express their feelings by acting out roles along with other patient-actors on a stage. After a scene has been presented, the audience (composed of other patients) is asked to make comments and offer interpretations about what they have observed.

Hypnosis. A **trance** (state of altered consciousness) is created to increase the speed of psychotherapy or to help recovery of deeply repressed memories.

Play Therapy. Therapy in which a child, through play, uses toys to express conflicts and feelings that she or he is unable to communicate in a direct manner.

Psychoanalysis. Developed by Sigmund Freud, this long-term and intense form of psychotherapy seeks to influence behavior and resolve internal conflicts by allowing patients to bring their unconscious emotions to the surface. Through techniques such as **free association** (speaking one's thoughts one after another without censorship), **transference** (relating to the therapist as one had to a person who figured prominently in early childhood, such as a parent or sibling), and **dream interpretation,** the patient is able to bring to awareness his or her unconscious emotional conflicts and thus can overcome these problems.

Sex Therapy. This form of therapy helps individuals to overcome sexual dysfunctions such as **frigidity** (inhibited sexual response in women), **impotence** (inability of a man to achieve and/or maintain an erection), and **premature ejaculation** (release of semen before coitus can be achieved).

Electroconvulsive Therapy (ECT)

A treatment in which an electric current is applied to the brain while the patient is anesthetized, paralyzed, and being ventilated. This produces convulsions (involuntary muscular contractions) which, with modern techniques, are usually observable only in the form of a twitching of the toe. It is used chiefly for serious depression and the depressive phase of bipolar (manic-depressive) disorder. With the introduction of antidepressant drug therapy, there are fewer indications for electroconvulsive therapy, although it can be life saving when a rapid response is needed.

Drug Therapy

The following are categories of drugs used to treat psychiatric disorders. Figure 22–4 reviews these groups and lists specific drugs in each category.

- **Antianxiety and antipanic agents.** These drugs lessen anxiety, tension, and agitation, especially when they are associated with panic attacks. Examples are **benzodiazepines (BZDs),** which act as antianxiety agents, sedatives, or anticonvulsants (clonazepam). Benzodiazepines directly affect the brain to slow down the transmission of nerve impulses. Other antianxiety and antipanic agents are **selective serotonin reuptake inhibitors (SSRIs).** These agents prevent the movement of serotonin (a neurotransmitter) into nerve endings, allowing it to remain in the spaces surrounding nerve endings.

- **Antidepressants.** These drugs gradually reverse depressive symptoms and produce feelings of well-being. The basis of depression is thought to be an imbalance in the levels of neurotransmitters in the brain. There are several groups of drugs that are used as antidepressants. These include:

  1. **SSRIs** (selective serotonin reuptake inhibitors) such as fluoxetine (Prozac). They improve mood, mental alertness, physical acitivity, and sleep patterns.
  2. **Monoamine oxidase (MAO) inhibitors.** These drugs suppress an enzyme (monoamine oxidase) that normally degrades neurotransmitters. MAO inhibitors are not as widely prescribed as other antidepressants because serious cardiovascular and liver complications can occur with their use.
  3. **Tricyclic antidepressants.** These drugs contain three fused rings (tricyclic) in their chemical structure. They block the reuptake of neurotransmitters at nerve endings.
  4. **Atypical antidepressants.** These are antidepressants that do not fit in the previous categories.

- **Antiobsessive-compulsive disorder (OCD) agents.** These drugs are prescribed to relieve the symptoms of obsessive-compulsive disorder. Tricyclic antidepressants and SSRIs are examples of these agents.

- **Antipsychotics (neuroleptics).** These drugs modify psychotic symptoms and behavior (neur/o = nerve, -leptic = taking hold). Examples are **phenothiazines,** which are tranquilizers that reduce the anxiety, tension, agitation, and aggressiveness associated with psychoses and modify psychotic symptoms such as delusions and hallucinations. Atypical drugs are examples of antipsychotics other than phenothiazines.

  An important side effect of taking neuroleptic drugs is **tardive dyskinesia** (tardive means late and dyskinesias are abnormal movements). This is a potentially irreversible condition marked by uncontrollable movements.

- **Hypnotics.** These drugs are used to produce sleep (hypn/o = sleep) and relieve insomnia. Examples are sedatives and benzodiazepines.

- **Mood stabilizers.** These drugs treat the manic episodes of bipolar illness. **Lithium (Eskalith, Lithane)** is commonly used to reduce the levels of manic symptoms, such as rapid speech, hyperactive movements, grandiose ideas, poor judgment, aggressiveness, and hostility. It is also used as an adjunct in the treatment of depression. Lithium is a simple salt that is thought to stabilize nerve membranes. Other drugs used as mood stabilizers are anticonvulsants.

- **Stimulants.** These drugs **(amphetamines)** are prescribed for **attention-deficit hyperactivity disorder (ADHD)** in children. Common symptoms of ADHD are having a short attention span and being easily distracted, emotionally unstable, impulsive, and moderately to severely hyperactive.

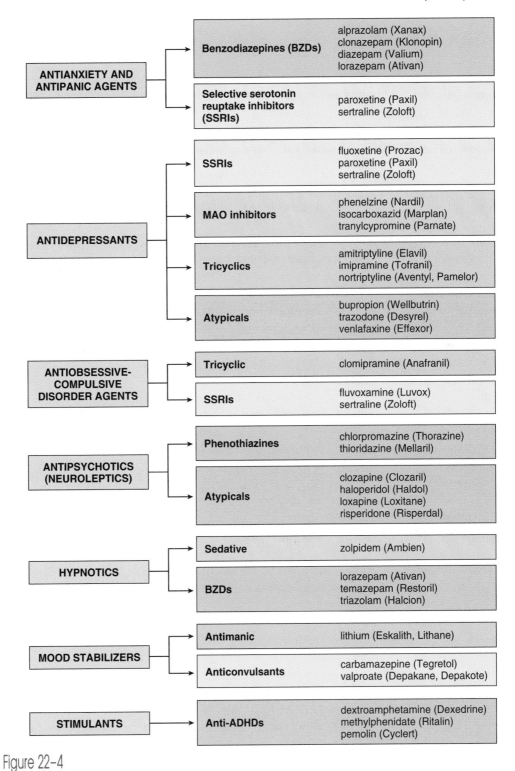

Figure 22-4

Psychiatric drug therapies and specific drugs.

V. Vocabulary

This list will help you review many of the new terms introduced in the text. Short definitions will reinforce your understanding of the terms. See Section XI of this chapter for help in pronouncing the more difficult terms.

Psychiatric Symptoms and Disorders

affect	The expression of emotion, or emotional response.
amnesia	Loss of memory.
anorexia nervosa	An eating disorder of excessive dieting and refusal to maintain a normal body weight.
anxiety disorders	Characterized by unpleasant tension, distress, and avoidance behavior; examples are phobias, obsessive-compulsive disorder, and post-traumatic stress disorder.
apathy	Absence of emotions; lack of interest or emotional involvement.
autism	Severe lack of response to other people; withdrawal, inability to interact, and retarded language development.
bipolar disorder	Alternating periods of mania and depression.
bulimia nervosa	An eating disorder of binge eating followed by vomiting, purging, and depression.
compulsion	Uncontrollable urge to perform an act repeatedly.
conversion disorder	A physical symptom, with no organic basis, that appears as a result of anxiety and conflict.
defense mechanism	Unconscious technique a person uses to resolve or conceal conflicts and anxiety.
delirium	Confusion in thinking; faulty perceptions and irrational behavior. Delirium tremens is associated with alcohol withdrawal.
delusion	Fixed, false belief that cannot be changed by logical reasoning or evidence.
dementia	Loss of intellectual abilities with impairment of memory, judgment, and reasoning as well as changes in personality.
depression	Major mood disorder with chronic sadness, loss of energy, hopelessness, worry, and discouragement and, commonly, suicidal impulses and thoughts.

dissociative disorder	Chronic or sudden disturbance of memory, identity, or consciousness; dissociative identity disorder, amnesia, and fugue.
ego	The central coordinating branch of the personality.
fugue	Amnesia with flight from customary surroundings.
gender identity disorder	Strong and persistent cross-gender identification with the opposite sex.
hallucination	False sensory perception.
id	The major unconscious part of the personality; energy from instinctual drives and desires.
labile	Unstable; undergoing rapid emotional change.
mania	Extreme excitement, hyperactivity, inflated self-esteem.
mood disorders	Prolonged emotion dominates a person's life; examples are bipolar and depressive disorders.
mutism	Nonreactive state; stupor.
obsessive-compulsive disorder	An anxiety disorder in which recurrent thoughts and repetitive acts dominate behavior.
paranoia	Delusions of persecution or grandeur or combinations of the two.
paraphilia	Recurrent intense sexual urge, fantasy, or behavior that involves unusual objects, activities, or situations.
personality disorders	Lifelong personality patterns marked by inflexibility and impairment of social functioning.
phobia	Irrational or disabling fear of an object or situation.
post-traumatic stress disorder	Anxiety-related symptoms appear following exposure to personal experience of a traumatic event.
psychosis	Impairment of mental capacity to recognize reality, communicate, and relate to others.
reality testing	Ability to perceive fact from fantasy; severely impaired in psychoses.
repression	Defense mechanism by which unacceptable thoughts, feelings, and impulses are automatically pushed into the unconscious.
schizophrenia	Withdrawal from reality into an inner world of disorganized thinking and conflict.

sexual disorders	Disorders of paraphilias and sexual dysfunctions.
somatoform disorders	Having physical symptoms that cannot be explained by any actual physical disorder or other well-described mental disorder such as depression.
substance-related disorders	Regular use of psychoactive substances (alcohol, amphetamines, cannabis, cocaine, hallucinogens, opioids, and sedatives) that affect the central nervous system.
superego	Internalized conscience and moral part of the personality.

Therapy

amphetamines	Central nervous system stimulants that may be used to treat depression and attention-deficit hyperactivity disorder.
behavior therapy	Conditioning (changing behavior patterns by training and repetition) is used to relieve anxiety and improve symptoms of illness.
benzodiazepines	Drugs that lessen anxiety, tension, and agitation and panic attacks.
electroconvulsive therapy	Electric current is used to produce convulsions in the treatment of depression. Modern techniques use anesthesia, so the convulsion is not observable.
family therapy	Treatment of an entire family to resolve and understand conflicts.
free association	A psychoanalytic technique in which the patient verbalizes, without censorship, the passing contents of his or her mind.
group therapy	A group of patients with similar problems gain insight into their personalities through discussion and interaction with each other.
hypnosis	Trance (state of altered consciousness) is used to increase the pace of psychotherapy.
lithium	A medication used to treat the manic stage of manic-depressive illness.
neuroleptic drug	Any drug that favorably modifies psychotic symptoms. Examples are phenothiazines.
phenothiazines	Tranquilizers used to treat psychoses.
play therapy	Treatment in which a child, through use of toys in a playroom setting, expresses conflicts and feelings unable to be communicated in a direct manner.
psychoanalysis	A treatment that allows the patient to explore inner emotions and conflicts so as to understand and change current behavior.

psychopharmacology	Treatment of psychiatric disorders with drugs.
psychodrama	Group therapy in which a patient expresses feelings by acting out roles with other patients.
sedatives	Drugs that lessen anxiety.
transference	Psychoanalytic process in which the patient relates to the therapist as he or she had to a prominent childhood figure.
tricyclic antidepressants	Drugs used to treat severe depression; three-ringed fused structure.

VI. Combining Forms, Suffixes, Prefixes, and Terminology

Write the meanings of the medical terms in the spaces provided.

Combining Forms

Combining Form	Meaning	Terminology	Meaning
anxi/o	uneasy, anxious, distressed	anxiolytic _____ *This type of drug relieves anxiety.*	
hallucin/o	hallucination, to wander in the mind	hallucinogen _____ *A hallucination is a sensory perception in the absence of any external stimuli, and an illusion is an error in perception in which sensory stimuli are present but incorrectly interpreted.*	
hypn/o	sleep	hypnosis _____ *The Greek god of sleep (Hypnos) put people to sleep by touching them with his magic wand or by fanning them with his dark wings.*	
iatr/o	treatment	psychiatrist _____	
ment/o	mind	mental _____	
neur/o	nerve	neurosis _____ *A term formerly used to describe mental disorders in which symptoms are distressing but reality testing is intact.*	
phil/o	attraction to, love	paraphilia _____ *para- means abnormal.*	

phren/o	mind	schizophrenia _____	

schiz/o means split.

psych/o	mind	psychosis _____	

Significant impairment of reality testing with symptoms such as delusions, hallucinations, and bizarre behavior.

psychopharmacology _____

psychotherapy _____

schiz/o	split	schizoid _____	

Used to describe a mild form of schizophrenia or a withdrawn, introverted personality.

somat/o	body	psychosomatic _____	

somatoform disorder _____

-form means resembling. Symptoms of these disorders resemble those of actual physical disease, but the origins are in the mind (psychogenic).

Suffixes			
Suffix	**Meaning**	**Terminology**	**Meaning**
-genic	produced by	psychogenic _____	
-leptic	to seize hold of	neuroleptic drugs _____	
-mania	obsessive preoccupation	kleptomania _____	

klept/o means to steal.

pyromania _____

pyr/o means fire, heat.

-phobia	fear (irrational and often disabling)	agoraphobia _____	

agora- means marketplace. Agoraphobics fear being left alone and feel anxious when away from familiar surroundings.

xenophobia _____

xen/o means stranger. Table 22–2 lists other phobias.

Table 22-2. PHOBIAS

Phobia	Medical Term
Air	Aerophobia
Animals	Zoophobia
Bees	Apiphobia, melissophobia
Blood or bleeding	Hematophobia, hemophobia
Books	Bibliophobia
Cats	Ailurophobia
Corpses	Necrophobia
Crossing a bridge	Gephyrophobia
Darkness	Nyctophobia, scotophobia
Death	Thanatophobia
Dogs	Cynophobia
Drugs	Pharmacophobia
Eating	Phagophobia
Enclosed places	Claustrophobia
Hair	Trichophobia, trichopathophobia
Heights	Acrophobia
Insects	Entomophobia
Light	Photophobia
Marriage	Gamophobia
Men	Androphobia
Needles	Belonephobia
Sexual intercourse	Coitophobia, cypridophobia
Sleep	Hypnophobia
Snakes	Ophidiophobia
Spiders	Arachnophobia
Traveling	Hodophobia
Vomiting	Emetophobia
Women	Gynephobia
Worms	Helminthophobia
Writing	Graphophobia

-phoria	feeling, bearing	euphoria _____
		dysphoria _____
-thymia	mind	cyclothymia _____

cycl/o means circle, recurring. Alternating periods of hypomania and depression.

dysthymia _____

Depressed mood that is not as severe as major depression.

Prefixes Prefix	Meaning	Terminology	Meaning
a-, an-	no, not	apathy _____	
cata-	down	catatonic stupor _____	

ton/o means tension. A type of schizophrenia in which the patient has a decrease in activity and reactivity to the environment.

hypo-	deficient, less than, below	hypomania _____	
		hypochondriasis _____	

chondr/o means cartilage. The Greeks believed that the liver and spleen (under the cartilage of the ribs) were the seat of melancholy or sadness.

para-	abnormal	paranoia _____	

no- comes from the Greek word nous, *meaning mind.*

VII. ABBREVIATIONS

AD	Alzheimer disease (dementia)	**M.A.**	mental age (as determined by psychological tests)
ADHD	attention-deficit hyperactivity disorder	**MAO**	monoamine oxidase
C.A.	chronological age	**MMPI**	Minnesota Multiphasic Personality Inventory
CNS	central nervous system		
DSM	Diagnostic and Statistical Manual of Mental Disorders	**OCD**	obsessive-compulsive disorder
		SAD	seasonal affective disorder
DT	delirium tremens	**SSRI**	selective serotonin reuptake inhibitor (Prozac, Paxil, Zoloft)
ECT	electroconvulsive therapy		
I.Q.	intelligence quotient. The average person is considered to have an I.Q. of between 90 and 110. Those who score below 70 are considered mentally retarded.	**TAT**	Thematic Apperception Test
		THC	delta-9-tetrahydrocannabinol (active ingredient in marijuana)
		WAIS	Wechsler Adult Intelligence Scale
LSD	lysergic acid diethylamide (hallucinogen)	**WISC**	Wechsler Intelligence Scale for Children

VIII. Practical Applications

Major Depression: Case Report

Mrs. C, a 58-year-old widow, was brought to an emergency ward by her daughter, who found her at home in bed in the middle of the day. For a period of months, Mrs. C had become increasingly withdrawn and dysphoric, without any precipitating events. She had become progressively less active and even required encouragement to eat and perform her daily tasks. Her daughter and son-in-law became alarmed but did not know what to do. Mrs. C's medical history was unremarkable, but her psychiatric history revealed an episode of postpartum depression following the birth of one of her children.

On examination, the ER physician noted that Mrs. C was withdrawn and negativistic, refusing to cooperate with the examination, and even refusing to open her mouth. There were signs of acute dehydration and decline in personal hygiene and grooming.

Further questioning of Mrs. C's daughter revealed that Mrs. C had become increasingly paranoid and had delusions of sinfulness and guilt. Recently, she had shown signs of increasing mutism.

The physician recognized signs of major depression and arranged for immediate hospitalization. Mrs. C responded favorably to combined use of an antipsychotic and an antidepressant drug. An alternative treatment would have been a course of electroconvulsive therapy, which also produces favorable results.

Somatoform Disorder: Case Report

A 35-year-old man presented with a 6-year history of abdominal pain that he was convinced was cancer. For most of his life, the patient had been dominated by a tyrannical father who never gave him the love he craved. When the patient was 29, his father died of carcinoma of the colon, and soon afterward, the patient developed abdominal pain. His complaints gradually increased as his identification with his father, as well as his unconscious hostility toward him, increased. The patient began to present to the clinic almost daily with complaints of bloody stools (the feces were found to be free of blood) and the belief that he had cancer. He felt that none of the clinic doctors listened to him, just as his father had not.

Treatment included a long-standing, trusting, positive relationship with one of the clinic physicians who allowed the patient time to talk about the illness. His hypochondriasis gradually subsided during a 12-month period of a supportive physician-patient relationship.

IX. Exercises

Remember to check your answers carefully with those given in Section X, Answers to Exercises.

A. Give the terms for the following definitions.

1. a physician specializing in treating mental illness: _____

2. a nonphysician trained in the treatment of mental illness: _____

3. a therapist who practices psychoanalysis: _____

4. branch of psychiatry dealing with legal matters: _____ psychiatry

5. unconscious part of the personality: _____

6. conscious, coordinating part of the personality: _____

7. conscience or moral part of the personality: _____

8. the ability to perceive fact from fantasy: _____ testing

9. unconscious technique used to resolve or conceal conflicts and anxiety:

_____ mechanism

10. branch of psychology dealing with patient care: _____ psychology

B. Match the following psychiatric symptoms with their meanings as given below.

delusion	conversion	autism
compulsion	mutism	mania
hallucination	amnesia	apathy
dissociation	anxiety	obsession

1. a nonreactive state; stupor _____

2. state of excessive excitability; agitation _____

3. loss of memory _____

4. uncontrollable urge to perform an act repeatedly _____

5. persistent idea, emotion, or urge _____

6. feelings of apprehension, uneasiness, dread _____

7. uncomfortable feelings are separated from their real object and redirected toward a second object

   or behavior pattern _____

8. anxiety becomes a bodily symptom that has no organic basis _____

9. lack of responsiveness to others _____

10. absence of emotions _____

11. fixed false belief that cannot be changed by logical reasoning or evidence _____

12. false or unreal sensory perception _____

C. Give the meanings of the following terms.

1. dysphoria _____

2. euphoria _____

3. amnesia _____

4. paranoia _____

5. psychosis _____

6. neurosis _____

7. phobia _____

8. agoraphobia _____

9. labile _____

10. affect _____

D. Select from the following terms to complete the sentences below.

anxiety disorders   dissociative disorders   substance-related disorders
mood disorders   eating disorder   delirium
sexual disorders   personality disorder   dementia
somatoform disorders

1. Mental symptoms (disturbances of memory and identity) that hide the anxiety of unconscious conflicts are _____.

2. Troubled feelings, unpleasant tension, distress, and avoidance behavior are hallmarks of

    _____.

3. Illnesses related to regular use of drugs and alcohol are _____.

4. Bulimia nervosa is an example of a (an) _____.

5. Disorders involving paraphilias are _____.

6. Illnesses marked by prolonged emotions (mania and depression) are _____.

7. Mental disorders in which physical symptoms cannot be explained by an actual physical disorder

    are _____.

8. A lifelong personality pattern that is inflexible and causes impairment of social functioning,

    distress, and conflict is a (an) _____.

9. Loss of intellectual abilities with impairment of memory, judgment, and reasoning is known as

    _____.

10. Confusion in thinking with faulty perceptions and irrational behavior is _____.

E. Give the meanings of the following terms.

1. obsessive-compulsive disorder _____

2. post-traumatic stress disorder _____

3. bipolar disorder _____

4. fugue _____

5. paranoia _____

6. amphetamines _____

7. cannabis _____

8. schizophrenia _____

9. sexual sadism _____

10. hypochondriasis _____

F. Match the general psychiatric disorder in column I with its example in column II. Write the letter of the answer in the space provided.

Column I

1. somatoform disorder   _____

2. sexual disorder   _____

3. anxiety disorder   _____

4. mood disorder   _____

5. substance-related disorder   _____

6. schizophrenia   _____

7. dissociative disorder   _____

8. personality disorder   _____

Column II

A. conversion disorder
B. cocaine abuse
C. phobia
D. catatonia
E. pedophilia
F. fugue
G. bipolar I and II
H. narcissism

G. Give the meanings of the following terms.

1. anorexia nervosa _____

2. bulimia nervosa _____

3. repression _____

4. dementia _____

5. hypomania _____

6. hallucinogen _____

7. opioids _____

8. cocaine _____

9. cyclothymic disorder _____

10. dysthymia _____

H. Identify the personality disorder based on its description as given below.

1. flamboyant, theatrical, emotionally immature _____

2. no loyalty or concern for others; does not tolerate frustration and blames others when he or she is

   at fault _____

3. has fantasies of success and power and a grandiose sense of self-importance _____

4. pervasive, unwarranted suspiciousness and mistrust of people _____

5. emotionally cold, aloof, indifferent to praise or criticism or to the feelings of others _____

6. instability in personal relationships and sense of self; alternating overinvolvement with and rejec-

   tion of people _____

I. Identify the psychotherapeutic technique based on its description as given below.

1. patients express feelings by acting out roles with other patients _____

2. a trance helps patients recover deeply repressed feelings _____

3. long-term and intense exploration of unconscious feelings uses techniques such as transference

   and free association _____

4. toys help a child express conflicts and feelings _____

5. conditioning changes actual behavior patterns rather than focusing on subconscious thoughts and

   feelings _____

6. techniques help patients overcome sexual dysfunctions _____

7. electric current is applied to the brain to reverse major depression _____

8. agents (chemicals) relieve symptoms of psychiatric disorders _____

J. Select from the following terms to complete the sentences below.

amphetamines   tricyclic antidepressants   kleptomania
MAO inhibitors   benzodiazepines   agoraphobia
phenothiazines   pyromania   dysthymia
cyclothymia   lithium   xenophobia

1. Fear of strangers is _____.

2. Obsessive preoccupation with stealing is _____.

3. Antidepressant agents that work by blocking the action of a specific enzyme are

 _____.

4. A mood disorder marked by depressive periods that are milder than major depression is

 _____.

5. Antipsychotic (neuroleptic) tranquilizers such as Thorazine are _____.

6. Fear of being left alone in unfamiliar surroundings is _____.

7. Stimulants that are used as therapy for mood disorders or for treatment of children with

 attention-deficit hyperactivity disorder are _____.

8. A mild form of bipolar disorder in which hypomanic episodes alternate with depression is

 _____.

9. An obsessive preoccupation with fire is _____.

10. Drugs (containing three fused rings) used to elevate mood and increase physical activity and

 mental alertness are _____.

11. Anxiolytic agents that lessen the anxiety associated with panic attacks are _____.

12. A drug that treats the manic episodes of bipolar disorder is _____.

K. Give the meanings of the following word parts.

1. phren/o _____   5. iatr/o _____

2. hypn/o _____   6. schiz/o _____

3. somat/o _____   7. -mania _____

4. phil/o _____   8. -phobia _____

9. -thymia _____   12. para- _____

10. -tropic _____   13. hypo- _____

11. -genic _____   14. cata- _____

L. Circle the term that best completes the meaning of the sentence.

1. Robin fluctuated between bouts of depression and mania and was finally diagnosed as having a **(xenophobic, histrionic, bipolar)** disorder.

2. Although the root of Jon's problems could hardly be addressed simply with medication, his personality disorder and his depression were treated with a selective serotonin reuptake inhibitor (SSRI) called **(lithium, Prozac, Valium).**

3. Hillary had an enormous fear of open-air markets, shopping malls, and stadiums. She was diagnosed as having **(agoraphobia, xenophobia, pyromania).**

4. When Sam was admitted to the hospital after his automobile accident his physicians were told of his alcoholism. They needed to know Sam's history so that they could prevent **(dementia, dysthymia, delirium tremens).**

5. Hanna was afraid of everyone she met. She had the **(paranoid, narcissistic, schizoid)** delusion that everyone was out to get her.

6. Bill was told that an important potential side effect of taking neuroleptic drugs such as phenothiazines was **(amnesia, gender identity disorder, tardive dyskinesia).**

X. Answers to Exercises

A

1. psychiatrist	4. forensic	8. reality
2. psychologist, psychiatric nurse, licensed clinical social worker	5. id	9. defense
3. psychoanalyst	6. ego	10. clinical
	7. superego	

B

1. mutism	5. obsession	9. autism
2. mania	6. anxiety	10. apathy
3. amnesia	7. dissociation	11. delusion
4. compulsion	8. conversion	12. hallucination

C

1. sadness, hopelessness, despair
2. exaggerated feeling of well-being ("high")
3. loss of memory
4. delusions of grandeur or persecution
5. severe mental disorder in which the patient withdraws from reality into a world of disorganized thinking and

feeling or cannot function in basic ways owing to severe impairment of mood
6. emotional disorder, such as anxiety or fear, that disturbs a person's ability to function or impairs a person's physical health

7. an irrational fear of an object or a situation
8. fear of being alone or in open, public places from which escape may be difficult
9. unstable; undergoing rapid emotional change
10. a person's external emotional reactions

D

1. dissociative disorders
2. anxiety disorders
3. substance-related disorders
4. eating disorder
5. sexual disorders
6. mood disorders
7. somatoform disorders
8. personality disorder
9. dementia
10. delirium

E

1. recurrent thoughts and repetitive acts that dominate a person's behavior
2. anxiety-related symptoms appear following exposure to personal experience of a traumatic event
3. alternating periods of mania and depression
4. amnesia with flight from customary surroundings
5. delusions of persecution or grandeur
6. CNS stimulants
7. marijuana, hashish; derived from the cannabis plant and possessing psychoactive properties
8. withdrawal from reality into an inner world of disorganized thinking and conflict
9. achievement of sexual gratification by

inflicting physical or psychological pain
10. preoccupation with bodily aches, pains, and discomforts (in the absence of real illness)

F

1. A
2. E
3. C
4. G
5. B
6. D
7. F
8. H

G

1. eating disorder marked by excessive dieting because of emotional factors
2. eating disorder characterized by binge eating followed by vomiting, purging, and depression
3. a defense mechanism by which unacceptable thoughts, feelings, and impulses are pushed into the unconscious
4. loss of higher mental functioning, memory, judgment, and reasoning
5. mood disorder resembling mania (exaggerated excitement, hyperactivity) but of lesser intensity
6. drug that produces hallucinations (false sensory perceptions)
7. drugs that are derived from opium (morphine and heroin)
8. stimulant drug that causes euphoria and hallucinations
9. two years of hypomania and depressive episodes
10. depressed mood persisting over a 2-year period but not as severe as a major depression

H

1. histrionic
2. antisocial
3. narcissistic
4. paranoid
5. schizoid
6. borderline

I

1. psychodrama
2. hypnosis
3. psychoanalysis
4. play therapy
5. behavioral therapy
6. sexual therapy
7. electroconvulsive therapy
8. psychopharmacology, or drug therapy

J

1. xenophobia
2. kleptomania
3. MAO inhibitors
4. dysthymia
5. phenothiazines
6. agoraphobia
7. amphetamines
8. cyclothymia
9. pyromania
10. tricyclic antidepressants
11. benzodiazepines
12. lithium

K

1. mind
2. sleep
3. body
4. love, attraction to
5. treatment
6. split
7. obsessive preoccupation
8. fear
9. mind
10. to influence, turn
11. produced by
12. abnormal
13. deficient, less than, below
14. down

L

1. bipolar
2. Prozac
3. agoraphobia
4. delirium tremens
5. paranoid
6. tardive dyskinesia

XI. Pronunciation of Terms

Pronunciation Guide

ā as in āpe   ă as in ăpple
ē as in ēven   ĕ as in ĕvery
ī as in īce   ĭ as in ĭnterest
ō as in ōpen   ŏ as in pŏt
ū as in ūnit   ŭ as in ŭnder

To test your understanding of the terminology in this chapter, write the meaning of each term in the space provided. In addition, you may wish to cover the terms and write them by looking at your definitions. Make sure your spelling is correct. The page number after each term indicates where it is defined or used in the text so you can easily check your responses.

Term	Pronunciation	Meaning
affect (858)	ĂF-fĕkt	
agoraphobia (862)	ăg-ŏ-ră-FŌ-bē-ă	
amnesia (858)	ăm-NĒ-zē-ă	
amphetamines (860)	ăm-FĔT-ă-mēnz	
anorexia nervosa (858)	ăn-ō-RĔK-sē-ă nĕr-VŌ-să	
antisocial personality (850)	ăn-tē-SŌ-shăl pĕr-sŏ-NĂL-ĭ-tē	
anxiety disorders (858)	ăng-ZĪ-ĕ-tē dĭs-ŎR-derz	
anxiolytic (861)	ăng-zī-ō-LĬT-ik	
apathy (858)	ĂP-ă-thē	
autism (858)	ĂW-tĭzm	
behavior therapy (860)	bē-HĀV-yŏr THĔR-ă-pē	
benzodiazepines (860)	bĕn-zō-dī-ĂZ-ĕ-pēnz	
bipolar disorder (858)	bī-PŌ-lăr dĭs-ŎR-dĕr	
borderline personality (850)	BŎR-dĕr-līn pĕr-sŏ-NĂL-ĭ-tē	
bulimia nervosa (858)	bū-LĒ-mē-ă nĕr-VŌ-să	
cannabis (853)	KĂ-nă-bis	
catatonic stupor (864)	kăt-ă-TŎN-ĭk STOO-pĕr	
claustrophobia (848)	klaws-trō-FŌ-bē-ă	
compulsion (858)	kŏm-PŬL-shŭn	
conversion disorder (858)	kŏn-VĔR-zhŭn dĭs-ŎR-dĕr	

cyclothymia (863)   sī-klō-THĪ-mē-ă   _____

defense mechanism (858)   dē-FĔNS mĕ-kăn-NĬ-zm   _____

delirium (858)   dĕ-LĬR-ē-ŭm   _____

delirium tremens (848)   dĕ-LĬR-ē-ŭm TRĒ-mĕnz   _____

delusion (858)   dĕ-LŪ-zhŭn   _____

dementia (858)   dē-MĔN-shē-ă   _____

depression (858)   dē-PRĔ-shŭn   _____

dissociative disorder (859) dĭs-SŌ-shē-ă-tĭv dĭs-ŌR-der   _____

dysphoria (863)   dĭs-FŌR-ē-ă   _____

dysthymia (863)   dīs-THĪ-mē-ă   _____

ego (859)   Ē-gō   _____

electroconvulsive   ē-lĕk-trō-kŏn-VŬL-sĭv   _____
   therapy (860)   THĔR-ă-pē

euphoria (863)   ū-FŌR-ē-ă   _____

exhibitionism (851)   ĕk-sĭ-BĬSH-ŭ-nĭzm   _____

family therapy (860)   FĂM-ĭ-lē THĔR-ă-pē   _____

fetishism (851)   FĔT-ĭsh-ĭzm   _____

free association (860)   frē ă-sō-shē-Ā-shŭn   _____

fugue (859)   fūg   _____

gender-identity   GĔN-dĕr ī-DĔN-tĭ-te   _____
   disorder (859)   dĭs-ŌR-dĕr

group therapy (860)   groop THĔR-ă-pē   _____

hallucination (859)   hă-lū-sĭ-NĀ-shŭn   _____

hallucinogen (861)   hă-LŪ-sĭ-nō-jĕn   _____

histrionic   hĭs-trē-ŎN-ĭk   _____
   personality (850)   pĕr-sŏn-ĂL-ĭ-tē

hypnosis (860)   hĭp-NŌ-sĭs   _____

hypochondriasis (864)   hī-pō-kŏn-DRĪ-ă-sĭs   _____

hypomania (864)   hī-pō-MĀ-nē-ă   _____

id (859)	ĭd	_____
kleptomania (862)	klĕp-tō-MĀ-nē-ă	_____
labile (859)	LĀ-bĭl	_____
lithium (860)	LĬTH-ē-ŭm	_____
mania (859)	MĀ-nē-ă	_____
mental (861)	MĔN-tăl	_____
mood disorders (859)	MOOD dĭs-ŎR-dĕrz	_____
mutism (859)	MŪ-tĭzm	_____
narcissistic personality (850)	năr-sĭ-SĬS-tik pĕr-sĕ-NĂL-ĭ-tē	_____
neuroleptic drug (860)	nū-rō-LĔP-tik drŭg	_____
neurosis (861)	nū-RŌ-sĭs	_____
obsession (846)	ŏb-SĔSH-ŭn	_____
obsessive-compulsive disorder (859)	ŏb-SĔS-ĭv cŏm-PŬL-sĭv dĭs-ŎR-dĕr	_____
opioid (853)	Ō-pē-ŏyd	_____
paranoia (859)	păr-ă-NŎY-ă	_____
paranoid personality (850)	PĂR-ă-nŏyd pĕr-sĕ-NĂL-ĭ-tē	_____
paraphilia (859)	păr-ă-FĬL-ē-ă	_____
pedophilia (851)	pē-dō-FĬL-ē-ă	_____
personality disorders (859)	pĕr-sĕ-NĂL-ĭ-tē dĭs-ŎR-dĕrz	_____
phenothiazines (860)	fē-nō-THĪ-ă-zēnz	_____
phobia (859)	FŌ-bē-ă	_____
play therapy (860)	plā THĔR-ă-pē	_____
post-traumatic stress disorder (859)	pōst-trăw-MĂT-ĭk strĕs dĭs-ŎR-der	_____
psychiatrist (861)	sī-KĪ-ă-trĭst	_____
psychiatry (844)	sī-KĪ-ă-trē	_____

psychoanalysis (860)	sī-kō-ă-NĂL-ĭ-sĭs	_____
psychodrama (861)	sī-kō-DRĂ-mă	_____
psychogenic (862)	sī-kō-JĔN-ĭk	_____
psychologist (844)	sī-KŌL-ō-jĭst	_____
psychopharmacology (861)	sī-kō-făr-mă-KŎL-ō-jē	_____
psychosis (859)	sī-KŌ-sĭs	_____
psychosomatic (862)	sī-kō-sō-MĂT-ĭk	_____
psychotherapy (862)	sī-kō-THĔR-ă-pē	_____
pyromania (862)	pī-rō-MĀ-nē-ă	_____
reality testing (859)	rē-ĂL-ĭ-tē TĔS-tĭng	_____
repression (859)	rē-PRĔ-shŭn	_____
schizoid personality (850)	SKĬZ-ŏyd or SKĬT-sŏyd pĕr-sĕ-NĂL-ĭ-tē	_____
schizophrenia (859)	skĭz-ō-FRĒ-nē-ă or skĭt-sō-FRĒ-nē-ă	_____
sedatives (861)	SĔD-ă-tĭvz	_____
sexual disorders (860)	SĔX-ū-ăl dĭs-ŎR-dĕrz	_____
sexual masochism (851)	SĔX-ū-ăl MĂS-ō-kĭzm	_____
sexual sadism (851)	SĔX-ŭ-ăl SĀ-dĭzm	_____
somatoform disorders (860)	sō-MĂT-ō-fŏrm dĭs-ŎR-dĕrz	_____
superego (860)	sū-pĕr-Ē-gō	_____
tolerance (852)	TŎL-ĕr-ănz	_____
transference (861)	trăns-FŬR-ĕns	_____
transvestic fetishism (851)	trăns-VĔS-tĭk FĔT-ĭsh-ĭzm	_____
tricyclic antidepressants (861)	trī-SĬK-lĭk ăn-tĭ-dĕ-PRĔ-săntz	_____
voyeurism (851)	VŎY-yĕr-ĭzm	_____
xenophobia (862)	zĕn-ō-FŌ-bē-ă	_____

XII. Review Sheet

Write the meanings of the word parts in the spaces provided and test yourself. Check your answers with the information in the chapter or in the glossary (Medical Terms—English) at the back of the book.

COMBINING FORMS

Combining Form	Meaning	Combining Form	Meaning
anxi/o	_____	phil/o	_____
cycl/o	_____	phren/o	_____
hallucin/o	_____	psych/o	_____
hypn/o	_____	pyr/o	_____
iatr/o	_____	schiz/o	_____
klept/o	_____	somat/o	_____
ment/o	_____	ton/o	_____
neur/o	_____	xen/o	_____

SUFFIXES

Suffix	Meaning	Suffix	Meaning
-form	_____	-pathy	_____
-genic	_____	-phobia	_____
-kinesia	_____	-phoria	_____
-leptic	_____	-somnia	_____
-mania	_____	-thymia	_____
-oid	_____	-tropic	_____

PREFIXES

Prefix	Meaning	Prefix	Meaning
a-, an-	_____	dys-	_____
agora-	_____	hypo-	_____
cata-	_____	para-	_____

GLOSSARY

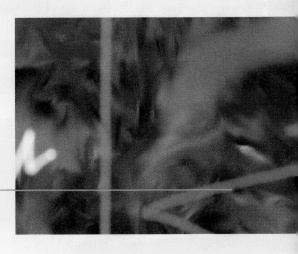

Medical Word Parts—English

Combining Form, Suffix, or Prefix	Meaning
a-, an-	no; not; without
ab-	away from
abdomin/o	abdomen
-ac	pertaining to
acanth/o	spiny; thorny
acetabul/o	acetabulum (hip socket)
acous/o	hearing
acr/o	extremities; top; extreme point
acromi/o	acromion (extension of shoulder bone)
actin/o	light
acu/o	sharp; severe; sudden
-acusis	hearing
ad-	toward
aden/o	gland
adenoid/o	adenoids
adip/o	fat
adren/o	adrenal gland
adrenal/o	adrenal gland
aer/o	air
af-	toward
agglutin/o	clumping; sticking together
-agon	to assemble, gather
agora-	marketplace
-agra	excessive pain
-al	pertaining to
alb/o	white
albin/o	white
albumin/o	albumin (protein)
alges/o	sensitivity to pain
-algesia	sensitivity to pain
-algia	pain
all/o	other
alveol/o	alveolus; air sac; small sac
ambly/o	dim; dull
-amine	nitrogen compound
amni/o	amnion (sac surrounding the embryo)
amyl/o	starch
an/o	anus
-an	pertaining to
ana-	up; apart; backward
andr/o	male
aneurysm/o	aneurysm (widened blood vessel)
angi/o	vessel (blood)
anis/o	unequal
ankyl/o	crooked; bent; stiff
ante-	before; forward
anter/o	front
anthrac/o	coal
anti-	against
anxi/o	uneasy; anxious
aort/o	aorta (largest artery)
-apheresis	removal
aphth/o	ulcer
apo-	off, away

879

Combining Form, Suffix, or Prefix	Meaning	Combining Form, Suffix, or Prefix	Meaning
aponeur/o	aponeurosis (type of tendon)	**bunion/o**	bunion
append/o	appendix	**burs/o**	bursa (sac of fluid near joints)
appendic/o	appendix	**byssin/o**	cotton dust
aque/o	water		
-ar	pertaining to		
-arche	beginning	**cac/o**	bad
arter/o	artery	**calc/o**	calcium
arteri/o	artery	**calcane/o**	calcaneus (heel bone)
arteriol/o	arteriole (small artery)	**calci/o**	calcium
arthr/o	joint	**cali/o**	calyx
-arthria	articulate (speak distinctly)	**calic/o**	calyx
articul/o	joint	**capillar/o**	capillary (tiniest blood vessel)
-ary	pertaining to	**capn/o**	carbon dioxide
asbest/o	asbestos	**-capnia**	carbon dioxide
-ase	enzyme	**carcin/o**	cancerous; cancer
-asthenia	lack of strength	**cardi/o**	heart
atel/o	incomplete	**carp/o**	wrist bones (carpals)
ather/o	plaque (fatty substance)	**cata-**	down
-ation	process; condition	**caud/o**	tail; lower part of body
atri/o	atrium (upper heart chamber)	**caus/o**	burn; burning
audi/o	hearing	**cauter/o**	heat; burn
audit/o	hearing	**cec/o**	cecum (first part of the colon)
aur/o	ear	**-cele**	hernia
auricul/o	ear	**celi/o**	belly; abdomen
auto-	self, own	**-centesis**	surgical puncture to remove fluid
axill/o	armpit	**cephal/o**	head
azot/o	urea; nitrogen	**cerebell/o**	cerebellum (posterior part of the brain)
		cerebr/o	cerebrum (largest part of the brain)
		cerumin/o	cerumen
bacill/o	bacilli (bacteria)	**cervic/o**	neck; cervix (neck of uterus)
bacteri/o	bacteria	**-chalasia**	relaxation
balan/o	glans penis	**-chalasis**	relaxation
bar/o	pressure; weight	**cheil/o**	lip
bartholin/o	Bartholin glands	**chem/o**	drug; chemical
bas/o	base; opposite of acid	**-chezia**	defecation; elimination of wastes
bi-	two	**chir/o**	hand
bi/o	life	**chlor/o**	green
bil/i	bile; gall	**chlorhydr/o**	hydrochloric acid
bilirubin/o	bilirubin	**chol/e**	bile; gall
-blast	embryonic; immature	**cholangi/o**	bile vessel
blephar/o	eyelid	**cholecyst/o**	gallbladder
bol/o	cast; throw	**choledoch/o**	comon bile duct
brachi/o	arm	**cholesterol/o**	cholesterol
brachy-	short	**chondr/o**	cartilage
brady-	slow	**chore/o**	dance
bronch/o	bronchial tube	**chori/o**	chorion (outermost membrane of the fetus)
bronchi/o	bronchial tube		
bronchiol/o	bronchiole	**chorion/o**	chorion
bucc/o	cheek	**choroid/o**	choroid layer of eye

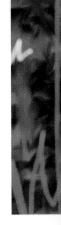

Combining Form, Suffix, or Prefix	Meaning
chrom/o	color
chron/o	time
chym/o	to pour
cib/o	meal
-cide	killing
-cidal	pertaining to killing
cine/o	movement
cirrh/o	orange-yellow
cis/o	to cut
-clasis	to break
-clast	to break
claustr/o	enclosed space
clavicul/o	clavicle (collar bone)
-clysis	irrigation; washing
coagul/o	coagulation (clotting)
-coccus	berry-shaped bacterium
(-cocci, pl.)	
coccyg/o	coccyx (tailbone)
col/o	colon (large intestine)
coll/a	glue
colon/o	colon (large intestine)
colp/o	vagina
comat/o	deep sleep
comi/o	to care for
con-	together, with
coni/o	dust
conjunctiv/o	conjunctiva (lines the eyelids)
-constriction	narrowing
contra-	against; opposite
cor/o	pupil
core/o	pupil
corne/o	cornea
coron/o	heart
corpor/o	body
cortic/o	cortex, outer region
cost/o	rib
crani/o	skull
cras/o	mixture; temperament
crin/o	secrete
-crine	secrete; separate
-crit	to separate
cry/o	cold
crypt/o	hidden
culd/o	cul-de-sac
-cusis	hearing
cutane/o	skin
cyan/o	blue
cycl/o	ciliary body of eye; cycle; circle
-cyesis	pregnancy

Combining Form, Suffix, or Prefix	Meaning
cyst/o	urinary bladder; cyst; sac of fluid
cyt/o	cell
-cyte	cell
-cytosis	condition of cells; slight increase in numbers
dacry/o	tear
dacryoaden/o	tear gland
dacryocyst/o	tear sac; lacrimal sac
dactyl/o	fingers; toes
de-	lack of; down; less; removal of
dem/o	people
dent/i	tooth
derm/o	skin
-derma	skin
dermat/o	skin
desicc/o	drying
-desis	to bind, tie together
dia-	complete; through
diaphor/o	sweat
-dilation	widening; stretching; expanding
dipl/o	double
dips/o	thirst
dist/o	far; distant
dors/o	back (of body)
dorsi-	back
-dote	to give
-drome	to run
duct/o	to lead, carry
duoden/o	duodenum
dur/o	dura mater
-dynia	pain
dys-	bad; painful; difficult; abnormal
-eal	pertaining to
ec-	out; outside
echo-	reflected sound
-ectasia	stretching; dilation; expansion
-ectasis	stretching; dilation; expansion
ecto-	out; outside
-ectomy	removal; excision; resection
-edema	swelling
-elasma	flat plate
electr/o	electricity
em-	in
-ema	condition
-emesis	vomiting

Combining Form, Suffix, or Prefix	Meaning	Combining Form, Suffix, or Prefix	Meaning
-emia	blood condition	fung/i	fungus; mushroom
-emic	pertaining to blood condition	furc/o	forking; branching
emmetr/o	in due measure	-fusion	to pour
en-	in; within		
encephal/o	brain		
endo-	in; within	galact/o	milk
enter/o	intestines (usually small intestine)	ganglion/o	ganglion; collection of nerve cell bodies
eosin/o	red; rosy; dawn-colored	gastr/o	stomach
epi-	above; upon; on	-gen	producing; forming
epididym/o	epididymis	-genesis	producing; forming
epiglott/o	epiglottis	-genic	produced by or in
episi/o	vulva (external female genitalia)	ger/o	old age
epitheli/o	skin; epithelium	gest/o	pregnancy
equin/o	horse	gester/o	pregnancy
-er	one who	gingiv/o	gum
erg/o	work	glauc/o	gray
erythem/o	flushed; redness	gli/o	glue; neuroglial tissue (supportive tissue of nervous system)
erythr/o	red		
-esis	condition	-globin	protein
eso-	inward	-globulin	protein
esophag/o	esophagus	glomerul/o	glomerulus
esthes/o	nervous sensation (feeling)	gloss/o	tongue
esthesi/o	nervous sensation	gluc/o	glucose; sugar
-esthesia	nervous sensation	glyc/o	glucose; sugar
estr/o	female	glycogen/o	glycogen; animal starch
ethm/o	sieve	glycos/o	glucose; sugar
eti/o	cause	gnos/o	knowledge
eu-	good; normal	gon/o	seed
-eurysm	widening	gonad/o	sex glands
ex-	out; away from	goni/o	angle
exanthemat/o	rash	-grade	to go
exo-	out; away from	-gram	record
extra-	outside	granul/o	granule(s)
		-graph	instrument for recording
		-graphy	process of recording
faci/o	face	gravid/o	pregnancy
fasci/o	fascia (membrane supporting muscles)	-gravida	pregnant woman
femor/o	femur (thigh bone)	gynec/o	woman; female
-ferent	to carry		
fibr/o	fiber		
fibros/o	fibrous connective tissue	hallucin/o	hallucination
fibul/o	fibula	hem/o	blood
-fication	process of making	hemat/o	blood
-fida	split	hemi-	half
flex/o	to bend	hemoglobin/o	hemoglobin
fluor/o	luminous	hepat/o	liver
follicul/o	follicle; small sac	herni/o	hernia
-form	resembling; in the shape of	-hexia	habit

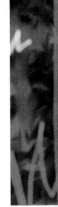

Combining Form, Suffix, or Prefix	Meaning
hidr/o	sweat
hist/o	tissue
histi/o	tissue
home/o	sameness; unchanging; constant
hormon/o	hormone
humer/o	humerus (upper arm bone)
hydr/o	water
hyper-	above; excessive
hypn/o	sleep
hypo-	deficient; below; under
hypophys/o	pituitary gland
hyster/o	uterus; womb
-ia	condition
-iac	pertaining to
-iasis	abnormal condition
iatr/o	physician; treatment
-ic	pertaining to
-ical	pertaining to
ichthy/o	dry; scaly
-icle	small
idi/o	unknown; individual; distinct
ile/o	ileum
ili/o	ilium
immun/o	immune; protection; safe
in-	in; into; not
-in, -ine	a substance
-ine	pertaining to
infra-	below; inferior to; beneath
inguin/o	groin
inter-	between
intra-	within; into
iod/o	iodine
ion/o	ion; to wander
-ion	process
-ior	pertaining to
ipsi-	same
ir-	in
ir/o	iris (colored portion of eye)
irid/o	iris (colored portion of eye)
is/o	same; equal
isch/o	to hold back; back
ischi/o	ischium (part of hip bone)
-ism	process; condition
-ist	specialist
-itis	inflammation
-ium	structure; tissue

Combining Form, Suffix, or Prefix	Meaning
jaund/o	yellow
jejun/o	jejunum
kal/i	potassium
kary/o	nucleus
kerat/o	horny, hard; cornea
kern-	nucleus (collection of nerve cells in the brain)
ket/o	ketones; acetones
keton/o	ketones; acetones
kines/o	movement
kinesi/o	movement
-kinesia	movement
-kinesis	movement
klept/o	to steal
kyph/o	humpback
labi/o	lip
lacrim/o	tear; tear duct; lacrimal duct
lact/o	milk
lamin/o	lamina (part of vertebral arch)
lapar/o	abdominal wall; abdomen
-lapse	to slide, fall, sag
laryng/o	larynx (voice box)
later/o	side
leiomy/o	smooth (visceral) muscle
-lemma	sheath, covering
-lepsy	seizure
lept/o	thin, slender
-leptic	to seize, take hold of
leth/o	death
leuk/o	white
lex/o	word; phrase
-lexia	word; phrase
ligament/o	ligament
lingu/o	tongue
lip/o	fat; lipid
-listhesis	slipping
lith/o	stone; calculus
-lithiasis	condition of stones
-lithotomy	incision (for removal) of a stone
lob/o	lobe
log/o	study of
-logy	study of
lord/o	curve; swayback
-lucent	to shine

Combining Form, Suffix, or Prefix	Meaning	Combining Form, Suffix, or Prefix	Meaning
lumb/o	lower back; loin	**-motor**	movement
lute/o	yellow	**muc/o**	mucus
lux/o	to slide	**mucos/o**	mucous membrane (mucosa)
lymph/o	lymph	**multi-**	many
lymphaden/o	lymph gland (node)	**mut/a**	genetic change
lymphangi/o	lymph vessel	**mutagen/o**	causing genetic change
-lysis	breakdown; separation; destruction; loosening	**my/o**	muscle
		myc/o	fungus
-lytic	to reduce, destroy	**mydr/o**	wide
		myel/o	spinal cord; bone marrow
		myocardi/o	myocardium (heart muscle)
macro-	large	**myom/o**	muscle tumor
mal-	bad	**myos/o**	muscle
-malacia	softening	**myring/o**	tympanic membrane (eardrum)
malleol/o	malleolus	**myx/o**	mucus
mamm/o	breast		
mandibul/o	mandible (lower jaw bone)		
-mania	obsessive preoccupation	**narc/o**	numbness; stupor; sleep
mast/o	breast	**nas/o**	nose
mastoid/o	mastoid process (behind the ear)	**nat/i**	birth
maxill/o	maxilla (upper jaw bone)	**natr/o**	sodium
meat/o	meatus (opening)	**necr/o**	death
medi/o	middle	**nect/o**	to bind, tie, connect
mediastin/o	mediastinum	**neo-**	new
medull/o	medulla (inner section); middle; soft, marrow	**nephr/o**	kidney
		neur/o	nerve
mega-	large	**neutr/o**	neither; neutral
-megaly	enlargement	**nid/o**	nest
melan/o	black	**noct/i**	night
men/o	menses; menstruation	**norm/o**	rule; order
mening/o	meninges (membranes covering the spinal cord and brain)	**nos/o**	disease
		nucle/o	nucleus
meningi/o	meninges	**nulli-**	none
ment/o	mind; chin	**nyct/o**	night
meso-	middle		
meta-	change; beyond		
metacarp/o	metacarpals (hand bones)	**obstetr/o**	midwife
metatars/o	metatarsals (foot bones)	**ocul/o**	eye
-meter	measure	**odont/o**	tooth
metr/o	uterus (womb); measure	**odyn/o**	pain
metri/o	uterus (womb)	**-oid**	resembling
mi/o	smaller; less	**-ole**	little; small
micro-	small	**olecran/o**	olecranon (elbow)
-mimetic	mimic; copy	**olig/o**	scanty
-mission	to send	**om/o**	shoulder
mon/o	one; single	**-oma**	tumor; mass; fluid collection
morph/o	shape; form	**omphal/o**	umbilicus (navel)
mort/o	death	**onc/o**	tumor
-mortem	death	**-one**	hormone

Combining Form, Suffix, or Prefix	Meaning	Combining Form, Suffix, or Prefix	Meaning
onych/o	nail (of fingers or toes)	**-partum**	birth; labor
o/o	egg	**patell/a**	patella
oophor/o	ovary	**patell/o**	patella
-opaque	obscure	**path/o**	disease
ophthalm/o	eye	**-pathy**	disease; emotion
-opia	vision	**pector/o**	chest
-opsia	vision	**ped/o**	child; foot
-opsy	view of	**pelv/i**	pelvic bone; hip
opt/o	eye; vision	**pend/o**	to hang
optic/o	eye; vision	**-penia**	deficiency
-or	one who	**-pepsia**	digestion
or/o	mouth	**per-**	through
orch/o	testis	**peri-**	surrounding
orchi/o	testis	**perine/o**	perineum
orchid/o	testis	**peritone/o**	peritoneum
-orexia	appetite	**perone/o**	fibula
orth/o	straight	**-pexy**	fixation; to put in place
-ose	full of; pertaining to; sugar	**phac/o**	lens of eye
-osis	condition, usually abnormal	**phag/o**	eat; swallow
-osmia	smell	**-phage**	eat; swallow
ossicul/o	ossicle (small bone)	**-phagia**	eating; swallowing
oste/o	bone	**phak/o**	lens of eye
-ostosis	condition of bone	**phalang/o**	phalanges (fingers and toes)
ot/o	ear	**phall/o**	penis
-otia	ear condition	**pharmac/o**	drug
-ous	pertaining to	**pharmaceut/o**	drug
ov/o	egg	**pharyng/o**	throat (pharynx)
ovari/o	ovary	**phas/o**	speech
ovul/o	egg	**-phasia**	speech
ox/o	oxygen	**phe/o**	dusky; dark
-oxia	oxygen	**-pheresis**	removal
oxy-	swift; sharp; acid	**phil/o**	like; love; attraction to
oxysm/o	sudden	**-phil**	attraction for
		-philia	attraction for
		phim/o	muzzle
pachy-	heavy; thick	**phleb/o**	vein
palat/o	palate (roof of the mouth)	**phob/o**	fear
palpebr/o	eyelid	**-phobia**	fear
pan-	all	**phon/o**	voice; sound
pancreat/o	pancreas	**-phonia**	voice; sound
papill/o	nipple-like; optic disc (disk)	**-phor/o**	to bear
par-	other than; abnormal	**-phoresis**	carrying; transmission
para-	near; beside; abnormal; apart from; along the side of	**-phoria**	to bear, carry; feeling (mental state)
-para	to bear, bring forth (live births)	**phot/o**	light
-parous	to bear, bring forth	**phren/o**	diaphragm; mind
parathyroid/o	parathyroid glands	**-phthisis**	wasting away
-paresis	slight paralysis	**-phylaxis**	protection
-pareunia	sexual intercourse	**physi/o**	nature; function
		-physis	to grow

Combining Form, Suffix, or Prefix	Meaning	Combining Form, Suffix, or Prefix	Meaning
phyt/o	plant	pub/o	pubis (anterior part of hip bone)
-phyte	plant	pulmon/o	lung
pil/o	hair	pupill/o	pupil (dark center of the eye)
pineal/o	pineal gland	purul/o	pus
pituitar/o	pituitary gland	py/o	pus
-plakia	plaque	pyel/o	renal pelvis
plant/o	sole of the foot	pylor/o	pylorus; pyloric sphincter
plas/o	development; formation	pyr/o	fever; fire
-plasia	development; formation; growth	pyret/o	fever
-plasm	formation	pyrex/o	fever
-plastic	pertaining to formation		
-plasty	surgical repair		
ple/o	more; many	quadri-	four
-plegia	paralysis; palsy		
-plegic	paralysis; palsy		
pleur/o	pleura	rachi/o	spinal column; vertebrae
plex/o	plexus; network (of nerves)	radi/o	x-rays; radioactivity; radius (lateral lower arm bone)
-pnea	breathing		
pneum/o	lung; air; gas	radicul/o	nerve root
pneumon/o	lung; air; gas	re-	back; again; backward
pod/o	foot	rect/o	rectum
-poiesis	formation	ren/o	kidney
-poietin	substance that forms	reticul/o	network
poikil/o	varied; irregular	retin/o	retina
pol/o	extreme	retro-	behind; back; backward
polio-	gray matter (of brain or spinal cord)	rhabdomy/o	striated (skeletal) muscle
poly-	many; much	rheumat/o	watery flow
polyp/o	polyp; small growth	rhin/o	nose
pont/o	pons (a part of the brain)	roentgen/o	x-rays
-porosis	condition of pores (spaces)	-rrhage	bursting forth of blood
post-	after; behind	-rrhagia	bursting forth of blood
poster/o	back (of body); behind	-rrhaphy	suture
-prandial	meal	-rrhea	flow; discharge
-praxia	action	-rrhexis	rupture
pre-	before; in front of	rrhythm/o	rhythm
presby/o	old age		
primi-	first		
pro-	before; forward	sacr/o	sacrum
proct/o	anus and rectum	salping/o	fallopian tube; auditory (eustachian) tube
pros-	before; forward		
prostat/o	prostate gland	-salpinx	fallopian tube; oviduct
prot/o	first	sarc/o	flesh (connective tissue)
prote/o	protein	scapul/o	scapula; shoulder blade
proxim/o	near	-schisis	to split
prurit/o	itching	schiz/o	split
pseudo-	false	scint/i	spark
psych/o	mind	scirrh/o	hard
-ptosis	droop; sag; prolapse; fall	scler/o	sclera (white of eye)
-ptysis	spitting	-sclerosis	hardening

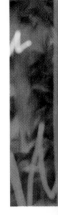

Combining Form, Suffix, or Prefix	Meaning
scoli/o	crooked; bent
-scope	instrument for visual examination
-scopy	visual examination
scot/o	darkness
seb/o	sebum
sebace/o	sebum
sect/o	to cut
semi-	half
semin/i	semen; seed
seps/o	infection
sial/o	saliva
sialaden/o	salivary gland
sider/o	iron
sigmoid/o	sigmoid colon
silic/o	glass
sinus/o	sinus
-sis	state of; condition
-sol	solution
somat/o	body
-some	body
somn/o	sleep
-somnia	sleep
son/o	sound
-spadia	to tear, cut
-spasm	sudden contraction of muscles
sperm/o	spermatozoa; sperm cells
spermat/o	spermatozoa; sperm cells
sphen/o	wedge; sphenoid bone
spher/o	globe-shaped; round
sphygm/o	pulse
-sphyxia	pulse
spin/o	spine (backbone)
spir/o	to breathe
splen/o	spleen
spondyl/o	vertebra (backbone)
squam/o	scale
-stalsis	contraction
staped/o	stapes (middle ear bone)
staphyl/o	clusters; uvula
-stasis	stop; control; place
-static	pertaining to stopping; controlling
steat/o	fat, sebum
-stenosis	tightening; stricture
ster/o	solid structure; steroid
stere/o	solid; three-dimensional
stern/o	sternum (breastbone)
steth/o	chest
-sthenia	strength

Combining Form, Suffix, or Prefix	Meaning
-stitial	to set; pertaining to standing or positioned
stomat/o	mouth
-stomy	new opening (to form a mouth)
strept/o	twisted chains
styl/o	pole or stake
sub-	under; below
submaxill/o	mandible (lower jaw bone)
-suppression	to stop
supra-	above, upper
sym-	together; with
syn-	together; with
syncop/o	to cut off, cut short
syndesm/o	ligament
synov/o	synovia; synovial membrane; sheath around a tendon
syring/o	tube
tachy-	fast
tars/o	tarsus; hindfoot or ankle (7 bones between the foot and the leg)
tax/o	order; coordination
tel/o	complete
tele/o	distant
ten/o	tendon
tendin/o	tendon
-tension	pressure
terat/o	monster; malformed fetus
test/o	testis (testicle)
tetra-	four
thalam/o	thalamus
thalass/o	sea
the/o	put; place
thec/o	sheath
thel/o	nipple
therapeut/o	treatment
-therapy	treatment
therm/o	heat
thorac/o	chest
-thorax	chest; pleural cavity
thromb/o	clot
thym/o	thymus gland
-thymia	mind (condition of)
-thymic	pertaining to mind
thyr/o	thyroid gland; shield
thyroid/o	thyroid gland
tibi/o	tibia (shin bone)
-tic	pertaining to

Combining Form, Suffix, or Prefix	Meaning	Combining Form, Suffix, or Prefix	Meaning
toc/o	labor; birth	**uter/o**	uterus (womb)
-tocia	labor; birth (condition of)	**uve/o**	uvea, vascular layer of eye (iris, choroid, ciliary body)
-tocin	labor; birth (a substance for)	**uvul/o**	uvula
tom/o	to cut		
-tome	instrument to cut		
-tomy	process of cutting	**vag/o**	vagus nerve
ton/o	tension	**vagin/o**	vagina
tone/o	to stretch	**valv/o**	valve
tonsill/o	tonsil	**valvul/o**	valve
top/o	place; position; location	**varic/o**	varicose veins
tox/o	poison	**vas/o**	vessel; duct; vas deferens
toxic/o	poison	**vascul/o**	vessel (blood)
trache/o	trachea (windpipe)	**ven/o**	vein
trans-	across; through	**ventr/o**	belly side of body
-tresia	opening	**ventricul/o**	ventricle (of heart or brain)
tri-	three	**venul/o**	venule (small vein)
trich/o	hair	**-verse**	to turn
trigon/o	trigone (area within the bladder)	**-version**	to turn
-tripsy	to crush	**vertebr/o**	vertebra (backbone)
troph/o	nourishment; development	**vesic/o**	urinary bladder
-trophy	nourishment; development	**vesicul/o**	seminal vesicle
-tropia	to turn	**vestibul/o**	vestibule of the inner ear
-tropic	turning	**viscer/o**	internal organs
-tropin	stimulate; act on	**vit/o**	life
tympan/o	tympanic membrane (eardrum); middle ear	**vitr/o**	vitreous body (of the eye)
-type	classification; picture	**vitre/o**	glass
		viv/o	life
		vol/o	to roll
-ule	little; small	**vulv/o**	vulva (female external genitalia)
uln/o	ulna (medial lower arm bone)		
ultra-	beyond; excess		
-um	structure; tissue; thing	**xanth/o**	yellow
umbilic/o	umbilicus (navel)	**xen/o**	stranger
ungu/o	nail	**xer/o**	dry
uni-	one	**xiph/o**	sword
ur/o	urine; urinary tract		
ureter/o	ureter		
urethr/o	urethra	**-y**	condition; process
-uria	urination; condition of urine		
urin/o	urine		
-us	structure; thing	**zo/o**	animal life

English—Medical Word Parts

Meaning	Combining Form, Prefix, or Suffix	Meaning	Combining Form, Prefix, or Suffix
abdomen	abdomin/o (use with -al, -centesis)	appendix	append/o (use with -ectomy) appendic/o (use with -itis)
	celi/o (use with -ac)	appetite	-orexia
	lapar/o (use with -scope, -scopy, -tomy)	arm	brachi/o
abdominal wall	lapar/o	arm bone, lower, lateral	radi/o
abnormal	dys-	arm bone, lower, medial	uln/o
	par-	arm bone, upper	humer/o
	para-	armpit	axill/o
abnormal condition	-iasis	arteriole	arteriol/o
	-osis	artery	arter/o
above	epi-		arteri/o
	hyper-	articulate (speak distinctly)	-arthria
	supra-		
acetabulum	acetabul/o	asbestos	asbest/o
acetones	ket/o	assemble	-agon
	keton/o	atrium	atri/o
acid	oxy-	attraction for	-phil
acromion	acromi/o		-philia
across	trans-	attraction to	phil/o
action	-praxia	auditory tube	salping/o
act on	-tropin	away from	ab-
adrenal glands	adren/o		apo-
	adrenal/o		ex-
after	post-		exo-
again	re-		
against	anti-	back	re-
	contra-		retro-
air	aer/o	back, lower	lumb/o
	pneum/o	back portion of body	dorsi-
	pneumon/o		dors/o
air sac	alveol/o		poster/o
albumin	albumin/o	backbone	spin/o (use with -al)
all	pan-		spondyl/o (use with -itis, -listhesis, -osis, -pathy)
along the side of	para-		vertebr/o (use with -al)
alveolus	alveol/o	backward	ana-
amnion	amni/o		retro-
aneurysm	aneurysm/o	bacteria	bacteri/o
angle	goni/o	bacterium (berry-shaped)	-coccus (-cocci, pl.)
animal life	zo/o	bacilli (rod-shaped bacteria)	bacill/o
animal starch	glycogen/o		
ankle	tars/o	bad	cac/o
anus	an/o		dys-
anus and rectum	proct/o		mal-
anxiety	anxi/o	barrier	claustr/o
apart	ana-	base (not acidic)	bas/o
apart from	para-		

Meaning	Combining Form, Prefix, or Suffix	Meaning	Combining Form, Prefix, or Suffix
bear (to)	-para	**blood condition**	-emia
	-parous		-emic
	-phoria	**blood vessel**	angi/o (use with -ectomy,
	phor/o		-genesis, -gram, -graphy,
before	ante-		-oma, -plasty, -spasm)
	pre-		vas/o (use with
	pro-		-constriction, -dilation,
	pros-		-motor)
beginning	-arche		vascul/o (use with -ar, -itis)
behind	post-	**blue**	cyan/o
	poster/o	**body**	corpor/o
	retro-		somat/o
belly	celi/o		-some
belly side of body	ventr/o	**bone**	oste/o
below, beneath	hypo-	**bone condition**	-ostosis
	infra-	**bone marrow**	myel/o
	sub-	**brain**	encephal/o
bend (to)	flex/o		cerebr/o
bent	ankyl/o	**branching**	furc/o
	scoli/o	**break**	-clasis
beside	para-		-clast
between	inter-	**breakdown**	-lysis
beyond	hyper-	**breast**	mamm/o (use with -ary,
	meta-		-gram, -graphy, -plasty)
	ultra-		mast/o (use with -algia,
bile	bil/i		-dynia, -ectomy, -itis)
	chol/e	**breastbone**	stern/o
bile vessel	cholangi/o	**breathe**	spir/o
bilirubin	bilirubin/o	**breathing**	-pnea
bind	-desis	**bring forth**	-para
	nect/o		-parous
birth	nat/i	**bronchial tube**	bronch/o
	-partum	**(bronchus)**	bronchi/o
	toc/o	**bronchiole**	bronchiol/o
	-tocia	**bunion**	bunion/o
birth (substance for)	-tocin	**burn**	caus/o
births (live)	-para		cauter/o
black	anthrac/o, melan/o	**bursa**	burs/o
bladder (urinary)	cyst/o (use with -ic, -itis,	**bursting forth of blood**	-rrhage
	-cele, -gram, -scopy,		-rrhagia
	-stomy, -tomy)		
	vesic/o (use with -al)		
blood	hem/o (use with -dialysis,	**calcaneus**	calcane/o
	-globin, -lysis, -philia,	**calcium**	calc/o
	-ptysis, -rrhage, -stasis,		calci/o
	-stat)	**calculus**	lith/o
	hemat/o (use with -crit,	**calyx**	cali/o
	-emesis, -logist, -logy,		calic/o
	-oma, -poiesis, -uria)	**cancerous**	carcin/o

Meaning	Combining Form, Prefix, or Suffix	Meaning	Combining Form, Prefix, or Suffix
capillary	capillar/o	common bile duct	choledoch/o
carbon dioxide	capn/o	complete	dia-
	-capnia		tel/o
care for (to)	comi/o	condition	-ation
carry	duct/o		-ema
	-ferent		-esis
	-phoria		-ia
carrying	-phoresis		-ism
cartilage	chondr/o		-sis
cast; throw	bol/o		-y
cause	eti/o	condition, abnormal	-iasis
cecum	cec/o		-osis
cell	cyt/o	connect	nect/o
	-cyte	connective tissue	sarc/o
cells, condition of	-cytosis	constant	home/o
cerebellum	cerebell/o	control	-stasis, -stat
cerebrum	cerebr/o	contraction	-stalsis
cerumen	cerumin/o	contraction of muscles,	-spasm
cervix	cervic/o	sudden	
change	meta-	coordination	tax/o
cheek	bucc/o	copy	-mimetic
chemical	chem/o	cornea (of the eye)	corne/o
chest	pector/o		kerat/o
	steth/o	cortex	cortic/o
	thorac/o	cotton dust	byssin/o
	-thorax	crooked	ankyl/o
child	ped/o		scoli/o
chin	ment/o	crush (to)	-tripsy
cholesterol	cholesterol/o	curve	lord/o
chorion	chori/o	cut	cis/o
	chorion/o		sect/o, -section
choroid layer (of the eye)	choroid/o		tom/o
ciliary body (of the eye)	cycl/o	cut off	syncop/o
circle or cycle	cycl/o	cutting, process of	-tomy
clavicle (collar bone)	clavicul/o	cycle	cycl/o
clot	thromb/o	cyst (sac of fluid)	cyst/o
clumping	agglutin/o		
clusters	staphyl/o	dance	chore/o
coagulation	coagul/o	dark	phe/o
coal dust	anthrac/o	darkness	scot/o
coccyx	coccyg/o	dawn-colored	eosin/o
cold	cry/o	death	leth/o
collar bone	clavicul/o		mort/o, -mortem
colon	col/o (use with -ectomy, -itis, -pexy, -stomy)		necr/o
	colon/o (use with -ic, -pathy, -scope, -scopy)	defecation	-chezia
		deficiency	-penia
color	chrom/o	deficient	hypo-

Meaning	Combining Form, Prefix, or Suffix	Meaning	Combining Form, Prefix, or Suffix
destroy	-lytic	**eating**	-phagia
destruction	-lysis	**egg cell**	o/o
development	plas/o		ov/o
	-plasia		ovul/o
	troph/o	**elbow**	olecran/o
	-trophy	**electricity**	electr/o
diaphragm	phren/o	**elimination of wastes**	-chezia
difficult	dys-	**embryonic**	-blast
digestion	-pepsia	**enlargement**	-megaly
dilation	-ectasia	**enzyme**	-ase
	-ectasis	**epididymis**	epididym/o
dim	ambly/o	**epiglottis**	epiglott/o
discharge	-rrhea	**equal**	is/o
disease	nos/o	**esophagus**	esophag/o
	path/o	**eustachian tube**	salping/o
	-pathy	**excess**	ultra-
distant	dist/o	**excessive**	hyper-
	tele/o	**excision**	-ectomy
distinct	idi/o	**expansion**	-ectasia
double	dipl/o		-ectasis
down	cata-	**extreme**	pol/o
	de-	**extreme point**	acr/o
droop	-ptosis	**extremities**	acr/o
drug	chem/o	**eye**	ocul/o (use with -ar, -facial, -motor)
	pharmac/o		
	pharmaceut/o		ophthalm/o (use with -ia, -ic, -logist, -logy, -pathy, -plasty, -plegia, -scope, -scopy)
dry	ichthy/o		
	xer/o		
drying	desicc/o		opt/o (use with -ic, -metrist)
duct	vas/o		optic/o (use with -al, -ian)
dull	ambly/o		
duodenum	duoden/o	**eyelid**	blephar/o (use with -chalasis, -itis, -plasty, -plegia, -ptosis, -tomy)
dura mater	dur/o		
dusky	phe/o		
dust	coni/o		palpebr/o (use with -al)
ear	aur/o (use with -al, -icle)	**face**	faci/o
	auricul/o (use with -ar)	**fall**	-ptosis
	ot/o (use with -algia, -ic, -itis, -logy, -mycosis, -rrhea, -sclerosis, -scope, -scopy)	**fallopian tube**	salping/o
			-salpinx
		false	pseudo-
ear (condition of)	-otia	**far**	dist/o
eardrum	myring/o (use with -ectomy, -itis, -tomy)	**fascia**	fasci/o
		fast	tachy-
		fat	adip/o (use with -ose, -osis)
	tympan/o (use with, -ic, -metry, -plasty)		lip/o (use with -ase, -cyte, -genesis, -oid, -oma)
eat	phag/o		steat/o (use with -oma, -rrhea)
	-phage		

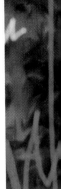

Meaning	Combining Form, Prefix, or Suffix	Meaning	Combining Form, Prefix, or Suffix
fear	phob/o	gas	pneum/o
	-phobia		pneumon/o
feeling	esthesi/o	gather	-agon
	-phoria	genetic change	mut/a
female	estr/o (use with -gen, -genic)		mutagen/o
		give (to)	-dote
	gynec/o (use with -logist, -logy, -mastia)	given (what is)	-dote
		gland	aden/o
femur	femor/o	glans penis	balan/o
fever	pyr/o	glass	silic/o
	pyret/o		vitre/o
	pyrex/o	globe-shaped	spher/o
fiber	fibr/o	glomerulus	glomerul/o
fibrous connective tissue	fibros/o	glucose	gluc/o
fibula	fibul/o (use with -ar)		glyc/o
	perone/o (use with -al)		glycos/o
finger and toe bones	phalang/o	glue	coll/a
fingers	dactyl/o		gli/o
fire	pyr/o	glycogen	glycogen/o
first	prot/o	go (to)	-grade
fixation	-pexy	good	eu-
flat plate	-elasma	granule(s)	granul/o
flesh	sarc/o	gray	glauc/o
flow	-rrhea	gray matter	poli/o
fluid collection	-oma	green	chlor/o
flushed	erythem/o	groin	inguin/o
foot	pod/o	grow	-physis
foot bones	metatars/o	growth	-plasia
forking	furc/o	gum	gingiv/o
form	morph/o		
formation	plas/o		
	-plasia	habit	-hexia
	-plasm	hair	pil/o
	-poiesis		trich/o
forming	-genesis	half	hemi-
forward	ante-, pro-, pros-		semi-
four	quadri-	hallucination	hallucin/o
front	anter/o	hand	chir/o
full of	-ose	hand bones	metacarp/o
fungus	fung/i (use with -cide, -oid, -ous, -stasis)	hang (to)	pend/o
		hard	kerat/o
	myc/o (use with -logist, -logy, -osis, -tic)		scirrh/o
		hardening	-sclerosis
		head	cephal/o
gall	bil/i (use with -ary)	hearing	acous/o
	chol/e (use with -lithiasis)		audi/o
gallbladder	cholecyst/o		audit/o
ganglion	gangli/o		-acusis
	ganglion/o		-cusis

Meaning	Combining Form, Prefix, or Suffix	Meaning	Combining Form, Prefix, or Suffix
heart	cardi/o (use with -ac, -graphy, -logy, -logist, -megaly, -pathy, -vascular)	**intestine, small**	enter/o
		iodine	iod/o
		ion	ion/o
	coron/o (use with -ary)	**iris**	ir/o
			irid/o
heart muscle	myocardi/o	**iron**	sider/o
heat	cauter/o	**irregular**	poikil/o
	therm/o	**irrigation**	-clysis
heavy	pachy-	**ischium**	ischi/o
heel bone	calcane/o	**itching**	prurit/o
hemoglobin	hemoglobin/o		
hernia	-cele		
	herni/o	**jaw, lower**	mandibul/o
hidden	crypt/o		submaxill/o
hip	pelv/i	**jaw, upper**	maxill/o
hold back	isch/o	**joint**	arthr/o
hormone	hormon/o		articul/o
	-one		
horny	kerat/o		
horse	equin/o	**ketones**	ket/o
humerus	humer/o		keton/o
humpback	kyph/o	**kidney**	nephr/o (use with -algia, -ectomy, -ic, -itis, -lith, -megaly, -oma, -osis, -pathy, -ptosis, -sclerosis, -stomy, -tomy)
hydrochloric acid	chlorhydr/o		
			ren/o (use with -al, -gram, -vascular)
ileum	ile/o		
ilium	ili/o		
immature	-blast		
immune	immun/o	**killing**	-cidal
in, into	em-		-cide
	en-	**knowledge**	gnos/o
	endo-		
	in-, intra-		
	ir-	**labor**	-partum
in due measure	emmetr/o		toc/o
in front of	pre-		-tocia
incomplete	atel/o	**labor (substance for)**	-tocin
increase in numbers (blood cells)	-cytosis	**lack of**	de-
		lack of strength	-asthenia
individual	idi/o	**lacrimal duct**	dacry/o
infection	seps/o		lacrim/o
inferior to	infra-	**lacrimal sac**	dacryocyst/o
inflammation	-itis	**lamina**	lamin/o
instrument for recording	-graph	**large**	macro-
instrument for visual examination	-scope		mega-
		larynx	laryng/o
instrument to cut	-tome	**lead**	duct/o
internal organs	viscer/o	**lens of eye**	phac/o
intestine, large	col/o		phak/o

Meaning	Combining Form, Prefix, or Suffix	Meaning	Combining Form, Prefix, or Suffix
less	de-	meatus	meat/o
	mi/o	mediastinum	mediastin/o
life	bi/o	medulla oblongata	medull/o
	vit/o	meninges	mening/o
	viv/o		meningi/o
ligament	ligament/o	menstruation; menses	men/o
	syndesm/o	metacarpals	metacarp/o
like	phil/o	metatarsals	metatars/o
lip	cheil/o	middle	medi/o
	labi/o		medull/o
lipid	lip/o		meso-
little	-ole	middle ear	tympan/o
	-ule	midwife	obstetr/o
liver	hepat/o	milk	galact/o
lobe	lob/o		lact/o
location	top/o	mimic	-mimetic
loin	lumb/o	mind	ment/o
loosening	-lysis		phren/o
love	phil/o		psych/o
luminous	fluor/o		-thymia
lung	pneum/o (use with -coccus, -coniosis, -thorax)		-thymic
	pneumon/o (use with -ectomy, -ia, -ic, -itis, -lysis)	mixture	cras/o
		monster	terat/o
		more	ple/o
	pulmon/o (use with -ary)	mouth	or/o (use with -al)
			stomat/o (use with -itis)
lymph	lymph/o	movement	cine/o
lymph gland	lymphaden/o		kines/o
lymph vessel	lymphangi/o		kinesi/o
			-kinesia
			-kinesis
make (to)	-fication		-motor
male	andr/o	much	poly-
malformed fetus	terat/o	mucous membrane	mucos/o
malleolus	malleol/o	mucus	muc/o
mandible	mandibul/o		myx/o
	submaxill/o	muscle	muscul/o (use with -ar, -skeletal)
many	multi-		
	ple/o		my/o (use with -algia, -ectomy, -oma, -neural, -pathy, -rrhaphy, -therapy)
	poly-		
marketplace	agora		
marrow	medull/o		
mass	-oma		myos/o (use with -in, -itis)
mastoid process	mastoid/o	muscle, heart	myocardi/o
maxilla	maxill/o	muscle, smooth (visceral)	leiomy/o
meal	cib/o		
	-prandial	muscle, striated (skeletal)	rhabdomy/o
measure	-meter	muscle tumor	myom/o
	metr/o	muzzle	phim/o

Meaning	Combining Form, Prefix, or Suffix	Meaning	Combining Form, Prefix, or Suffix
nail	onych/o	one's own	aut/o
	ungu/o		auto-
narrowing	-constriction	one who	-er
	-stenosis		-or
nature	physi/o	opening	-tresia
navel	omphal/o	opening (new)	-stomy
	umbilic/o	opposite	contra-
near	para-	optic disc (disk)	papill/o
	proxim/o	orange-yellow	cirrh/o
neck	cervic/o	order	norm/o
neither	neutr/o		tax/o
nerve	neur/o	organs, internal	viscer/o
nerve root	radicul/o	ossicle	ossicul/o
nest	nid/o	other	all/o
new	neo-	other than	par-
network	reticul/o	out, outside	ec-
network of nerves	plex/o		ex-
neutral	neutr/o		exo-
night	nocti/i		extra-
	nyct/o	outer region	cortic/o
nipple	thel/o	ovary	oophor/o (use with -itis, -ectomy, -pexy)
nipple-like	papill/o		
nitrogen	azot/o		ovari/o (use with -an)
nitrogen compound	-amine	oxygen	ox/o
no, not	a-		-oxia
	an-		
none	nulli-		
normal	eu-	pain	-algia
nose	nas/o (use with -al)		-dynia
	rhin/o (use with -itis, -rrhea, -plasty)		odyn/o
		pain, excessive	-agra
nourishment	troph/o	pain, sensitivity to	-algesia
	-trophy		algesi/o
nucleus	kary/o	painful	dys-
	nucle/o	palate	palat/o
nucleus (collection of nerve cells in the brain)	kern-	palsy	-plegia
			-plegic
numbness	narc/o	pancreas	pancreat/o
		paralysis	-plegia
			-plegic
obscure	-opaque	paralysis, slight	-paresis
obsessive preoccupation	-mania	patella	patell/a (use with -pexy)
off	apo-		patell/o (use with -ar, -ectomy, -femoral)
old age	ger/o		
	presby/o	pelvic bone, pelvis	pelv/i
olecranon (elbow)	olecran/o		pelv/o
on	epi-	penis	balan/o
one	mon/o		phall/o
	mono-	people	dem/o
	uni-	perineum	perine/o

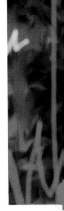

Meaning	Combining Form, Prefix, or Suffix	Meaning	Combining Form, Prefix, or Suffix
peritoneum	peritone/o	process	-ation
pertaining to	-ac (cardiac)		-ion
	-al (inguinal)		-ism
	-an (ovarian)		-y
	-ar (palmar)	produced by or in	-genic
	-ary (papillary)	producing	-gen
	-eal (pharyngeal)		-genesis
	-iac (hypochondriac)	prolapse	-ptosis
	-ic (nucleic)	prostate gland	prostat/o
	-ical (neurological)	protection	immun/o
	-ine (equine)		-phylaxis
	-ior (superior)	protein	-globin
	-ose (adipose)		-globulin
	-ous (mucous)		prote/o
	-tic (necrotic)	pubis	pub/o
phalanges	phalang/o	pulse	sphygm/o
pharynx (throat)	pharyng/o		-sphyxia
phrase	-lexia	puncture to remove fluid	-centesis
physician	iatr/o	pupil	cor/o
pineal gland	pineal/o		core/o
pituitary gland	hypophys/o		pupill/o
	pituit/o	pus	py/o, purul/o
	pituitar/o	put	the/o
place	-stasis	put in place	-pexy
	the/o	pyloric sphincter, pylorus	pylor/o
	top/o		
plant	phyt/o	radioactivity	radi/o
	-phyte	radius (lower arm bone)	radi/o
plaque	ather/o	rapid	oxy-
	-plakia	rash	exanthemat/o
pleura	pleur/o	rays	radi/o
pleural cavity	-thorax	record	-gram
plexus	plex/o	recording, process of	-graphy
poison	tox/o	rectum	rect/o
	toxic/o	recurring	cycl/o
pole	styl/o	red	eosin/o
polyp	polyp/o		erythr/o
pons	pont/o		
pores (condition of)	-porosis	redness	erythem/o
position	top/o		erythemat/o
potassium	kal/i	reduce	-lytic
pour	chym/o	relaxation	-chalasia, -chalasis
	-fusion	removal	-apheresis
pregnancy	-cyesis		-ectomy
	gest/o		-pheresis
	gester/o	renal pelvis	pyel/o
	gravid/o	repair	-plasty
	-gravida	resembling	-form
pressure	bar/o		-oid
	-tension	retina	retin/o

Meaning	Combining Form, Prefix, or Suffix	Meaning	Combining Form, Prefix, or Suffix
rib	cost/o	**sheath**	thec/o
roll (to)	vol/o	**shield**	thyr/o
rosy	eosin/o	**shin bone**	tibi/o
round	spher/o	**shine**	-lucent
rule	norm/o	**short**	brachy-
run	-drome	**shoulder**	om/o
rupture	-rrhexis	**side**	later/o
		sieve	ethm/o
		sigmoid colon	sigmoid/o
sac, small	alveol/o	**single**	mon/o
	follicul/o	**sinus**	sinus/o
sac of fluid	cyst/o	**skin**	cutane/o (use with -ous)
sacrum	sacr/o		derm/o (use with -al)
safe	immun/o		-derma (use with erythr/o,
sag (to)	-ptosis		leuk/o)
saliva	sial/o		dermat/o (use with -itis,
salivary gland	sialaden/o		-logist, -logy, -osis)
same	ipsi-		epitheli/o (use with -al,
	is/o		-lysis, -oid, -oma,
sameness	home/o		-um)
scaly	ichthy/o	**skull**	crani/o
scanty	olig/o	**sleep**	hypn/o
sclera	scler/o		somn/o
scrotum	scrot/o		-somnia
sea	thalass/o	**sleep (deep)**	comat/o
sebum	seb/o	**slender**	lept/o
	sebace/o	**slide (to)**	-lapse
	steat/o		lux/o
secrete	crin/o	**slipping**	-listhesis
	-crine	**slow**	brady-
seed	gon/o	**small**	-icle
	semin/i		micro-
seizure	-lepsy		-ole
seize (to); take hold of	-leptic		-ule
self	aut/o	**small intestine**	enter/o
	auto-	**smaller**	mi/o
semen	semin/i	**smell**	-osmia
seminal vesicle	vesicul/o	**sodium**	natr/o
send (to)	-mission	**soft**	medull/o
sensation (nervous)	-esthesia	**softening**	-malacia
separate	-crine	**sole (of the foot)**	plant/o
separation	-lysis	**solution**	-sol
set (to)	-stitial	**sound**	echo-
severe	acu/o		phon/o
sex glands	gonad/o		-phonia
sexual intercourse	-pareunia		son/o
shape	-form	**spark**	scint/i
	morph/o	**specialist**	-ist
sharp	acu/o	**speech**	phas/o
	oxy-		-phasia

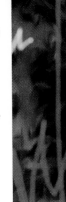

Meaning	Combining Form, Prefix, or Suffix	Meaning	Combining Form, Prefix, or Suffix
sperm cells (spermatozoa)	sperm/o spermat/o	surgical repair surrounding	-plasty peri-
spinal column	rachi/o	suture	-rrhaphy
spinal cord	myel/o	swallow	phag/o
spinal column (spine)	spin/o	swallowing	-phagia
	rachi/o	swayback	lord/o
	vertebr/o	sweat	diaphor/o (use with -esis)
spiny	acanth/o		hidr/o (use with -osis)
spitting	-ptysis	swift	oxy-
spleen	splen/o	sword	xiph/o
split	-fida	synovia (fluid)	synov/o
	schiz/o	synovial membrane	synov/o
split (to)	-schisis		
stake (pole)	styl/o		
stapes	staped/o	tail	caud/o
starch	amyl/o	tailbone	coccyg/o
state of	-sis	tear	dacry/o (use with -genic, -rrhea)
steal	klept/o		
sternum	stern/o		lacrim/o (use with -al, -ation)
steroid	ster/o		
sticking together	agglutin/o	tear (to cut)	-spadia
stiff	ankyl/o	tear gland	dacryoaden/o
stimulate	-tropin	tear sac	dacryocyst/o
stomach	gastr/o	temperament	cras/o
stone	lith/o	tendon	ten/o
stop	-suppression		tend/o
stopping	-stasis		tendin/o
	-static	tension	ton/o
straight	orth/o	testis	orch/o (use with -itis)
stranger	xen/o		orchi/o (use with -algia, -dynia, -ectomy, -pathy, -pexy, -tomy)
strength	-sthenia		
stretch	tone/o		
stretching	-ectasia		orchid/o (use with -ectomy, -pexy, -plasty, -ptosis, -tomy)
	-ectasis		
stricture	-stenosis		
structure	-ium		test/o (use with -sterone)
	-um, -us	thick	pachy-
structure, solid	ster/o	thigh bone	femor/o
study of	log/o	thin	lept/o
	-logy	thing	-um
stupor	narc/o		-us
substance	-in	thirst	dips/o
	-ine	thorny	acanth/o
substance that forms	-poietin	three	tri-
sudden	acu/o	throat	pharyng/o
	oxysm/o	through	dia-
sugar	gluc/o		per-
	glyc/o		trans-
	glycos/o	throw (to)	bol/o
	-ose	thymus gland	thym/o

Meaning	Combining Form, Prefix, or Suffix	Meaning	Combining Form, Prefix, or Suffix
thyroid gland	thyr/o	**unchanging**	home/o
	thyroid/o	**under**	hypo-
tibia	tibi/o	**unequal**	anis/o
tie	nect/o	**unknown**	idi/o
tie together	-desis	**up**	ana-
tightening	-stenosis	**upon**	epi-
time	chron/o	**urea**	azot/o
tissue	hist/o	**ureter**	ureter/o
	histi/o	**urethra**	urethr/o
	-ium	**urinary bladder**	cyst/o (use with cele,
	-um		-ectomy, -itis, -pexy,
toes	dactyl/o		-plasty, -plegia, -scope,
together	con-		-scopy, -stomy, -tomy)
	sym-		vesic/o (use with -al)
	syn-	**urinary tract**	ur/o
tongue	gloss/o (use with -al, -dynia,	**urination**	-uria
	-plasty, -plegia, -rrhaphy,	**urine**	ur/o
	-spasm, -tomy)		-uria
	lingu/o (use with -al)		urin/o
tonsil	tonsill/o	**uterus**	hyster/o (use with -ectomy,
tooth	dent/i		-graphy, -gram,
	odont/o		-tomy)
top	acr/o		metr/o (use with -rrhagia,
toward	ad-		-rrhea, -rrhexis)
	af-		metri/o (use with -osis)
trachea	trache/o		uter/o (use with -ine)
transmission	-phoresis	**uvea**	uve/o
treatment	iatr/o	**uvula**	uvul/o (use with -ar, -itis,
	therapeut/o		-ptosis)
	-therapy		staphyl/o (use with -ectomy,
trigone	trigon/o		-plasty, -tomy)
tube	syring/o		
tumor	-oma		
	onc/o	**vagina**	colp/o (use with -pexy,
turn	-tropia		-plasty, -scope, -scopy,
	-verse		-tomy)
	-version		vagin/o (use with -al,
turning	-tropic		-itis)
twisted chains	strept/o	**vagus nerve**	vag/o
two	bi-	**valve**	valv/o
tympanic membrane	myring/o		valvul/o
	tympan/o	**varicose veins**	varic/o
		varied	poikil/o
		vas deferens	vas/o
ulcer	aphth/o	**vein**	phleb/o (use with -ectomy,
ulna	uln/o		-itis, -tomy)
umbilicus, navel	omphal/o (use with -cele,		ven/o (use with -ous,
	-ectomy, -rrhagia,		-gram)
	-rrhexis)	**vein, small**	venul/o
	umbilic/o (use with -al)	**ventricle**	ventricul/o

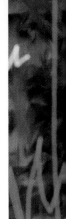

Meaning	Combining Form, Prefix, or Suffix	Meaning	Combining Form, Prefix, or Suffix
vertebra	rachi/o (use with -itis, -tomy)	**wedge**	sphen/o
		weight	bar/o
	spondyl/o (use with -itis, -listhesis, -osis, -pathy)	**white**	alb/o
			albin/o
	vertebr/o (use with -al)		leuk/o
vessel	angi/o (use with -ectomy, -genesis, -gram, -graphy, -oma, -plasty, -spasm)	**wide**	mydr/o
		widening	-dilation
			-ectasia
	vas/o (use with -constriction, -dilation, -motor)		-ectasis
			-eurysm
		windpipe	trache/o
	vascul/o (-ar, -itis)	**with**	con-
view of	-opsy		sym-
vision	-opia		syn-
	-opsia	**within**	en-
	opt/o		endo-
	optic/o		intra-
visual examination	-scopy	**woman**	gynec/o
vitreous body	vitr/o	**womb**	hyster/o
voice	phon/o		metr/o
	-phonia		metri/o
voice box	laryng/o		uter/o
vomiting	-emesis	**word**	-lexia
vulva	episi/o (use with -tomy)	**work**	erg/o
	vulv/o (use with -ar)	**wrist bone**	carp/o
wander	ion/o	**x-rays**	radi/o
washing	-clysis		
wasting away	-phthisis		
water	aque/o	**yellow**	lute/o
	hydr/o		jaund/o
watery flow	rheumat/o		xanth/o

APPENDIX I

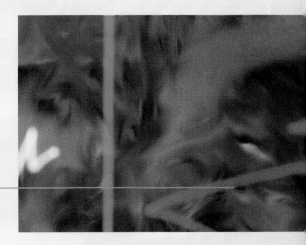

Plurals

The rules commonly used to form plurals of medical terms are as follows:

1. For words ending in **a,** retain the **a** and add **e:**
Examples:

Singular	Plural
vertebra	vertebrae
bursa	bursae
bulla	bullae

2. For words ending in **is,** drop the **is** and add **es:**
Examples:

Singular	Plural
anastomosis	anastomoses
metastasis	metastases
epiphysis	epiphyses
prosthesis	prostheses
pubis	pubes

3. For words ending in **ix** and **ex,** drop the **ix** or **ex** and add **ices:**
Examples:

Singular	Plural
apex	apices
varix	varices

4. For words ending in **on,** drop the **on** and add **a:**
Examples:

Singular	Plural
ganglion	ganglia
spermatozoon	spermatozoa

5. For words ending in **um,** drop the **um** and add **a:**
Examples:

Singular	Plural
bacterium	bacteria
diverticulum	diverticula
ovum	ova

6. For words ending in **us,** drop the **us** and add **i:**
Examples:

Singular	Plural
calculus	calculi
bronchus	bronchi
nucleus	nuclei

   Two exceptions to this rule are viruses and sinuses.

7. Examples of other plural changes are:

Singular	Plural
foramen	foramina
iris	irides
femur	femora
anomaly	anomalies
biopsy	biopsies
adenoma	adenomata

APPENDIX II

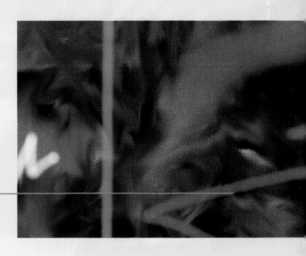

Abbreviations and Symbols

Abbreviations

Many of these abbreviations may appear with or without periods and with either a capital or a lowercase first letter.

ā	before
A2 or A₂	aortic valve closure (heart sound)
AAA	abdominal aortic aneurysm
AAL	anterior axillary line
AB	abortion
ab	antibody
abd	abdomen; abduction
ABG	arterial blood gas
a.c.	before meals *(ante cibum)*
ACE	angiotensin-converting enzyme (ACE inhibitors are used to treat hypertension)
ACh	acetylcholine (neurotransmitter)
ACTH	adrenocorticotropic hormone (secreted by the anterior pituitary gland)
AD	right ear *(auris dextra);* Alzheimer disease
ADD	attention deficit disorder
add	adduction
ADH	antidiuretic hormone; vasopressin (secreted by the posterior pituitary gland)
ADHD	attention-deficit hyperactivity disorder
ADL	activities of daily living
ADT	admission, discharge, transfer
ad lib	as desired
AF	atrial fibrillation
AFB	acid-fast bacillus (bacilli)
AFO	ankle foot orthosis (device for stabilization)
AFP	alpha-fetoprotein
AHF	antihemophilic factor (coagulation factor XIII)
AI	aortic insufficiency; artificial insemination
AIDS	acquired immunodeficiency syndrome
AIHA	autoimmune hemolytic anemia
AKA	above-knee amputation
alb	albumin (protein)
alk phos	alkaline phosphatase (elevated in liver disease)
ALL	acute lymphocytic leukemia
ALS	amyotrophic lateral sclerosis (Lou Gehrig disease)
ALT	alanine aminotransferase (elevated in liver and heart disease); formerly SGPT
Amb	ambulate, ambulatory (walking)
AML	acute myelocytic (myelogenous) leukemia
ANC	absolute neutrophil count
AODL	activities of daily living
AP, A.P., or A/P	anteroposterior
A&P	auscultation and percussion
aq.	water *(aqua);* aqueous
ARDS	adult respiratory distress syndrome
ARF	acute renal failure

ARMD	age-related macular degeneration
AROM	active range of motion
AS	left ear *(auris sinistra);* aortic stenosis
ASA	acetylsalicylic acid (aspirin)
ASD	atrial septal defect
ASH	asymmetrical septal hypertrophy
ASHD	arteriosclerotic heart disease
AST	aspartate aminotransferase (elevated in liver and heart disease); formerly SGOT
AU	both ears *(auris uterque)*
Au	gold
AV	arteriovenous; atrioventricular
AVM	arteriovenous malformation
AVR	aortic valve replacement
A&W	alive and well
Ba	barium
bands	banded neutrophils
baso	basophils
BBB	bundle branch block
BC	bone conduction
B cells	lymphocytes produced in the bone marrow
BE	barium enema
bid, b.i.d.	twice a day *(bis in die)*
BKA	below-knee amputation
BM	bowel movement
BMR	basal metabolic rate
BMT	bone marrow transplant
BP	blood pressure
BPH	benign prostatic hyperplasia (hypertrophy)
BRBPR	bright red blood per rectum; hematochezia
BSE	breast self-examination
BSO	bilateral salpingo-oophorectomy
BSP	bromsulphalein (dye used in liver function test; its retention is indicative of liver damage or disease)
BT	bleeding time
BUN	blood urea nitrogen
Bx, bx	biopsy
C	Celsius or centigrade; calorie
c̄	with *(cum)*
C1, C2	first, second cervical vertebra
CA	chronological age; cardiac arrest
Ca	calcium; cancer
CABG	coronary artery bypass graft
CAD	coronary artery disease
CAO	chronic airway obstruction
CAPD	continuous ambulatory peritoneal dialysis
cap	capsule
Cath	catheter; catheterization

CAT scan	computed (axial) tomography
CBC, c.b.c.	complete blood count
CC	chief complaint
cc	cubic centimeter (unit of volume; 1/1000 liter)
CCU	coronary care unit
CDH	congenital dislocated hip
CEA	carcinoembryonic antigen
cf.	compare
CF	cystic fibrosis
cGy	centigray (one hundredth of a gray; a rad)
CHD	coronary heart disease
chemo	chemotherapy
CHF	congestive heart failure
chol	cholesterol
chr	chronic
μCi	microcurie
CIN	cervical intraepithelial neoplasia
CIS	carcinoma *in situ*
CK	creatine kinase
Cl	chlorine
CLD	chronic liver disease
CLL	chronic lymphocytic leukemia
cm	centimeter (1/100 meter)
CMG	cystometrogram
CML	chronic myelogenous leukemia
CMV	cytomegalovirus
CNS	central nervous system
Co	cobalt
C/O	complains of
CO₂	carbon dioxide
COPD	chronic obstructive pulmonary disease
CP	cerebral palsy; chest pain
CPA	costophrenic angle
CPD	cephalopelvic disproportion
CPK	creatine phosphokinase
CPR	cardiopulmonary resuscitation
CR	complete response
CRF	chronic renal failure
CS	cesarean section
C&S	culture and sensitivity
C-section	cesarean section
CSF	cerebrospinal fluid
C-spine	cervical spine films
ct.	count
CTA	clear to auscultation
CTS	carpal tunnel syndrome
CT scan	computed tomography (x-ray images in a cross-sectional view)
CVA	cerebrovascular accident; costovertebral angle
CVP	central venous pressure
CVS	cardiovascular system; chorionic villus sampling

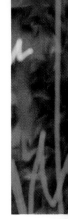

c/w	compare with; consistent with
CX (CXR)	chest x-ray
Cx	cervix
cysto	cystoscopy
D/C	discontinue; discharge
D&C	dilatation (dilation) and curettage
DCIS	ductal carcinoma *in situ*
DD	discharge diagnosis
Decub.	decubitus (lying down)
Derm.	dermatology
DES	diethylstilbestrol; diffuse esophageal spasm
DI	diabetes insipidus; diagnostic imaging
DIC	disseminated intravascular coagulation
diff.	differential count (white blood cells)
DIG	digoxin; digitalis
dL, dl	deciliter (1/10 liter)
DLE	discoid lupus erythematosus
DM	diabetes mellitus
DNA	deoxyribonucleic acid
DNR	do not resuscitate
D.O.	Doctor of Osteopathy
DOA	dead on arrival
DOB	date of birth
DOE	dyspnea on exertion
DPT	diphtheria, pertussis, tetanus (vaccine)
DRE	digital rectal exam
DRG	diagnosis-related group
DSA	digital subtraction angiography
DSM	Diagnostic and Statistical Manual of Mental Disorders
DT	delirium tremens (caused by alcohol withdrawal)
DTR	deep tendon reflexes
DUB	dysfunctional uterine bleeding
DVT	deep venous thrombosis
Dx	diagnosis
EBV	Epstein-Barr virus
ECC	endocervical curettage; extracorporeal circulation
ECF	extended-care facility
ECG	electrocardiogram
ECHO	echocardiography
ECMO	extracorporeal membrane oxygenation
ECT	electroconvulsive therapy
ED	emergency department
EDC	estimated date of confinement
EEG	electroencephalogram
EENT	eyes, ears, nose, and throat
EGD	esophagogastroduodenoscopy
EKG	electrocardiogram

ELISA	enzyme-linked immunosorbent assay (AIDS test)
EM	electron microscope
EMB	endometrial biopsy
EMG	electromyogram
ENT	ear, nose, and throat
EOM	extraocular movement; extraocular muscles
eos.	eosinophil (type of white blood cell)
Epo	erythropoietin
ER	emergency room; estrogen receptor
ERCP	endoscopic retrograde cholangiopancreatography
ERT	estrogen replacement therapy
ESR	erythrocyte sedimentation rate
ESRD	end-stage renal disease
ESWL	extracorporeal shock wave lithotripsy
ETOH	ethyl alcohol
ETT	exercise tolerance test
F	Fahrenheit
FACP	Fellow, American College of Physicians
FACS	Fellow, American College of Surgeons
FB	fingerbreadth; foreign body
FBS	fasting blood sugar
FDA	Food and Drug Administration
Fe	iron
FEF	forced expiratory flow
FEV	forced expiratory volume
FH	family history
FHR	fetal heart rate
FROM	full range of movement/motion
FSH	follicle-stimulating hormone
F/u	follow-up
5-FU	5-fluorouracil (used in cancer chemotherapy)
FUO	fever of undetermined origin
F_x, Fx	fracture
μg	microgram (one-millionth of a gram)
G	gravida (pregnant)
g, gm	gram
Ga	gallium
GABA	gamma-aminobutyric acid (neurotransmitter)
GB	gallbladder
GBS	gallbladder series (x-rays)
GC	gonorrhea
G-CSF	granulocyte colony stimulating factor
GERD	gastroesophageal reflux disease
GFR	glomerular filtration rate
GH	growth hormone

GI	gastrointestinal
Grav. 1, 2, 3	first, second, third pregnancy
GTT	glucose tolerance test
gt, gtt	drop (*gutta*), drops (*guttae*)
GU	genitourinary
Gy	gray (unit of radiation and equal to 100 rads)
GYN	gynecology
H	hydrogen
h, hr	hour
H2 blocker	H2 (histamine) receptor antagonist (inhibitor of gastric acid secretion)
HBV	hepatitis B virus
HCG (hCG)	human chorionic gonadotropin
HCl	hydrochloric acid
HCO₃	bicarbonate
Hct (HCT)	hematocrit
HCV	hepatitis C virus
HCVD	hypertensive cardiovascular disease
HD	hemodialysis (artificial kidney machine)
HDL	high-density lipoprotein
He	helium
HEENT	head, eyes, ears, nose, and throat
Hg	mercury
Hgb	hemoglobin
hGH	human growth hormone
H&H	hematocrit and hemoglobin
HIV	human immunodeficiency virus
HLA	histocompatibility locus antigen (identifies cells as "self")
HNP	herniated nucleus pulposus
h/o	history of
H₂O	water
hpf	high-power field (microscope)
HPI	history of present illness
HPV	human papillomavirus
HRT	hormone replacement therapy
h.s.	at bedtime (*hora somni*)
HSG	hysterosalpingography
HSV	herpes simplex virus
ht	height
HTN	hypertension (high blood pressure)
Hx	history
I	iodine
¹³¹I	radioactive isotope of iodine
IBD	inflammatory bowel disease
ICP	intracranial pressure
ICSH	interstitial cell-stimulating hormone
ICU	intensive care unit
I&D	incision and drainage

ID	infectious disease
IDDM	insulin-dependent diabetes mellitus (type 1)
IgA, IgD, IgE, IgG, IgM	immunoglobulins
IHD	ischemic heart disease
IHSS	idiopathic hypertrophic subaortic stenosis
IM	intramuscular; infectious mononucleosis
IMV	intermittent mandatory ventilation
inf.	infusion; inferior
INH	isoniazid (drug used to treat tuberculosis)
inj.	injection
I&O	intake and output (measurement of patient's fluids)
IOL	intraocular lens (implant)
IOP	intraocular pressure
I.Q.	intelligence quotient
IUD	intrauterine device
IUP	intrauterine pregnancy
IV	intravenous (injection)
IVP	intravenous pyelogram
K	potassium
kg	kilogram (1000 grams)
KJ	knee jerk
KS	Kaposi sarcoma
KUB	kidney, ureter, and bladder (x-ray exam)
L, l	liter; left; lower
L1, L2	first, second lumbar vertebra
LA	left atrium
LAD	left anterior descending (coronary artery)
lat	lateral
LAVH	laparoscopic assisted vaginal hysterectomy
LB	large bowel
LBBB	left bundle branch block (heart block)
LD	lethal dose
LDH	lactate dehydrogenase (elevation associated with heart attacks)
LDL	low-density lipoprotein (high levels associated with heart disease)
L-dopa	levodopa (used to treat Parkinson disease)
L.E.	lupus erythematosus
LEEP	loop electrocautery excision procedure
LES	lower esophageal sphincter
LFTs	liver function tests
LH	luteinizing hormone
LLL	left lower lobe (lung)
LLQ	left lower quadrant (abdomen)
LMP	last menstrual period
LOC	loss of consciousness

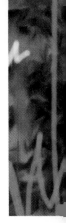

LOS	length of stay
LP	lumbar puncture
lpf	low-power field (microscope)
LPN	licensed practical nurse
LS	lumbosacral spine
LSD	lysergic acid diethylamide
LSK	liver, spleen, and kidneys
LTB	laryngotracheal bronchitis
LTC	long-term care
LTH	luteotropic hormone (prolactin)
LUL	left upper lobe (lung)
LUQ	left upper quadrant (abdomen)
LV	left ventricle
L&W	living and well
lymphs	lymphocytes
lytes	electrolytes
MA	mental age
MAI	*Mycobacterium avium intracellulare*
MAOI	monoamine oxidase inhibitor (antidepressant drug)
MBD	minimal brain dysfunction
mcg	microgram
MCH	mean corpuscular hemoglobin (average amount in each red blood cell)
MCHC	mean corpuscular hemoglobin concentration (average concentration in a single red cell)
mCi	millicurie
μCi	microcurie
MCP	metacarpophalangeal joint
MCV	mean corpuscular volume (average size of a single red blood cell)
M.D.	Doctor of Medicine
MED	minimum effective dose
mEq	milliequivalent
mEq/L	milliequivalent per liter (measurement of the concentration of a solution)
mets	metastases
Mg	magnesium
mg	milligram (1/1000 gram)
mg/cc	milligram per cubic centimeter
mg/dl	milligram per deciliter
μg	microgram (one-millionth of a gram)
MH	marital history; mental health
MI	myocardial infarction; mitral insufficiency
mL, ml	milliliter (1/1000 liter)
mm	millimeter (1/1000 meter; 0.039 inch)
mmHg	millimeters of mercury
MMPI	Minnesota Multiphasic Personality Inventory
MMR	measles-mumps-rubella (vaccine)
MMT	manual muscle testing

mμ	millimicron (1/1000 micron; a micron is 10^{-3} mm)
μm	micrometer (one-millionth of a meter)
mono	monocyte (white blood cell)
MR	mitral regurgitation
MRI	magnetic resonance imaging
mRNA	messenger RNA
MS	multiple sclerosis; mitral stenosis
MSL	midsternal line
MTX	methotrexate
MUGA	multiple-gated acquisition scan (of heart)
multip	multipara; multiparous
MVP	mitral valve prolapse
N	nitrogen
Na	sodium
NB	newborn
NBS	normal bowel or breath sounds
ND	normal delivery; normal development
NED	no evidence of disease
neg.	negative
NG tube	nasogastric tube
NHL	non-Hodgkin lymphoma
NIDDM	non–insulin-dependent diabetes mellitus (type 2)
NK cells	natural killer cells
NKDA	no known drug allergies
NPO	nothing by mouth *(non per os)*
NSAID	nonsteroidal anti-inflammatory drug
NSR	normal sinus rhythm (of heart)
NTP	normal temperature and pressure
O	oxygen
OA	osteoarthritis
OB/GYN	obstetrics and gynecology
OCPs	oral contraceptive pills
O.D.	Doctor of Optometry; overdose; right eye *(oculus dexter)*
OR	operating room
ORIF	open reduction internal fixation
ORTH; Ortho.	orthopedics
O.S.	left eye *(oculus sinister)*
os	opening; mouth; bone
O.T.	occupational therapy
O.U.	each eye *(oculus uterque)*
oz.	ounce
P	phosphorus; posterior; pressure; pulse; pupil
p̄	after
P2 or P$_2$	pulmonary valve closure (heart sound)

PA	pulmonary artery; posteroanterior	preop	preoperative
P-A	posteroanterior	prep	prepare for
P&A	percussion and auscultation	PR	partial response
PAC	premature atrial contraction	primip	primipara
$PaCO_2$, pCO_2	partial pressure of carbon dioxide (in blood)	PRL	prolactin
		p.r.n.	as required (*pro re nata*)
palp.	palpable; palpation	procto	proctoscopy
PALS	pediatric advanced life support	prot.	protocol
PaO_2, pO_2	partial pressure of oxygen	Pro. time	prothrombin time (test of blood clotting)
Pap smear	Papanicolaou smear (cells from cervix and vagina)	PSA	prostate-specific antigen
		PT	prothrombin time; physical therapy
Para 1, 2, 3	unipara, bipara, tripara (number of viable births)	PTA	prior to admission (to hospital)
		PTC	percutaneous transhepatic cholangiography
p.c.	after meals (*post cibum*)		
PCP	*Pneumocystis carinii* pneumonia; phencyclidine (hallucinogen)	PTCA	percutaneous transluminal coronary angioplasty
PCR	polymerase chain reaction (process allows making copies of genes)	PTH	parathyroid hormone
		PTT	partial thromboplastin time (test of blood clotting)
PD	peritoneal dialysis		
PDA	patent ductus arteriosus	PU	pregnancy urine
PDR	Physicians' Desk Reference	PUVA therapy	psoralen ultraviolet A (treatment for psoriasis)
PE	physical examination; pulmonary embolism		
		PVC	premature ventricular contraction
PEEP	positive end-expiratory pressure	PVD	peripheral vascular disease
PEG	percutaneous endoscopic gastrostomy (a feeding tube)	PWB	partial weight bearing
PEJ	percutaneous endoscopic jejunostomy (a feeding tube)		
		q	every (*quaque*)
per os	by mouth	q.d.	every day (*quaque die*)
PERRLA	pupils equal, round, react to light and accommodation	q.h.	every hour (*quaque hora*)
		q.i.d.	four times daily (*quater in die*)
PET	positron emission tomography	q.n.	each night (*quaque nox*)
PE tube	ventilating tube for eardrum	q.s.	as much as suffices (*quantum sufficit*)
PFT	pulmonary function test	qt	quart
PG	prostaglandin		
PH	past history		
pH	hydrogen ion concentration (alkalinity and acidity measurement)	R	respiration; right
		RA	rheumatoid arthritis; right atrium
PI	present illness	Ra	radium
PID	pelvic inflammatory disease	rad	radiation absorbed dose
PIP	proximal interphalangeal joint	RBBB	right bundle branch block
PKU	phenylketonuria	RBC, rbc	red blood cell (corpuscle); red blood count
p.m.	afternoon (post meridian)	R.D.D.A.	recommended daily dietary allowance
PMH	past medical history	RDS	respiratory distress syndrome
PMN	polymorphonuclear leukocyte	REM	rapid eye movement
PMS	premenstrual syndrome	RF	rheumatoid factor
PND	paroxysmal nocturnal dyspnea	Rh	rhesus (monkey) factor in blood
p/o	postoperative	RIA	radioimmunoassay (minute quantities are measured)
p.o.	by mouth (*per os*)		
poly	polymorphonuclear leukocyte	RIND	reversible ischemic neurologic deficit/defect
postop	postoperative (after surgery)		
PPBS	postprandial blood sugar	RLL	right lower lobe (lung)
PPD	purified protein derivative (test for tuberculosis)	RLQ	right lower quadrant (abdomen)
		RML	right middle lobe (lung)

RNA	ribonucleic acid	**T**	temperature; time
R/O	rule out	**T1, T2**	first, second thoracic vertebra
ROM	range of motion	**T$_3$**	triiodothyronine test
ROS	review of systems	**T$_4$**	thyroxine test
RRR	regular rate and rhythm (of the heart)	**TA**	therapeutic abortion
RT	right; radiation therapy	**T&A**	tonsillectomy and adenoidectomy
RUL	right upper lobe (lung)	**TAH**	total abdominal hysterectomy
RUQ	right upper quadrant (abdomen)	**TAT**	Thematic Apperception Test
RV	right ventricle	**TB**	tuberculosis
Rx	treatment; therapy; prescription	**Tc**	technetium
		T cells	lymphocytes produced in the thymus gland
s̄	without *(sine)*	**TEE**	transesophageal echocardiogram
S1, S2	first, second sacral vertebra	**TENS**	transcutaneous electrical nerve stimulation
S-A node	sinoatrial node (pacemaker of heart)	**TFT**	thyroid function test
SAD	seasonal affective disorder	**TIA**	transient ischemic attack
SBE	subacute bacterial endocarditis	**t.i.d.**	three times daily *(ter in die)*
SBFT	small bowel follow-through (x-rays of small intestine)	**TLC**	total lung capacity
		TM	tympanic membrane
sed. rate	sedimentation rate (rate of erythrocyte sedimentation)	**TMJ**	temporomandibular joint
		TNM	tumor, nodes, and metastases
segs	segmented neutrophils; polys	**tPA**	tissue plasminogen activator
SERM	selective estrogen receptor modifier	**TPN**	total parenteral nutrition
SGOT (AST)	serum glutamic-oxaloacetic transaminase	**TPR**	temperature, pulse, and respiration
		TRUS	transrectal ultrasound
SGPT (ALT)	serum glutamic-pyruvic transaminase	**TSH**	thyroid-stimulating hormone
		TSS	toxic shock syndrome
SIADH	syndrome of inappropriate antidiuretic hormone	**TUR, TURP**	transurethral resection of the prostate
SIDS	sudden infant death syndrome	**TVH**	total vaginal hysterectomy
sig.	let it be labeled	**Tx**	treatment
SLE	systemic lupus erythematosus		
SMA 12	twelve blood chemistries		
SOAP	subjective, objective, assessment, and plan	**U**	unit
SOB	shortness of breath	**UA**	urinalysis
s.o.s.	if necessary *(si opus sit)*	**UAO**	upper airway obstruction
S/P	status post (previous disease condition)	**UC**	uterine contractions
SPECT	single-photon emission computed tomography	**UE**	upper extremity
		UGI	upper gastrointestinal
sp. gr.	specific gravity	**umb.**	navel *(umbilicus)*
SSRI	selective serotonin reuptake inhibitor (antidepressant)	**U/O**	urinary output
		URI	upper respiratory infection
Staph.	staphylococci (berry-shaped bacteria in clusters)	**U/S**	ultrasound
		UTI	urinary tract infection
stat.	immediately *(statim)*	**UV**	ultraviolet
STD	sexually transmitted disease		
STH	somatotropin (growth hormone)		
Strep.	streptococci (berry-shaped bacteria in twisted chains)	**VA**	visual acuity
		VC	vital capacity (of lungs)
Subcu	subcutaneous	**VCUG**	voiding cystourethrogram
SVC	superior vena cava	**VF**	visual field
SVD	spontaneous vaginal delivery	**vis à vis**	as compared with; in relation to
Sx	symptoms	**V/Q scan**	ventilation-perfusion scan

V/S	vital signs; versus	**WISC**	Wechsler Intelligence Scale for Children
VSD	ventricular septal defect	**WNL**	within normal limits
VT	ventricular tachycardia (abnormal heart rhythm)	**wt**	weight
		XRT	radiation therapy
WAIS	Wechsler Adult Intelligence Scale		
WBC, wbc	white blood cell; white blood count		
WDWN	well developed, well nourished	**y/o, yrs**	year(s) old

Symbols

=	equal	%	percent
≠	unequal	°	degree; hour
+	positive	:	ratio; "is to"
−	negative	±	plus or minus (either positive or negative)
↑	above, increase	′	foot
↓	below, decrease	″	inch
♀	female	∴	therefore
♂	male	@	at, each
→	to (in direction of)	c̄	with
>	is greater than	s̄	without
<	is less than	#	pound
1°	primary to	≅	approximately, about
2°	secondary to	Δ	change
ℨ	dram	**p**	short arm of a chromosome
℥	ounce	**q**	long arm of a chromosome

APPENDIX III

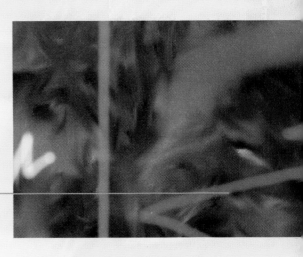

Normal Hematological Reference Values and Implications of Abnormal Results

The implications of abnormal results are major ones in each category. SI units are the International System of Units that are generally accepted for all scientific and technical uses.

cu mm = cubic millimeter (mm³)
dL = deciliter (1/10 liter or 100 mL)
g = gram
L = liter
mg = milligram (1/1000 gram)
mL = milliliter
mEq = milliequivalent

mill = million
mm = millimeter (1/1000 meter)
mmol = millimole
thou = thousand
U = unit
μmol = micromole (one-millionth of a mole)

Cell Counts

	Conventional Units	SI Units	Implications
Erythrocytes (RBC)			
Females	4.2–5.4 million/mm³	$4.2-5.4 \times 10^{12}$/L	*High* ■ Polycythemia
Males	4.6–6.2 million/mm³	$4.6-6.2 \times 10^{12}$/L	■ Dehydration
Children	4.5–5.1 million/mm³	$4.5-5.1 \times 10^{12}$/L	*Low* ■ Iron deficiency anemia
			■ Blood loss
Leukocytes (WBC)			
Total	4500–11,000/mm³	$4.5-11.0 \times 10^{9}$/L	*High* ■ Bacterial infection
			■ Leukemia
Differential	%		■ Eosinophils high in allergy
Neutrophils	54–62		*Low* ■ Viral infection
Lymphocytes	20–40		■ Aplastic anemia
Monocytes	3–7		■ Chemotherapy
Eosinophils	1–3		
Basophils	0–1		
Platelets	200,000–400,000/mm³	$200-400 \times 10^{9}$/L	*High* ■ Hemorrhage
			■ Infections
			■ Malignancy
			■ Splenectomy
			Low ■ Aplastic anemia
			■ Chemotherapy
			■ Hypersplenism

Coagulation Tests

	Conventional Units	SI Units	Implications
Bleeding Time (template method)	2.75–8.0 min	2.75–8.0 min	*Prolonged* ■ Aspirin ingestion ■ Low platelet count
Coagulation Time	5–15 min	5–15 min	*Prolonged* ■ Heparin therapy
Prothrombin Time (PT)	12–14 sec	12–14 sec	*Prolonged* ■ Vitamin K deficiency ■ Hepatic disease ■ Oral anticoagulant therapy

Red Blood Cell Tests

	Conventional Units	SI Units	Implications
Hematocrit (Hct)			
Females	37–47%	0.37–0.47	*High* ■ Polycythemia
Males	40–54%	0.40–0.54	■ Dehydration
			Low ■ Loss of blood
			■ Anemia
Hemoglobin (Hgb)			
Females	12.0–14.0 gm/dL	1.86–2.48 mmol/L	*High* ■ Polycythemia
Males	14.0–16.0 gm/dL	2.17–2.79 mmol/L	■ Dehydration
			Low ■ Anemia
			■ Blood loss

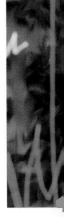

Serum Tests

	Conventional Units	SI Units	Implications
Alanine aminotransferase (ALT, SGPT)	5–30 U/L	5–30 U/L	*High* ■ Hepatitis
Albumin	3.5–5.5 gm/dL	35–55 g/L	*Low* ■ Hepatic disease ■ Malnutrition ■ Nephritis and nephrosis
Alkaline phosphatase (ALP)	20–90 U/L	20–90 U/L	*High* ■ Bone disease ■ Hepatitis or tumor infiltration of liver ■ Biliary obstruction
Aspartate aminotransferase (AST, SGOT)	10–30 U/L	10–30 U/L	*High* ■ Hepatitis ■ Cardiac and muscle injury
Bilirubin			*High* ■ Hemolysis
Total	0.3–1.1 mg/dL	5.1–19 μmol/L	■ Neonatal hepatic immaturity
Neonates	1–12 mg/dL	17–205 μmol/L	■ Cirrhosis ■ Biliary tract obstruction
Blood urea nitrogen (BUN)	8–20 mg/dL	3.0–7.1 mmol/L	*High* ■ Renal disease ■ Reduced renal blood flow ■ Urinary tract obstruction *Low* ■ Hepatic damage ■ Malnutrition
Calcium	9.0–11.0 mg/dL	2.23–2.75 mmol/L	*High* ■ Hyperparathyroidism ■ Multiple myeloma ■ Metastatic cancer *Low* ■ Hypoparathyroidism ■ Total parathyroidectomy
Cholesterol			
Desirable range	<200 mg/dL	<5.18 mmol/L	*High* ■ High fat diet
LDL cholesterol	60–80 mg/dL	600–1800 mg/L	■ Inherited hypercholesterolemia
HDL cholesterol	30–80 mg/dL	300–800 mg/L	*Low* ■ Starvation
Creatine phosphokinase (CPK)			
Females	30–135 U/L	30–135 U/L	*High* ■ Myocardial infarction
Males	55–170 U/L	55–170 U/L	■ Muscle disease
Creatinine	0.6–1.2 mg/dL	53–106 μmol/L	*High* ■ Renal disease
Glucose (fasting)	70–115 mg/dL	3.89–6.38 mmol/L	*High* ■ Diabetes mellitus *Low* ■ Hyperinsulinism ■ Fasting ■ Hypothyroidism ■ Addison disease ■ Pituitary insufficiency
Lactate dehydrogenase (LDH)	100–190 U/L	100–190 U/L	*High* ■ Tissue necrosis ■ Myocardial infarction ■ Liver disease ■ Muscle disease
Phosphate (–PO₄)	3.0–4.5 mg/dL	1.0–1.5 mmol/L	*High* ■ Renal failure ■ Bone metastases ■ Hypoparathyroidism *Low* ■ Malnutrition ■ Malabsorption ■ Hyperparathyroidism

	Conventional Units	SI Units	Implications
Potassium (K)	3.5–5.0 mEq/L	3.5–5.0 mmol/L	*High* ■ Burn victims ■ Renal failure ■ Diabetic ketoacidosis *Low* ■ Cushing syndrome ■ Loss of body fluids
Sodium (Na)	136–145 mEq/L	136–145 mmol/L	*High* ■ Inadequate water intake ■ Water loss in excess of sodium *Low* ■ Adrenal insufficiency ■ Inadequate sodium intake ■ Excessive sodium loss
Thyroxine (T_4)	4.4–9.9 μg/dL	57–128 nmol/L	*High* ■ Graves disease (hyperthyroidism) *Low* ■ Hypothyroidism
Uric acid			
Females	1.5–7.0 mg/dL	0.09–0.42 mmol/L	*High* ■ Gout
Males	2.5–8.0 mg/dL	0.15–0.48 mmol/L	■ Leukemia

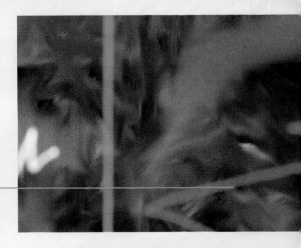

INDEX

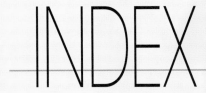

Note: Page numbers in *italics* indicate figures; those followed by t indicate tables.

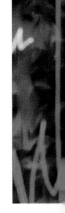

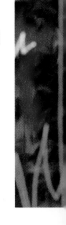

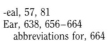

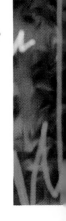

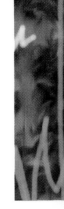

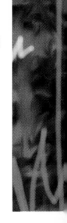

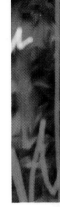

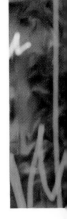

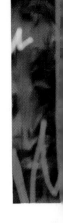

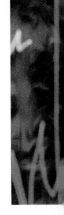

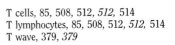

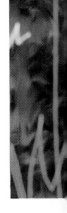

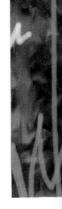

Multimedia CD-ROM
Single User License Agreement

1. NOTICE. WE ARE WILLING TO LICENSE THE MULTIMEDIA PROGRAM PRODUCT TITLED "CD-ROM TO ACCOMPANY THE LANGUAGE OF MEDICINE, SIXTH EDITION" ("MULTIMEDIA PROGRAM") TO YOU ONLY ON THE CONDITION THAT YOU ACCEPT ALL OF THE TERMS CONTAINED IN THIS LICENSE AGREEMENT. PLEASE READ THIS LICENSE AGREEMENT CAREFULLY BEFORE OPENING THE SEALED DISK PACKAGE. BY OPENING THAT PACKAGE YOU AGREE TO BE BOUND BY THE TERMS OF THIS AGREEMENT. IF YOU DO NOT AGREE TO THESE TERMS WE ARE UNWILLING TO LICENSE THE MULTIMEDIA PROGRAM TO YOU, AND YOU SHOULD NOT OPEN THE DISK PACKAGE. IN SUCH CASE, PROMPTLY RETURN THE UNOPENED DISK PACKAGE AND ALL OTHER MATERIAL IN THIS PACKAGE, ALONG WITH PROOF OF PAYMENT, TO THE AUTHORIZED DEALER FROM WHOM YOU OBTAINED IT FOR A FULL REFUND OF THE PRICE YOU PAID.

2. **Ownership and License.** This is a license agreement and NOT an agreement for sale. It permits you to use one copy of the MULTIMEDIA PROGRAM on a single computer. The MULTIMEDIA PROGRAM and its contents are owned by us or our licensors, and are protected by U.S. and international copyright laws. Your rights to use the MULTIMEDIA PROGRAM are specified in this Agreement, and we retain all rights not expressly granted to you in this Agreement.

   • You may use one copy of the MULTIMEDIA PROGRAM on a single computer.

   • After you have installed the MULTIMEDIA PROGRAM on your computer, you may use the MULTIMEDIA PROGRAM on a different computer only if you first delete the files installed by the installation program from the first computer.

   • You may not copy any portion of the MULTIMEDIA PROGRAM to your computer hard disk or any other media other than printing out or downloading nonsubstantial portions of the text and images in the MULTIMEDIA PROGRAM for your own internal informational use.

   • You may not copy any of the documentation or other printed materials accompanying the MULTIMEDIA PROGRAM.

   Neither concurrent use on two or more computers nor use in a local area network or other network is permitted without separate authorization and the payment of additional license fees.

3. **Transfer and Other Restrictions.** You may not rent, lend, or lease this MULTIMEDIA PROGRAM. You may not and you may not permit others to (a) disassemble, decompile, or otherwise derive source code from the software included in the MULTIMEDIA PROGRAM (the "Software"), (b) reverse engineer the Software, (c) modify or prepare derivative works of the MULTIMEDIA PROGRAM, (d) use the Software in an on-line system, or (e) use the MULTIMEDIA PROGRAM in any manner that infringes on the intellectual property or other rights of another party.

   However, you may transfer this license to use the MULTIMEDIA PROGRAM to another party on a permanent basis by transferring this copy of the License Agreement, the MULTIMEDIA PROGRAM, and all documentation. Such transfer of possession terminates your license from us. Such other party shall be licensed under the terms of this Agreement upon its acceptance of this Agreement by its initial use of the MULTIMEDIA PROGRAM. If you transfer the MULTIMEDIA PROGRAM, you must remove the installation files from your hard disk and you may not retain any copies of those files for your own use.

4. **Limited Warranty and Limitation of Liability.** For a period of sixty (60) days from the date you acquired the MULTIMEDIA PROGRAM from us or our authorized dealer, we warrant that the media containing the MULTIMEDIA PROGRAM will be free from defects that prevent you from installing the MULTIMEDIA PROGRAM on your computer. If the disk fails to conform to this warranty, you may, as your sole and exclusive remedy, obtain a replacement free of charge if you return the defective disk to us with a dated proof of purchase. Otherwise the MULTIMEDIA PROGRAM is licensed to you on an "AS IS" basis without any warranty of any nature.

WE DO NOT WARRANT THAT THE MULTIMEDIA PROGRAM WILL MEET YOUR REQUIREMENTS OR THAT ITS OPERATION WILL BE UNINTERRUPTED OR ERROR-FREE. WE EXCLUDE AND EXPRESSLY DISCLAIM ALL EXPRESS AND IMPLIED WARRANTIES NOT STATED HEREIN, INCLUDING THE IMPLIED WARRANTIES OF MERCHANTABILITY AND FITNESS FOR A PARTICULAR PURPOSE.

WE SHALL NOT BE LIABLE FOR ANY DAMAGE OR LOSS OF ANY KIND ARISING OUT OF OR RESULTING FROM YOUR POSSESSION OR USE OF THE MULTIMEDIA PROGRAM (INCLUDING DATA LOSS OR CORRUPTION), REGARDLESS OF WHETHER SUCH LIABILITY IS BASED IN TORT, CONTRACT OR OTHERWISE AND INCLUDING, BUT NOT LIMITED TO, ACTUAL, SPECIAL, INDIRECT, INCIDENTAL OR CONSEQUENTIAL DAMAGES. IF THE FOREGOING LIMITATION IS HELD TO BE UNENFORCEABLE, OUR MAXIMUM LIABILITY TO YOU SHALL NOT EXCEED THE AMOUNT OF THE LICENSE FEE PAID BY YOU FOR THE MULTIMEDIA PROGRAM. THE REMEDIES AVAILABLE TO YOU AGAINST US AND THE LICENSORS OF MATERIALS INCLUDED IN THE MULTIMEDIA PROGRAM ARE EXCLUSIVE.

Some states do not allow the limitation or exclusion of implied warranties or liability for incidental or consequential damages, so the above limitations or exclusions may not apply to you.

5. **United States Government Restricted Rights.** The MULTIMEDIA PROGRAM and documentation are provided with Restricted Rights. Use, duplication, or disclosure by the U.S. Government or any agency or instrumentality thereof is subject to restrictions as set forth in subdivision (c)(1)(ii) of the Rights in Technical Data and Computer Software clause at 48 C.F.R. 252.277-7013, or in subdivision (c)(1) and (2) of the Commercial Computer Software-Restricted Rights Clause at 48 C.F.R. 52.277-19, as applicable. Manufacturer is the W.B. Saunders Company, the Curtis Center, Suite 300, Independence Square West, Philadelphia, PA 19106.

6. **Termination.** This license and your right to use this MULTIMEDIA PROGRAM automatically terminate if you fail to comply with any provisions of this Agreement, destroy the copy of the MULTIMEDIA PROGRAM in your possession, or voluntarily return the MULTIMEDIA PROGRAM to us. Upon termination you will destroy all copies of the MULTIMEDIA PROGRAM and documentation.

7. **Miscellaneous Provisions.** This Agreement will be governed by and construed in accordance with the substantive laws of the Commonwealth of Pennsylvania. This is the entire agreement between us relating to the MULTIMEDIA PROGRAM, and supersedes any prior purchase order, communications, advertising or representations concerning the contents of this package. No change or modification of this Agreement will be valid unless it is in writing and is signed by us.

A HISTORY OF THE
ROMAN PEOPLE